AF736767

FOOD SUPPLEMENTS AND DIETARY FIBER IN HEALTH AND DISEASE

AAP Advances in Nutraceuticals

FOOD SUPPLEMENTS AND DIETARY FIBER IN HEALTH AND DISEASE

Edited by

Bhushan R. Rane, PhD, MPharm

Raj K. Keservani, MPharm

Durgesh Singh, DPhil

Nayan A. Gujarathi, PhD

Ashish S. Jain, PhD

AAP | APPLE ACADEMIC PRESS

First edition published 2024

Apple Academic Press Inc.
1265 Goldenrod Circle, NE,
Palm Bay, FL 32905 USA

760 Laurentian Drive, Unit 19,
Burlington, ON L7N 0A4, CANADA

CRC Press
2385 NW Executive Center Drive,
Suite 320, Boca Raton FL 33431

4 Park Square, Milton Park,
Abingdon, Oxon, OX14 4RN UK

© 2024 by Apple Academic Press, Inc.

Apple Academic Press exclusively co-publishes with CRC Press, an imprint of Taylor & Francis Group, LLC

Reasonable efforts have been made to publish reliable data and information, but the authors, editors, and publisher cannot assume responsibility for the validity of all materials or the consequences of their use. The authors are solely responsible for all the chapter content, figures, tables, data etc. provided by them. The authors, editors, and publishers have attempted to trace the copyright holders of all material reproduced in this publication and apologize to copyright holders if permission to publish in this form has not been obtained. If any copyright material has not been acknowledged, please write and let us know so we may rectify in any future reprint.

Except as permitted under U.S. Copyright Law, no part of this book may be reprinted, reproduced, transmitted, or utilized in any form by any electronic, mechanical, or other means, now known or hereafter invented, including photocopying, microfilming, and recording, or in any information storage or retrieval system, without written permission from the publishers.

For permission to photocopy or use material electronically from this work, access www.copyright.com or contact the Copyright Clearance Center, Inc. (CCC), 222 Rosewood Drive, Danvers, MA 01923, 978-750-8400. For works that are not available on CCC please contact mpkbookspermissions@tandf.co.uk

Trademark notice: Product or corporate names may be trademarks or registered trademarks and are used only for identification and explanation without intent to infringe.

Library and Archives Canada Cataloguing in Publication

Title: Food supplements and dietary fiber in health and disease / edited by Bhushan R. Rane, PhD, MPharm, Raj K. Keservani, MPharm, Durgesh Singh, DPhil, Nayan A. Gujarathi, PhD, Ashish S. Jain, PhD.
Names: Rane, Bhushan R., editor. | Keservani, Raj K., 1981- editor. | Singh, Durgesh, editor. | Gujarathi, Nayan A., 1980- editor. | Jain, Ashish S., editor.
Series: AAP advances in nutraceuticals.
Description: First edition. | Series statement: AAP advances in nutraceuticals | Includes bibliographical references and index.
Identifiers: Canadiana (print) 2023047182X | Canadiana (ebook) 20230471870 | ISBN 9781774913369 (hardcover) | ISBN 9781774913376 (softcover) | ISBN 9781003386308 (ebook)
Subjects: LCSH: Dietary supplements. | LCSH: Dietary supplements—Therapeutic use. | LCSH: Fiber in human nutrition. | LCSH: Food—Fiber content.
Classification: LCC RM258.5 .F66 2024 | DDC 613.2—dc23

Library of Congress Cataloging-in-Publication Data

CIP data on file with US Library of Congress

ISBN: 978-1-77491-336-9 (hbk)
ISBN: 978-1-77491-337-6 (pbk)
ISBN: 978-1-00338-630-8 (ebk)

ABOUT THE BOOK SERIES: AAP ADVANCES IN NUTRACEUTICALS

In the modern era, mankind has witnessed a paradigm shift with respect to fundamental eating behavior. The lack of physical workouts and busy schedules at offices and in households have promoted the consumption of junk foods, which eventually results in numerous diseases and disorders since the nutritional content from fast food is inadequate. Plumpness and obesity have become a global health threat. The leading causes of death from most developing nations are noncommunicable diseases such as cardiovascular diseases, cancer, arthritis, osteoporosis, and liver toxicity. Patients suffering from such lifestyle ailments are a bit apprehensive towards prolonged use of costly modern therapeutics, which encourages instead the use of alternative approaches for management of such diseases and disorders.

The emerging sector of the nutraceutical industry encompasses products derived from nature, dietary supplements, and functional foods. Nutraceuticals are used for treatment and prevention of a broad range of diseases, such as the common cold, arthritis, sleep-related disorders, cancers, cardiovascular complications, metabolic disorders, and others.

The research on nutraceuticals is increasing day by day, considering the beneficial effects of food or food supplements in the management of diverse diseases. The issue of paramount concern is standardization and establishment of clinical efficacy of nutraceuticals, which is in fact a challenge for researchers around the globe.

This book series aims at realizing the significance of the variety of nutraceuticals for human well-being. The books in the series will also emphasize the role of dieticians and nutritionists for the prescription of judicious eating habits. The key food components such as carbohydrates, proteins, and lipids as well as micronutrients (vitamins, minerals) are demonstrated to maintain good health, obviating the need for medicines. Thus, nutraceuticals that are indeed derived from food ingredients are believed to be potential alternative therapeutics.

Asymptomatic diseases/disorders necessitate proper diagnosis. Stressed circumstances have been reported to cause weight loss. Workplace stress is a key variable in the genesis and propagation of metabolic disorders. The nuances of the underlying mechanisms are still to be deciphered. Poor lifestyle trends have been attributed along with the consumption of junk foods in several such instances. Sugar-rich carbonated beverages, the use of contraband drugs, and the consumption of liquor in excess are assigned as risk factors. This book series will cover advances and applications in addition to providing the basics of nutraceuticals.

The books in this series may be valuable resources for industry professionals to design and develop quality products for end users. In addition, the book series will be fortified by ideas of innovation, concept building, manufacturing aspects, quality control, and regulatory status of nutraceuticals.

Ostensibly, business has seen a rise in the nutraceutical consumption in recent years. Pure, safe, efficacious products are the need of the hour globally. There are a number of books on nutraceuticals in the market, yet these are only a few books presenting certain aspects of nutraceuticals therein. This book series aims to offer a holistic view of this promising strategy, which is picking up pace with time. This book series will be a unique endeavor to bring manufacturing, research and development, and marketing strategies under a single umbrella.

CURRENT BOOKS IN THE SERIES

- **Micronutrients and Macronutrients as Nutraceuticals**
  Editors: Prakash Chandra Gupta, PhD, Sayan Bhattacharyya, MBBS, MD, Nisha Sharma, PhD, MPharm, Rajesh K. Kesharwani, PhD, and Raj K. Keservani, MPharm
- **Formulations, Regulations, and Challenges of Nutraceuticals**
  Editors: Tingirikari Jagan Mohan Rao, PhD, Rajesh K. Kesharwani, PhD, Raj. K. Keservani, MPharm, and Anil K. Sharma, PhD
- **Food Supplements and Dietary Fiber in Health and Disease**
  Editors: Bhushan R. Rane, PhD, MPharm, Raj K. Keservani, M Pharm, Durgesh Singh, DPhil, Nayan A. Gujarathi, PhD, and Ashish S. Jain, PhD
- **Nutraceuticals in Cancer Prevention, Management, and Treatment**
  Editors: Raj K. Keservani, MPharm, Bui Thanh Tung, PhD, Sippy Singh, DPhil, and Rajesh K. Kesharwani, PhD
- **Advances in Flavonoids for Human Health and Prevention of Diseases**
  Editors: Nisha Sharma, PhD, Deepika Saini, PhD, Rajesh K. Kesharwani, PhD, Prakash Chandra Gupta, and Raj. K. Keservani, MPharm

- **The Flavonoids: Extraction and Applications**
  Editors: Deepika Saini, PhD, Rajesh K. Kesharwani, PhD, and Raj K. Keservani, MPharm
- **Immune-Boosting Nutraceuticals for Better Human Health: Novel Applications**
  Editors: Urmila Jarouliya, PhD, Raj K. Keservani, MPharm, Rajesh K. Kesharwani, PhD, Virendra K. Patel, PhD, and Adi D. Bharti
- **Applications of Functional Foods in Disease Prevention**
  Editors: Raj K. Keservani, MPharm, and Eknath D. Ahire, MSPharm
- **Plant Metabolites and Vegetables as Nutraceuticals**
  Editors: Raj K. Keservani, MPharm, Bui Thanh Tung, PhD, Rajesh K. Kesharwani, PhD, MPharm, and Eknath D. Ahire
- **Preventive and Therapeutic Role of Vitamins as Nutraceuticals**
  Editors: Khemchand R. Surana, Eknath D. Ahire, Raj K. Keservani, MPharm, and Rajesh K. Kesharwani, PhD
- **Nutraceuticals and Bone Health**
  Editors: Deepak Sharma, PhD, Madan Mohan Gupta, PhD, Anil K. Sharma, PhD, MPharm, Raj K. Keservani, MPharm, and Rajesh K. Kesharwani, PhD
- **Flavonoids as Nutraceuticals**
  Editors: Rajesh K. Kesharwani, PhD, MTech, Deepika Saini, PhD, Raj K. Keservani, MPharm, and Anil Kumar Sharma, PhD, MPharm
- **Herbals as Nutraceuticals: Their Role in Healthcare**
  Editors: Raj K. Keservani, MPharm, Rajeshwar Kamal Kant Arya, PhD, MPharm, and Rajesh K. Kesharwani, PhD, MTech
- **Nutraceutical Fruits: Overview and Disease Prevention**
  Editor: Raj K. Keservani, MPharm
- **Nutrigenomics and Nutraceuticals**
  Editors: Raj K. Keservani, MPharm, Eknath D. Ahire, Shubham J. Khainar, PhD, Sanjay J. Kshirsagar, PhD, and Rajesh K. Kesharwani, PhD
- **The Nature of Nutraceuticals: History, Properties, Sources, and Nanotechnology**
  Editors: Rajesh K. Kesharwani, PhD, Prashant Kumar, PhD, and Raj K. Keservani, MPharm

- **Nutraceuticals for the Treatment and Prevention of Sexual Disorders**
  Editors: Raj K. Keservani, MPharm, Sharangouda J. Patil, PhD, and Ivan Aranha, PhD
- **Antioxidants as Nutraceuticals**
  Editors: Nayan A. Gujaratih, PhD, Raj K. Keservani, MPharm, Rajesh K. Kesharwani, PhD, Bhushan R. Rane, PhD, and Yogeeta Sameer Goyal, PhD

ABOUT THE EDITORS

Bhushan R. Rane, PhD
Shri. D.D. Vispute, College of Pharmacy and Research Center, New Panvel, Navi Mumbai, Maharashtra, India

Bhushan R. Rane, PhD, MPharm, is presently a Professor and Head of the Department of Pharmaceutics, Shri. D.D. Vispute, College of Pharmacy and Research Center, New Panvel, Navi Mumbai, affiliated to Mumbai University, Maharashtra, India. He has over 14 years of teaching experience at the UG and PG Levels. To date, he has guided more than 50 students for MPharm. He has published more than 75 peer-reviewed research and review articles in national and international journals. He has co-authored eight books at the national level and more than 15 book chapters at the international level published by Taylor and Francis Group and Bentham Science worldwide. He is a reviewer for several scientific and international journals. He received a grant of Rs. 20 Lakhs from various apex bodies for research, such as AICTE, New Delhi. He is a lifetime member of APTI, MSPC, and IPGA. His research interests are focused around plan, improvement, and the portrayal of vesicular, microparticulate, and nanoparticulate systems and the advancement of different solid dosage forms for oral conveyance.

Raj K. Keservani, PhD, MPharm
Associate Professor, Faculty of BPharmacy, CSM Group of Institutions, Prayagraj, Uttar Pradesh, India

Raj K. Keservani, PhD, MPharm, is working as Associate Professor in the Faculty of B. Pharmacy at the CSM Group of Institutions, Prayagraj, India. He has more than 12 years of academic (teaching) experience from various institutes of India in pharmaceutical education. He has supervised more than 25 undergraduate students for their research work. He has published over 30 peer-reviewed papers in the field of pharmaceutical sciences in national and international journals, six patents, over 70 book chapters, three co-authored books, and over 40 edited books. He is also active as a reviewer for several international scientific journals. His research interests include nutraceutical and functional foods, novel drug delivery systems (NDDS), transdermal drug delivery/drug delivery, health science, cancer biology, and neurobiology. Dr. Keservani graduated with a pharmacy degree from the Department of Pharmacy, Kumaun University, Nainital, Uttarakhand, India. He received his Master of Pharmacy (MPharm) (specialization in pharmaceutics) from the School of Pharmaceutical Sciences, Rajiv Gandhi Proudyogiki Vishwavidyalaya, Bhopal, India. He earned his PhD degree from IKG Punjab Technical University, Jalandhar, Punjab, India. Dr. Keservani is a life member of the Society of Pharmaceutical Education and Research (SPER).

Durgesh Singh, DPhil
Assistant Professor at Department of Zoology, S.S. Khanna Girls' Degree College, Prayagraj (A Constituent College of the University of Allahabad), Prayagraj, Uttar Pradesh, India.

Durgesh Singh, DPhil, is an Assistant Professor at the Department of Zoology, S.S. Khanna Girls' Degree College, Prayagraj (A Constituent College of the University of Allahabad, Prayagraj). Dr. Singh has completed his DPhil in Zoology with specialization in Neurobiology from the University of Allahabad. He has completed his PG with specialization in Cytogenetics. He was awarded UGC-BSR fellowship in Science for meritorious student during his DPhil. Dr. Singh has 19 publications in the form of research papers, book chapters, and review articles in international and national journals of high repute. His papers have been cited in international and national journals of high-impact factors. He is a life member of scientific bodies such as ISCA, IAN, and ABRF. He is the recipient of three national awards, including "Nasi-Swarna Jayanti Puraskar" by NASI for presentation. His research interest includes neurobiology, cell biology, cytogenetics, and nutraceuticals.

Nayan A. Gujarathi, PhD
Assistant Professor, Department of Pharmaceutics, Shri Vile Parle Kelavani Mandal's Institute of Pharmacy, Dhule, Maharashtra, India

Nayan A. Gujarathi, PhD, MPharm, is an Assistant Professor at the Department of Pharmaceutics, Shri Vile Parle Kelavani Mandal's Institute of Pharmacy, Dhule, India. He has 13 years of academic experience in pharmaceutical science. He has published over 30 peer-reviewed papers in the field of pharmaceutical sciences in national and international journals as well as several book chapters. He has presented his research work at an international conference organized by the Controlled Release Society and delivered several expert talks on outcome-based education for the accreditation process. His research interest encompasses novel drug delivery systems, polymer science, nanotechnology, and nutraceuticals.

Ashish S. Jain, PhD
Shri. D.D. Vispute, College of Pharmacy and Research Center, New Panvel, Navi Mumbai, Maharashtra, India

Ashish S. Jain, PhD, is one of the best minds in the field of pharmacy research management and administration. Presently, he is offering his services as the Principal at Shri. D.D. Vispute College of Pharmacy and Research Center, New Panvel. He is one of the key persons at the Adarsh Scientific Research Center and Testing Lab Pvt. Ltd., Panvel. He also works as a consultant for pharma industries and food testing laboratories. His biographical note has been published in *Who's Who of Asian Americans,* Vol. VIII. He received honorary doctorates from the University of South America. He is the recipient of Dr. A.P.J. Abdul Kalam's national award for remarkable achievement in the field of teaching, research, and publications. He is the co-author of many books, which include Nanotechnology: A Recent Trend, Modern Method for Solubility Enhancement, CRC Press, London, and A Glimpse of Novel Vesicular Drug Delivery System, Nirali Publication, Pune. As of now, he has published 48 research and review papers in several national and international journals. He has a keen interest in the area of phytoformulation research.

CONTENTS

CONTRIBUTORS

Surendra Agrawal
Shobhaben Pratapbhai Patel School of Pharmacy and Technology Management, SVKM's NMIMS, Vile Parle, Mumbai, Maharashtra, India; Datta Meghe College of Pharmacy, DMIHER, Sawangi Meghe, Wardha, India

Pratiksha R. Aher
Gokhale Education Society's Sir Dr. M. S. Gosavi College of Pharmaceutical Education and Research, Nashik, Maharashtra, India

Rajesh A. Ahirrao
PG College of Pharmaceutical Science and Research, Nandurbar, Maharashtra, India

Punam D. Bagad
Gokhale Education Society's Sir Dr. M. S. Gosavi College of Pharmaceutical Education and Research, Maharashtra, India

Shashikant B. Bagade
Department of Pharmaceutical Chemistry, SVKM's NMIMS School of Pharmacy and Technology Management, Shirpur, Maharashtra, India

Mangesh S. Bansod
Shri D.D. Vispute College of Pharmacy and Research Center, Panvel, Maharashtra, India

Kedar R. Bavaskar
Shri D.D. Vispute College of Pharmacy and Research Center, Devad-Vichumbe, Panvel, Navi Mumbai, Maharashtra, India

Pushkar Y. Chavan
Shri D.D. Vispute College of Pharmacy and Research Center, Panvel, Maharashtra, India

Amitkumar R. Dhankani
P.S.G.V.P. Mandal's College of Pharmacy, Shahada, Nandurbar, Maharashtra, India

Mansi A. Dhankani
P.S.G.V.P. Mandal's College of Pharmacy, Shahada, Nandurbar, Maharashtra, India

Sanket Dharashivkar
Dr. L.H. Hiranandani College of Pharmacy, Ulhasnagar, Maharashtra, India

Madhuri Gaikwad
AIKTC School of Pharmacy, Panvel, Maharashtra, India

Shiv Garg
Maharishi Arvind College of Pharmacy, Ambabari Circle, Ambabari, Jaipur, Rajasthan, India

Trunali Ghude
Dr. L. H. Hiranandani College of Pharmacy, Ulhasnagar, Maharashtra, India

Nayan A. Gujarathi
Department of Pharmaceutics, Shri Vile Parle Kelvani Mandal's Institute of Pharmacy, Dhule, Maharashtra, India

Richa Gupta
Amar Shaheed Baba Ajit Singh Jujhar Singh Memorial College of Pharmacy (An Autonomous College), Bela, Ropar, Punjab, India

Pravina Gurjar
Sharadchandra Pawar College of Pharmacy, Otur, Pune, Maharashtra, India

Y. Hasni Sayyed Hamid
Poojya Sane Guruji Vidya Prasarak Mandal's College of Pharmacy, Shahada, Nandurbar, Maharashtra, India

Akash S. Jain
P.S.G.V.P. Mandal's College of Pharmacy, Shahada, Nandurbar, Maharashtra, India

Ashish S. Jain
Shri D.D. Vispute College of Pharmacy and Research Center, Devad-Vichumbe, Panvel, Navi Mumbai, Maharashtra, India

Rajan V. Kalamkar
Vivekanand Education Society's College of Pharmacy, Chembur, Mumbai, Maharashtra, India

Ashish A. Karle
Shri D.D. Vispute College of Pharmacy and Research Center, Devad-Vichumbe, Panvel, Maharashtra, India

Raj K. Keservani
Faculty of B. Pharmacy, CSM Group of Institutions, Prayagraj, Uttar Pradesh, India

Ajay Singh Kushwah
Amar Shaheed Baba Ajit Singh Jujhar Singh Memorial College of Pharmacy (An Autonomous College), Bela, Ropar, Punjab, India

Hitendra S. Mahajan
Department of Pharmaceutics, R. C. Patel, Institute of Pharmaceutical Education and Research, Shirpur, Maharashtra, India

Amul Mishra
B. N. University, Udaipur, Rajasthan, India

Dilip O. Morani
Shri D.D. Vispute College of Pharmacy and Research Center, Panvel, Maharashtra, India

Jayvadan K. Patel
Department of Pharmaceutics, Nootan College of Pharmacy, Visnagar, Gujarat, India

Mukesh R. Patel
Assistant Registrar, Shri Govind Guru University, Godhra, Gujarat, India

Divakar R. Patil
P.S.G.V.P. Mandal's College of Pharmacy, Shahada, Nandurbar, Maharashtra, India

Javesh Kashinath Patil
Poojya Sane Guruji Vidya Prasarak Mandal's College of Pharmacy, Shahada, Nandurbar, Maharashtra, India

Mukesh S. Patil
PhD Research Scholar, R.C. Patel Institute of Pharmaceutical Education and Research, Shirpur, Maharashtra, India

Pramod N. Patil
RCP, Institute of Technology, Shirpur, Maharashtra, India

Pravin O. Patil
H.R. Patel Institute of Pharmaceutical Education and Research, Shirpur, Maharashtra, India

Rupali A. Patil
Gokhale Education Society's Sir Dr. M. S. Gosavi College of Pharmaceutical Education and Research, Nashik, Maharashtra, India

Sunila A. Patil
P.S.G.V.P. Mandal's College of Pharmacy, Shahada, Nandurbar, Maharashtra, India

Sarvesh S. Pawar
Shri D.D. Vispute College of Pharmacy and Research Center, Panvel, Maharashtra, India

Prashant L. Pingale
Gokhale Education Society's Sir Dr. M. S. Gosavi College of Pharmaceutical Education and Research, Nashik, Maharashtra, India

Rupesh A. Pingale
NCRD Sterling Institute of Pharmacy, Nerul, Navi Mumbai, Maharashtra, India

Ramsaneh Raghuwanshi
Professor, Department of Pharmaceutical Chemistry, Corporate Institute of Pharmacy, Bhopal, Madhya Pradesh, India

Bhushan R. Rane
Shri D.D. Vispute College of Pharmacy and Research Center, Devad-Vichumbe, Panvel, Navi Mumbai, Maharashtra, India

Savita Rathore
Maharishi Arvind College of Pharmacy, Ambabari Circle, Ambabari, Rajasthan, India

Bhawana Sharma
Maharishi Arvind College of Pharmacy, Ambabari Circle, Ambabari, Jaipur, Rajasthan, India

Piush Sharma
Maharishi Arvind College of Pharmacy, Ambabari Circle, Ambabari, Jaipur, Rajasthan, India

A. A. Shirkhedkar
Department of Chemistry, R.C. Patel Institute of Pharmaceutical Education and Research, Shirpur, Maharashtra, India

Parikshit R. Shirode
Department of Shalyatantra, Parul Institute of Ayurveda, Parul University, Vadodara, Gujarat, India

Nitin Rajendra Shirsath
H.R. Patel Institute of Pharmaceutical Education and Research, Karwand Naka, Shirpur, Maharashtra, India

Hemant P. Suryawanshi
PG College of Pharmaceutical Science and Research, Chaupale, Maharashtra, India

Rina H. Suryawanshi
NTV'S Sharada Junior College, Joganipada, Maharashtra, India

Sandip A. Tadvi
P.S.G.V.P. Mandal's College of Pharmacy, Shahada, Nandurbar, Maharashtra, India

Tejas S. Telange
Shri D.D. Vispute College of Pharmacy and Research Center, Panvel, Maharashtra, India

Payal Tiwari
Shobhaben Pratapbhai Patel School of Pharmacy and Technology Management, SVKM's NMIMS, Vile Parle, Mumbai, Maharashtra, India

Bui Thanh Tung
VNU University of Medicine and Pharmacy, Vietnam National University, Hanoi, Vietnam

Pranit S. Waghchaure
Shri D.D. Vispute College of Pharmacy and Research Center, Devad-Vichumbe, Panvel, Navi Mumbai, Maharashtra, India

Gautami Warghade
Dr. L. H. Hiranandani College of Pharmacy, Ulhasnagar, Maharashtra, India

Laxmikant R. Zawar
H.R. Patel Institute of Pharmaceutical Education and Research, Karwand Naka, Shirpur, Maharashtra, India

ABBREVIATIONS

AACC	American Association of Cereal Chemists
ACE	angiotensin-changing enzyme
ACs	anthocyanosides
AGE	advanced glycation end products
AI	adequate intake
AICR	American Institute for Cancer Research
ALA	alpha lipoic acid
ALA	alpha-linolenic acid
AND	Academy of Nutrition and Dietetics
AOAC	Association of Official Analytical Chemists
AOM	azoxymethane
AX	arabinoxylan
BMI	body mass index
BP	blood pressure
BPH	benign prostatic hyperplasia
BRCA	BReast CAncer
C/EBPδ	CCAAT/enhancer-binding protein
CAD	charged aerosol detector
CAD	coronary artery disease
CAM	complementary alternative medicine
CBC	complete blood count
CCPs	critical control points
CD20	cluster of differentiate 20
CD52	cluster of differentiation 52
CDA	Canadian Diabetes Association
CDC	Centers for Disease Control and Prevention
CEA	carcinoembryonic antigen
CFR	Code of Federal Regulations
CFSAN	Center for Food Safety and Applied Nutrition
CHD	coronary heart disease
CL	consumer laboratory
CLA	conjugated linoleic acid
CMC	carboxy methyl cellulose
CMV	cytomegalovirus

CO_2	carbon dioxide
CP	cell-penetrating
CTLA-4	cytotoxic T-lymphocyte–associated antigen-4
CVD	cardiovascular disease
DASH	dietary approaches to stop hypertension
DCM	diabetic cardiomyopathy
DF	dietary fiber
DHA	docosahexaenoic acid
DHSEA	dietary supplement health and education
DLLME	dispersive liquid-liquid microextraction
DM	diabetes mellitus
DMAB	3, 2'- dimethyl-4-aminobiphenyl
DMSPE	dispersive micro solid phase extraction
DNA	deoxyribonucleic acid
DPA	docosapentaenoic acid
DRI	dietary reference intake
DSHEA	Dietary Supplement Health and Education Act
DSPE	dispersive solid phase extraction
EASD	European Association for the Study of Diabetes
EDs	endocrine disruptors
EFSA	European Food Safety Authority
EGCG	epigallocatechin gallate
EGFR	epidermal growth factor receptor
EPA	eicosapentaenoic acid
ER	estrogen receptor
ER-	estrogen receptor-negative
EU	European Union
FAK	focal adhesion kinase
FDA	Food and Drug Administration
FHS	Framingham heart study
FID	flame ionization detector
FOS	fructo oligosaccharides
FSSA	Financial Services and Markets Authority
FSSA	Food Safety Standard and Standards Act
FSSAI	Food Safety and Standard Authority of India
FTC	Federal Trade Commission
FTIR	Fourier transform infrared spectroscopy
FT-NIR	Fourier transform near infra-red spectroscopy
GC	gas chromatography

GERD	gastroesophageal reflux disease
GI	gastrointestinal
GIP	gastric inhibitory polypeptide
GISTs	gastrointestinal stromal tumors
GJIC	gap junction intercellular communication
GLUT-2	glucose transporter
GM	gut microbiota
GMP	good manufacturing practices
GPx	glutathione peroxidase
GRAS	generally recognized as safe
HACCP	hazard analysis and critical control point
HCl	hydrochloric acid
HDL-C	high density lipoprotein cholesterol
HER	human epidermal growth factor receptor-2
HFD	high-fat diet
HIF-1	hypoxia-inducible factor
HIV	human immunodeficiency virus
HOMA	homeostasis model assessment
HPLC	high performance liquid chromatography
HPLC-MS	high performance liquid chromatography-mass spectrometry
HPTLC	high performance thin layer chromatography
HRMS	high resolution mass spectrometry
HT29	human colon adenocarcinoma cells
IBD	inflammatory bowel disease
IBS	irritable bowel syndrome
ICC	interstitial cells of Cajal
ICH	International Conference on Harmonization
ICP-MS	inductively coupled plasma-mass-spectrometry
IDDM	insulin-dependent
IDF	insoluble dietary fiber
IDF	International Diabetes Federation
IHD	ischemic heart diseases
IL	interleukin
INS-IR	inactivates the insulin-receptor
ISO	International Standard Organization
JACN	Journal of the American College of Nutrition
LC	liquid chromatography

LC-CAD	liquid chromatography method with charged aerosol detection
LC-HRMS	liquid chromatography-high resolution mass spectrometry
LC-MS/MS	liquid chromatography-tandem mass spectrometry
LDL	low density lipoprotein
LLE	liquid-liquid extraction
LLME	liquid-liquid microextraction
mAbs	monoclonal antibodies
MAE	microwave-assisted extraction
Mg	magnesium
MIPs	molecularly imprinted polymers
MNT	medical nutrition therapy
MPT	mycobacterium tuberculosis
MS	mass spectrometry
MSM	methyl sulfonyl methane
MUC2	oligomeric mucus gel-forming
MUFAs	saturated polyunsaturated fatty acids
MW	molecular weight
NADPH	nicotinamide adenine dinucleotide phosphate
NAM	National Academy of Medicine
NCD	non-communicable diseases
NCI	National Cancer Institute
NDI	new dietary ingredient
NDIN	NDI notification
NETs	neuroendocrine tumors
NF-κB	nuclear factor-kappa B
NGR-hTNF	asparagine–glycine–arginine–human tumor necrosis factor
NIDDM	noninsulin-dependent diabetic mellitus
NMR	nuclear magnetic resonance
NPLC	normal phase liquid chromatography
NSPs	non-starch polysaccharides
ODI	old dietary ingredient
OMCL	official medicines control laboratory
OTC	over the counter
PDA/ UV	photodiode array ultraviolet
PDE-5	phosphodiesterase-5
PET	positron emission tomography

PPAR-γ	proliferator-activated receptor-γ
PTP	protein tyrosine phosphatases
PUFAs	polyunsaturated fatty acid
RBP	retinol-binding protein
RCTs	randomized controlled trials
RD	registered dietitian
RDA	recommended dietary allowance
RDN	registered dietitian nutritionist
RNA	ribonucleic acid
ROS	reactive oxygen species
RP-LC	reverse phase liquid chromatography
RS	resistant starch
RWPs	red wine polyphenols
SCFA	short-chain fatty acids
SDF	soluble dietary fiber
SDME	single-drop microextraction
SERS	surface enhance Raman spectroscopy
SFAs	saturated fatty acids
SFC	supercritical fluid chromatography
SLE	solid-liquid extraction
SOPs	standard operating procedures
SPE	solid phase extraction
SRB	sulfate-reducing bacteria
SSP	sessile serrated polyps
T1D	type 1 diabetes
T2DM	type 2 diabetes mellitus
TBARS	thio-barbituric acid reactive substances
TDF	total dietary fiber
TLC	thin-layer chromatography
TLC-MS	thin-layer chromatography-mass spectrometry
TLC-SERS	thin-layer chromatography-surface enhanced Raman spectroscopy
TNF-α	tumor necrosis factor
UHPLC	ultra-high-performance liquid chromatography
UHPLC-HRMS	ultra-high-performance liquid chromatography-HRMS
UHPLC-MS	ultra-performance liquid chromatography-tandem mass spectrometer

UHPLC-Q-TOF-MS	ultra-high performance liquid chromatography-quadrupole time-of-flight mass spectrometry
UHPSFC	ultra-high-performance supercritical fluid chromatography
UK	United Kingdom
ULs	upper intake levels
US	United States
USDA	U.S. Department of Agriculture
USFDA	US Food and Drug Administration
VEGF	vascular endothelial growth factor
VEGFR	vascular endothelial growth factor receptor
VLDL	very-low-density lipoprotein
WCRF	World Cancer Research Foundation
WHO	World Health Organization

PREFACE

Food supplements, also called nutritional supplements or dietary supplements, deliver nutrients that may not be consumed in sufficient quantities. Food supplements include minerals, vitamins, fatty acids, amino acids, and other substances that can be consumed in the form of tablets, capsules, pills, liquid, etc. The worldwide health food supplements market size was estimated at USD 310.4 billion in the year 2020 and is required to increment at a yearly development pace of 6.2%. Also, the COVID-19 pandemic has improved health awareness among consumers. Furthermore, consumers are moving towards nutritional dietary supplements to improve health. According to WHO, a healthy diet with food supplements is necessary for improving the immune system, and it is an important approach for speedy recovery from several viruses, including SARS-CoV-2 infection.

The term "dietary fibers" refers to indigestible carbohydrates of plant origin that include a wide range of diverging compounds that differentially affect many systemic and gastrointestinal processes. However, consuming dietary fibers is important for a healthy gut. Also, dietary fibers can prevent or relieve constipation and help waste to smoothly move through the body. The world dietary fibers market size was valued at USD 39.8 billion in 2019 and is expected to increase at a compound yearly growth rate of 8.9%.

Thus, consumers prefer fiber-based food products with added health benefits due to increased chances of various diseases like heart disease, cancer, and diabetes and become more health consciousness.

Food supplements play an important role in the treatment of various diseases and infections by maintaining health. It was reported that an unbalanced diet or non-nutritious food uptake was responsible for poor health. Food supplements are considered as concentrated sources of nutrients or other substances that have a physiological or nutritional impact and whose function is to supplement a normal diet because of their presumed health advantages. The sales of food supplements worldwide especially plant extracts and botanicals which are most popular as they are considered to be healthier and safer compared to synthetic drugs. Also, they are considered to be free of any side effects. Food supplements are regulated the same as food, and current legislations are concentrated on minerals and vitamins that are contained in food supplements in European Union (EU) (Directive,

2002). While in United States (US), the Food Drug Administration (FDA) has defined dietary supplements as the official term.

In the present book, the reader will understand the concept of food supplements and dietary fibers, definitions, role of food supplements and dietary fibers in various diseases such as cancer, diabetes, obesity, etc. Current market and future trends of nutraceutical products and regulatory guidelines are elaborated in this book which will be beneficial for the entrepreneurs, industries, etc.

This book *Food Supplements and Dietary Fiber in Health and Disease*, comprises 15 chapters in three parts that describe the use of food supplements and dietary fiber in the management, prevention, and treatment of different diseases and its regulation.

Part I: Dietary Fiber

Dietary fiber classifications, physiological features, and food sources are reviewed in Chapter 1, "Introduction of Dietary Fibers," written by Mukesh S. Patil and his team.

Health-conscious citizens around the globe will benefit from the wealth of knowledge on traditional Indian and Ayurvedic health foods as well as nutraceuticals based on innovative formulations, thanks to the globalization of the population and the international trade of food, as discussed in Chapter 2, "Formulation-Based Approaches for the Delivery of Food Supplements and Dietary Fibers," written by Tejas S. Telange and his associates.

The purpose of Chapter 3, "Role of Dietary Fibers in Diabetes," by Bhawana Sharma et al., is to show how dietary fiber plays a role in diabetes. When dietary fiber is included in a meal, it reduces postprandial glycemic and insulinemic excursions, hence altering plasma lipid levels in type 2 diabetes patients.

Dietary fiber has a number of functions in the body, one of which is to aid in the control of energy intake and the prevention of obesity, which is described by Hemant P. Suryawanshi et al. in Chapter 4, "Role of Dietary Fibers in Obesity."

Many marketed nutritional fiber products are available. Nutritional fibers help in reducing the risk of congenital heart defects (CHDs). Research shows that the probable interactions among other dietary compounds, drug treatments, and nutritional fibers interact with dietary macro- and micro-nutrients, as discussed in Chapter 5, "Role of Dietary Fiber in Coronary Heart Disease (CHD)" written by Ashish A. Karle and his associates.

Chapter 6, "Role of Dietary Fiber in Gut Health," written by Sanket Dharashivkar et al., covers the beneficial effect of dietary fibers in different diseases, such as constipation, diarrhea, inflammatory bowel diseases, hiatal hernias, gastroesophageal reflux disease, Barrett's esophagus, diverticular disease, hemorrhoids, peptic ulcer, gastritis, celiac disease, irritable bowel syndrome, gallstone, and colon cancer.

Part II: Food Supplements

Consumers are becoming more health conscious and prefer food supplements with added health benefits to combat the chances of various diseases like heart disease, cancer, and diabetes. Chapter 7 provides an "Introduction and Overview of Food Supplements," written by Dilip O. Morani and his colleagues.

Chapter 8, "Role of Food Supplement in Diabetes," written by Javesh K. Patil and his friends, reports that diet and supplements have an important role in the prevention as well as management of diabetes; even the long-term complications of diabetes can be prevented or delayed with food supplements.

Chapter 9, "Role of Food Supplements in Obesity," written by Hemant P. Suryawanshi et al., summarizes food intake and weight control with a focus on diet recommendations that can help prevent obesity and its further complications.

Most people can use supplements safely as long as they don't take too much. When supplements are overused, they are not safe and can have risks, especially for people who are receiving treatment for cancer. Some supplements may interact with medications used before and after surgery, as discussed in Chapter 10, "Role of Food Supplement in Cancer," written by Prashant L. Pingale and his associates.

Amitkumar R. Dhankani et al. discuss the role of food supplements in the management and prevention of coronary heart disease (CHD) in Chapter 11, "Role of Food Supplements in CHD."

Laxmikant R. Zawar and Nitin Rajendra Shirsath describe the role of various dietary food supplements that help in maintaining normal gut health in Chapter 12, "Role of Food Supplement in Gut Health."

A HELGA cohort case study and research outcomes, presented in Chapter 13, "Role of Dietary Fibers in Colorectal Cancer," by Surendra Agrawal and his team, outline and conclude that dietary fibers are effective in the treatment of colorectal cancer.

Part III: Regulation and Miscellaneous

Chapter 14, "Botanicals in Dietary Supplements and Fibers," written by Ajay Singh Kushwah et al., describes botanicals that are rich in fiber. These include fruits, vegetables, whole grains, nuts, and dry fruits.

Chapter 15, "Regulatory Guidance on Food Supplement and Dietary Fiber," written by Ashish A. Karle et al., discusses the many current statutes and regulations addressing dietary ingredients, manufacturing standards, safety, labeling, and claims, all of which promote the safe use of dietary supplements and preserve continued consumer access.

PART I
Dietary Fiber

CHAPTER 1

INTRODUCTION TO DIETARY FIBERS

MUKESH S. PATIL,[1] KEDAR R. BAVASKAR,[2] BHUSHAN R. RANE,[2] ASHISH S. JAIN,[2] and A. A. SHIRKHEDKAR[3]

[1]PhD Research Scholar, R.C. Patel Institute of Pharmaceutical Education and Research, Shirpur, Maharashtra, India

[2]Shri D.D. Vispute College of Pharmacy and Research Center, Devad-Vichumbe, Panvel, Navi Mumbai, Maharashtra, India

[3]Department of Chemistry, R.C. Patel Institute of Pharmaceutical Education and Research, Shirpur, Maharashtra, India

ABSTRACT

Food scientists, nutritionists, and food processors are interested in dietary fiber because of their role in promoting health through illness prevention and control. Dietary fiber has been related to a lower incidence of colon cancer, gastrointestinal problems, type 2 diabetes, and coronary heart disease. Dietary fibers are a significant segment of the functional foods market due to their health benefits. Soluble dietary fiber and insoluble dietary fiber are the two types of dietary fiber classified by their water solubility. β-glucan, pectin, gums, and insulin are examples of soluble dietary fibers, while cellulose, hemicelluloses, lignin, cutin, suberin, chitin, chitosan, and starch are examples of insoluble dietary fibers. In general, dietary fiber sources contain both types of dietary fiber, but in different proportions. Cereals, legumes, fruits, and vegetables are excellent sources of dietary fiber. Dietary fiber physicochemical qualities are linked to physiological functions in human metabolism and play a significant role in their functionality. Solubility,

Food Supplements and Dietary Fiber in Health and Disease. Bhushan R. Rane, Raj K. Keservani, Durgesh Singh, Nayan A. Gujarathi, and Ashish S. Jain, (Eds.)
© 2024 Apple Academic Press, Inc. Co-published with CRC Press (Taylor & Francis)

viscosity, water-holding, binding capacity, fermentability, mineral, and bile acid binding ability, oil-binding ability, particle size, and porosity are all essential features of dietary fibers. Dietary fiber classification, physiological features, and food sources are reviewed in this chapter.

1.1 INTRODUCTION

Dietary fibers (Keservani et al., 2010a, b) are food components that cannot be broken down by human digestive enzymes in the small intestine, notably carbohydrates. Hippocrates observed in 430 BC that course wheat flour was more laxative than refined wheat flour. J. H. Kellogg wrote about the health benefits of wheat bran in 1920, suggesting a laxative action and a rise in stool weight (Slavin, 1987). Hispley coined the phrase "dietary fiber" to describe cell wall components, including cellulose, hemicellulose, and lignin for the first time in literature (Hispley, 1953). Because of its relevance in human nutrition, dietary fiber became a prominent topic of research in the 1980s. Following this time, the field of dietary fiber research continued to expand at a rapid pace. On various elements of dietary fibers, several scientific publications and books have been published. Dietary fibers are also known as "roughage" material because they help to bulk up the amount of food expelled in the stool. When derived from plants, these indigestible carbohydrates are referred to as "functional fiber," and they provide advantages in terms of physical health when ingested. Based on their water solubility or insolubility, fermentability in the human large intestine, and physiological activities in human metabolism, dietary fibers can be categorized into numerous classes. Non-starch polysaccharides, certain oligosaccharides, lignin, phytic acid, cutin, suberin, and other dietary fibers are included in dietary fiber (Champ et al., 2003). Because they are indigestible in the human gastrointestinal tract, resistant starches are another family of molecules that fall under the notion of dietary fibers (Ferguson, Chavan, & Harris, 2001). Based on their sources and qualities, resistant starches are divided into distinct types. Resistant starches can be found in whole or partially milled grains, legumes, cornflakes, and cooked potatoes. Traditional sources of dietary fiber include cereals, legumes, oilseeds, fruits, vegetables, and other plant parts. Whole grains, cereals, and legumes are high in dietary fiber. According to research, cereal bran is also an abundant source of dietary fiber. Wheat bran can be used to make bread in baking industries (Hemdane et al., 2016). The amount of plant fiber consumed, as well as storage, ripening, and processing methods, all influence dietary fiber level in plant foods. All of these factors have an impact on the natural dietary fiber content. Cellulose is the main component of dietary fiber in cereals and vegetables. Lignin is the main component of dietary fiber in fruits and matured root vegetables. The greatest dietary fiber, hemicellulose, is found in wholegrain cereals and cereal bran. Pectin, a primary component of dietary fiber, is found in fruits (apples, oranges, etc.). Soluble dietary fiber can be found in oats and dried beans like guar (Mudgil & Barak, 2013). In the last few decades, extensive research studies have been conducted to examine the characteristics and effects of dietary fibers on a variety of human physiological conditions, such as blood cholesterol levels, gastrointestinal function, postprandial blood glucose levels, and insulin levels, among others. Dietary fibers interact with other food components and may affect the uptake and metabolism of nutrients in human physiology (Buttriss & Stokes, 2008). Dietary fibers are divided into two categories based on their ability to dissolve in water: soluble dietary fiber and insoluble dietary fiber (Mudgil & Barak, 2013). Dietary fiber sources may contain both forms of dietary fiber in various quantities. Components such as cellulose, hemicellulose, and lignin make up insoluble dietary fibers. Shortening colon transit time, increasing fecal size, and resulting in softer stool are all advantages of insoluble fibers in the human digestive system. Decreasing stomach emptying, slowing glucose absorption, and lowering serum cholesterol levels are all physiological actions of soluble dietary fibers. They ferment in the human colon producing short-chain fatty acids (SCFA), which limit cholesterol synthesis and, as a result, lower blood serum cholesterol levels. Food products contain a mixture of soluble and insoluble dietary fibers in varying proportions. The health benefits of dietary fiber are linked to physicochemical properties, which are responsible for dietary fiber's ultimate functional behavior and contribute to specific health benefits after consumption (Redgwell & Fischer, 2005; Kaczmarczyk, Miller, & Freund, 2012; Anderson et al., 2009).

1.2 CLASSIFICATION

Dietary fiber is categorized according to its origin, solubility, fermentability, digestion site, digestion products, as well as physiological consequences. Classification of dietary fibers is based on their water solubility (soluble and insoluble) and fermentability (fermentable and non-fermentable). Non-fermentable or least-fermentable dietary fibers are water-insoluble in nature, whereas fermentable dietary fibers are water soluble in nature (Tungland & Meyer, 2002). Both have different effects on human metabolism (Table 1.1).

TABLE 1.1 Dietary Fiber Classification

Category	Hydrophilic Dietary Fiber	Hydrophobic Dietary Fiber
Examples	β-glucan, pectin, gums, inulin, etc.	Non-starch polysaccharides, celluloses, hemicelluloses, lignins, resistant starches

1.2.1 SOLUBLE DIETARY FIBER

Dietary fibers that are soluble in water resist digestion in the small intestine and are fermented by intestinal microorganisms in the large intestine. Soluble dietary fiber can be found in fruits, vegetables, legumes, and other foods (Mudgil & Barak, 2013). Based on their ability to generate viscous gel when dissolved in water, soluble fibers are divided into two categories: viscous fiber and non-viscous fiber. Soluble dietary fibers lengthen transit time in the human digestive tract and cause stomach emptying to be delayed, resulting in a slower rate of absorption. β-glucan, pectin, gums, and inulin are examples of soluble dietary fibers.

1.2.1.1 β-GLUCAN

β-glucans generated from cereals are usually composed of glucose units linked byβ (1→3), β (1→4), and β (1→6). It can be identified in a various types of foods, including oats, barley, mushrooms, and microorganisms. It is most commonly found in the bran part of cereal grains. β-glucans produced from cereals are normally made up of glucose units that are connected by a sugar molecules β(1→3), β (1→4), and β (1→5). β-glucans generated from yeast and fungus, on the other hand, include cereal-glucan components present in endosperm, the cell wall portion of grains (oats and barley), are linear chain molecules with between 30% (1→3) and 70% (1→4) linkages (Bacic & Stone, 1981). The molecular weight of β-glucan obtained from oats is considered to be higher than that of glucan derived from barley (Lazaridou & Biliaderis, 2004; Lazaridou, Biliadirs, & Izydorczyk, 2003). β-Glucan has a strong proclivity for hydrating in the presence of water, resulting in a viscous solution. The rheological properties of β-glucan are influenced by the molecular weight, degree of polymerization chain association, proportion, and arrangement of cellotriosyl/cellotetraosyl units (Cui & Wood, 2000; Tosh, Wood, Wang, & Weis 2004).

1.2.1.2 PECTIN

Pectin is a component of a fibrous structure of plant cells that can be found in both the cell walls and internal layers of the cells. The most popular sources are apples and citrus fruits. Apple peel and pulp, as well as the peel component of citrus fruits, contain this substance. Apple pomace has a pectin level ranging from 10% to 15% by dry weight, but citrus peel has a pectin content ranging from 20% to 30% by dry weight (May, 1990). Pectin is a polymer containing a galacturonic acid backbone and a (1→4) glycosidic link between monomer units. This backbone chain is changed with a (1→2) rhamnopyranose unit at various points in the pectin molecule, resulting inside chains containing mannose, glucose, galactose, and xylose. In pectin molecules, galacturonic acid molecules are methyl esterified. Based on methyl esterification, pectin is divided into two types: high methoxyl pectin and low methoxyl pectin. Pectin with a high methoxyl content has more than 50% galacturonic acid esterified, whereas pectin with a low methoxyl content has less than 50%. Pectin molecules have a molecular weight of 50,000 to 1,50,000 Dalton. Pectin is a high-classified soluble dietary fiber because of its water-soluble nature. In the small intestine, it resists digestion by human digestive enzymes, but it is digested by bacteria in the large intestine. Due to their proclivity to gel in aqueous systems, pectins are assumed to have a hypocholesterolemic impact; however, they can only be supplemented in food products up to a certain extent before interfering with the sensory features of the product (Chen et al., 2015).

1.2.1.3 GUMS

Gums are a form of polymer that is naturally water-soluble and produces a viscous solution when mixed with water. Plant exudates, plant seeds, microbial fermentation products, and seaweed extracts all contain this gum. Acacia gum, guar gum, locust bean gum, tragacanth gum, carrageenan, alginate, xanthan gum, pullulan gum, gellan gum, and others are some of the gums used (Islam, Phillips, Sljivo, Snowden, & Williams, 1997; Garcia Ochoa, Santos, Casas, & Gomez, 2000; Leathers, 2003; Bajaj, Survase, Saudagar, & Singhal, 2007;

Campo, Kawano, Da Silva, & Carvalho, 2009; Saha & Bhattacharya, 2010; Barak & Mudgil, 2014; Mudgil & Barak, 2013; Modgil, Barak, & Khatkar, 2014). The content and concentration of plant-based gums varies by species. Gums' polymeric content varies depending on the type. Some bacteria create gum, such as xanthan gum and pullulan gum, as a byproduct of their fermentation process. This gum can be used as dietary fiber sources because they are resistant to enzymatic digestion and act as functional dietary fiber. When it is added to a food product, it boosts the dietary fiber level. They are employed as food additives due to their ability to generate viscous solutions in water, as well as their dietary fiber properties. Enzymatic hydrolysis was recently employed to produce partially hydrolyzed guar gum, which can be used as a soluble dietary fiber source (Mudgil, Barak, & Khatkar, 2012; Mudgil, Barak, & Khatkar, 2014b). It improves the sensory and textural aspects of a dish while also increasing the dietary fiber content when added to it (Mudgil, Barak, & Khatkar, 2016a, b, c).

1.2.1.4 INULIN

The fructans family of indigestible carbohydrate polymers includes inulin, which is a water-soluble polymer. In the United States, it has GRAS (generally recognized as safe) status. In the wild, it's found in roughly 36,000 plant species (Shoaib et al., 2016). The most prevalent source of inulin is chicory roots, which are utilized in the commercial manufacture of inulin. Dahlia and Jerusalem, in the addition to chicory roots, are used in the commercial synthesis of inulin (Flamm, Glinsmann, Kritchershy, Procky, & Roberfroid, 2001). The fructose units in inulin are connected together by the β (2→1) D-frutosyl fructose linkage. No, the small intestine, anomeric carbon with a β-configuration is indigestible, but it is fermentable by microbial flora in the large intestine (Apolinario et al., 2014). Chicory-derived inulin may contain 2–60 fructose units HTV (Roberfroid 2005). Inulin's functioning is directly proportional to its degree of polymerization and branching. Bacterial inulin has a high degree of polymerization (more than 10,000). Inulin obtained from bacteria has a more branching structure than inulin derived from plants (Cho & Samuel, 2009). Inulin has been shown to have prebiotic properties and can be used to substitute fat and affect the texture of meals. It can also be used to develop unique functional foods with special health benefits for the human digestive system (Shoaib et al., 2016).

1.2.2 INSOLUBLE DIETARY FIBER

Insoluble dietary fibers are water-insoluble and so do not form gels. Microflora in the large intestine does not ferment insoluble food fibers. When consumed, they increase feces volume, aid in waste clearance, and reduce intestinal transit time. Celluloses and hemicelluloses are insoluble dietary fibers. Lignin, cutin, suberin, chitin, and chitosan are some of the proteins found in plants.

1.2.2.1 CELLULOSE

Cellulose, which is the main component of plant cell walls, is the most abundant organic material found in nature. Its molecules, along with other polysaccharides and lignins, can be found in plant cell walls. Algae and bacteria can also make cellulose (Iwamoto, Nakagaito, & Yano, 2007; Klemm et al., 2006). It's made up of glucose monomers organized in a straight line with no branching. The β-D-1,4-glycosidic links connect glucose units in cellulose molecules. In its natural condition, cellulose is made up of 10,000–15,000 units per chain. The ability of these cellulose linear chains to form hydrogen bonds with one another results in the formation of rigid, nonflexible, and crystalline micro-fibrils (McDougall, Morrison, Stewart, & Hillman, 1996). This fiber structure gives cellulose its strength, density, crystalline structure, chemical, and enzymatic resistance. The remaining 10% of cellulose is amorphous, with 90% of it being crystalline. In dilute acid and basic solutions, cellulose is similarly insoluble. Cellulose has a high-water absorption capacity due to its fibrous nature. Cellulose is resistant to human digestive enzymes in the small intestine, but microorganisms in the large intestine may break it down. This microflora's cellulose enzymes can degrade cellulose by breaking the -D-1,4-glycosidic linkages.

1.2.2.2 HEMICELLULOSE

In comparison to cellulose, hemicellulose has a more complicated structure. Hemicelluloses have a backbone chain made up of several monosaccharide units that can be found singly or in combination. Aside from that, hemicelluloses can have a variety of side chains attached to the backbone chain, making their structure more complex. In contrast to cellulose, hemicelluloses are soluble in dilute basic solutions. Hemicelluloses, like cellulose, are water and dilute acid solutions insoluble. These hemicelluloses can be recovered from plant cell walls using a standard extraction method once the pectin is removed (base solution) (McDougall et al., 1996). Hemicelluloses have a complicated structure because to their changeable monomer backbone chain, which is generally made up of glucose, galactose, xylose, mannose, and arabinose (singly or in combination) joined through 714 glycosides linkages. Hemicellulose polysaccharide molecules can have anywhere from 50 to 200 monomer units. Uronic acids may make up the side chain that connects the backbone chain to the side chain. The presence of monosaccharide units and the suffix "an" establish the nomenclature of hemicellulose molecules, such as xylan, arabinan, and so on. Under this structure-based classification, all glucans should be classified as hemicelluloses. Glucans, on the other hand, do not match the criterion for hemicellulose based on solubility, hence they are not included in this category. Because curdlan (β-1,3 glucan) is water-insoluble in nature and in dilute acid solutions, it is categorized as hemicelluloses (McIntosh, Stone, & Stanisich, 2005). Water soluble β-glucans generated from barley and oats that have both types of linkages (i.e., β-1,3 and β-1,4) are not considered hemicellulose. Because extracting and eliminating their related components, as well as isolating pure hemicellulose, is difficult and expensive, pure hemicelluloses are not commercially accessible.

1.2.2.3 LIGNIN

Lignin, commonly known as nature's most abundant aromatic polymer, is the second most abundant raw material on the globe (Gosselink et al., 2004; Lora & Glasser, 2002). It acts as a cellulose fiber cementing material in plant cells. Rather than being a polysaccharide, it is a polyphenyl-propane polymer. It contains a highly branched three-dimensional phenolic structure made up of phenyl-propane units such as p-coumaryl alcohol, coniferyl alcohol, and sinapyl alcohol. Lignin, like cellulose, is insoluble in aqueous solutions. Because of their inclination to create cross-links with other saccharide molecules, it aids in the interaction of plant cell wall components. Lignin molecules are resistant to enzymatic and chemical destruction in a way that no other molecule is. It also has a good bacterial degradation resistance. Lignin is more resistant to human digestive juices than other natural compounds. It is responsible for the structural strength of the wood due to its rigid structure. Some high-fiber components, such as oats, fiber, and cellulose, are processed to remove lignin due to their insoluble nature. Even boiling water is incapable of dissolving or softening lignin molecules. Despite the fact that lignin is not commercially isolated as a high-fiber ingredient, it is always found in conjunction with other fiber substances, especially those originating from plant cells. Because of the condensation and oxidation events that occur during the process, isolating lignin from lignocellulosic material is difficult (Hon, 1996). Lignin, a dietary fiber that is insoluble, has been demonstrated to benefit gastrointestinal physiology (Anderson & Bridges, 1988). Lignin-rich foods include celery, carrots, and other vegetables.

1.2.2.4 CUTIN AND SUBERIN

Cutin and suberin are complex polymers found in plant cell walls. The hydroxy fatty acid polyesters are what they're called. These, together with waxes that make up the hydrocarbon chain, can be found in plant cells. Both cutin and suberin are insoluble in water Insoluble dietary fibers make up a small percentage of plant-based fibers and are classed as such. Despite their modest concentration, they have a significant impact on the prevention of colorectal cancer (Ferguson & Harris, 1998). These are not commercially removed for use as fiber components, like lignin. Cutin produces the cuticle in plant cells, which can be found on both sides of the outer-epidermal walls of leaves and fruits, along with associated waxes. Suberin is a biopolymer generated from ferulic acid that has polyaliphatic and polyaromatic domains. Suberin is found in the cork cell wall of a number of root crops and tubers, and it is responsible for skin production (e.g., potatoes). Potato peels have been used as special culinary ingredients in cookies and pastry items after processing because of their unique baking qualities (Arora & Camire, 1994). In the colon, cutin and suberin have been demonstrated to protect cell-wall polysaccharides against bacterial enzymes (Harris & Ferguson, 1993). Cutin and suberin make the plant cell wall hydrophobic due to their high water insolubility. As a result, carcinogens that are hydrophobic in nature may be able to absorb them (Harris, Triggs, Roberton, Watson, & Ferguson, 1996).

1.2.2.5 CHITIN AND CHITOSAN

Chitin and chitosan are biological polymers composed of glucosamine and N-acetylated glucosamine monomers linked by β-1-4-glycosidic bonds

(Hamed, Ozogul, & Regenstein, 2016). Crabs and shrimp, for example, have them in their shells (Champ et al., 2003). Exopolysaccharides are also produced by some fungi and brown algae. Chitin and chitosan are identical except for their levels of acetylation and solubility. The chitosan molecule is deacetylated, but the chitin molecule is considerably acetylated. Chitin has high water insolubility, whereas chitosan has lower water insolubility. Chitosan molecules dissolve in acid. Human blood cholesterol levels are considerably reduced when chitosan is ingested as part of a diet. Clinical experiments show that chitosan decreases total serum cholesterol and raises serum HDL cholesterol when eaten in enriched biscuits at a dose of 6 g/day by healthy adult males (Maczaki et al., 1993). In the human gastrointestinal tract, chitosan molecules containing at least six glucosamine units and a low degree of deacetylation are adequate to prevent fat and cholesterol absorption. Chitosan's ability to form gels in the alimentary canal has been related to a reduction in cholesterol absorption (Deuchi, Kunauchi, Imasato, & Kobayashi, 1995). Ascorbic acid has also been demonstrated to increase chitosan's gel-forming capability, which leads to an increase in its ability to bind lipids and a decrease in plasma cholesterol levels.

1.2.2.6 RESISTANT STARCH

Starch is a polysaccharide made up of glucose monomers that can be found in plant cells. Glucose molecules are found in two polymeric forms in starch granules: Amylose and Amylopectin. Amylose is made up of glucose units connected by α-(1-4) glycosidic connections, whereas amylopectin is made up of glucose units connected by α-(1-4) and α-(1-6) glycosidic links: α-(1-6) linkages are crucial for starch granule branching. Amylases hydrolyze plant-derived starch molecules in the small intestine, rendering them digestible by human digestive enzymes. The term "resistant starch" refers to a group of starch molecules that, like other dietary fibers, resist amylase enzyme action in the human small intestine while showing some bacterial degradation in the large intestine. They can be classified as dietary fiber because of this feature (Fuentes-Zaragoza et al., 2010). RS1, RS2, RS3, and RS4 are the four varieties of resistant starches, respectively (Sajilata, Singhal, & Kulkarni, 2006). RS1 refers to starch molecules that are physically unavailable or inaccessible, suggesting that starches embedded or entrapped in plant parts (such as seeds and partially milled grains) are unavailable and resistant to enzymatic activity. These starches become digestible or available for digestion when their enclosing coating or structure is physically dissolved. Another type of starch is intact starch granules, often known as RS2 starches. There hasn't been any gelatinization of these starches. Amylase has no ability to break them down. Unripe bananas, undercooked peas, and potatoes are all high in these carbohydrates. After gelatinization, RS3 starches undergo retrogradation and lose their granular structure. This type of starch has a crystalline network in its structure and is resistant to amylase action in the human small intestine during digestion. Amylase enzymes can only hydrolyze gelatinized starch; they are unable to hydrolyze retrograded starch due to their network structure. Some of its sources are cooked, cooled potatoes, ready-to-eat cereals, and bread that has had its starches retrograded during production (Yue & Waring, 1998). RS4 type starches are chemically modified starches that have been finely changed: The best example of chemical modification is the crosslinking reaction, which changes the structure of starches and allows them to resist enzyme action during digestion.

1.3 PHYSICOCHEMICAL PROPERTIES

Dietary fiber's solubility, viscosity, and water-holding capacity, as well as bulking and fermentability, are significant physicochemical properties that are responsible for the physiological activities it provides.

1.3.1 SOLUBILITY

Dietary fiber's most important feature is its solubility, which is directly related to the physiological impacts it has. Based on their solubility, dietary fibers are classed as soluble or insoluble. Dietary fibers that are soluble have a physiological influence on plasma lipids and have been related to a lower risk of cardiovascular disease (Keservani et al., 2016a). When insoluble dietary fibers are ingested, they have been associated with positive effects on the human digestive system, such as better laxation and protection against colon cancer. The link between dietary fiber solubility and action is convoluted and ambiguous. Instead of being a single component, soluble fiber is a mixture of different types of polysaccharides with varying molecular weights. Dietary fiber solubility refers to the ability of the fiber to hydrate readily in water. Under the correct circumstances, they can also lead to the formulation of genuine solutions. The molecular structure of a polysaccharide impacts its water solubility (Morris & Norton, 1983). Polymers made consisting of monomer units made up of monosaccharides are known as polysaccharides (e.g., glucose, galactose, mannose, xylose, arabinose, etc.). The polysaccharide chain's monosaccharide units undergo structural changes in solution. They undergo reversible intramolecular chemical interactions between the dCHO and dOH groups, resulting in the formation of the hemiacetal structure. The dOH groups of other monosaccharide units can form a glycosidic bond with this hemiacetal, resulting in the formation of final polysaccharide and intermediate disaccharide. When D-glucose is used as the monosaccharide unit, a glycosidic bond can form between the first carbon of one glucose molecule and the first, second, third, fourth, or sixth carbon of another glucose molecule, resulting in a variety of configurations. As a result, the structure of the polysaccharide can be determined by the type of monosaccharide molecules present, as well as the type of connections between the monosaccharide units. The type of bonds or linkages present in monosaccharide units, on the other hand, has a bigger impact on polysaccharide solubility than the monosaccharide units themselves (Morris, 1979). Consider the similarities and differences between cellulose and barley-glucans, which are both made up of the same monomer units but have different types of connections between them, notably glucose units. Because of the different sorts of connections present, both have differing solubility properties in water. β-glucan, on the other hand, is water soluble in nature, but cellulose is not. Cellulose molecules have 1→4) links, whereas β-glucan molecules have both (1→4) and (1→3) linkages, resulting in their differing solubility. The insoluble property of cellulose is owing to the crystalline structure of cellulose chains linked via hydrogen bonds, which is attributable to comparable types of connections and regularity (Morris, 1989; Rees, 1977). Because β-glucans can't form organized crystalline structures due to their irregular structure, they're water soluble in nature and classified as soluble dietary fiber. The branching structure of polysaccharides is also responsible for their water-soluble characteristic. For example, arabinoxylans in wheat have a branched structure because they are unable to form organized crystalline structures and are hence water soluble in nature. The presence of charged groups on polysaccharides, such as COO- or SO-3, results in water solubility due to an electrostatic repulsive force between the charged groups, which prevents them from forming organized structures by packing of molecules, such as pectin's and carrageenan (Morris, 1989). As a result, several structural properties of polysaccharides, such as branching, the presence of ionizing groups, the bonding pattern, and structural nonuniformity, are clearly responsible for their solubility behavior (Glass, 1986).

Dietary fiber solubility has an impact on both physiological and technological functions in food (Jimenez-Escrig & Sanchez-Muniz, 2000). Consumption of soluble dietary fiber raises aqueous phase viscosity while lowering plasma cholesterol levels and glycemic response (McCarty, 2005; Slavin & Greenberg, 2003). Insoluble dietary fibers have a particular porosity and low density, which helps to increase feces volume and reduce intestinal transit time (Olson, Gray, & Chiu, 1987). Soluble and insoluble dietary fibers have different impacts on human physiology. On the other hand, functional food manufacturers seek to create soluble dietary fiber products.

1.3.2 VISCOSITY

One of the most important characteristics of soluble dietary fiber is its viscosity, which is defined as a fluid's resistance to its own flow (Dikeman & Fahey, 2006). When soluble dietary fiber (e.g., glucan, guar gum, psyllium, pectins, etc.) is distributed in the aqueous phase, it generates viscous solutions. The ability of dietary fibers to form gels is related to their predisposition for absorbing water, resulting in gelatinous bulk or viscous or gel-like solutions. Dietary fibers increase not just the volume but also the viscosity of the contents of the gastrointestinal system when consumed (Olson et al., 1987). Stomach emptying is delayed because of the increased viscosity and volume of digest, resulting in enhanced fullness. It also has an effect on lipid emulsification and can be used as a model. Dietary fiber makes food viscous in the stomach, resulting in a viscous gel-like substance that behaves like a solid rather than a semisolid or liquid. The digestion process is slowed by lowering the pace at which digestive enzymes diffuse toward their substrate. It also reduces the rate at which hydrolysis products are released for absorption on the mucosal surface. Intrinsic viscosity refers to the amount of space or volume that a dietary fiber molecule occupies (Morris, 1990). In the upper intestine, these components do not change as they do in other parts of the gut. Although they may be destroyed later, such as pectin, which is soluble at acidic pH in the stomach but not at neutral pH in the small intestine, the viscosity of a digest including dietary fiber components differs from that of, even if they may be destroyed later. Dietary fiber degradation may have a nutritional effect as a result of decreased viscosity, which is linked to physiological activity. The ionic environment and pH of the gastrointestinal tract influence the viscosity and solubility of dietary fiber components in the gastrointestinal system. It's been shown in polyelectrolytes like alginate, which gels in the stomach but hydrolyzes in the GI tract's small intestine. The concentration, content, molecular weight, and structure of dietary fiber components all play a role in determining their viscosity values in the gastrointestinal tract, and hence the physiological activity they cause. Water-soluble polysaccharides form viscous solutions in the majority of cases. The fundamental reason of polysaccharide viscosity in aqueous solutions is physical interactions, such as polysaccharide molecule entanglements in aqueous solutions (Glicksman, 1969; Graessley, 1974). Understanding the concept of polymer space or volume in aqueous solutions can help identify the characteristics of polysaccharide solutions (Morris et al., 1981). Polysaccharides are most typically seen in disordered conformation forms in solution. Brownian movements cause random fluctuating forms in polysaccharide molecules, which are referred to as random coils. In dilute solutions, there is a lot of free space between polysaccharide molecules. Polysaccharide molecules 1 are free to roam about. In concentrated solutions, polysaccharide molecules have no free space or volume: they overlap, interpenetrate, and become entangled with one another: The viscosity of the solution increases as the concentration of polysaccharides increases. As a result, the viscosity of polysaccharide solutions is affected by polysaccharide content. Another factor that affects the viscosity of polysaccharide solutions is shear rate. The entangled chain of polysaccharide molecules opens as a result of the shear rate, decreasing the viscosity of the concentrated polysaccharide solution. These characteristics are known as polysaccharide shear thinning behavior. In dilute liquids, the shear rate has an effect on viscosity. Temperature is another factor that determines the viscosity of polysaccharide solutions, however due to the constant temperature of the human body (37°C), this factor is less important in the case of dietary fiber for human intake. As a result, viscosity values for polysaccharide solutions should be reported alongside concentration, shear rate, and other viscosity-related factors. Under precise concentration, temperature, pH, shear rate, and other conditions, rotational-type viscometers and rheometers can be used to determine the viscosity of food-based compositions. These gadgets employ a spring to detect the resistance force on a rotating spindle and work on the resistance to flow idea.

1.3.3 WATER HOLDING AND BINDING CAPACITY

The interaction of dietary fiber with water can be described using terms like hydration, water-adsorption, water-binding, water-holding, water-uptake, and others. All of these phrases have similar meanings or have very little variance in meaning depending on the circumstances. The most frequent word used to define dietary fibers is water-holding and water-binding capacity. In the literature, there are certain definitions for these terms that can be used to distinguish between water-holding and water-binding capacity. Researchers developed a definition based on the polysaccharide gel formation concept, which can be applied to dietary fibers as well (Rey & Labuza, 1981). According to them, the amount of water in the gel structure that it can keep after being exposed to external force or stress is called water-binding capability. An example of an external force is centrifugal force. The water-binding capacity of dietary fiber is thought more relevant since different processing techniques of food products containing dietary fiber require exposure to external force or stress. Extrusion (cereal products), homogenization (liquid products), and high-speed mixing or kneading (bakery products) are only a few examples. Binding and water-holding characteristics. The capacity of dietary fibers is determined by numerous elements, the most important of which is the source of dietary fiber, which determines its chemical makeup. Water holding and water-binding capacity of dietary fibers are influenced by microstructure, processing conditions, and the method used to measure water holding and water-binding capacity. The water-binding or retention capacity of dietary technique fibers, according to some researchers, is a function of the fiber's origin or source, as well as the method used to quantify it. They also claimed that dietary fiber's shape is more important than its chemical composition (Robertson & Eastwood, 1981). The length, particle size, and porosity behavior of dietary fiber determine its microstructure. Both the supply of dietary fiber and the circumstances of processing processes have an impact on the microstructure of dietary fiber. As a result, producers can change the above-mentioned parameters to change dietary fiber's water-holding and binding capability and create custom-made dietary fiber. The conditions or ingredients used to meet the needs of specific food processors are also factors that influence dietary fiber's water-holding and binding capabilities. As a result, producers can vary these above-mentioned parameters to change the water-holding and binding capability of dietary fiber and create custom-made dietary fiber. The conditions or ingredients to meet the needs of specific food processors environment of the food system in which dietary fiber is incorporated are also elements that influence its water-holding and binding capabilities. All of these variables obstruct the ability of dietary fiber to bind water. The interaction of soluble dietary fibers with water molecules is influenced by pH and ionic behavior. This is especially true for soluble dietary fibers. The methods for determining the water-holding or binding property of dietary fibers have an impact on their value. There are several methods for measuring dietary fibers' water-holding and binding capacity; however, there is no universally accepted or approved approach. This makes comparing data on water-holding and binding capacity from different sources challenging. A recent article advocated choosing the best centrifugation method for water-binding capacity based on the hydration characteristics of dietary fibers (Robertson et al., 2000). According to the researchers, resistant starch and other dietary fibers such as apple pulp, pea hull, and citrus pulp produced statistically significant results. Dietary fibers made consisting of primary cell walls have a higher hydration capacity than secondary cell wall fibers (Thibault, Lahaye, & Guillon, 1992; Thibault, Renard, & Guillon, 1994). To measure the water-binding capacity of dietary fibers, a known volume of water is added to a known weight of the dietary fiber sample, which is then separated using filtration or centrifugation. Temperature, soaking time, centrifugation speed, and duration should all be addressed when determining the water binding capability of dietary fibers. When measuring the water-holding or binding capacity of dietary fiber, a small amount of soluble fiber is frequently lost, affecting the results (Fleury & Lahaye, 1991). The literature includes both direct and indirect methods for determining dietary fiber's water retention and water-binding ability (Cho, DeVries, & Prosky, 1997). Several updated methods for determining dietary fibers' water-holding and water-binding capacity have also been reported (Dreher, 1987; Thibault et al., 1992). Un-fermentable insoluble dietary fibers (cellulose, lignin, etc.) swell and have a high water-holding and water-binding capacity, resulting in an increase in fecal volume (Elleuch et al., 2011). Insoluble dietary fiber bulks up the colon by absorbing and entrapping water in its porous structure, which causes swelling. The water-binding property of insoluble dietary fiber allows it to dilute dangerous chemicals in the human large intestine, reducing their potency.

1.3.4 FERMENTABILITY

Dietary fibers are resistant to enzymatic action in the gastrointestinal tract, and they are slightly degraded by colonic microbial fermentation (Topping & Illman, 1986). Ferment ability is a critical characteristic of dietary fiber that permits it to act as a substrate in the fermentation process. According to the literature, a low-fiber diet results in normal excretion of 50 g per day with

800 k joules per day, but a high-fiber diet results in normal excretion of 88 g per day with 1700 k joules per day (Langkilde & Andersson, 1998) Dietary fibers that have not been fermented, such as lignin, and those that have been fully fermented, such as pectins, have various degrees of fermentation. Soluble dietary fiber is generally more fermentable by bacteria in the colon than insoluble dietary fiber. The fermentability and pattern of dietary fiber fermentation influence a variety of bowel functions, including fecal weight, stool frequency, colon pH, and energy from non-digestible meals (Edwards, 1995). Dietary fiber is classified as fast fermentable, slowly fermentable, or non-fermentable depending on its capacity to ferment in the colon. Dietary fibers derived from fruits and vegetables are an example of quickly fermentable dietary fibers. These variations do not add considerably to fecal bulk when compared to other types of dietary fibers. Dietary fibers generated from psyllium, wheat bran, and other sources are slowly fermentable. They also contribute to stool weight after fermentation. No fermentable or poorly fermentable dietary fibers have been associated with an increase in fecal size and weight in the human large intestine, resulting in a lower risk of constipation and colon cancer. Because of the formation of metabolites as a result of colonic fermentation, fermentable dietary fibers cause physiological changes in the colon mucosa (Bingham, 1990). Fast-fermenting dietary fibers have a post-absorption effect on the liver and other organ tissues (Topping & Pant, 1995). A few dietary fibers have also been connected to the activation of beneficial bacteria (bifidobacteria, lactobacilli, and others) in the human alimentary canal, which operate as a protective barrier and improve human immune response (Salminen et al., 1998). The fiber supply structure, which is further linked to bacterial interaction with the fermentation substrate, has a substantial impact on the rate and degree of fermentation (Guillon & Champ, 2000). Fruits and vegetables with a higher number of parenchyma tissues, such as the hull and bran components of grains and legumes, are more prone to fermentation than fiber sources with a higher number of secondary tissues. Soluble polysaccharides have a faster rate of fermentation than insoluble polysaccharides located in the cell wall. Dietary fibers having a quick fermentation characteristic (e.g., pectin and guar gum) are not protective against colon cancer, according to animal studies: In contrast, dietary fibers with a moderate fermentation rate (such as wheat bran) have been shown to protect against colon cancer (Young, 1991). Polysaccharides with a blocked branched structure aid fermentation in polysaccharides with larger and random branching. In contrast to the human microflora, which varies from person to person, the fermentation process, as well as the

densities of major taxonomic groups' cell populations, are strongly reliant on it (Macfarlane & Macfarlane, 1993). *Bacteria that may hydrolyze polysaccharides include Bifidobacterium, Ruminococcus Bacteroides, Clostridium,* and *Eubacterium.* In the colon, fructo-oligosaccharides, and inulin have the ability to increase the growth and activity of one or more bacteria kinds. Non-digestible oligosaccharides known as prebiotics promote the growth of beneficial microorganisms in the human stomach (Mudgil, Barak, Patel, & Shah, 2018). Short-chain fatty acids like acetate, butyrate, and others, as well as gases that are beneficial to humans, are end products of these fermentation activities in the human colon.

1.3.5 BINDING ABILITY OF MINERALS AND BILE ACIDS

In addition to water, dietary fiber components have been demonstrated to bind polar and ionic substances such as bile acids and minerals. Mineral availability and ionic component absorption are reduced when dietary fiber is included, as it has the ability to bind ions and polar molecules (Schneeman, 1986). The existence of free carboxylic groups and the amount of uronic acid present in the diet regulate the minerals and ion-binding ability of dietary fiber components. In the colon, where some dietary fibers are degraded, these metal ions and polar molecules may be released and absorbed. Wheat bran fiber, on the other hand, hinders absorption due to the presence of phytate, whereas sugar beet fiber promotes iron and zinc absorption (Fairweather-Tait & Wright, 1990). The adsorption and trapping of bile acids by dietary fibers from diverse food sources has been found to boost bile acid synthesis in human feces, which is regarded to be beneficial to human health (Eastwood & Hamilton, 1968; Kritchevsky & Story, 1974). When soluble dietary fiber comes into touch with water, it forms gel-like formations that are evacuated in the feces. According to these gel structures, the binding and entrapment of bile acids from the gallbladder is thrown out with the feces. In the terminal region of the ileum, where bile acids from the digest and are normally reabsorbed, the binding of bile acids by soluble dietary fiber gel structures is thought to be particularly important (Elleuch et al., 2011). Increased bile acid output in human feces causes the body to consume more cholesterol for bile acid synthesis, resulting in lower cholesterol levels in the body. The exact mechanism by which dietary fiber binds to bile acids remains a mystery. Some researchers suggest that ionic and hydrophobic interactions between bile acids and dietary fiber components promote bile acid binding and adsorption by dietary fiber (Thibault et al., 1992). The ability of dietary fibers to bind is also affected by their composition. The binding ability of fiber components improves when they comprise more courses and lignified tissues (Robertson, 1998). The adsorption ability of dietary fiber for different components can be determined using a variety of methods for measuring water-binding ability. Due to entrapment and adsorption, these components are maintained in dietary fiber cell matrices. A multitude of factors can affect the adsorption and binding ability of dietary fiber components. The two conditions are the pH of the digest in the small intestine and the behavior of digest, including dietary fiber in the small intestine: As a result, conditions should be controlled and reported when evaluating the binding ability of the dietary fiber.

1.3.6 OIL-BINDING ABILITY

Dietary fiber components have the ability to bind oil due to their structure. The chemical composition and structure of dietary fiber components determine oil-binding capacity. In determining oil-binding ability, dietary fiber structure porosity is a more essential determinant than chemical makeup or affinity for oil molecules. Chemical makeup or affinity plays a major impact in dietary fiber molecules ability to bind water. Dietary fiber components are porous, which permits them to bind oil in their pores. Simple pre-processing processes, such as soaking dietary fiber components in water, can reduce their oil-binding potential. Because water molecules occupy pores, pre-soaking products containing dietary-fiber components in water before adding oil helps to minimize oil uptake by fiber components. In the manufacturing of fried dishes, this is a crucial stage. As a result, the fat content of fried dishes is lowered, which is beneficial to one's health. The fat molecules are preserved in emulsified meat products when dietary fiber ingredients are added to comminuted meat products, resulting in emulsification. In the creation of low-fat meat products, this property of dietary fiber components is extremely important: the molecules of fiber: bond the formulation's low-fat content, resulting in improved textures in the finished product (Nelson, 2001).

1.3.7 PARTICLE SIZE AND POROSITY

The size of dietary fiber particles influences a number of essential physiological activities in the human colon, including digestion transit time, digestion fermentation rate, and fecal excretion. The surface area of dietary fiber is linked to the rate of dietary fiber fermentation. By expanding the surface area of dietary fiber, the fermentation process is accelerated, more bacteria attach to the substrate, making the fermentation process easier (Cherbut, 1995). Wheat bran coarse particles have a greater impact on digestion transit time than fine wheat bran particles. Dietary fiber reduces transit time in the human colon, shielding it from cytotoxic substances that are harmful to one's health. The kind of plant cell wall and the degree of processing define the particle size of dietary fiber. The particle size of dietary fiber is significantly affected by grinding, comminution, mincing, and other processing processes. Colonic bacteria can break down the fiber matrix, causing the particles to almost totally disintegrate. Dietary fiber activity in the colon isn't necessarily proportional to the particle size of dietary fiber consumed (Guillon & Champ, 2000). Dietary fiber porosity is another key property that influences bacterial and enzymatic degradation, and it varies depending on the types of cells, dietary fiber composition, and degree of processing. Pectins are hypothesized to have a major role in establishing cell wall porosity (Guillon et al., 1998).

1.4 IMPORTANT SUSTAINABLE SOURCES OF DIETARY FIBER

1.4.1 CEREALS AS A SOURCE OF DIETARY FIBER

Cereal grain consists of a variety of tissues with different compositions and capabilities. The outer grain tissues' cell walls are thick and act as a protective barrier in grain. These cell walls are made up of cellulose and complex xylans, with a little lignin thrown in for good measure. However, arabinoxylans and Beta-glucan make up the bulk of aleurone and endosperm cell walls, with cellulose, heteromannans, protein, and esterifies phenolic acids coming in second and third place, respectively (Fincher, 1986; Hemery et al., 2007; Saulnier & Quemener, 2009) (Table 1.2).

TABLE 1.2 Dietary Fiber Sources with Examples

Sources	Cereals	Legumes	Fruits	Vegetables
Examples	Wheat, rice, barley, oats, rye pseudocereals	Cluster beans, broad beans, chickpeas, lentils, soybeans, lentils, lupins, mung beans, lotus bean, sprouts, dry beans, green beans, peas	Oranges, kiwi fruit, apples, citrus fruits, prunes	Tomatoes, cabbage, alfalfa, carrots, potatoes, and lady fingers

1.4.1.1 WHEAT

Wheat is the second most often consumed cereal by humans, following rice. Wheat is a nutrient-dense grain that contains proteins and minerals. B-vitamins (Singh et al., 2017a) and dietary fiber (Keservani et al., 2020; Keservani et al., 2015d), to name a few (Sarwar, Qadri, & Moghal, 2013). The fiber content of whole wheat grains ranges from 11.6% to 12.7% (dry weight). Wheat bran, which accounts for 13–17% of the total weight of the wheat grain, is the majority of the fiber found in the outer layers of the grain. Although the composition of bran varies widely between crops, it mostly contains nutritional fiber, vitamins, and minerals (Stevenson. Phillips, Osullivan, & Walton, 2012). Wheat bran is a high-fiber food, with non-starch polysaccharide accounting for the majority of it (NSP) Arabinoxylan, cellulose, and glucan are the three main NSPs present in bran, accounting for 70%, 24%, and 6% of the total NSP, respectively (Maes & Delcour, 2002), Wheat bran soluble dietary fiber makes up 5% of total dietary fiber and is made up of glucan and xylans, which is substantially less than barley (3–11%) and oats (3–7%) (Wood, 1997). The water-insoluble fiber in wheat bran is made up of Arabinoxylan (19%–25%), Starch (17–29%), Protein (14–18%), Lignin (3%), β-glucans (1%), Phytic acid (3–5%), and Ferulic acid (0.3–5%). β-glucans are highly viscous and soluble in water. β-glucans make up about 2.2% to 2.7% of the dry weight of wheat bran. Wheat bran has long been recommended as part of a healthy diet to help prevent constipation and cancer caused by fiber deficiency. Wheat bran has been used to increase the nutritional value of cereal-based foods for a long time. Wheat bran is a good source of nutrients and fiber. The health benefits of B vitamins and bioactive substances have all been discovered (Onipe, Jideani, & Beswa, 2015). Dietary fibers have been shown to improve gut health, hunger control, and satiety duration. As a result of fiber fermentation, increased stool size, reduced gut transit time, increased viscosity in the small intestine, and short-chain fatty acid (SCFA) synthesis in the colon occur (Brouns, Hemery, Price, & Anson, 2012) are all variables that lead to extended satiety (Brouns, Hemery, Price, & Anson, 2012). Although there has been little research published on the influence of wheat bran dietary fiber on human weight regulation, there is insufficient evidence to support its use as a weight regulator. Arahinoxylans, which make up around 64% of the cell walls in wheat bran, have been demonstrated to minimize the risk of type 2 diabetes by reducing postprandial glycemic response by retaining gut viscosity. Wheat bran is a food additive that aids in the making of dough and the baking of bread (Anson, Hemery, Bast, & Haenen, 2012).

1.4.1.2 RICE

Rice is a starchy cereal grain consumed by a large section of the world's population, especially in East and Southeast Asia, where rice is the sole food supply. Rice has long been a source of food for mankind, with humans consuming nearly all of the rice produced worldwide. Rice is a nutritious food that is especially high in vitamins and fiber. Because each layer includes various levels of fat, carbohydrate, protein, and fiber, the nutritional quality of rice is modified by the removal of different layers during the milling process. There's a layer of bran on the outside. The seed coat, aleuronic layer, and anthocyanin layer are all lost during brown rice milling. Milled rice loses a lot of fat, crude protein, and neutral detergent fiber as a result of this process. Rice bran, which contains a lot of crude fiber, produces two tractions when the rice is milled. Another choice is white rice, which is high in carbs. The majority of rice bran fiber is made up of no cellulosic polysaccharide (24%), cellulose (10.3%), and lignin (10.7%) (Sera et al., 2005). SDF (soluble dietary fiber) (Rao & Muralikrishna, 2004) is made up of arabinoxylans and a small amount of ß-D-glucans found in rice bran as well as rhamnose, xylose, mannose, galactose, and glucose, while IDF (insoluble dietary fiber) is made up of cellulose, hemicellulose, Insolubleβ-glucan, and arabinoxylans (Lai, Lu, He, & Chen, 2007). The number and amount of these non-starch polysaccharides are influenced by rice cultivar, degree of milling, and water solubility. Rice bran has about 25.3 g of dietary fiber per 100 g, which could be adequate to meet an adult's daily dietary fiber need of roughly 27 gm. The majority of the dietary fiber in rice bran is made up of insoluble fibers, such as cellulose, hemicellulose (13%), and pentosans (6.5%). Additionally, it contains roughly 2% soluble dietary fiber. The role of dietary fiber in the prevention of diabetes and heart disease has been well-proven in the literature. Despite the fact that rats and hamsters have been extensively studied in this field, only a few human studies have been conducted to demonstrate the anti-diabetic and hypocholesterolemic effects of rice bran dietary fiber (Kahlon, Chow, Sayre, & Betschart, 1992). In a human investigation (Hegsted, Windhauser, Morris, & Lester, 1993), Rice bran has been found to lower plasma cholesterol levels by 100 grams per day, making it comparable to oat bran. About 30 grams of rice bran, on the other hand, had no discernible effect. Rice bran, both full-fat and defatted, is high in dietary fiber, with the latter having a higher fiber content (30%). Rice bran can be found in a number of meals, including prepared foods, nutraceuticals, and functional foods, and contains oryzanol and phytosterols, which may contribute to its hypocholesterolemic effect. Snack items, baked goods, pasta, gluten-free cuisine, and beverages are all available (Faccin, Miotto, do Nascimento Vieria, Barreto, & Amante, 2009), and animal products are just a few examples (Huang, Shiau, Liu, Chu, & Hwang, 2005).

1.4.1.3 BARLEY

Barley (Hordeum vulgare) contributes considerably to the nutritional requirements of the human population. While barley is an excellent source of some nutrients, it may be lacking in others (Newman & Newman, 2006). However, the barley grain is well-known for its high levels of dietary fiber and polyphenols. Because of its nutritional content and nutraceutical properties, whole-grain barley is suggested (Lahouar et al., 2014). The soluble fiber β-glucan has a nutraceutical characteristic. β-glucan is a polymer found mostly in barley kernel cell walls, aleurone layer, and endosperm. The amount of β-glucan in the extract depends on the cultivar, the viscosity of the extract, and the amount and type of starch in the extract (Andersson et al., 2004). β-glucan, a soluble fiber, helps to prevent hypercholesterolemia, hypoglycemia, and colon cancer caused by chemicals (Newman & Newman, 2008). Fiber, after starch, is the second most essential component of the grain, and it may be found all over the kernel (Brownlee, 2011). Soluble and insoluble fibers are the two forms of fiber. Barley has a total fiber content ranging from 11–34%. Soluble dietary fiber, usually in the form of β-glucan, make up around 3%–20% of the total content (Jalili, Wildman, & Medeiros, 2000; Makeri, Mkama, & Badau, 2013). The β-glucan concentration of barley ranges from 2% to 11%, which is greater than the β-glucan content of oats (2.2–708) and wheat (2.2–708) (0.4%–1.4%). Two of the health benefits of consuming glucan-rich foods include lower blood glucose levels and lower serum total and LDL cholesterol levels. Hashemi (2015); Smith, Queenan, Thomas, Fulcher, & Salvin (2008) attribute the above-mentioned health benefits of β-glucan to the increased viscosity of intestinal material, which is dependent on the molecular weight solubility of β-glucan. A portion of barley escapes digestion and absorption in the small intestine and is fermented into short-chain fatty acids in the large intestine (Wong & Jenkins, 2007). Resistant starch (RS) is a starch fraction that has been associated to a lower glycemia index, decreased cholesterol absorption, and colon cancer prevention (Le Leu, Brown, Hu, & Young, 2003). As a functional element, RS may be found in a wide range of culinary items.

Barley's RS concentration rises after processing. The heating and cooling cycles that occur during barley processing promote starch retrogradation, which increases the concentration of RS. Another method for making RS is gelatinization of starch, enzymatic disbranching of the gelatinized polymer, inactivation of the disbranching enzyme, and separation of the resultant product by drying, extrusion, or crystallization. The indigestibility of the small intestine is thought to be one of its health benefits. It is fermented in the large intestine by the intestinal microflora, and it has a prebiotic effect by changing the ecology of the microbial flora in the large intestine. As resistant starch and probiotics are taken together, a symbiotic effect develops in which the prebiotic RS shields a portion of the ingested organisms from digestion in the colon, thereby increasing the initial levels of the desired species when they reach the colon (Salvin, 2013; Topping, Fukushima, & Bird, 2003).

1.4.1.4 OATS

Oats are abundant in dietary fiber, proteins, and minerals, which are all good for your health (Butt et al., 2008). Food manufacturers can market goods containing 1 gm-glucan/portion with claims of decreasing blood cholesterol and lowering postprandial glycemic response under the European Union's health claims. Furthermore, ingesting oat and barley grain fiber has been associated to increased stool volume and the prevention of metabolic syndrome (Clotens et al., 2012). The bulk of mixed-linkage (13) and (14)-D-glucan, which is also found in the starchy endosperm, is located in the innermost layer of aleuronic layer of oat grains, showing that -D-glucan is predominantly found in the sub-aleurone area. The primary dietary fiber components of oats are mixed-linkage (13) and (14) β-D-glucan (β-glucan) and arabinoxylan (AX) (Khan et al., 2016). The bran portion has a higher concentration of β-glucan and AX than the starch-rich endosperm part. β-glucan makes up about a third of the insoluble fiber in oats, whereas it makes up the majority of the soluble fiber (Manthey, Hareland, & Huseby, 1999). The percentage of protein in whole-grain oats ranges from 65 to 9% (Shewry et al., 2008). In oats, the glucan is a linear polymer composed of -D-glucopyranose units connected by (14) and (13) connections (Parrish, Perlin, & Reese, 1960). Approximately 90% of (14) linked D-glucopyronoses are found in groups of three (cellotriose) or four (cellotetraose) units separated by one (1→3) linkage, with a 70:30 ratio of (1→4) to (1→3) connections (Doublier & Wood, 1995). The β–(1→3) bonds increase the flexibility of the chain, preventing cellulose molecules from aggregating and enhancing the solubility of β-glucan in water (Buliga, Brants, & Fincher, 1986). The molecular weight (MW) of oat glucan ranges from 1000 to 3100 kDa (Sikora, Tosh, & Olsson, 2013). In multiple trials and meta-analyzes, oat-glucan was found to successfully decrease LDL cholesterol levels (low density lipoprotein) in hypercholesterolemia individuals (Othman, Moghadasian, & Jones, 2011; Ripsin et al., 1992). According to research by Othman et al. (2011), consuming 3 g of oat-glucan on a daily basis can lower blood total LDL cholesterol levels by 5% to 10% in normal and hypercholesterolemic people.

1.4.1.5 RYE

Rye is one of the heartiest grains and is said to be more nutritious than wheat. In Central Asia, rye was initially grown as a wild plant. Rye has a magnesium-to-calcium ratio of 4:1 and is strong in dietary fiber, phosphorus, magnesium, and vitamin B1. Rye, with its high avoids blood sugar increases and is therefore useful for diabetics. Irritable bowel syndrome sufferers have been demonstrated to benefit from rye's fiber content, which has been shown to alleviate symptoms. Rye's ability to create more soluble and insoluble fiber, as well as increase colonic butyric acid production, may help to prevent colon cancer. Rye can assist regular bowel function and improve the sensation of fullness by providing water-binding, non-cellulose polysaccharides (Aman, Anderrson, Rakha, & Andersson, 2010).

1.4.1.6 PSEUDOCEREALS

Amaranth, quinoa, and buckwheat are dicotyledonous plants, whereas wheat, rice, and barley are monocotyledonous. Psuedocereals are seeds that function and compositionally resemble those of actual cereals. It is well accepted that consuming foods naturally high in dietary fiber is beneficial to one's health (Champ et al., 2003). In a gluten-free diet, physicians advocate consuming more fiber-rich whole-grain cereals rather than refined grains, as a gluten-free diet's fiber intake is considered insufficient (Hopman et al., 2006; Kupper, 2005; Pagano, 2006; Thompson et al., 2005). In research, the pseudocereals amaranth, quinoa, and buckwheat have been shown to be good sources of dietary fiber. Buckwheat seeds, for example, have far higher dietary fiber than amaranth and quinoa, which have fiber levels comparable to those found in common cereals (Alvarez-Lubete, Arendt, & Gallagher,

2009). As a consequence, adding these seeds in the diets of celiac disease patients should help to alleviate, at least in part, the population's fiber shortage.

1.4.1.7 LEGUMES AS A SOURCE OF DIETARY FIBER

Legumes are one of the world's oldest food crops, having been grown for more than 10,000 years. The legume family comprises pod-bearing, common food plants such dry beans, broad beans, dry beans, chickpeas, lentils, soybeans, lupine, mung beans, lotus, sprouts, alfalfa, green beans, peas, and peanuts. The phrases "legumes" and "pulses" are used interchangeably since all pulses are legumes, but not all legumes are pulses. According to the Food and Agriculture Organization, pulses are "crops harvested solely for the dry seed of leguminous plants." Legumes are high in protein, low glycemic carbohydrates, dietary fiber, minerals, and vitamins. Peas and beans have a protein content of 17–20% dry weight, whereas legumes have a protein content of 38–40% dry weight. Legumes are high in protein (17–20% dry weight in peas and beans, 38–40% dry weight in soybeans and lupines) and dietary fiber (5–37% dry weight) (Kouris-Blazos & Belski, 2016). Beans, chickpeas, and peas have the largest dietary fiber content, with 60–85% insoluble and 40–15% soluble, followed by lentils, which have the lowest. Because of the great range of legume species grown in different places, the DF content of each pulse described in the literature varies. The impact of cooking on the dietary fiber level of common legumes was researched by Xuan & Azlan (2017), who discovered that kidney beans, chickpeas, and mung beans had total dietary fiber content of 27.66%, 15.88%, and 19.38%, respectively. Cooking also reduced the fiber level of the various legumes evaluated, according to the researchers. Eashwarage (2017) investigated the level of dietary fiber and resistant starch in Sri Lankan legumes. Cow peas had dietary fiber levels of 13.07% to 15.99%, soybeans had 18.51%, horse beans had 21.38%, lentils had 14%, and peas had 6%. The most resistant starch is found in horse gram (10.68%), followed by cowpea (9.62%). Chavan, Kute, and Kadam (1989) found that the crude fiber content of Faba beans ranged from 5.0 to 8.5%, whereas Pritchaed, Dryburgh, and Wilson (1973) and Hove, King, and Hill (1973) found dietary fiber values of 15 to 30% (1978). The various types used in the study might have led to the differences in fiber content. Beach bean (*Canavalia maritime*), marama bean (*Tylosema esculentum*), rice bean (*Vigna umbellate*), winged bean

(*Phosphocarpus tetragonolobus*), bambara nut (*Vigna subterranean*), and tepary bean (*Phaseolus acutifolius*) are some of the underutilized legumes that have recently gained attention as highly nutritive (Katoch, 2013). The nutritional fiber content of these underutilized legumes has been studied by researchers from all over the world. The overall dietary fiber content of the Tepary bean is 9.8%, with 9.2% insoluble dietary fiber and 0.6% soluble dietary fiber. Beach bean has 2.26% dietary fiber, marama bean has 18–24% (Holse, Husted, & Hansen, 2010), rice bean has 12.23% (Holse, Husted, & Hansen, 2010), rice bean has 5.22–7.43% (Rodriguez & Mendoza, 1991), and winged bean has 12.23% (Holse, Husted, & Hansen, 2010), rice bean has 5.22–7.43% (Rod (Holse, Husted, & Hansen, 2010) (Amoo, Adebayo, & Oyeleye, 2006). In general, hemicelluloses and cellulose make up the majority of insoluble dietary fiber in legumes; however, the main polysaccharides in chickpea and lentil IDF are Arabians and cellulose (Martin-Cabrejas et al., 2006), whereas cellulose and peptic polysaccharides are the main polysaccharides in pea IDF (Martin-Cabrejas et al., 2006) (Martin-Cabrejas et al., 2003). Soluble dietary fiber in beans, peas, and chickpeas, on the other hand is mostly made up of pectin polysaccharides, but SDF fractions in lentils and cowpeas have reduced pectin polysaccharide content (Benitez et al., 2013). Legume fibers have a number of benefits over grain fibers. Legume fibers had a higher concentration of soluble components, resulting in the formation of more volatile fatty acids such as acetic acid, prop-ionic acid, and butyric acid. Butyric acid has been found to reduce the incidence of colorectal cancer (Fechner, Kiehntopf, & Jahreis, 2014; Fechner, Fenske, & Jahreis, 2013). Furthermore, new study suggests that acetic acid increases the experience of satiation from fiber through modifying brain (Keservani et al., 2015b, 2016b) homeostatic systems as well as its well-known effect on gastrointestinal baro-receptors (Frost et al., 2014).

1.4.2 THE EFFECT OF DIFFERENT TREATMENTS ON LEGUMES DIETARY FIBER CONTENT

Because raw beans have anti-nutritional components that can damage enzyme function, digestion, nutrition, and health, they are rarely taken. Cooking, soaking, and roasting, for example, may change the amount of dietary fiber and phenolics in legumes (Guillon & Champ, 2000). Cooking is one of the most common ways people prepare legumes. Germination has been proposed as a method of removing antinutritive components from legumes by mobilizing secondary metabolic products that serve as reserve nutrients (e.g., phyates and galactosides). Vidal et al. (1998) looked into the effects of Faba bean processing on the nutrients and anti-nutrients in the beans. Cooking the presoaked Faba beans marginally decreased carbohydrate, dietary fiber, calcium, and phytic acid levels. Germination resulted in a considerable drop in galatoside and phytic acid concentrations after 6 days, but only a little reduction in carbohydrate and dietary fiber. Uncooked and cooked germinated seeds of the wild legume canavailia maritime produced on the southwest coast of India's coastal sand dunes were evaluated by D'Cunha, Sridhar, and Bhatt (2009). Cooking lowered the crude fiber content of un-germinated legume seeds from 2.26% to 1.70%, while germination slightly reduced the crude fiber content. De Almmeida Costa, Da Silva Queiroz-Monici, Reis, and De Oliveria studied the influence of heating and freeze-drying on the delivery fiber content of traditional legumes (2006). The amount of dietary fiber in raw and processed beans did not differ significantly. Kutos, Golob, Kac, and Plestenjak (2003) found a significant decrease in IDF and TDF content after canning and boiling beans. The IDF content of the beans reduced whereas the SDF level increased during soaking. The SDF content of soaked beans was reduced by cooking and canning. When compared to raw legumes, Marconi, Ruggeri, Cappelloni, Leonardi, & Carnovale (2000) discovered that boiling and microwave heating did not modify the total non-starch polysaccharides content of beans and chickpeas, but both methods increased SDF and decreased IDF. These changes were produced by partial solubilization and de-polymerization of hemicelluloses and insoluble pectin polysaccharides. As a result of the cooking and microwave heating, plant tissues were softened (Pena, Vergara, & Carpita, 2001). Aldwairji, Chu, Burley, and Orfila (2014) investigated the fiber content of boiled and canned beans commonly consumed in the United Kingdom. TDF levels in boiling legumes were higher (3.6% in green beans to 11.2% in red kidney beans) as compared to raw legumes (TDF values of 2.7% in canned beans to 7.4% for canned chickpeas). As a result, canned beans were found to have significantly lower TDF levels than cooked legumes. When compared to boiled legumes, however, canning had no significant effect on the percentage of IDF to SDF. Germination increases the IDF to SDF fractions as well as the TDF concentration in general (Lee, Oh, Yang, & Kim 2006). Furthermore, the TDF concentration of bean DF decreases as a result of both natural and microbial fermentation (Martin-Cabrejas et al., 2004).

1.4.3 FRUITS AND VEGETABLES AND THEIR WASTE AS SOURCE OF DIETARY FIBER

According to worldwide nutrition standards, consumers should eat a variety of fruits, vegetables, and whole grains to meet their daily dietary fiber intake objectives. Cereal fibers include barley, corn germ, rice bran, rye bran, sorghum bran, corn bran, lignin, wheat bran, wheat starch, arabinoxylan, barley bran flour, oat bran, resistant starch, and soluble corn fiber, while vegetables fiber includes tomatoes, alfalfa, cabbage, carrot fiber, fructo-oligosaccharides (FOS), insulin, and potatoes. Fruit fiber may be found in oranges, kiwi fruit, apples, citrus pectin, and prunes. The fruit and vegetables processing sector, one of the most well-known in the world, generates a great number of byproducts, such as fruit peel, pomance, and other byproducts. Fruit peels make for 20% to 40% of the overall weight of the fruit, according to recent research. The byproducts are commonly used as animal feed and fertilizers, but they may also be turned into more valuable culinary goods to save money on shipping and disposal. As a result, there's been a boom in interest in incorporating the health-promoting components and other key compounds found in fruit and vegetable peels into functional meals. Fruit peels include significant amounts of non-starch polysaccharide and lignin, both of which are important components of the plant's cell wall. Insoluble food fibers such as non-starch polysaccharides and lignin are not digested or absorbed in the human small intestine. As a result, researchers from all over the world have attempted to convert banana (Emaga Andraianaivo, Wathelet, Tchango, & Paquot, 2007), mango (Koubala et al., 2008), citrus (Figuerola, Hurtado, Estevez, Chiffelle, & Asenjo, 2005), and lime (Figuerola, Hurtado, Estevez, Chiffelle, & Asenjo, 2005) peels into (Ubando-Rivera, Navarro-Ocana & Valdidvia-Lopez, 2005). According to the literature, the residue of apple (Grigelmo-Miguel & Martin-Belloso, 1999) and citrus fruit, such as grapefruit, lemon, and orange (Figierola et al., 2005), as well as citrus peels, such as Valencia orange, Persa lime, Maxicanlime, lemon, and sweet orange, from juice extraction, as well as citrus peels, such as Valencia orange, Persa lime, Maxi can (Marin, Soler-Rivas, Benavente-Garcia, Castillo). Furthermore, due to the presence of associated bioactive components with antioxidant qualities such as flavonoids (Singh et al., 2017a; Keservani & Sharma, 2014), polyphenols, and carotene, the dietary fiber from citrus peels is of better quality than other fiber sources (Marin et al., 2017). Lim & Ra (2013) The proximate analysis of three apple species found that water makes up 83.28% to 89.92% of the apple, whereas dietary fiber makes up only 0.86%

to 1.81%. The total dietary fiber content of apple pomace extracted after processing, on the other hand, is reported to be 51.10 g/100 g (dry matter basis). Insoluble dietary fiber is 36.50 g/100 g, whereas DM is 14.60 g/100 g soluble. The quantity of pressing, the use of enzymes, and subsequent extraction with water and other solvents, among other things, have an impact on the outcomes. Nilnakara, Chiewchan, and Devahastin (2009) studied the crude fiber content of cabbage leaves and discovered that it ranged from 19.92 to 47.47 g/100 g DM. Tanongkankit, Chiewchan, and Devahastin (2010) discovered that cabbage leaves contain 40.89 g/100 g DM of total dietary fiber, which is similar to Tanongkankit, Chiewchan, and Devahastin's results (2009). Carrots are another commonly used vegetable in the food industry, although their peels or pomance are typically thrown away or given to animals. Carrot peels contain 45.45 g/100 g DM of dietary fiber and have a high antioxidant capacity of 94.67%, according to Chan taro, Devahastin, and Chiewchan (2008). According to the researchers, blanching increases total dietary fiber (TDF) yield and the ratio of insoluble dietary fiber (IDF) to soluble dietary fiber (SDF), while having no effect on total phenolic content. Murthy & Naidu (2012) looked into the coffee bean's byproducts and discovered that coffee pulp, husk, silver skin, and spent coffee are high in natural antioxidant compounds connected to dietary fiber. These byproducts have a total dietary fiber content ranging from 28% to 80%. Guava (*Psidium guajava* L) is a tropical fruit that is widely consumed both fresh and processed in the form of drinks, syrups, ice cream, and jams (Jimenez-Escrig, Rincon, Pulido, & Saura-Calixto, 2001). Guava fruit and byproducts have a high antioxidant capacity, which adds to their health benefits. According to Jimenez-Escrig et al. (2001); and Martinez et al. (2012) research, guava concentrate, and byproducts have a high dietary fiber content of up to 69.1 g/100 g DM. Vitis vinifera grapes are primarily produced for wine making. The total weights of grapes used are a consequence of the total weights of grapes used (Torres et al., 2002). Grape pomace contains seeds, skins, and steams, all of which may be used to manufacture grape seed oil. The dietary fiber content of grape pomace was studied by Saura-Calixto (1998). Dietary fiber content was reported to be 64.6% DM. Llobera & Canellas (2007), as well as Sanchez-Alonso, Jimenez-Escrig, Saura-Calixto, and Borderias (2007), evaluated the fiber content of red grapes and discovered that red grapes produced an even higher value of dietary fiber, ranging from 74% to 77.2% DM. White grape pomace and stem have a total dietary fiber content of 71.5–79.5 g/100 g Dm, according to Llobera & Canellas (2008), which validates these findings. Mango (Mangifera indica L) is a popular fruit that is produced all over the world, especially in the tropics. According to Vergara-Valencia et al. mango fiber concentrate (Martinez et al., 2012) and powder from mango peels (Ajila, Leelavathi, & Rao, 2008), have high dietary fiber content of 28.05–70.0 g/100 g DM (2007). Oranges are well-known for their high vitamin C and phenolic content. These bioactive compounds are abundant in orange juice, which helps to improve its antioxidant capabilities (Stella, Ferrarezi, dos Santos & Monteiro, 2011). The flavedo of oranges includes greater vitamin C, flavones, and carotenoid content than orange juice, according to Escobedo-Avellaneda, Gutierrez-Uribe, Valdez-Fragoso, Torres, and Welti-Chanes (2014), while the albino contains phenolics, flavanones, and antioxidant activity. According to Fernandez-Lopez et al. the orange peel has a high dietary fiber level of 71.62 g/100 g DM (2009). Martinez et al. (2012) found that dietary fiber concentrate produced from Passiflora byproducts contained 81.5 g/100 g DM of total dietary fiber. In a comparable research, Lopez-Vargas, Fernandez-Lopez, Perez-Alvarez, and Viuda-Martos (2013) discovered 53.52–71.79 g/100 g DM total dietary fiber from yellow passion fruit co-products, pulp, seed, and albedo. Martinez et al. (2012) investigated pineapple fiber concentrate, which is a waste product from industrial operations, and discovered that it has an abnormally high amount of total dietary fiber (75.8 g/100 g DM). Pomegranates are one of the oldest edible fruits on the planet. Pomegranate is a native of Persia and its environs, with juice, pulp, and seeds accounting for 65–75% of the total weight of the fruit (Tehranifar, Zarei, Nemati, Esfandiyari, & Vazifesenas, 2010). Pomegranates are high in dietary fiber. Total dietary fiber in various varieties of pomegranates ranged from 0.57 g/100 g to 1.15 g/100 g, with an average of 0.82 g/100 g. Insoluble dietary fiber was the most prevalent portion detected in pomegranate dietary fiber concentrates, with an average of 0.64 g/100 g. As a result, fruits, vegetables, and even their waste may be used as a rich source of dietary fiber.

1.5 OPPORTUNITIES AND CHALLENGES

Despite evidence of the health benefits of eating carbohydrates (Singh et al., 2017b) that resist digestion in the small intestine, fiber intakes in the UK are now much below recommended levels. Some of the health benefits of fiber consumption are well-known (for example, promoting regular bowel movements), whereas others are still being studied. New evidence, especially from animal research, is always emerging, but it must be backed up by consistent evidence from human studies. Although there is a lot of overlap, the advantages of the various non-digestible components that are commonly referred to as dietary fiber are not necessarily interchangeable. As a result, getting your fiber from a range of sources is crucial for getting the maximum health benefits. The majority of customers, on the other hand, are likely to be unaware of recent developments and the overlapping qualities of various types of carbohydrate that resist digestion in the small intestine, as well as their specific origins. This shows that a consumer education campaign focusing on carbohydrates, namely the health benefits of fiber, is long overdue. The question of whether extra fiber, whether as a dietary element or as a supplement, is as useful as fiber found intact in whole foods is a major problem. Although there is currently little research on this topic, it has been discovered in other areas of nutrition that fruits and vegetables, for example, are more effective than the antioxidants they contain when taken as dietary supplements in preventing cardiovascular disease and cancer. Other considerations include the structure of the item (e.g., food vs. liquid) and the physiological effects of various fiber components. The ability to make claims about such features will necessitate robust and extensive documentation that follows the structure of the new Regulation. As scientific knowledge of insulin and oligo-fructose/insulin-type fructans' physiological benefits in humans has grown, so has their use. Long-chain insulin has been used for a variety of purposes, including as a fat substitute (owing to its ability to replicate the mouth feel of fat) and to improve the stability of foams and emulsions (Alexiou & Franck, 2008). Oligo-fructose is utilized as a sugar substitute since it is fairly sweet. In both cases, these folks have the same vitality.

1.6 CONCLUSION

Dietary fibers are divided into two categories based on their ability to dissolve in water: soluble and insoluble. Textural and sensory features of food products are also linked to dietary fiber. Solubility, viscosity, water-holding ability, oil-holding ability, particle size, porosity, and other properties of dietary fibers are all significant. Dietary fibers can be found in a variety of foods, including cereals (wheat, rice, barley, oats), legumes (dry beans, broad beans, drybeans, chickpeas, lentils, soybean, lupins), fruits (orange, kiwis, apples), and vegetables (tomatoes, carrots) while the recovery of dietary fibers to summaries, dietary fibers are key food ingredients that can be used to provide health benefits as well as desirable sensory and textural changes.

KEYWORDS

- **arabinoxylan**
- **dietary fibers**
- **fructo-oligosaccharides**
- **molecular weight**
- **physiological properties**
- **resistant starch**
- **short-chain fatty acids**

REFERENCES

Ajila, C. M., Leelavathi, K. U. J. S., & Rao, U. P., (2008). Improvement of dietary fiber content and antioxidant properties in soft dough biscuits with the incorporation of mango peel powder. *Journal of Cereal Science, 48*(2), 319–326.

Aldwairji, M. A., Chu, J., Burley, V. J., & Orfila, C., (2014). Analysis of dietary fiber of boiled and canned legumes commonly consumed in the United Kingdom. *Journal of Food Composition and Analysis, 36*(1, 2), 111–116.

Alexiou, A., & Franck, A., (2008). Prebiotic inulin-type fructans: Nutritional benefits beyond dietary fiber source. *Nutri. Bulle., 33*, 227–233.

Alvaez-Jubete, L., Arendt, E. K., & Gallagher, E., (2009). Nutritive value and chemical composition of psuedocereals as gluten-free ingredients. *International Journal of Food Sciences and Nutrition, 60*(suppl 4), 240–257.

Amado, R., Amaea-Collaco, M. T., Andersson, H., Asp, N. G., Bach, K. K. E., Champ, M., Mathers, J., Robertson, J. A., Rowland, I., & Van, L. J., (eds.), *Functional Properties of Nondigestible Carbohydrates* (pp. 140–142).

Aman, P., Andersson, A. A. M., Rakha, A., & Andersson, R., (2010). Rye, a healthy cereal full of dietary fiber. *Cereal Foods World, 55*(5), 231–234.

Amoo, I. A., Adebayo, O. T., & Oyeleye, A. O., (2006). Chemical evaluation of winged beans (*Psophocarpus tetragonolobus*), Pitanga cherries (*Eugenia uniflora*) and orchid fruit (orchid fruit myristic a). *African Journal of Food Agriculture, Nutrition and Development, 6*(2).

Anderson, J. W., & Baird, P., Davis, R. H., Ferreri, S., Knudtson, M., Koraym, A., et al., (2009). Health benefits of dietary fiber. *Nutrition Reviews, 67*(4), 188–205.

Anderson, J. W., & Bridges, S. R., (1988). Dietary fiber content of selected foods. *The American Journal of Clinical Nutrition, 47*(3), 40–447.

Andersson, A. A., Armo, E., Grangeon, E., Fredriksson, H., Andersson, R., & Aman, P., (2004). Molecular weight and structure units of (1! 3, 1! 4)-β-glucans in dough and bread made from hull – less barley milling fractions. *Journal of Cereal Science, 40*(3), 195–204.

Anson, N. M., Hemery, Y. M., Bast, A., & Haenen, G. R., (2012). Optimizing the bioactive potential of wheat bran by processing. *Food & Function, 3*(4), 362–375.

Apolinario, A. C., Damasceno, B. P. G. L., De Macedo, B. N. E., Pessoa, A., Converti, A., & Da Silva, J. A., (2014). Inulin – type fructans: A review on different aspects of biochemical and pharmaceutical technology. *Carbo-Hydrate Polymers, 101*, 368–378.

Arora, A., & Camire, M. E., (1994). Performance of potato peels in muffins and cookies. *Food Research International, 27*(1), 15–22.

Bacic, A., & Stone, B. A., (1981). Isolation and ultrastructure of aleurone cell walls from wheat and barley. *Australian Journal of Plant Physiology, 8*(5), 453–474.

Bajaj, I. B., Survase, S. A., Saudagar, P. S., & Singhal, R. S., (2007). Gellan gum: Fermentative production, downstream processing and application. *Food Technology and Biotechnology, 45*(4), 341–354.

Barak, S., & Mudgil, D., (2014). Locust bean gum: Processing, properties and food applications a review. *International Journal of Biological Macromolecules, 66*, 74–80.

Benitez, V., Cantera, S. A., Saudagar, P. S., & Singhal, R. M., Esteban, R. M., Diaz, M. F., et al., (2013). Impact of germination on starch, dietary fiber and physiochemical properties in non-conventional legumes. *Food Research International, 50*(1), 64–69.

Bingham, S. A., (1990). Mechanisms and experimental and epidemiological evidence relating dietary fiber (non-starch polysaccharides) and starch to protection against large bowel cancer. *Proceedings of the Nutrition Society, 49*(2), 153–171.

Brouns, F., Hemery, Y., Price, R., & Anson, N. M., (2012). Wheat aleurone: Separation, composition, health aspects and potential food use. *Critical Reviews in Food Science and Nutrition, 52*(6), 553–568.

Brownlee, I. A., (2011). The physiological roles of dietary fiber. *Food Hydrocolloids, 25*(2), 238–250.

Buliga, G. S., Brant, D. A., & Fincher, G. B., (1986). The sequence statistics and solution conformation of the barley (1 3, 1)-β-d- glucan. *Carbohydrates Research, 157*, 139–156.

Butt, M. S., Tahir – Nadeem, M., Khan, M. K. I., Shabir, R., & Butt, M. S., (2008). Oats: Unique among the cereals. *European Journal of Nutrition, 47*(2), 68–79.

Buttriss, J. L., & Stokes, C. S., (2008). Dietary fiber and health: An overview. *Nutrition Bulletin, 33*(3), 186–200.

Campo, V. L., Kawano, D. F., Da Silva, Jr. D. B., & Carvalho, I., (2009). Carrageenans: Biological properties, chemical modifications and structural analysis: A review. *Carbohydrates Polymers, 77*(2), 167–180.

Champ, M., Landkilde, A. M., Brouns, F., Kettlitz, B., & Collect, Y. L. B., (2003). Advances in dietary fiber characterization. 1. Definition of dietary fiber, physiological relevance, health benefits and analytical aspects. *Nutrition Research Reviews, 16*(1), 71–82.

Chantaro, P., Devahastin, S., & Chiewchan, N., (2008). Production of antioxidant high dietary fiber powder from carrot peels. *LWT –Food Science and Technology, 441*(10), 1987–1994.

Chavan, J. K., Kute, L. S., & Kadam, S. S., (1989). Broad bean. In: *Handbook of World Food Legumes: Nutritional, Processing, Technology & Utilization* (Vol. 1, pp. 223–245). Boca Raton, F1: CRC Press.

Chen, J., Liu, C. M., Li, T., Liang, R. H., & Luo, S. J., (2015). Pectin modification: A review. *Critical Reviews in Food Science and Nutrition, 55*(12), 1684–1698.

Cherbut, C., (1995). Fermentation and colonic digestive function. *Nutrition and Diet Notebooks, 30*(3), 143–147.

Cho, S. S., & Samuel, P., (2009). *Fiber Ingredients: Food Applications and Health Benefits*. Boca Raton, FL, USA: CRC Press.

Cloetens, L., Ulmius, M., Johansson-Persson, A., Akesson, B., & Onning, G., (2012). Role of dietary beta-glucans in the prevention of the metabolic syndrome. *Nutrition Reviews, 70*(8), 444–458.

Cui, W., & Wood, P. J., (2000). Relationship between Structural Features, Molecular Weight and Rheological Properties of Cereal β-Glucan. In: Nishinari, K., (ed.), *Hydrocolloids Physical Chemistry and Industrial Applications of Gels, Polysaccharides and Proteins* (Vol. 1, pp. 363–384). Nova Science Publishers Inc.

D'Cunha, M., Sridhar, K. R., & Bhat, R., (2009). Nutritional quality of germinated seeds of Canavalia maritime of coastal sand dunes. In: *Food Processing Methods, Techniques and Trends* (pp. 363–384). New York: Nova Science publishers INC.

De Almeida, C. G. E., Da Queiroz-Monici, K. S., Reis, S. M. P. M., & De Oliveira, A. C., (2006). Chemical composition, dietary fiber and resistant starch content of raw and cooked pea, common bean, chickpea and lentil legumes. *Food Chemistry, 94*(3), 327–330.

Deuchi, K., Kanauchi, O., Imasato, Y., & Kobayashi, E., (1995). Effect of the viscosity or deacetylation degree of chitosan on fecal fat excreted from rats fed on a high-fat diet. *Bioscience, Biotechnology and Biochemistry, 39*(5), 781–785.

Deuchi, K., Kanauchi, O., Shizukuishi, M., & Kobayashi, E., (1995). Continuous and massive intake of chitosan affects mineral and fat-soluble vitamin status in rats fed on a high-fat diet. *Bioscience Biotechnology and Biochemistry, 39*(7), 1211–1216.

Dikeman, C. L., & Fabey, G. C. Jr., (2006). Viscosity as related to dietary fiber a review. *Critical Reviews in Food Science and Nutrition, 46*(8), 649–663.

Doublier, J. L., & Wood, P. J., (1995). Rheological properties of aqueous solutions of (113) (114)-B-D-glucan from outs (*Vena sativa* L.). *Cereal Chemistry, 72*(4), 335–340.

Dreher, M. L., (1987). *Handbook of Dietary Fiber: An Applied Approach*. New York: Marcel Dekker.

Eashwarage, I. S., (2017). Dietary fiber, resistant starch and eleven commonly consumed legumes horse gram. *Research Journal of Chemical, 7*(2), 1–7.

Eastwood, M. A., & Hamilton, D., (1968). Studies on the adsorption of bile salts to non-absorbed components of diet. *Biochimica et Biophysica Acta (BBA) – Lipids and Lipid Metabolism, 152*(1), 165–173.

Edwards, C., (1995). Dietary fiber, fermentation and the colon. In: Cherbut, C., Barry, J. L., Lairon, D., & Durand, M., (eds.), *Dietary Fiber: Mechanisms of Action in Human Physiology and Metabolism* (pp. 51–60).

Elleuch, M., Bedigian, D., Roiseux, O., Besbes, S., Blecker, C., & Attia, H., (2011). Dietary fiber and fiber-rich by-products of food processing: Characterization, technological functionality and commercial applications: A review. *Food Chemistry, 124*(2), 411–421. Paris: John Libbey Eurotex.

Emaga, T. H., Andrianaivo, R. H., Wathelet, B., Tchango, J. T., & Paquot, M., (2007). Effects of the stage of maturation and varieties on the chemical composition of banana and plantain peels. *Food Chemistry, 103*(2), 590–600.

Escobedo-Avellaneda, Z., Gutierrez-Uribe, J., Valdez-Fragoso, A., Torres, J. A., & Welti-Chanes, J., (2014). Phytochemicals and antioxidant activity of juice, flavedo, albedo and comminuted orange. *Journal of Functional Foods, 6*, 470–481.

Faccin, G. L., Miotto, L. A., Do Nascimento, V. L., Barreto, P. L. M., & Amante, E. R., (2009). Chemical, sensorial and rheological properties of a new organic rice bran beverage. *Rice Science, 16*(3), 226–234.

Fairweather-Tait, S. J., & Wright, A. J. A., (1990). The effects of sugar – beet: Fiber and wheat bran on iron and zinc absorption in rats. *British Journal of Nutrition, 64*(2), 547–552.

Fechner, A., Fenske, K., & Jahreis, G., (2013). Effects of legume kernel fibers and citrus fiber on putative risk factors for colorectal cancer: A randomized, double blind, crossover human intervention trial. *Nutrition Journal, 12*(1), 101.

Fechner, A., Kiehntopf, M., & Jahreis, G., (2014). The formation of short-chain fatty acids is positively associated with the blood lipid – lowering effect of Lupin kernel fiber in moderately hypercholesterolemic adults-3. *The Journal of Nutrition, 144*(5), 599–607.

Ferguson, L. R., & Harris, P. J., (1998). Suberized plant cell walls suppress formation of heterocyclic amine-induced aberrant crypts in a rat model. *Chemico – Biological Interactions, 114*(3), 191–209.

Ferguson, L. R., Chavan, R. R., & Harris, P. J., (2001). Changing concepts of dietary fiber: Implications for carcinogenesis. *Nutrition and Cancer, 39*(2), 155–169.

Fernandez-Lopez, J., Sendra-Navarro, C., Sayas, E., Viuda-Martos, M., & Alvarez, J. A. P., (2009). Storage stability of a high dietary fiber powder from range by-products. *International Journal of Food Science & Technology, 44*(4), 748–756.

Figuerola, F., Hurtado, M. L., Estevez, A. M., Chiffelle, I., & Asenjo, F., (2005). Fiber concentrates from apple pomace and citrus peel as potential fiber sources for food enrichment. *Food Chemistry, 91*(3), 395–401.

Fincher, G. B., (1986). Cell walls and their components in cereal grain technology. *Advances in Cereal Science and Technology, 8,* 207–295.

Flamm, G., Glinsmann, W., Kritchevsky, D., Prosky, L., & Roberfroud, M., (2001). Inulin and oligofructose as dietary fiber: A review of the evidence. *Critical Reviews in Food Science and Nutrition, 41*(5), 353–362.

Fleury, N., & Lahaye, M., (1991). Chemical and physico-chemical characterization of fibers from *Laminaria digitata* (kombu Breton): A physiological approach. *Journal of the Science of Food and Agriculture, 55*(3), 389–400.

Frost, G., Sleeth, M. L., Sahuri-Arisoylu, M., Lizarbe, B., Cerdan, S., Brody, L., et al., (2014). The short-chain fatty acid acetate reduces appetite via a central homeostatic mechanism. *Nature Communications, 5,* 3611.

Fuentes-Zaragoza, E., Riquelme-Navarrete, M. J., Sanchez-Zapata, E., & Perez-Alvarez, J. A., (2010). Resistant starch as functional ingredient: A review. *Food Research International, 43*(4), 931–942.

Garcia-Ochoa, F., Santos, V. E., Casas, J. A., & Gomez, E., (2000). Xanthan gum: Production, recovery, and properties. *Biotechnology Advances, 18*(7), 549–579.

Glass, J. E., (1986). Water solubility in carbohydrate polymers. In: Glass, J. E., (ed.), *Advances in Chemistry Series 213. Water Soluble Polymers – Beauty with Performance* (pp. 3–27). Washington, DC: American Chemical Society.

Glicksman, M., (1969). *Gum Technology in the Food Industry.* New York: Academic press.

Gosselink, R. J. A., De Jong, E., Guran, B., & Abacherli, A., (2004). Co-ordination network for lignin-Standardization, production and applications adapted to market requirements (EUROLIGNIN). *Industrial Crops and Products, 20*(2), 121–129.

Graessley, W. W., (1974). The entanglement concept in polymer rheology. In: *Advances in Polymer Science: The Entanglement Concept in Polymer Rheology* (Vol. 16). Berlin, Heidelberg: Springer.

Grigelmo-Miguel, N., & Martin-Belloso, O., (1999). Comparison of dietary fiber from by-products of processing fruits and greens and from cereals. *LWT-Food Science and Technology, 32*(8), 503–508.

Guillon, F., & Champ, M., (2002). Structural and physical properties of dietary fibers, and consequences of processing on human physiology. *Food Research International, 33*(3, 4), 233–245.

Guillon, F., Auffret, A., Robertson, J. A., Thibault, J. F., & Barry, J. L., (1998). Relationships between physical characteristics of sugar – beet fiber and its fermentability by human faecal flora. *Carbohydrate Polymers, 37*(2), 185–197.

Hamed, I., Ozogul, F., & Regentein, J. M., (2016). Industrial applications of crustacean by-products (chitin, chitosan, and chitooligosaccharides): A review. *Trends in Food Science & Technology, 48*, 40–50.

Harris, P. J., & Ferguson, L. R., (1993). Dietary fiber: Its composition and role in protection against colorectal cancer. *Mutation Research/Fundamental and Molecular Mechanisms of Mutagenesis, 290*(1), 97–110.

Harris, P. J., Triggs, C. M., Roberton, A. M., Watson, M. E., & Ferguson, L. R., (1996). The adsorption of heterocyclic aromatic amines by model dietary fibers with contrasting compositions. *Chemico – Biological Interaction, 100*(1), 13–25.

Hashemi, J. M., (2015). Biomedical effects of barley: A review. *New York Science Journal, 8*(3), 52–55.

Hegsted, M., Windhauser, M. M., Morris, S. K., & Lester, S. B., (1993). Stabilized rice bran and oat bran lower cholesterol in humans. *Nutrition Research, 13*(4), 387–398.

Hemdane, S., Jacobs, P. J., Dornez, E., Veerspreet, J., Delcour, J. A., & Courtin, C. M., (2016). Wheat *(Triticum aestivum L.)* bran in bread making: A critical review. *Comprehensive Reviews in Food Science and Food Safety, 15*(1), 28–42.

Hemery, Y., Rouau, X., Lullien-Pellerin, V., Barron, C., & Abecassis, J., (2007). Dry processes to develop wheat fractions and products with enhanced nutritional quality. *Journal of Cereal Science, 46*(3), 327–347.

Hispley, E. H., (1953). Dietary "fiber" and pregnancy toxaemia. *British Medical Journal, 2*(4833), 420–422.

Holse, M., Husted, S., & Hansen, (2010). Chemical composition of marama bean (*Tylosema esculentum)* – a wild African bean with unexploited potential. *Journal of Food Composition and Analysis, 23*(6), 648–657.

Hon, D. N. S., (1996). Cellulose and its derivatives: Structures, reactions, and medical uses. In: *Polysaccharides in Medicinal Applications* (pp. 87–105). New York, USA: Marcel Dekker.

Hopman, E. G., Le Cessie, S., Von, B. B. M. E., & Mearin, M. L., (2006). Nutritional management of the gluten – free diet in young people with celiac disease in the Netherlands. *Journal of Pediatric Gastroenterology and Nutrition, 43*(1), 102–108.

Hove, E. L., King, S., & Hill, G. D., (1978). Composition, protein quality, and toxins of seeds of the grain legumes *Glycine max, Lupinus spp. Phaseolus spp. Pisum sativum, and Vicia faba. New Zealand Journal of Agricultural Research, 21*(3), 457–462.

Huang, S. C., Shiau, C. Y., Liu, T. E., Chu, C. L., & Hwang, D. F., (2005). Effects of rice bran on sensory and physico – chemical properties of emulsified pork meatballs. *Meat Science, 70*(4), 613–619.

Islam, A. M., Phillips, G. O., Sljivo, A., Snowden, M. J., & Williams, P. A., (1997). A review of recent developments on the regulatory, structural and functional aspects of gum Arabic. *Food Hydrocolloids, 11*(4), 493–505.

Iwamoto, S., Nakagaito, A. N., & Yano, H., (2007). Nano-fibrillation of pulp fibers for the processing of transparent nanocomposites. *Applied Physics A, 89*(2), 461–466.

Jalili, T., Wildman, R. E., & Medeiros M., (2000). Nutraceutical roles of dietary fiber. *Journal of Nutraceutical, Functional & Medical Foods, 2*(4), 19–34.

Jimenez-Escrig, A., & Sa'nchez-Muniz, F. J., (2000). Dietary fiber from edible seaweeds: Chemical structure, physico – chemical properties and effects on cholesterol metabolism. *Nutrition Research, 20*(4), 585–598.

Jimenez-Escrig, A., Rincon, M., Polido, R., & Saura-Calixto, F., (2001). Guava fruit (*Psidium guajava* L.) as a new source of antioxidant dietary fiber. *Journal of Agricultural and Food Chemistry, 49*(11), 5489–5493.

Kaczmarczyk, M. M., Miller, M. J., & Freund, G. G., (2012). The health benefits of dietary fiber: Beyond the usual suspects of type 2 diabetes mellitus, cardiovascular disease and colon cancer. *Metabolism, 61*(8), 1058–1066.

Kahlon, T. S., Chow, F. I., Sayre, R. N., & Betschart, A. A., (1992). Cholesterol – lowering in hamsters fed rice barn at various levels, defatted rice bran and rice bran oil. *The Journal of Nutrition, 122*(3), 513–519.

Katoch, R., (2013). Nutritional potential of rice bean (*Vigna umbellate*): An underutilized legume. *Journal of Food Science, 78*(1), C8–C16.

Keservani, R. K., & Sharma, A. K., (2014). Flavonoids: Emerging trends and potential health benefits. *Journal of Chinese Pharmaceutical Sciences, 23*(12), 815.

Keservani, R. K., Kesharwani, R. K., Sharma, A. K., & Jarouliya, U., (2015d). Dietary supplements, nutraceutical and functional foods in immune response (immunomodulators). In: Debasis, B., Harry, G. P., & Anand, S., (eds.), *Nutraceutical and Functional Foods in Human Life and Disease Prevention* (pp. 343–358). Boca Raton, Fl. CRC Press, Taylor and Francis, Chapter 20. ISBN: 9781482237214.

Keservani, R. K., Kesharwani, R. K., Sharma, A. K., Vyas, N., & Chadoker, A., (2010b). Nutritional supplements: An overview. *International Journal of Current Pharmaceutical Review and Research, 1*(1), 59–75.

Keservani, R. K., Kesharwani, R. K., Vyas, N., Jain, S., Raghuvanshi, R., & Sharma, A. K., (2010a). Nutraceutical and functional food as future food: A review. *Der Pharmacia Lettre, 2*(1), 106–116.

Keservani, R. K., Sharma, A. K., & Kesharwani, R. K., (2016a). Nutraceutical and functional foods for cardiovascular health. In: *Food Process Engineering* (pp. 257–278, 291–312). Apple Academic Press, CRC Press. ISBN: 9781771884020.

Keservani, R. K., Sharma, A. K., & Kesharwani, R. K., (2016b). Medicinal effect of nutraceutical fruits for the cognition and brain health. *Scientifica* (p. 10). Article ID 3109254. doi: 10.1155/2016/3109254.

Keservani, R. K., Sharma, A. K., & Kesharwani, R. K., (2020). *Nutraceuticals and Dietary Supplements: Applications in Health Improvement and Disease Management*. CRC Press. ISBN: 9781771888738.

Keservani, R. K., Singh, S., Singh, V., Kesharwani, R. K., & Sharma, A. K., (2015b). Nutraceuticals and functional foods in the prevention of mental disorder. In: Debasis, B., Harry, G. P., & Anand, S., (eds.), *Nutraceutical and Functional Foods in Human Life and Disease Prevention* (pp. 255–268). Boca Raton, Fl. CRC Press, Taylor and Francis, Chapter 15b. ISBN: 9781482237214.

Khan, M. A., Nadeem, M., Rakha, A., Shakoor, S., Shehzad, A., & Khan, M. R., (2016). Structural characterization of oat bran-β-D-glucans by lichenase hydrolysis through high–performance anion exchange chromatography with pulsed amperometric detection. *International Journal of Food Properties, 19*(4), 929–935.

Klemm, D., Schumann, D., Kramer, F., Hebler, N., Hornung, M., Schmauder, H. P., et al., (2006). Nanocellulose as innovative polymers in research and application. In: Klemm, D., (ed.), *Polysaccharides II Advances in Polymer Science* (pp. 49–96).

Koubala, B. B., Kansci, G., Mbome, L. I., Crepeau, M. J., Thibault, J. F., & Ralet, M. C., (2008). Effect of extraction conditions on some physicochemical characteristics of pectins from "amelioree" and "mango" mango peels. *Food Hydrocolloids, 22*(7), 1345–1351.

Kouris-Blazos, A., & Belski, R., (2016). Health benefits of legumes and pulses with a focus on Australian sweet lupins. *Asia Pacific Journal of Clinical Nutrition, 25*(1), 1–17.

Kritchevsky, D., & Story, J. A., (1974). Binding of bile salts *in vitro* by nonnutritive fiber. *The Journal of Nutrition, 104*(4), 458–462.

Kupper, C., (2005). Dietary guidelines and implementation for celiac disease. *Gastroenterology, 128*(4), S121–S127.

Kutos, Y., Golob, T., Kac, M., & Plestenjak, A., (2003). Dietary fiber content of dry and processed beans. *Food Chemistry, 80*(2), 231–235.

Lahouar, L., Ghrairi, F., El Arem, A., Sghaeir, W., El Felah, M., Salem, H. B., et al., (2014). Attenuation of histopathological alterations of colon, liver and lung by dietary fiber of barley Rihane in azoxymethane treated rats. *Food Chemistry, 149*, 271–276.

Lai, V. M., Lu, S., He, W. H., & Chen, H. H., (2007). Non-starch polysaccharide compositions of rice grains with respect to rice variety and degree of milling. *Food Chemistry, 101*(3), 1205–1210.

Langkilde, A. M., & Andersson, H., (1998). Amount and composition of substrate entering the colon. In: Guillon,

Lazaridou, A., & Biliaderis, C. G., (2004). Cryogelation of cereal β-glucans: Structure and molecular size effects. *Food Hydrocolloids, 18*(6), 933–947.

Lazaridou, A., Biliaderis, C. G., & Izydorczyk, M. S., (2003). Molecular size effects on rheological properties of oat β-glucans in solution and gels. *Food Hydrocolloids, 17*(5), 693–712.

Le Leu, R. K., Brown, I. L., Hu, Y., & Young, G. P., (2003). Effect of resistant starch on genotoxin–induced apoptosis, colonic epithelium, and luminal contents in rats. *Carcinogenesis, 24*(8), 1347–1352.

Leathers, T. D., (2003). Biotechnological production and application of pullulan. *Applied Microbiology and Biotechnology, 62*(5, 6), 468–473.

Lee, C. H., Oh, S. H., Yang, E. J., & Kim, Y. S., (2006). Effects of raw, cooked, and germinated small black soybean powders on dietary fiber content and gastrointestinal functions. *Food Science and Biotechnology, 15*(4), 635–638.

Lim, A. S. L., & Rabeta, M. S., (2013). Proximate analysis, mineral content and antioxidant capacity of milk apple, malay apple and water apple. *International Food Research Journal, 20*(2).

Llober, A., & Canellas, J., (2008). Antioxidant activity and dietary fiber of Prensal Blanc white grape (*Vitis vinifera*) byproducts. *International Journal of Food Science & Technology, 43*(11), 1953–1959.

Llobera, A., & Canellas, J., (2007). Dietary fiber content and antioxidant activity of Manto Negro red grape (*Vitis vinifera*): Pomace and stem. *Food Chemistry, 101*(2), 659–666.

Lopez-Vargas, J. H., Fernandez-Lopez, J., Perez-Alvarez, J. A., & Viuda-Martos, M., (2013). Chemical, physicochemical technological, antibacterial and antioxidant properties of dietary fiber powder obtained from yellow passion fruit (*Passiflora edulis* var. flavicarpa) co-products. *Food Research International, 51*(2), 756–763.

Lora, J. H., & Glasser, W. G., (2002). Recent industrial applications of lignin: A sustainable alternative to nonrenewable materials. *Journal of Polymers and the Environment, 10*(1, 2), 39–48.

Macfarlane, G. T., & Macfarlane, S., (1993). Factors affecting fermentation reactions in the large bowel. *Proceedings of the Nutrition Society, 52*(2), 367–373.

Maes, C., & Delcour, J. A., (2002). Structural characterization of water–extractable and water–unextractable arabinoxylans in wheat bran. *Journal of Cereal Science, 35*(3), 315–326.

Maezaki, Y., Tsuji, K., Nakagawa, Y., Kawai, Y., Akimoto, M., Tsugita, T., et al., (1993). Hypocholesterolemic effect of chitosan in adult males. *Bioscience Biotechnology and Biochemistry, 57*(9), 1439–1444.

Makeri, M. U., Nkama, I., & Badau, M. H., (2013). Physicochemical, malting and biochemical properties of some improved Nigerian barely cultivars and their malts. *International Food Research Journal, 20*(4).

Manthey, F. A., Hareland, G. A., & Huseby, D. J., (1999). Soluble and insoluble dietary fiber content and composition in oat. *Cereal Chemistry, 76*(3), 417–420.

Marconi, E., Ruggeri, S., Cappelloni, M., Leonardi, D., & Carnovale, E., (2000). Physicochemical, nutritional, and microstructural characteristics of chickpeas (*Cicer arietinum* L.) and common beans (*Phaseolus vulgaris* L.) following microwave cooking. *Journal of Agricultural and Food Chemistry, 48*(12), 5986–5994.

Marin, F. R., Soler-Rivas, C., Benavente-Garcia, O., Castillo, J., & Perez-Alvarez, J. A., (2007). By-products from different citrus processes as a source of customized functional fibers. *Food Chemistry, 100*(2), 736–741.

Martin-Cabrejas, M. A., Aguilera, Y., Benitez, V., Molla, E., Lopez-Andreu, F. J., & Esteban, R. M., (2006). Effect of industrial dehydration on the soluble carbohydrates and dietary fiber fractions in legumes. *Journal of Agricultural and Food Chemistry, 54*(20), 7652–7657.

Martin-Cabrejas, M. A., Ariza, N., Esteban, R., Molla, E., Waldron, K., & Lopez-Andreu, F. J., (2003). Effect of germination on the carbohydrate composition of the dietary fiber of peas (*Pisum sativum* L.). *Journal of Agriculture and Food Chemistry, 51*(5), 1254–1259.

Martin-Cabrejas, M. A., Sanfiz, B., Vidal, A., Molla, E., Esteban, R., & Lopez-Andreu, F. J., (2004). Effect of fermentation and autoclaving on dietary fiber fractions and antinutritional factors of beans (*Phaseolus vulgaris* L.). *Journal of Agricultural and Food Chemistry, 52*(2), 261–226.

Martinez, R., Torres, P., Meneses, M. A., Figueroa, J. G., Perez-Alvarez, J. A., & Viuda-Martos, M., (2012). Chemical, technology and *in vitro* antioxidant properties of mango, guava, pineapple and passion fruit dietary fiber concentrate. *Food Chemistry, 135*(3), 1520–1526.

May, C. D., (1990). Industrial pectins: Sources, production and applications. *Carbohydrate Polymers, 12*(1), 79–99.

McCarty, M. F., (2005). Nutraceuticals resources for diabetes prevention–an update. *Medical Hypothesis, 64*(1), 151–158.

McDougall, G. J., Morrison, I. M., Stewart, D., & Hillman, J. R., (1996). Plant cell walls as dietary fiber: Range, structure, processing and function. *Journal of the Science of Food and Agriculture, 70*(2), 133–150.

McIntosh, M., Stone, B. A., & Stanisich, V. A., (2005). Curdlan and other bacterial (1 3)-β-D-glucans. *Applied Micro-Biology and Biotechnology, 68*(2), 163–173.

Morris, E. R., (1979). Polysaccharide structure and conformation in solutions and gels. In: Blanshard, J. M. V., & Mitchell, J. R., (eds.), *Polysaccharides in Food* (pp. 15–31). London: Butterworth.

Morris, E. R., (1989). Polysaccharide solution properties: Origin, rheological characterization and implications for food systems. In: Millane, R. P., BeMiller, J. N., & Chandrasekaran, R., (eds.), *Frontiers in Carbohydrate Research–1: Food Applications* (pp. 132–163). London: Elsevier.

Morris, E. R., (1990). Shear–thinning of 'random coil' polysaccharides: Characterization by two parameters from a simple linear plot. *Carbohydrate Polymers, 13*(1), 85–96.

Morris, E. R., & Norton, I. T., (1983). Polysaccharide aggregation in solutions and gels. In: Wyn-Jones, E., & Gormally, J., (eds.), *Aggregation Process in Solution* (pp. 549–593). New York: Elsevier.

Morris, E. R., Cutler, A. N., Ross-Murphy, S. B., Rees, D. A., & Price, J., (1981). Concentration and shear rate dependence of viscosity in random coil polysaccharide solutions. *Carbohydrate Polymers, 1*(1), 5–21.

Mudgil, D., & Barak, S., (2013). Composition, properties and health benefits of indigestible carbohydrate polymers as dietary fiber: A review. *International Journal of Biological Macromolecules, 61*, 1–6.

Mudgil, D., Barak, S., & Khatkar, B. S., (2012). Process optimization of partially hydrolyzed guar gum using response surface methodology. *Agro Food Industry Hi Tech, 23*(1), 13–15.

Mudgil, D., Barak, S., & Khatkar, B. S., (2012a). Gaur gum: Processing, properties and food applications: A review. *Journal of Food Science and Technology, 51*(3), 409–418.

Mudgil, D., Barak, S., & Khatkar, B. S., (2014b). Optimization of enzymatic hydrolysis of guar gum using response surface methodology. *Journal of Food Science and Technology, 51*(8), 1600–1605.

Mudgil, D., Barak, S., & Khatkar, B. S., (2016a). Development of functional yoghurt via soluble fiber fortification utilizing enzymatically hydrolyzed guar gum. *Food Bioscience, 14*, 28–33.

Mudgil, D., Barak, S., & Khatkar, B. S., (2016b). Optimization of bread firmness, specific loaf volume and sensory acceptability of bread with soluble fiber and different water levels. *Journal of Cereal of Cereal Science, 70,* 186–191.

Mudgil, D., Barak, S., & Khatkar, B. S., (2016c). Effect of partially hydrolyzed guar gum on pasting, thermo–mechanical and rheological properties of wheat dough. *International Journal of Biological Macromolecules, 93,* 131–135.

Mudgil, D., Barak, S., Patel, A., & Shah, N., (2018). Partially hydrolyzed guar gum as a potential prebiotic source. *International Journal of Biological Macromolecules, 112*, 207–210.

Murthy, P. S., & Naidu, M. M., (2012). Recovery of phenolic antioxidants and functional compounds from coffee industry by–products. *Food and Bioprocess Technology, 5*(3), 897–903.

Nelson, A. L., (2001). *High Fiber Ingredients.* St. Paul, Minnesota, USA: Eagan Press.

Newman, C. W., & Newman, R. K., (2006). A brief history of barley foods. *Cereal Foods World, 51*(1), 4–7.

Newman, R. K., & Newman, C. W., (2008). *Barley for Food and Health: Science, Technology, and Production.* John Wiley & Sons.

Nilnakara, S., Chiewchan, N., & Devahastin, S., (2009). Production of antioxidant dietary fiber powder from cabbage outer leaves. *Food and Bioproducts Processing, 87*(4), 301–307.

Olson, A., Gray, G. M., & Chiu, M., (1987). Chemistry and analysis of soluble dietary fiber. *Food Technology, 41*, 71–80.

Onipe, O. O., Jideani, A. I., & Beswa, D., (2015). Composition and functionality of wheat bran and its application in some cereal food products. *International Journal of Food Science & Technology, 50*(12), 2509–2518.

Othman, R. A., Moghadasian, M. H., & Jones, P. J., (2011). Cholesterol–lowering effects of oat β–glucan. *Nutrition Reviews, 69*(6), 299–309.

Pagano, A. E., (2006). Whole grains and the gluten–free diet. *Practical Gastroenterology, 30*(10), 66.

Parrish, F. W., Perlin, A. S., & Reese, E. T., (1960). Selective enzymolysis of poly-β-D-glucans, and the structure of polymers. *Canadian Journal of Chemistry, 38*(11), 2094–2104.

Pena, M. J., Vergara, C. E., & Carpita, N. C., (2001). The structures and architectures of plant cell walls define dietary fiber composition and the textures of foods. *Advanced Dietary Fiber Technology*, 42–60.

Pritchard, P. J., Dryburgh, E. A., & Wilson, B. J., (1973). Carbohydrates of spring and winter field beans (*Vicia faba* L.). *Journal of the Science of Food and Agriculture, 24*(6), 663–668.

Rao, R. S. P., & Muralikrishna, G., (2004). Non-starch polysaccharide-phenolic acid complexes from native and germinated cereals and millet. *Food Chemistry, 84*(4), 527–531.

Redgwell, R. J., & Fischer, M., (2005). Dietary fiber as a versatile food component: An industrial perspective. *Molecular Nutrition & Food Research, 49*(6), 521–535.

Rees, D. A., (1977). *Polysaccharide Shapes.* London: Chapman and Hall.

Rehinan, Z. U., Rashid, M., & Shah, W. H., (2004). Insoluble dietary fiber components of food legumes as affected by soaking and cooking processes. *Food Chemistry, 85*(2), 245–249.

Rey, D. K., & Labuza, T. P., (1981). Characterization of the effect of solutes on the water–binding and gel strength properties of carrageenan. *Journal of Food Science, 46*(3), 786–789.

Ripsin, C. M., Keenan, J. M., Jacobs, D. R., Elmer, P. J., Welch, R. R., Van, H. L., et al., (1992). Oat products and lipid lowering: A meta–analysis. *JAMA, 267*(24), 3317–3325.

Roberfroid, M. B., (2005). Introducing inulin–type fructans. *British Journal of Nutrition, 93*(S1), S13–S25.

Robertson, J. A., (1998). Application of plant–based byproducts as fiber supplements in processed foods. *Recent Research and Development in Agricultural Food Chemistry, 2*, 705–717.

Robertson, J. A., & Eastwood, M. A., (1981). An examination of factors which may affect the water holding capacity of dietary fiber. *British Journal of Nutrition, 45*(1), 83–88.

Robertson, J. A., De Monredon, F. D., Dysseler, P., Guillon, F., Amado, R., & Thibault, J. F., (2000). Hydration properties of dietary fiber and resistant starch: A European collaborative study. *LWT–Food Science and Technology, 33*(2), 72–79.

Rodriguez, M. S., & Mendoza, E. M. T., (1991). Nutritional assessment of seed proteins in rice bean *Vigna umbellata* (Thumb.) Ohwi and Ohashi. *Plant Foods for Human Nutrition, 41*(1), 1–9.

Saha, D., & Bhattacharya, S., (2010). Hydrocolloids as thickening and gelling agents in food: A critical review. *Journal of Food and Technology, 47*(6), 587–597.

Sajilata, M. G., Singhal, R. S., & Kulkarni, P. R., (2006). Resistant starch–a review. *Comprehensive Reviews in Food Science and Food Safety, 5*(1), 1–17.

Salminen, S., Bouley, C., Boutron, M. C., Cummings, J. H., Franck, A., Gibson, G. R., et al., (1998). Functional food science and gastrointestinal physiology and function. *British Journal of Nutrition, 80*(1), 147–171.

Sanchez-Alonso, I., Jimenez-Escrig, A., Saura-Calixto, F., & Borderias, A. J., (2007). Effect of grape antioxidant dietary fiber on the prevention of lipid oxidation in minced fish: Evaluation by different methodologies. *Food Chemistry, 101*(1), 372–378.

Sarwar, M. H., Sarwar, M. F., Sawar, M., Qadri, N. A., & Moghal, S. (2013). The role of oilseeds nutrition in human health: A critical review, *4*(3), 32–35.

Saulnier, L., & Quemener, B., (2009). Enzymatic mapping of arabinoxylan structure. *Health Grain Methods: Analysis of Bioactive Components in Small Grain Cereals,* 191–201.

Saura-Calixto, F., (1998). Antioxidant dietary fiber product: A new concept and a potential food ingredient. *Journal of Agricultural and Food Chemistry, 46*(10), 4303–4306.

Schneeman, B. O., (1986). Dietary fiber: Physical and chemical properties, methods of analysis and physiological effects. *Food Technology, 40,* 104–110.

Sera, N., Morita, K., Nagasoe, M., Tokieda, H., Kituara, T., & Tokiwa, H., (2005). Binding effect of polychlorinated compounds and environmental carcinogens on rice bran fiber. *The Journal of Nutritional Biochemistry, 16*(1), 50–58.

Shewry, P. R., Piironem, V., Lampi, A. M., Nystrom, L., Li, L., Rakszegi, M., et al., (2008). Phytochemical and fiber components in oats varieties in the health grain diversity screen. *Journal of Agricultural and Food Chemistry, 56*(21). 9777–9784.

Shoaib, M., Shehzad, A., Omar, M., Rakha, A., Raza, H., Sharif, H. R., et al., (2016). Inulin: Properties, health benefits and food applications. *Carbohydrates Polymers, 147,* 444–454.

Sikora, P., Tosh, S. M., Brummer, Y., & Olsson, O., (2013). Identification of high β-glucan oat lines and localization and chemical characterization of their seed kernel β-glucans. *Food Chemistry, 137*(1–4), 83–91.

Singh, P., Kesharwani, R. K., & Keservani, R. K., (2017a). Antioxidants and vitamins: Roles in cellular function and metabolism. In: *Sustained Energy for Enhanced Human Functions and Activity* (pp. 385–407). Academic Press. ISBN:9780128054130.

Singh, P., Kesharwani, R. K., & Keservani, R. K., (2017b). Protein, carbohydrates, and fats: Energy metabolism. In: *Sustained Energy for Enhanced Human Functions and Activity* (pp. 103–115). Academic Press. ISBN:9780128054130.

Slavin, J. L., (1987). Dietary fiber: Classification, chemical analyses, and food sources. *Journal of the American Dietetic Association, 87*(9), 1164–1171.

Slavin, J. L., & Greenberg, N. A., (2003). Partially hydrolyzed guar gum: Clinical nutrition uses. *Nutrition, 19*(6), 549–552.

Slavin, J., (2013). Fiber and prebiotics: Mechanisms and health benefits. *Nutrients, 5*(4), 1417–1435.

Smith, K. N., Queenan, K. M., Thomas, W., Fulcher, R. G., & Slavin, J. L., (2008). Physiological effects of concentrated barley β-glucan in mildly hypercholesterolemic adults. *Journal of the American College of Nutrition, 27*(3), 434–440.

Stella, S. P., Ferrarezi, A. C., Dos, S. K. O., & Monteiro, M., (2011). Antioxidant activity of commercial ready-to-drink orange juice and nectar. *Journal of Food Science, 76*(3), C392–C397.

Stevenson, L., Phillips, F., O'sullivan, K., & Walton, J., (2012). Wheat bran: Its composition and benefits to health, a European perspective. *International Journal of Food Sciences and Nutrition, 63*(8), 1001–1013.

Tanongkankit, Y., Chiewchan, N., & Devahastin, S., (2010). Effect of processing on antioxidants and their activity in dietary fiber powder from cabbage outer leaves. *Drying Technology, 28*(9), 1063–1071.

Tehranifar, A., Zarei, M., Nemati, Z., Esfandiyari, B., & Vazifeshenas, M. R., (2010). Investigation of physico–chemical properties and antioxidant activity of twenty Iranian pomegranate (*Punica granatum* L.) cultivars. *Scientia Horticulturae, 126*(2), 180–185.

Thibault, J. F., Lahaye, M., & Guillon, F., (1992). Physicochemical properties of food plant cell walls. In: Schweizer, T. F., & Edwards, C., (eds.), *Dietary Fiber, a Component of Food: Nutritional Function in Health and Disease* (pp. 21–39). Berlin: Springer–Verlag. ILSI Europe.

Thibault, J. F., Renard, M. G. C., & Guillon, F., (1994). Physical and chemical analysis of dietary fibers in sugar–beet and vegetable. In: Jackson, J. F., & Linkens, H. F., (eds.), *Modern Methods of Plant Analysis* (Vol. XVI, pp. 23–55). Heidelberg: Springer–Verlag.

Thompson, T., Dennis, M., Higgins, L. A., Lee, A. R., & Sharrett, M. K., (2005). Gluten–free diet survey: Are Americans with coeliac disease consuming recommended amounts of fiber, iron, calcium and grain foods? *Journal of Human Nutrition and Dietetics, 18*(3), 163–169.

Topping, D. L., & Illman, R. J., (1986). Bacterial fermentation in the human large bowel. Time to change from the rough–age model of dietary fiber? *The Medical Journal of Australia, 144*(6), 307–309.

Topping, D. L., & Pant, I., (1995). Short-chain fatty acids and hepatic lipid metabolism: Experimental studies. In: Cummings, J. H., Rombeau, J. C., & Sakata, T., (eds.), *Physiological and Clinical Aspects of Short–Chain Fatty Acids* (pp. 496–508). Cambridge: Cambridge University Press.

Topping, D. L., Fukushima, M., & Bird, A. R., (2003). Resistant starch as a prebiotic and symbiotic: State of the art. *Proceedings of the Nutrition Society, 62*(1), 171–176.

Torres, J. L., Varela, B., Garc´ıa, M. T., Carilla, J., Matito, C., & Centelles, J. J. (2002). Antioxidant and biological properties of polyphenolic fractions differing in procyanidin composition and flavonol content. *Journal of Agricultural and Food Chemistry, 50*(26), 7548–7555.

Tosh, S. M., Wood, P. J., Wang, Q., & Weisz, J., (2004). Structural characteristics and rheological properties of partially hydrolyzed oat β-glucan: The effects of molecular weight and hydrolysis method. *Carbohydrate Polymers, 55*(4), 425–436.

Tungland, B. C., & Meyer, D., (2002). Nondigestible oligo – and polysaccharides (dietary fiber): Their physiology and role in human health and food. *Comprehensive Reviews in Food Science and Safety, 1*(3), 90–109.

Ubando-Rivera, J., Navarro-Ocana, A., & Valdivia-Lopez, M. A., (2005). Mexican lime peel: Comparative study on con-tents of dietary fiber and associated antioxidant activity. *Food Chemistry, 89*(1), 57–61.

Vergara-Valencia, N., Granados-Perez, E., Agama-Acevedo, E., Tovar, J., Ruales, J., & Bello-Perez, L. A., (2007). Fiber concentrate from mango fruit: Characterization, associated antioxidant capacity and application as a bakery product ingredient. *LWT–Food Science and Technology, 40*(4), 722–729.

Vidal-Valverde, C., Frias, J., Sotomayor, C., Diaz-Pollan, C., Fernandez, M., & Urbano, G., (1998). Nutrients and antinutritional factors in faba beans as affected by processing. *Journal of Food Examination and Research A, 207*(2), 140–145.

Wong, J. M., & Jenkins, D. J., (2007). Carbohydrate digestibility and metabolic effects. *The Journal of Nutrition, 137*(11), 2539S–2546S.

Wood, P., (1997). Functional foods for health: Opportunities for novel cereal processes and products. In: Campbell, G. M., Webb, C., & McKee, S. L., (eds.), *Cereals Novel Uses and Processes* (pp. 233–239). New York: Plenum Press.

Xuan, T. C., & Azlan, A., (2017). Effects of cooking on the dietary fiber and phenolic contents of selected beans and its combinations. *Journal of Food Science and Technology, 1*, 1–8.

Young, G. P., (1991). Dietary fiber and bowel cancer: Which fiber is best? In: *Cereals International Proceedings of an International Conference Held in Brisbane Australia* (pp. 379–383). Melbourne: Royal Australian Chemical Institute.

Yue, P., & Waring, S., (1998). Resistant start in food applications. *Cereal Foods World, 43*, 690–695.

CHAPTER 2

FORMULATION-BASED APPROACHES FOR THE DELIVERY OF FOOD SUPPLEMENTS AND DIETARY FIBERS

TEJAS S. TELANGE,[1] SARVESH S. PAWAR,[1] PUSHKAR Y. CHAVAN,[1] BHUSHAN R. RANE,[1] RUPESH A. PINGALE,[2] RAJ K. KESERVANI,[3] BUI THANH TUNG,[4] and RAMSANEH RAGHUWANSHI[5]

[1]Shri D.D. Vispute College of Pharmacy and Research Center, Panvel, Maharashtra, India

[2]NCRD Sterling Institute of Pharmacy, Nerul, Navi Mumbai, Maharashtra, India

[3]Faculty of B. Pharmacy, CSM Group of Institutions, Prayagraj, Uttar Pradesh, India

[4]VNU University of Medicine and Pharmacy, Vietnam National University, Hanoi, Vietnam

[5]Professor, Department of Pharmaceutical Chemistry, Corporate Institute of Pharmacy, Bhopal, Madhya Pradesh, India

ABSTRACT

Dietary fibers play a crucial role to modulate immunity and thus create a reduced risk of cardiovascular diseases, diabetes, obesity (Jarouliya & Keservani, 2019), and cancer. The most likely performance that is getting increasingly attention is fibers part in immune health. Global consumption of dietary fibers is projected to reach $21,672.9 million by 2030. Various industries, including pharmaceutical, animal feed, and cosmetics, increasingly use

Food Supplements and Dietary Fiber in Health and Disease. Bhushan R. Rane, Raj K. Keservani, Durgesh Singh, Nayan A. Gujarathi, and Ashish S. Jain, (Eds.)
© 2024 Apple Academic Press, Inc. Co-published with CRC Press (Taylor & Francis)

dietary fibers, which accelerates the global dietary fiber market's growth. The globalization of the population and the international trade of food will benefit health-conscious citizens around the world in regards to traditional Indian and Ayurvedic health foods and nutraceuticals.

2.1 INTRODUCTION

2.1.1 INTRODUCTION TO FOOD SUPPLEMENTS

The way humans eat and produce food has evolved slowly and steadily over the last few decades. A rise in chronic health issues such as diabetes, obesity, and metabolic syndrome has been attributed to highly processed and refined foods that have had much of their nutrients depleted.

The need for foods with improved health advantages is being driven by recent technological advancements, socioeconomic shifts, and population lifestyle changes around the world (Betoret et al., 2011; Keservani et al., 2015b, 2016b). According to this viewpoint, global demand for functional foods and dietary food supplements has risen fast. Foods nowadays are designed to do more than just satisfy hunger and deliver essential nutrients; they can also bring additional health benefits to humans, such as reducing nutrition-related maladies and boosting physical and mental well-being (Aluko et al., 2022).

Functional foods are foods that, when ingested as part of a regular diet, can deliver one or more bioactive chemicals in addition to nutrients, enhancing the traditional nutritional effects (Barauskaite et al., 2018). Functional foods are becoming more popular around the world, according to recent food industry trends, and they are becoming a component of the everyday diet of industrialized countries (Barauskaite et al., 2018). Bioactive chemicals, which can exist naturally, arise through industrial processing, or be derived from other sources and added to functional foods, provide health benefits. Whole grains, legumes, tubers, fruits, and vegetables are common food supplements that are concentrated and/or dehydrated. The vitamins are highly complex structures that incorporate a variety of nutrients such as enzymes, trace elements, coenzymes, antioxidants (Kesharwani et al., 2016; Singh et al., 2017a), and several other elements. Peptides, carotenoids, polyphenolic compounds, and iso-flavones, as well as proteins (Keservani et al., 2015) and amino acids, primarily fatty acids, provide health benefits, primarily in the areas of development and growth, metabolic regulation, oxidative stress defense, cardiovascular (Keservani et al., 2016a) and gastrointestinal physiology, and physical and cognitive performance (Butnariu, Sarac). When compared to comparable traditional items, these products targeted at maintaining well-being should have the highest quality criteria (Fibigr et al., 2022).

The term "food supplement" refers to a concentrated source of nutrients (such as minerals and vitamins) or other compounds with a nutritional or physiological effect, and are commonly available in "dose form" (e.g., capsules, pills, tablets, liquids in measured doses) rather than as a functional food product. Food supplements may contain a variety of nutrients and other components, including but not limited to vitamins, minerals, amino acids, essential fatty acids, fiber, and other plant and herbal extracts (Czepielewska et al., 2018; Keservani et al., 2020; Rane & Keservani, 2020; Rane et al., 2020a).

Food supplements are designed to address nutritional deficiencies, ensure appropriate nutrient intake, or support specific physiological processes. They aren't medicines; thus they can't have any pharmacological, immunological, or metabolic effects. As a result, their use is not meant to treat or prevent human diseases or to alter physiological functioning.

Food supplements are now widely available, and they are playing an increasingly essential role in consumer awareness. According to Euro monitor International, the current year sales of these food products in the European Union are close to 7 billion euros (Kowalska et al., 2019). Food supplements are utilized by the general public for a variety of reasons, including health maintenance, disease prevention, diet balancing, increasing attractiveness and wellness, and improving athletic performance (Colombo et al., 2020; Jha et al., 2017).

2.1.2 INTRODUCTION TO DIETARY FIBERS

Dietary fiber (DF) is a term that has been used to describe a group of plant-based cell wall components in the past. Fibers are found in all plant foods, including fruits (Keservani et al., 2016b), vegetables, legumes, and grains, and are the structural component of the plant. Dietary fiber, which includes "Non-Starch Polysaccharides" (NSPs), including cellulose, lignin, and pectin, is a type of carbohydrate found nearly exclusively in plants. It is a naturally occurring edible component of glucose and lignin found in plant food. The majority of dietary fibers are polysaccharides, which are carbohydrates that humans cannot digest. Starch is made up of a lengthy chain of glucose molecules joined by alpha bonds. Fiber is made up of a lengthy chain of glucose molecules joined by beta bonds (Jha et al., 2017). Fiber is not digested and absorbed because the human body lacks enzymes to dissolve beta bonds. The edible component of a plant or comparable carbohydrates that are resistant to digestion and absorption in the human intestine with complete or partial fermentation in the large intestine, according to the American Association of Cereal Chemists (AACC, 2000).

Dietary supplements are a vast range of ingestible products that are distinguishable from regular foods and pharmaceuticals that are consumed all over the world. Dietary supplements are classified in the United States as items (other than tobacco) that contain at least one of the following substances: vitamin, mineral, herb, or botanical (including extracts of herbs or botanicals), amino acid, metabolite, or any combination of these ingredients. Dietary supplements include products like multivitamins, garlic tablets, fish oil capsules, probiotics, natural weight-loss aids, and certain types of energy beverages, to name a few.

Diets that emphasize naturally high-fiber plant-based foods, including fruits, vegetables, and whole grains lessen the risk of chronic diseases like coronary heart disease (CHD), type 2 diabetes (T2DM), obesity, and certain types of cancer (Wong et al., 2017; Brennan & Tudorica, 2007).

Non-starch polysaccharides are the common name for fibers (NSPs). Based on their qualities and effects on the body, Dietary Fiber can be divided into two categories. Insoluble and soluble fibers are the two types. Water does not dissolve insoluble fibers like cellulose, hemicellulose, and lignin. Wheat bran, entire grains, and vegetables are all high in insoluble fibers. Insoluble fibers absorb water and add weight to the intestine, making it easier for it to operate properly. Gum and pectin are soluble fibers that dissolve in water and can be found in beans, oats, barley, and various fruits and vegetables. Soluble fibers may help to decrease blood cholesterol and regulate the body's sugar metabolism (Brennan & Tudorica, 2007).

Dietary fiber is only found in plant foods. Whole-grain bread and cereals, fruits and vegetables, and dried beans and peas are the finest sources of fiber. Both soluble and insoluble fibers are present in these meals (Schmeeman, 1999).

2.2 NEED OF FOOD SUPPLEMENTS AND DIETARY FIBERS GLOBALLY

Dietary supplements are used for a variety of reasons, including:

- Maintaining their general well-being;
- Assist mental and athletic performance;
- Support the immunological system;

- Normalizes bowel movements;
- Helps maintain bowel health;
- Lowers cholesterol levels;
- Helps control blood sugar levels;
- Aids in achieving a healthy weight;
- Helps you live longer.

However, certain people may require them more than others, such as:

1. **Women Who Are Pregnant or May Become Pregnant:** To protect against birth defects, women who are pregnant or may become pregnant should consume 400 micrograms of folate daily, either through food or supplements. Folate is a B vitamin that is required for the production of genetic elements such as DNA. It can be found in prenatal vitamins, which may also contain beneficial amounts of iron and calcium.
2. **Adults Over the Age of 50:** As we age, we may require more vitamins and minerals than younger people. Calcium and Vitamin D are crucial for bone strength, as is Vitamin B6, which aids in the formation of red blood cells, and Vitamin B12, which aids in the maintenance of neurons and red blood cells.
3. **Food Allergy Sufferers and People on Special Diets:** If you're a vegan have food allergies or lactose intolerance or have trouble digesting or absorbing nutrients, dietary supplements may be beneficial to you (How to Add More Fiber to Your Diet, 2022 https://www.mayoclinic.org/healthy-lifestyle/nutrition-and-healthy-eating/in-depth/fiber/art-20043983).

Polysaccharides, oligosaccharides, lignin, and other plant components make up dietary fibers. DF promotes beneficial properties such as laxation and/or lowering blood cholesterol levels (Anon., 2001). Clinical studies repeatedly suggest that consuming viscous DF lowers LDL cholesterol and postprandial glucose levels, as well as causing short-term satiety. Furthermore, only a few clinical investigations have shown that DF consumption improves diabetes and body weight management (Anderson et al., 2009).

2.3 ITS FUTURE PERSPECTIVE

The dietary fibers market is projected to grow at a CAGR of 11.1% between 2021 and 2030, according to a new report published by Allied Market Research. The research study is entitled, "Dietary fibers market by raw material, product, and application: global opportunity analysis and industry forecast, 2021–2030."

Global consumption of dietary fibers is projected to reach $21,672.9 million by 2030. As a result of the increasing demand for dietary supplements, dietary fibers are increasingly being used in various industries, such as pharmaceutical, animal feed, and cosmetics, which exponentially propels the growth of the dietary fibers market worldwide (Global Opportunity Analysis and Industry Forecast 2021–2027, 2022).

2.3.1 MARKET GROWTH FACTORS FOR DIETARY FIBERS

- As dietary fibers are increasingly used in fiber supplements, the market is expected to grow in a positive way.
- Due to an increasingly hectic lifestyle, consumers are spending less time on their diet, resulting in low fiber consumption.
- To meet their dietary fiber needs, consumers are increasingly turning to fiber supplements. This is expected to boost demand for fiber-based supplements, thereby contributing positively toward the growth of the dietary fibers market.
- As consumers become increasingly aware of the benefits of a healthy diet, the global market for dietary fibers will expand.
- Consumers are realizing the benefits of dietary fiber as a means to reduce diseases, such as hypertension, cardiovascular diseases, and obesity, resulting in an increase in demand for dietary fiber-based products.

2.3.2 KEY PLAYERS (FIGURE 2.1)

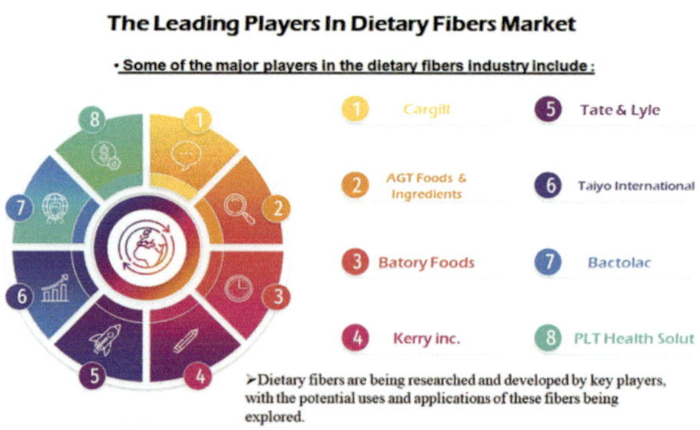
The Leading Players In Dietary Fibers Market
• Some of the major players in the dietary fibers industry include :
1 Cargill
2 AGT Foods & Ingredients
3 Batory Foods
4 Kerry inc.
5 Tate & Lyle
6 Taiyo International
7 Bactolac
8 PLT Health Solut
➢Dietary fibers are being researched and developed by key players, with the potential uses and applications of these fibers being explored.

FIGURE 2.1 The leading players in dietary fibers market.

2.3.3 MARKET DYNAMICS (FIGURE 2.2)

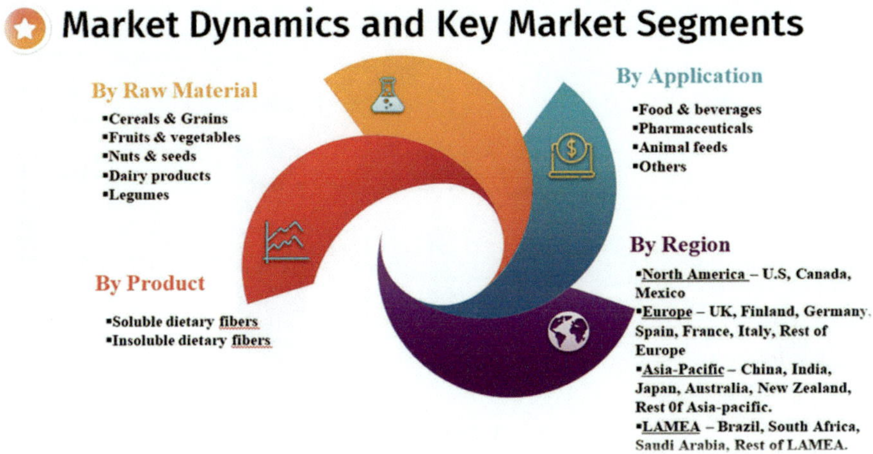

FIGURE 2.2 Market dynamics.

2.3.4 DIETARY FIBERS MARKET PLAYERS' KEY GROWTH STRATEGIES

- Product launches are the most important growth strategy for market players, followed by collaborations, agreements, expansion, joint ventures, and acquisitions.
- Diverse businesses have developed innovative products to broaden their market reach and serve international customers. Product launches are used by a variety of companies to broaden their market reach and service international customers.

In terms of dietary fibers market opportunities, the insoluble dietary fibers segment is expected to see the greatest growth, given the fact that insoluble dietary fibers are derived from oats, wheat, corn, potato, peas, rice, and legumes help prevent constipation, hypertension, and obesity (India Dietary Supplements Market Trends, Size, Growth, Opportunity, and Forecast, 2021–2026, 2022).

2.3.5 DIETARY SUPPLEMENTS MARKET SIZE, 2020 TO 2030 (USD BILLION) (FIGURE 2.3)

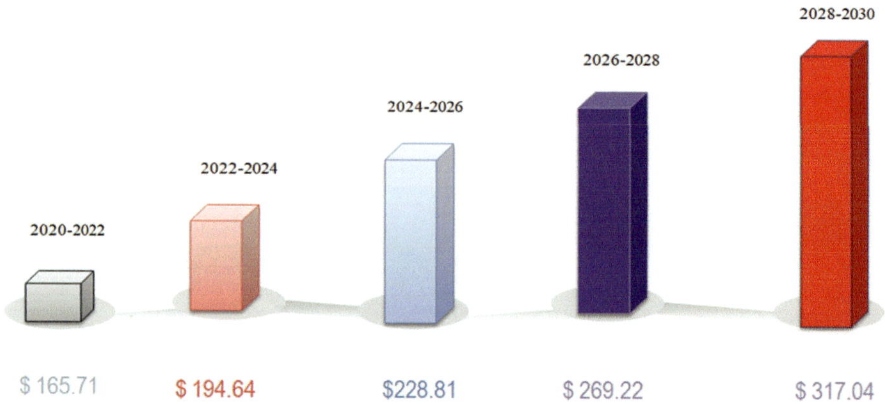

FIGURE 2.3 Dietary supplements market size, year 2020–2030 (USD billion).

2.3.6 MARKET CAPTURED BY FOOD SUPPLEMENTS AND DIETARY FIBERS

Among the regions, North America is the market leader due to the presence of major manufacturers, high disposable incomes, and an increased focus on physical appearance. The next highest stake was accounted for by Europe, mostly due to its large geriatric population and increasing prevalence of chronic illnesses.

As the largest market, Asia Pacific is expected to grow at the fastest CAGR owing to the popularity of social media, increasing health and well-being awareness, and the rise of the middle class. In the projected period, the Middle East, Latin America, and Africa region will show noteworthy growth (Figure 2.4).

In 2019, the global dietary fibers market size was over USD 5.3 billion. Globally, the Dietary Fiber and Functional Food Industry will see lucrative growth opportunities in the coming years as fiber-rich foods make their way into daily diets and functional foods are introduced. The global market for vitamins and dietary supplements grew at a compound annual growth rate of 6.3% (CAGR 2014–2018), driven mainly by the segment of food supplements.

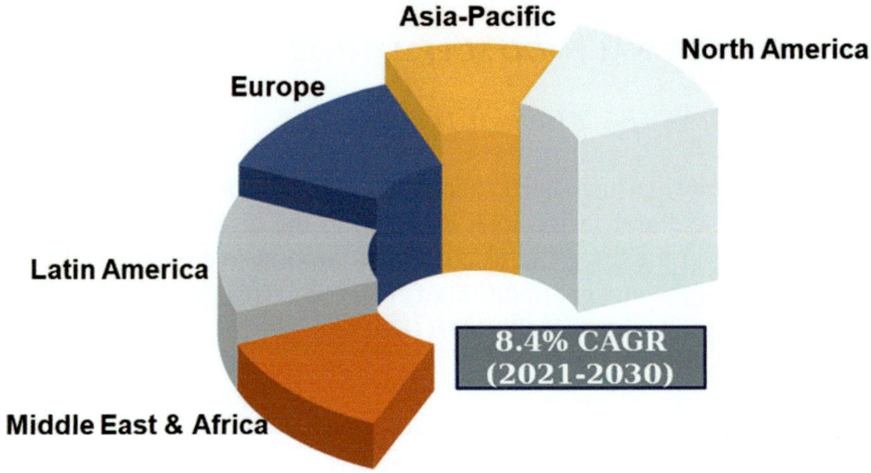

FIGURE 2.4 Market captured by food supplements and dietary fibers among the continental regions.

IMARC Group expects the global dietary fiber market to reach US$12.1 billion by 2027, with a value of US$7.8 billion in 2021.

Market research reports categorize dietary fibers by raw material, product, application, and geography. The market is divided into fruits and vegetables, cereals, and grains, legumes, nuts, and seeds, and other basic materials.

In dietary fibers, soluble, and insoluble dietary fiber is segmented based on product type. Soluble dietary fiber is expected to exceed USD 4 billion by 2026. According to dietary fibers market trends, the cereals and grains sector is the most dominant, accounting for 46.5% of the dietary fibers market share in 2020. Because of the fast-growing production and consumption of dietary fibers, the legumes category is predicted to grow the fastest (Dietary Fiber Market: Global Industry Trends, 2022).

An analysis of the dietary fibers market states that the insoluble dietary fibers segment is expected to grow at the fastest rate due to the fact that insoluble dietary fibers derived from grains such as oats, corn, wheat, potato, rice, peas, and legumes help to prevent high cholesterol, constipation, and obesity. Therefore, it is highly sought after all over the world (Dietary Supplements Are More Popular Than Ever, 2022).

2.4 FORMULATION-BASED APPROACHES

2.4.1 *TRADITIONAL FOOD SUPPLEMENTS*

2.4.1.1 INDIA'S TRADITIONAL FOODS

The Indian foodways have been characterized by a wide variety of seasonal variations and cultural factors that have led to the discovery of functional characteristics in the diet. The discovery of these characteristics led to the development of the ancient tradition of Ayurveda. This system of medicine is considered one of the world's oldest (Sarkar et al., 2015).

2.4.1.1.1 Cereals and Millets

Grains and millets fill in as the main wellspring of full-scale supplements. The two significant sorts of oat that are broadly consumed in India are rice and wheat, in spite of the fact that others like jowar (sorghum), bajra (pearl millet), and ragi (finger millets), and other minor millets are utilized as staples or substitutes in numerous locales.

They are generally utilized for making assortments of food arrangements that are eaten during all suppers of the day. Notwithstanding, the assortments of rice or wheat and the manner in which they are handled for utilization have changed throughout the long term. For example, cleaned rice is the most prevalently sold structure in both metropolitan and rustic settings.

Curiously, the rice used to be cleaned distinctly at a 2.5% level during the 1960s, while as of now the clean is around 10% for business purposes. Essentially, wheat is economically handled to make flour of two kinds, i.e., entire wheat flour (Atta) and refined wheat flour (Maida).

2.4.1.1.2 Legumes and Pulses

Legumes and Pulses have been a vital piece of the customary Indian food framework. They fill in as wellsprings of protein other than energy and micronutrients (nutrients and minerals). Heartbeats and vegetables are utilized to set up an enormous number of stews, and plans that are consumed as side dishes alongside a huge assortment of Indian bread (unleavened) level, for example, rotis and chapatis, rice arrangements, and breakfast things, for example, idli, dosa, apam, and so forth Many heartbeats and vegetables like dark gram, green gram, green peas, and rajmah (Kidney bean), soybeans track down a significant spot in the Indian food framework close by Bengal gram and red gram.

2.4.1.1.3 Dairy Products/Milk and Milk Products

The items solely got from cow or bison milk are significant conventional food sources in India. Milk is a significant wellspring of sustenance for babies and youngsters and is similarly universally drunk by grown-ups. It is utilized in that capacity and as a fixing in an assortment of drinks like tea/espresso, kheers (sweet porridge), and numerous provincial sweet arrangements like rosogolla, sandesh, and pedha.

Dahi (Indian yogurt) is a well-known matured item ready from milk utilizing lactic corrosive microbes. The bacterial movement brings about low pH which makes milk proteins coagulate, giving a trademark surface to dahi. It is utilized in an assortment of culinary arrangements, and furthermore as a supplement to plain rice.

Dahi is plentiful in B complex nutrients, folic corrosive, and riboflavin and gives a wide scope of medical advantages because of the presence of probiotic microorganisms (Sarkar et al., 2015). Other dairy items utilized in the Indian customary food framework are margarine, ghee (explained spread), and paneer (Indian curds).

There is, be that as it may, an ocean of progress in the manner in which milk and milk items are handled today contrasted with before times. Milk, as it was seen before, was just entire milk (new) that came from the udders of the milch cows. Every one of the healthful characteristics or useful properties of the milk were of that sort of milk, which was privately obtained and new all the time with practically no handling.

Today, homogenized and purified standard milk is accessible, in which fat rate is acclimated to meet the administrative necessities (FSSAI, 2011). Additionally, ghee accessible in the business sectors today is produced using the cream of new milk and not from the cream from curds or bubbled milk as in a conventional manner.

2.4.1.1.4 Fruits

These are rich wellsprings of flavonoids, minerals, nutrients, carotenoids, electrolytes, and other bioactive mixtures that affect human well-being.

While many organic products like apple, pineapple, papaya, bael (Aegle marmelos), citrus natural products, guava, and so forth structure part of customary Indian food, the most normally eaten natural products are mango and banana. They have consistently had a unique spot in Indian culture and custom and have been dealt with all the time as a basic piece of the conventional weight control plans.

2.4.1.1.5 Spices

One of the central points that put Indian food aside from the remainder of the world is the utilization of flavors and their mixes, which improve the fragrance of food. The zest altering given in singing hot oil gives Indian stews their trademark flavor and smell. Flavors are utilized in an enormous number of ways of getting ready stews and curries and to marinate different food arrangements.

Flavors usually utilized in India are turmeric, dark pepper, garlic, fenugreek seeds, ginger, cumin seeds, coriander seeds, cardamom, and nutmeg. They bring to food an enormous number of bio-actives that render food sources useful.

2.4.1.2 TRADITIONAL HEALTH FOODS BASED ON GRAINS

The literature discusses the use of grains in different civilizations of India. Grains are the primary staple food of the people of India. Grains are nutritionally rich products that provide the body with important nutrients.

We can find distinct grains used by our ancestors in Indian history. Beginning with the Yajurveda period, the urad (Vigna mungo), mung (Vigna radiata), and masoor (Lens culinaris) were the most widely used grains and legumes (Achaya, 1994). Grains contain good calorific value from starch and proteins; some grains, however, have antinutritional characteristics, such as trypsin inhibitors.

Traditionally processed foods such as fermented foods, soaked foods, and cooked foods can remove these antinutritional factors. In addition to its potential health benefits, resistant starch has also been studied because of its functional properties. In traditional Indian grain products, resistant starches may be present in greater amounts because whole grains are used more frequently and the processing is less intensive (Egounlety & Aworh, 2003; Nigudkar, 2002).

2.4.1.2.1 *Idli/Selroti/Dosas/Dhokla*

Rice and black gram batter are used to prepare idli batter, which is fermented (Agarwal and Bhasin, 2002). Rice and black gram are used in the ratio of 2:1 when preparing batter. Fermentation increases the nutritional and protein value of idli batter (Reddy et al., 1982). Idli batter is primarily leavened by heterofermentative lactic acid bacteria, Lactobacillus mesenteroides.

Probiotic bacteria such as Lactobacillus plantarum and Lactobacillus lactis are also present. In addition to producing vitamin B12 and an enzyme called bgalactosidase, these microorganisms increase the probiotic activity and promote health (Iyer et al., 2013). They also add a good amount of protein to the diet.

There are a number of microorganisms that are present in selroti, including Lactobacillus, Pediococci, Enterococci, and Leuconostocs. Selroti is comparable to idli in nutrition and contains a good amount of digestible proteins (Yonzan and Tamang, 2010). Dosas are easy to digest and nutritionally dense and are therefore appropriate for elderly people and children younger than 10.

A popular breakfast food in Gujarat state is the indigenous probiotic dish, Dhokla. An increase in oxidative stress is caused by free fatty acid intake and hyperglycemia in diabetic patients (Evans et al., 2002). Degenerative diseases caused by oxidative stress can be cured with Dhokla, due to its antioxidative property (Moktan et al., 2011).

2.4.1.2.2 *Ambali/Ragi-Hurihittu/Hawaiijar*

Ambali is a semiliquid finger millet-based fermented product of the states of Tamil Nadu and Karnataka in south India. Finger millet (ambali) contains a high level of calcium and has a low level of resistant starch, making it a health food for older adults (Mangala et al., 1999). As ambali is very cold in nature (endothermic), it should be avoided during the rainy season and winter. With sufficient calcium content, it is a healthy beverage for the elderly.

Using ragi hurihittu enhances palatable taste and aroma, decreases antinutritional factors, and improves digestibility and solubility of starch (Muralikrishna et al., 1986). Increases zinc and iron bioavailability. It is useful for the preparation of dietetic foods for patients with anemia and geriatric food formulations (Hemalatha et al., 2007).

Hawaiijar contains 26% to 27% soluble proteins (Thingom and Chhetry, 2011). Hawaiijar is a protein-rich food suitable for older children than 10 years and adults.

2.4.1.3 TRADITIONAL FOODS BASED ON FRUITS AND VEGETABLES

Several of the traditional Indian health foods prepared using fresh fruits and vegetables are discussed in subsections along with their health benefits. Fruits provide flavonoids, minerals, vitamins, carotenoids, electrolytes, and other bioactive compounds that affect human health.

2.4.1.3.1 Banana

In India, bananas are primarily used as Prasada (spiritual food). The banana plant, with its fruit, flower, and stem, is used as a medicinal herb for treating gastric problems. The alkaline nature of the banana fruit can neutralize acid conditions and help in the formation of a thick protective mucus layer.

Fruits like bananas contain iron, which is why women who suffer from anemia should consider eating them as they add flavor to hot foods and provide antioxidants such as epigallocatechin gallate. Health dishes made from banana plant parts include Bale Dandu Playa – made from banana plant stems, which is beneficial to diabetics and those suffering from stomach problems, Vazhai Poo Poriyal – made from banana plant flowers, which is useful for patients with diabetes or heartburn, and banana stem juice – taken in the morning on an empty stomach, which helps good skin health. The juice has 'hyperglycemic effects' and can be used for treating hypoglycemia (Singh et al., 2007).

2.4.1.3.2 Jackfruit

The jackfruit (*Artocarpus heterophyllus Lam. fam. Moraceae*) is an ancient fruit found in Southeast Asia. The edible part of jackfruit consists of both fruits and seeds. Phytonutrients and antioxidants contained in jackfruit, as well as carotenoids, provide the fruit and its seeds with increased medicinal value (Swami et al., 2012). Traditionally, jackfruit seeds are roasted/boiled and eaten in the Koorg region in the Karnataka state as jackfruit seed chutney, halasu beeja palya, and chekke kuru pajji.

2.4.1.3.3 Bael Fruit

Among Indian populations, bael fruit is traditionally used for the treatment of diarrhea due to its antimicrobial properties (Brijesh et al., 2009). Other uses include dietary supplementation with Angeline from bael tree leaves (Govindachari and Premila, 1983) as well as a beverage prepared from the pulp of bael fruit. Additionally, it is gut-friendly and has traditionally been used to treat constipation, diarrhea, and diabetes. It is known to act as a tonic for the heart and brain. It contains chemicals such as tannins, flavonoids, and coumarins, which help reduce inflammation.

2.4.1.3.4 Mango

Mango's nutraceutical value (Keservani et al., 2010a, b), particularly in terms of antioxidants and polyphenols, is widely recognized. Mangiferin, quercetin, kaempferol, gallic acid, and rhamnetin are just a few of the antioxidants found in mango. Mangiferin is an antioxidant that can be found in mango. It has the ability to chelate iron. Mango's functional qualities aid in the treatment of degenerative disorders (Masibo M and He Q, 2008).

Mango peel is a delectable delicacy. Dietary fibers and bioactive substances such as carotenoids, vitamin C, and vitamin E are abundant in mango peels (Ajila et al., 2007).

2.4.1.3.5 Jamun Fruit

Phytochemicals in this fruit make it a potentially valuable nutraceutical (Rane et al., 2020b). Phytochemicals in the tree are used in India as a treatment for diabetes (Kumar et al., 2015, 2008). Different parts of the tree, such as the leaf, bark, seed, and pulp, are used to treat diabetes, allergies, viral infection, inflammation, and gastric ulcers (Chaudhary et al., 2012). Moreover, all the parts of the Jamun tree offer medicinal benefits, and jamun seed powder has been shown to be particularly effective for diabetic patients.

2.4.1.3.6 *Papaya*

It is said that ripe papaya fruits relieve dyspepsia, ripe fruit juices treat bleeding piles, unripe fruits act as diuretics, and the paste of the young leaves relieves jaundice (Kirtikar and Basu, 1981). All parts of the papaya tree are used to treat diseases in one form or another.

2.4.1.3.7 *Bitter Gourd*

Medicinal properties are present in the vegetable. Despite its bitter flavor, bitter gourd holds antidiabetic properties thanks to its presence of chrantin, vicine, and polypeptide-p (Krawinkel & Keding, 2006). The juice of bitter gourd pulp may enhance glucose tolerance among diabetics (Raman and Lau, 1996). The health benefit of bharwan karela is that it can reduce blood sugar, possibly reduce cholesterol levels, and possibly fight cancer.

2.4.1.4 GREEN LEAFY VEGETABLE

Some of the health dishes used in Indian cuisine are based on foods rich in nutrients and antioxidants, like curry leaves, fenugreek, and Amaranthus (Gupta and Prakash, 2009). Many green leafy vegetables that are rich in vitamins and antioxidants are part of Indian culinary preparations. Read on for a list of Indian dishes that contain green leafy vegetables.

2.4.1.4.1 *Spinach Roti*

Spinach is a good source of iron and protein. It is recommended for women and girls who are menstruating and lactating.

2.4.1.4.2 *Gundruk*

Rayo-sag, mustard, or cauliflower leaves are fermented to form gundruk, a fermented food containing Lactic acid bacteria derived from Lactobacilli, Leuconostoc, and Pediococcus. Gundruk soup is also a good appetizer.

Among its many health benefits, Gundruk contains ascorbic acid, carotene, and lactic acid, which act as anticarcinogens (Tamang, 2010).

2.4.1.4.3 Basle Soppu Playa

Baselle soppu palya is made from the leaves of the *Baselle alba* L. plant, which are high in vitamin C, vitamin A, folic acid, and calcium. The flavonoid (Keservani & Sharma, 2014) kaempferol is found in the *Baselle alba* L. leaf. This dish has a cooling impact on the body and is beneficial for mouth ulcers and stomach disorders.

2.4.1.4.4 Saag

Saag is a dish made from leaves. Saag is made using green leafy vegetables such as spinach, basella, mustard leaf, and collard greens. Rich in antioxidants, a good source of iron, beneficial to eye health, aids in cholesterol control, and contains dietary fiber.

2.4.1.4.5 Batua Paratha

The plant's leaves contain ascaridole, a drug used to treat hookworm and roundworm infections. It has a variety of medical effects, such as laxative, blood purification, and antiscorbutic (Kirtikar & Basu, 1918). Batua paratha is a breakfast item offered only during the winter months.

In addition to India's traditional and nutritional dishes, there are numerous other dishes served in various sections of the nation with high nutritional content.

2.4.1.5 MILK-BASED HEALTH FOOD

Cattle played an important role in Vedic civilization. Cow, buffalo, and goat milk were drank either fresh or boiled in literature before 800 BCE. Sushrutha addresses human milk as well as cow, buffalo, goat, and sheep milk, detailing the differences between them. Ghee, curd, paneer, cheese, and buttermilk are some of the most common milk processing products. Buttermilk was widely used, and it was used to make saga, a seasoned food.

Rice and barley were served with curds. Colostrum became popular after 800 BCE, when it was blended with heated milk, crystal sugar, and fragrant plants (Achaya, 1994). Milk, according to the Ayurvedic philosophy, has nutrients that are not found in other foods. We'll go over the most important milk-based health foods here.

2.4.1.5.1 Dahi (Indian Yogurt)

It is consumed as a source of Bcomplex vitamins, folic acid, and riboflavin in the daily diet (Sharma & Lal, 1997). Dahi is high in lactic acid bacteria and has a probiotic effect, which benefits gut health. Children's diarrhea can be controlled with bacterial cultures (Agarwal & Bhasin, 2002).

2.4.1.5.2 Ginna

Ginna, also known as junnu, posu, or kharvas, is an Indian delicacy made with colostrum. Immune components such immunoglobulins and iron-binding lactoferrin protein, as well as nutrients like vitamin A (Singh et al., 2017a) and minerals, are abundant in colostrums (Uruakpa et al., 2002). Ginna is made from a cow's first day's thick milk (colostrum) after calving.

2.4.1.5.3 Sandesh

Sandesh is a protein-rich Indian milk product made by coagulating it with heat and acid. It has a distinctive scent and is high in the vitamins A and D. Sandesh is made from chhena, which is the main ingredient. Traditional sandesh is being studied to improve its nutritional content by integrating herbs that increase the product's antioxidant value (Bandyopadhyay et al., 2007).

2.4.1.5.4 Lassi

Lassi is a refreshing traditional milk beverage that is enjoyed during the summer months. Lassi is a probiotic product since it contains active cultures of Lactobacillus acidophilus and Streptococcus thermophilus. Lassi is characterized as salty lassi or sweet lassi depending on the ingredients used. Bhang lassi is a sort of lassi made using cannabis plant leaves as the main ingredient. The inclusion of cannabis plant components in bhang lassi provides health benefits, such as relief from digestive disorders, skin problems, fever, and sunstroke (Backes, 2014).

2.4.1.5.5 Buttermilk

Buttermilk is the liquid left over after the cream is churned into butter, and it can be eaten with or without salt and spices. When compared to ordinary milk or dahi, it contains less fat and calories. Buttermilk is a calcium and protein-rich alternative to milk. It's easier to digest and, because it contains live cultures, it promotes gut health. Buttermilk is recommended by the Ayurveda system to be consumed with meals (Pushpangadan et al., 2012).

2.4.1.6 AYURVEDIC LIQUID FOODS

2.4.1.6.1 Halu Kashaya

Ayurveda describes Kashaya as an herbal beverage that helps pitta dosha. It is sometimes called decoction of spices or herbs. This is an excellent remedy for colds and fevers. It can also help develop cranial nerves if taken on an empty stomach with milk (Hegde et al., 2013).

2.4.1.6.2 Jaljira Powder Juice

A cold beverage with cooling properties, this is typically drunk in the summer to keep cool. The basic ingredients in the powder are cumin, ginger, black pepper, black salt, and mint. Due to the presence of ginger and black pepper, this juice is recommended for those dealing with Kapha dosha. Cumin and black salt aid in digestion, while mint provides cooling properties and juice made from the powder can serve as an appetizer (Pushpangadan et al., 2012).

2.4.1.6.3 *Nannari Sharbat*

Ayurvedic medicine calls this plant Ananthamula; Nannari sharbat is a beverage based on the roots of *Decalepis hamiltonii*. It has good hepato-protective and stomach-nourishing properties. There is good antioxidant activity in the roots and pickles are prepared with them (Srivastava & Shiva-nandappa, 2010; Srivastava et al., 2006). Dehydrated patients would benefit from this beverage.

2.4.1.6.4 *Tambuli*

Typically an appetizer or starting food, tambuli has cooling properties, is recommended for those who have high pitta, and is recommended during the summer. The ingredients are further fried and added to buttermilk.

2.4.1.6.5 *Neem Flower Chutney*

Ayurvedic doctors recommend Neem products to young children who suffer from stomach problems because it effectively removes worms and gets rid of unwanted substances from the alimentary canal as well as reducing blood sugar levels. A possible benefit of Neem is its antioxidant and anti-inflammatory properties, which may help combat oxidative stress and, in turn, promote liver and kidney health.

2.4.1.6.6 *Bamboo Shoot Curry*

The medicinal qualities of bamboo shoots include low fat, high fiber content, as well as vitamins C and E (Srivastava et al., 2011). Bamboo shoots are recommended in Ayurvedic medicine for patients experiencing piles and urination discomfort, and the powdered shoot is taken with honey.

2.4.2 *NOVEL APPROACHES FOR NUTRACEUTICALS*

SL. No.	Name of Ingredients	Benefits	Types of Preparations
1.	➤ Spirulina https://ijmpronline.com/home/archive_show/2020/19/VOLUME-4-FEBRUARY-ISSUE-1 (Akao et al., 2009)	Antioxidant, anti-inflammatory effects, improvement of blood quality, prevention of anemia, reduction in blood pressure, elimination of heavy metals from the body, radioprotection, prevention of liver and renal poisonousness, resistance to cancer, and relief from unfavorably susceptible reactions.	➤ Tablets: • Parry's Wellness Organic Spirulina Tablets the Daily Superfood, 60 tablets of 500 mg each • Now Certified Organic Spirulina, 500 mg, 200 Tablets ➤ Capsules: • Himalayan Organics Spirulina, 2000 mg, 120 Vegetarian Capsules • Sunova Organic Spirulina Capsule, 500 mg, 60 Veg. Capsules ➤ Tinctures: • Secrets of the tribe spirulina alcohol-free tincture (glycerite), 2 fl oz • Hawaii Pharm Spirulina (*Arthrospira platensis*), 4 fl. Oz (120 ml) ➤ Powders: • Bioven Ingredients Spirulina Powder, Net wt. 125 g. • Heilen Biopharm Spirulina Powder Organic, 200 gm
2.	➤ Kava Kava (Kava Kava: Benefits, Side Effects & Dosage, 2022). https://www.healthline.com/nutrition/kava-kava#TOC_TITLE_HDR_2	Reduce anxiety, neurons are protected from damage, reduce the sensation of pain.	➤ Kava Tea: • Yogi Kava Stress Relief, 16 Tea Bags, Net wt. 1.27 OZ (36 g) • Celebration Herbals Kava Kava Blend, 24 tea bags, net weight 31 g 1.09 oz ➤ Kava Tincture or Liquid: • Herb Pharm Kava, 4 fluid ounces (120 ml) • The Herbal Toad Kava Tincture, 2 fl oz ➤ Kava Capsules: • NATROL Kava Kava, 200 mg, 30 Capsules • Natures Craft Kava Kava, 1400 mg Per Serving, 60 Gelatin Capsules

SL. No.	Name of Ingredients	Benefits	Types of Preparations
3.	➤ Beta-Sitosterol (BS) (Bouic et al., 1999) http://www.ijsit.com/admin/ijsit_files/BETA-SITOSTEROL%20MEDICINAL%20PROPERTIES_IJSIT_9.4.1.pdf (Paniagua-Pérez et al., 2005; Awad et al., 2007)	Primarily used for lowering cholesterol levels and improving the symptoms of benign prostatic hyperplasia (BPH). BS has antioxidant, antimicrobial, angiogenic, antioxidant, immunomodulatory, antidiabetic, anti-inflammatory, anticancer, and antinociceptive activities without major toxicity.	Tablets: • The Vitamin Shoppe Beta Sitosterol, 120 Tablets • Nature's Potent Beta-Sitosterol Advanced Formula, 500 mg, 90 Tablets ➤ Capsules: • Healthvit Beta-Sitosterol 160 mg, 60 capsules • Natures Craft Beta-Sitosterol, 500 mg complex, 30 capsules
4.	➤ Garlic as a Supplement (Amagase et al., 2022)	Garlic used as a solution for digestive issues, flatulence, worms, respiratory infections, skin diseases, wounds, symptoms of aging and numerous different infirmities. Utilization of garlic to treat wounds, hypolipidemic, antiplatelet, and pro-circulatory impacts seem to have hepatoprotective, immune enhancing, anticancer, and chemopreventive activities.	➤ Garlic Dehydrated Powder Forms: • Now Foods, Garlic 5000, 90 tablets. • Ranbaxy's Garlic Pearls (Soft gel capsules). ➤ Garlic Essential Oil Forms: • Sri Sri Tattva Garlic Oil Veg Capsule, 500 mg • Mason Natural, Garlic Oil, 1000 mg, 100 softgels ➤ Aged Garlic Extract (AGE) Forms: • Kyolic Aged Garlic Extract, Formula 101, 100 capsules

SL. No.	Name of Ingredients	Benefits	Types of Preparations
5.	➤ Alpha-Lipoic Acid (Mendoza-Núñez et al., 2022; Padmalayam et al., 2009; Shay et al., 2022; Smith et al., 2004)	Depicted as a powerful biological antioxidant, a detoxification agent, and a diabetes medication; it has been utilized to further develop age-associated cardiovascular, cognitive, and neuromuscular deficiencies.	➤ Tablet: • Himalayan Organics Alpha Lipoic Acid, 300 mg, 60 Tablets • Healthvit Alpha Lipoic Acid, 100 mg, 60 Tablets ➤ Capsules: • Nature's Bounty Alpha Lipoic Acid, 200 mg, 30 Capsules • ZeinPharma Alpha Liponsaure (Alpha Lipoic Acid), 300 mg, 90 Capsules ➤ Injection: • Relumins Alpha Lipoic Acid, 150 mg/6 ml, 10 diluent ampoules • Empower Pharmacy Alpha-Lipoic Acid, 30 ml Sterile Multi-Dose Vial, 25 mg/ml ➤ Oral Liquids: • Life Solutions Micro-Enhanced Alpha Lipoic Acid, 16 Fluid oz./473 ml • Dr's Advantage Liquid Alpha Lipoic Acid, 16 Fluid oz./473 ml ➤ Powders for Reconstitution: • Nutrabio Ala Alpha Lipoic Acid, 250G • Nutrija Ala Alpha Lipoic Acid, 50 Grams
6.	➤ Egg Shell Membrane Supplement (ESM) (Cordeiro & Hincke, 2022; Kondo & Yoshikawa, 2001; Jung et al., 2017; Jia et al., 2017; Vuong et al., 2017; Yoo et al., 2014; Nagamalli et al., 2017; Li et al., 2016; Shi et al., 2021	Addressing joint and connective tissue problems, such as pain, stiffness, wound healing, gut health, anti-inflammatory, and antioxidant activity, antibacterial activity after modification with inorganic compounds (e.g., silver nanoparticles)	➤ Tablet: • Natural Factors-NEM® Knee & Joint Formula 60 tab with glucosamine 1500 mg and NEM 500 mg • Wise Nutrition NEM Chewable Tablets, 60 Chewable Tablets ➤ Capsule: • Now Eggshell Membrane 500 mg, 60 veg capsules • 2-Healthy Origins Natural Eggshell Membrane, 500 mg, 30 veggie caps

SL. No.	Name of Ingredients	Benefits	Types of Preparations
7.	➤ Bromelain Supplement (Kwatra, B, 2020)	Numerous benefits it is known to inhibit platelet aggregation, sinusitis, surgical traumas, thrombophlebitis, pyelonephritis, bronchitis, and enhance absorption of medications, particularly antibiotics. *In-vitro* and *in-vivo* investigations have determined that bromelain displays anti-edematous, antithrombotic, and anti-inflammatory effects.	➤ Tablets: • Life Extension, Specially Coated Bromelain, 500 mg, 60 Enteric Coated Tablets • Jarrow Formulas, Bromelain, 1,000 GDU, 60 Tablets ➤ Capsules: • Doctor's Best, High Potency Bromelain 3000 GDU, 500 mg, 90 Veggie Caps • Now Foods, Bromelain, 2400 GDU/g, 500 mg, 120 Veg Capsules ➤ Oral Liquids: • Secrets of the Tribe Bromelain Alcohol-Free Tincture (Glycerite), 4 fl oz
8.	➤ Quercetin (Maalik et al., 2014)	Provides numerous health promoting benefits, including enhancement of cardiovascular health, anti-cancer, hypersensitivity disorders, arthritis, anti-inflammatory, antiviral, antibacterial, antioxidant, etc.	➤ Tablets: • Nature's Best High Potency Quercetin, 500 mg, 60 Tablets • super Smart Super Quercetin Natural Allergy Relief, 60 Tablets, 1000 mg Per Day ➤ Capsules: • Healthvit Quercetin, 100 mg, 60 capsules • A Squared Nutrition Quercetin 500 mg, 200 Capsules ➤ Oral Liquids: • Sub-lingual – Nutra Lingual Ionic Quercetin Ionized Nanoparticulate Liquid for Ultimate Absorption 1 FL OZ (30 ML) • Source Naturals NutraDrops Quercetin, 4 FL. OZ (118.28 ml) ➤ Intra-Oral Spray: • Quercetin Seasonal Extra Strength, 4 FL OZ/120 ML ➤ Powder: • Samsara Herbs Quercetin Net wt. 2 OZ (57 g)

SL. No.	Name of Ingredients	Benefits	Types of Preparations
9.	➤ Epigallocatechin Gallate Supplements (Pasrija & Anandharamakrishnan, 2015) (Dai et al., 2020; Mishra, 2022)	EGCG is a powerful antioxidant: it not only prevents the growth of cancer cells, but also kills them. It has been effective at lowering LDL cholesterol levels, inhibiting blood clot formations, preventing platelet aggregation, regulating lipids, and restricting the expansion of smooth muscle cells.	➤ Tablets: • Source Naturals EGCG, 700 mg, 120 Tablets • natures aid Green Tea Standardized to provide 297 mg of Polyphenols including 141 mg EGCG, 60 tablets) ➤ Capsules: • Now, EGCg, Green Tea Extract, 400 mg, 180 Veg Capsules • Healthy Hey Nutrition EGCG (epigallocatechin gallate), 500 mg/serving, 90 Vegetable Capsule
10.	➤ Lutein Supplements (Perrone et al., 2016; Nurul et al., 2020)	Zeaxanthin and oxidized lutein and zeaxanthin act as antioxidants; hence, the retina is protected. It is accepted that lutein's antioxidant properties are fundamental to its defensive role in the body.	➤ Tablets: • HealthAid Lutein, 20 mg, 30 Tablets Vegan. ➤ Capsules: • Healthvit Lutein, 20 mg, 60 Capsules. • Now Double Strength Lutein, 20 mg, 90 Veg Capsules. ➤ Oral Liquids: • Dr's Advantage Professional Formulas Liquid Lutein, 8 fluid oz./237 ml. ➤ Powders: • Lutein 5% Bulksupplements.com Clean and Pure Bulk Supplements, Lutein 20 mg (Standardized to 5%), 100 g [3.5 oz].

KEYWORDS

- **benign prostatic hyperplasia**
- **coronary heart disease**
- **dietary fiber**
- **dietary fibers market**
- **food supplements**
- **functional foods**
- **nutraceuticals**
- **traditional foods**

REFERENCES

Agarwal, K., & Bhasin, S., (2002). Feasibility studies to control acute diarrhoea in children by feeding fermented milk preparations Actimel and Indian Dahi. *European Journal of Clinical Nutrition, 56*(S4), S56–S59. doi: 10.1038/sj.ejcn.1601664.

Ajila, C., Bhat, S., & Prasada, R. U., (2007). Valuable components of raw and ripe peels from two Indian mango varieties. *Food Chemistry, 102*(4), 1006–1011. doi: 10.1016/j.foodchem.2006.06.036.

Akao, Y., Ebihara, T., Masuda, H., Saeki, Y., Akazawa, T., Hazeki, K., et al., (2009). Enhancement of antitumor natural killer cell activation by orally administered spirulina extract in mice. *Cancer Science, 100*(8), 1494–1501. doi: 10.1111/j.1349-7006.2009.01188.x.

Aluko, R. E. (2022). *Functional Foods and Nutraceuticals* | SpringerLink. Retrieved from: https://link.springer.com/book/10.1007%2F978-1-4614-3480-1 (accessed on 28 January 2023).

Amagase, H., Petesch, B. L., Matsuura, H., Kasuga, S., & Itakura, Y. (2001). Intake of garlic and its bioactive components. *The Journal of Nutrition, 131*(3s), 955S-62S. https://doi.org/10.1093/jn/131.3.955S.

American Association of Cereal Chemists (AACC), (2000). *Approved Methods of the AACC Method 44-15A (Moisture–Air Oven Methods)* (12th edn.). The Association, St. Paul, MN, USA.

Anderson, J. W., Baird, P., Davis, R. H. Jr., Ferreei, S., Knudtson, M., Koraym, A., Waters, V., & Williams, C. L., (2009). Health benefits of dietary fiber. *Nutrition Reviews, 67*(4), 188–205.

Anon. (2001). 'The definition of dietary fiber. *Cereal Foods World, 46*(3), 112–129.

Apte, M., Achaya, K. T., Khare, R. S., Toomey, P. M., & Lynch, O. M. (1996). Indian Food: A Historical Companion. *The Journal of Asian Studies, 55*(2), 478. doi:10.2307/2943406.

Awad, A., Chinnam, M., Fink, C., & Bradford, P., (2007). β-sitosterol activates Fas signaling in human breast cancer cells. *Phytomedicine, 14*(11), 747–754.

Bandyopadhyay, M., Chakraborty, R., & Raychaudhuri, U. (2007). *Incorporation of herbs into sandesh, an Indian sweet dairy product, as a source of natural antioxidants. International*

Journal of Dairy Technology, 60(3), 228–233. doi:10.1111/j.1471–0307.2007.00338.x (accessed on 28 February 2023).

Barauskaite, D., Gineikiene, J., Fennis, B., Auruskeviciene, V., Yamaguchi, M., & Kondo, N., (2018). Eating healthy to impress: How conspicuous consumption, perceived self–control motivation, and descriptive normative influence determine functional food choices. *Appetite, 131*, 59–67. doi: 10.1016/j.appet.2018.08.015.

Betoret, E., Betoret, N., Vidal, D., & Fito, P., (2011). Functional foods development: Trends and technologies. *Trends In Food Science & Technology, 22*(9), 498–508. doi: 10.1016/j.tifs.2011.05.004.

Bouic, P., Clark, A., Lamprecht, J., Freestone, M., Pool, E., & Liebenberg, R., et al., (1999). The effects of B-sitosterol (BSS) and B-sitosterol glucoside (BSSG) mixture on selected immune parameters of marathon runners: Inhibition of post marathon immune suppression and inflammation. *International Journal of Sports Medicine, 20*(04), 258–262. doi: 10.1055/s-2007-971127.

Brennan, C. S., & Tudorica, C. M., (2007). Pasta quality as affected by enrichment of non-starch polysaccharide. *Journal of Food Science, 72*(9), S659–S665.

Brijesh, S., Daswani, P., Tetali, P., Antia, N., & Birdi, T., (2009). Studies on the anti-diarrhoeal activity of *Aegle marmelos* unripe fruit: Validating its traditional usage. *BMC Complementary and Alternative Medicine, 9*(1). doi: 10.1186/1472-6882-9-47.

Butnariu, M., & Sarac, I., (2019). Functional food. *International Journal of Nutrition, 3*(3), 7–16. doi: 10.14302/issn.2379-7835.ijn-19-2615.

Cannabis Pharmacy, (2022). Retrieved from: https://books.google.com/books/about/Cannabis_Pharmacy.html?id=PTS7tAEACAAJ (accessed on 28 January 2023).

Chaudhary, B., & Mukhopadhyay, K., (2022). *Syzygium cumini* (L.) skeels a potential source of nutraceuticals. *International Journal of Pharmacy and Biological Sciences, 2*(1), 46–53. References – Scientific Research Publishing. Retrieved from: https://www.scirp.org/(S(i43dyn45teexjx455qlt3d2q))/reference/referencespapers.aspx?referenceid=528945 (accessed on 28 January 2023).

Chongtham, N., Bisht, M., & Haorongbam, S., (2011). Nutritional properties of bamboo shoots: Potential and prospects for utilization as a health food. *Comprehensive Reviews in Food Science and Food Safety, 10*(3), 153–168. doi: 10.1111/j.1541-4337.2011.00147.x.

Colombo, F., Restani, P., Biella, S., & Di Lorenzo, C., (2020). Botanicals in functional foods and food supplements: Tradition, efficacy and regulatory aspects. *Applied Sciences, 10*(7), 2387. doi: 10.3390/app10072387.

Cordeiro, C. M. M., & Hincke, M. T. (2011). Recent patents on eggshell: shell and membrane applications. *Recent Patents on Food, Nutrition & Agriculture, 3*(1), 1–8. https://doi.org/10.2174/2212798411103010001.

Czepielewska, E., Makarewicz-Wujec, M., Różewski, F., Wojtasik, E., & Kozłowska-Wojciechowska, M., (2018). Drug adulteration of food supplements: A threat to public health in the European Union?. *Regulatory Toxicology and Pharmacology, 97*, 98–102. doi: 10.1016/j.yrtph.2018.06.014.

Dai, W., Ruan, C., Zhang, Y., Wang, J., Han, J., Shao, Z., et al., (2020). Bioavailability enhancement of EGCG by structural modification and nano-delivery: A review. *Journal Of Functional Foods, 65*, 103732.

Dietary Fibers Market Size, Share & Trends Analysis Report By Raw Material (Fruits & Vegetables, Cereals & Grains), By Type (Soluble, Insoluble), By Application (Food & Beverages, Pharmaceuticals), By Region, and Segment Forecasts, 2022–2030. Retrieved from https://www.grandviewresearch.com/industry-analysis/dietary-fibers-market (accessed on 28 February 2023).

Egounlety, M., & Aworh, O., (2003). Effect of soaking, dehulling, cooking and fermentation with *Rhizopus oligosporus* on the oligosaccharides, trypsin inhibitor, phytic acid and tannins of soybean (Glycine max Merr.), cowpea (*Vigna unguiculata* L. Walp) and ground bean (*Macrotyloma geocarpa* Harms). *Journal Of Food Engineering, 56*(2, 3), 249–254. doi: 10.1016/s0260-8774(02)00262-5.

Evans, J., Goldfine, I., Maddux, B., & Grodsky, G., (2002). Oxidative stress and stress–activated signaling pathways: A unifying hypothesis of type 2 diabetes. *Endocrine Reviews, 23*(5), 599–622. doi: 10.1210/er.2001-0039.

Fibigr, J., Šatínský, D., & Solich, P. (2018). Current trends in the analysis and quality control of food supplements based on plant extracts. *Analytica Chimica Acta, 1036*, 1–15. https://doi.org/10.1016/j.aca.2018.08.017 (accessed on 28 January 2023).

Govindachari, T., & Premila, M., (1983). Some alkaloids from *Aegle marmelos. Phytochemistry, 22*(3), 755–757. doi: 10.1016/s0031-9422(00)86977-0.

Hegde, S., Yenagi, N., & Kasturiba, B., (2013). Indigenous knowledge of the traditional and qualified ayurveda practitioners on the nutritional significance and use of red rice in medications. *Indian Journals of Traditional Knowledge: IJTK, 12*(3), 506–511.

Hemalatha, S., Platel, K., & Srinivasan, K., (2006). Influence of germination and fermentation on bio-accessibility of zinc and iron from food grains. *European Journal of Clinical Nutrition, 61*(3), 342–348. doi: 10.1038/sj.ejcn.1602524.

How to Add More Fiber to Your Diet? (2022). Retrieved from: https://www.mayoclinic.org/healthy-lifestyle/nutrition-and-healthy-eating/in-depth/fiber/art-20043983 (accessed on 28 January 2023).

http://www.ijsit.com/admin/ijsit_files/BETA-SITOSTEROL%20MEDICINAL%20PROPERTIES_IJSIT_9.4.1.pdf (accessed on 28 January 2023).

https://www.researchgate.net/publication/342591176_Medicinal _uses_of_spices_used_in_our_traditional_culture_World_wide (accessed on 28 January 2023).

https://www.semanticscholar.org/paper/Nutritional-Analysis-of-Fermented-Soybean-Thingom Chhetry/92651ff95df9444a8793417e3debcf22d68c7aa1 (accessed on 28 January 2023).

https://www.semanticscholar.org/paper/Studies-on-Indian-Green-Leafy-Vegetables-for-Their-Gupta-Prakash/5966f997aa978b2eee9f4ced21e570e25ab17054 (accessed on 28 January 2023).

IJMPR. Archive View, (2022). Retrieved from: https://ijmpronline.com/home/archive_show/2020/19/VOLUME-4-FEBRUARY-ISSUE-1 (accessed on 28 January 2023).

India Dietary Supplements Market Trends, Size, Growth, Opportunity and Forecast 2021–2026, (2022). Retrieved from: https://www.linkedin.com/pulse/india-dietary-supplements-market-trends-size-growth-forecast-naagar (accessed on 28 January 2023).

Iyer, B., Singhal, R., & Ananthanarayan, L., (2011). Characterization and *in vitro* probiotic evaluation of lactic acid bacteria isolated from idli batter. *Journal Of Food Science and Technology, 50*(6), 1114–1121. doi: 10.1007/s13197-011-0445-6.

Jarouliya, U., & Keservani, R. K., (2019). Pathways leading to child obesity. In: Debasis, B., (ed.), *Global Perspectives on Childhood Obesity: Current Status, Consequences and Prevention* (2nd edn, pp. 137–146). Academic Press, Elsevier, chapter 12. ISBN: 9780128128404.

Jia, H., Hanate, M., Aw, W., Itoh, H., Saito, K., Kobayashi, S., et al., (2017). Eggshell membrane powder ameliorates intestinal inflammation by facilitating the restitution of epithelial injury and alleviating microbial dysbiosis. *Scientific Reports, 7*(1). doi: 10.1038/srep43993.

Jung, J., Yun, H., Kim, T., Joo, J., Song, I., Rah, Y., et al., (2017). Analysis of effect of eggshell membrane patching for moderate-to-large traumatic tympanic membrane perforation. *Journal Of Audiology and Otology, 21*(1), 39–43.

Kava, K., (2022). *Benefits, Side Effects, and Dosage.* Retrieved from: https://www.healthline.com/nutrition/kava-kava#TOC_TITLE_HDR_2 (accessed on 28 January 2023).

Keservani, R. K., & Sharma, A. K., (2014). Flavonoids: Emerging trends and potential health benefits. *Journal of Chinese Pharmaceutical Sciences, 23*(12), 815.

Keservani, R. K., Kesharwani, R. K., Sharma, A. K., Vyas, N., & Chadoker, A., (2010b). Nutritional supplements: An overview. *International Journal of Current Pharmaceutical Review and Research, 1*(1), 59–75.

Keservani, R. K., Sharma, A. K., & Jarouliya, U., (2015). Protein and peptide in drug targeting and its therapeutic approach. *Ars Pharmaceutica (Internet), 56*(3), 165–177.

Keservani, R. K., Sharma, A. K., & Kesharwani, R. K., (2016a). Nutraceutical and functional foods for cardiovascular health. In: *Food Process Engineering* (pp. 257–278, 291–312). Apple Academic Press, CRC Press. ISBN: 9781771884020.

Keservani, R. K., Sharma, A. K., & Kesharwani, R. K., (2016b). Medicinal effect of nutraceutical fruits for the cognition and brain health. *Scientifica,* 10. Article ID 3109254. doi: 10.1155/2016/3109254.

Keservani, R. K., Singh, S., Singh, V., Kesharwani, R. K., & Sharma, A. K., (2015b). Nutraceuticals and functional foods in the prevention of mental disorder. In: Debasis, B., Harry, G. P., & Anand, S., (eds.), *Nutraceutical and Functional Foods in Human Life and Disease Prevention* (pp. 255–268). Boca Raton, Fl. CRC Press, Taylor and Francis, Chapter 15b. ISBN: 9781482237214.

Kesharwani, R. K., Singh, P., & Keservani, R. K., (2016). Green coffee bean extract and chlorogenic acids: Chemistry and novel antioxidant benefits. In: Bagchi, D., Moriyama, H., & Swaroop, A., (eds.), *Green Coffee Bean Extract in Human Health* (pp. 1–17). Boca Raton, Taylor and Francis, USA. Chapter 1. ISBN: 9781498716376.

Kirtikar, K. R., & Basu, B. D., (1935). Indian medicinal plants. In: Lalit, M. B., (ed.), *Annonaceae* (2nd edn., Vol. 1, pp. 72, 73). Leader Road, Allahabad, India.

Kondo, Y., & Yoshikawa, M., (2001). Egg shell membranes for chiral separation. *Membrane, 26*(5), 228–230. doi: 10.5360/membrane.26.228.

Kowalska, A., Bieniek, M., & Manning, L., (2019). Food supplements' non-conformity in Europe-Poland: A case study. *Trends In Food Science & Technology, 93*, 262–270. doi: 10.1016/j.tifs.2019.09.022.

Krawinkel, M. B., & Keding, G. B., (2006). Bitter gourd (*Momordica charantia*) a dietary approach to hyperglycemia. *Nutrition Reviews, 64*, 331–337.

Kumar, A., Ilavarasan, R., Jayach, T., Deecaraman, R., Aravindan, P., Padmanabhan, N., & Krishan, M. V, (2022). *Research on Anti-diabetic Activity of Syzygium Cumini and its Isolated Compound Against Streptozotocin – Induced Diabetic Rats*. Retrieved from: https://www.internationalscholarsjournals.com/abstract/research-on-antidiabetic-activity-of-syzygium-rncumini-and-its-isolated-compound-against-rnstreptozotocin-induced-diabet-72336.html (accessed on 28 January 2023).

Kumar, A., Ilavarasan, R., Jayachandr, T., Decaraman, M., Aravindhan, P., Padmanabha, N., & Krishnan, M., (2008). Phytochemicals investigation on a tropical plant, *Syzygium cumini* from Kattuppalayam, Erode District, Tamil Nadu, South India. *Pakistan Journal of Nutrition, 8*(1), 83–85.

Kwatra, B., (2020). A review on potential properties and therapeutic applications of lycopene. *International Journal of Medical and Biomedical Studies, 4*(4). doi: 10.32553/ijmbs.v4i4.1081.

Li, J., Zhai, D., Lv, F., Yu, Q., Ma, H., Yin, J., et al., (2016). Preparation of copper-containing bioactive glass/eggshell membrane nanocomposites for improving angiogenesis, antibacterial activity and wound healing. *Acta Biomaterialia, 36*, 254–266. doi: 10.1016/j.actbio.2016.03.011.

Li, X., Cai, Z., Ahn, D., & Huang, X., (2019). Development of an antibacterial nanobiomaterial for wound–care based on the absorption of AgNPs on the eggshell membrane. *Colloids And Surfaces B: Biointerfaces, 183*, 110449.

Liu, M., Luo, G., Wang, Y., Xu, R., Wang, Y., He, W., et al., (2017). Nano–silver–decorated microfibrous eggshell membrane: Processing, cytotoxicity assessment and optimization, antibacterial activity and wound healing. *Scientific Reports, 7*(1). doi: 10.1038/s41598-017-00594-x.

Maalik, A., Khan, F., Mumtaz, A., Mehmood, A., Azhar, S., & Atif, M., et al., (2014). Pharmacological applications of quercetin and its derivatives: A short review. *Tropical Journal of Pharmaceutical Research, 13*(9), 1561.

Mangala, S., Malleshi, N., Tharanathan, R. N., Mahadevamma. Resistant starch from differently processed rice and ragi (finger millet). *Eur Food Res Technol., 209*, 32–37 (1999). https://doi.org/10.1007/s002170050452 (accessed on 28 February 2023).

Market Analysis: Dietary Supplements Are More Popular Than Ever, (2022). Retrieved from: http://enovatebiolife.com/blog/dietary-supplements-are-more-popular-than-ever/ (accessed on 28 January 2023).

Masibo, M., & He, Q., (2008). Major mango polyphenols and their potential significance to human health. *Comprehensive Reviews in Food Science and Food Safety, 7*(4), 309–319. doi: 10.1111/j.1541-4337.2008.00047.x.

Mendoza-Núñez, V. M., García-Martínez, B. I., Rosado-Pérez, J., Santiago-Osorio, E., Pedraza-Chaverri, J., Hernández-Abad, V. J. The Effect of 600 Mg Alpha-Lipoic Acid Supplementation on Oxidative Stress, Inflammation, and RAGE in Older Adults with Type 2 Diabetes Mellitus. *Oxidative Medicine and Cellular Longevity, 2019*, 1–12. https://doi.org/10.1155/2019/3276958 (accessed on 28 February 2023).

Mishra, H., (2022). *Review Green Tea: Health Benefits.* Retrieved from: https://www.academia.edu/71035440/REVIEW_Green_tea_Health_benefits (accessed on 28 January 2023).

Moktan, B., Roy, A., & Sarkar, P., (2010). Antioxidant activities of cereal–legume mixed batters as influenced by process parameters during preparation of dhokla and idli, traditional steamed pancakes. *International Journal of Food Sciences and Nutrition, 62*(4), 360–369. doi: 10.3109/09637486.2010.532116.

Muralikrishna, G., Malleshi, N., Desikachar, H., & Tharanathan, R., (1986). Effect of popping on the properties of some millet starches. *Starch – Stärke, 38*(2), 48–51. doi: 10.1002/star.19860380204.

Nagamalli, H., Sitaraman, M., Kandalai, K., & Mudhole, G., (2017). Chicken egg shell as a potential substrate for production of alkaline protease by *Bacillus altitudinis* GVC11 and its applications. *3 Biotech, 7*(3). doi: 10.1007/s13205-017-0801-y.

Nigudkar, M., (2014). Estimation of resistant starch content of selected routinely consumed Indian food preparations. *Current Research in Nutrition and Food Science Journal, 2*(2), 73–83. doi: 10.12944/crnfsj.2.2.03.

Nurul, F. N., Sekar, M., Gan, S., Lum, P., Vaijanathappa, J., & Ravi, S., (2020). Lutein: A comprehensive review on its chemical, biological activities and therapeutic potentials. *Pharmacognosy Journal, 12*(6s), 1769–1778. doi: 10.5530/pj.2020.12.239.

Ohto-Fujita, E., Shimizu, M., Sano, S., Kurimoto, M., Yamazawa, K., & Atomi, T., et al., (2018). Solubilized eggshell membrane supplies a type III collagen–rich elastic dermal papilla. *Cell And Tissue Research, 376*(1), 123–135. doi: 10.1007/s00441-018-2954-3.

Padmalayam, I., Hasham, S., Saxena, U., & Pillarisetti, S., (2009). Lipoic acid synthase (LASY). *Diabetes, 58*(3), 600–608. doi: 10.2337/db08-0473.

Paniagua-Pérez, R., Madrigal-Bujaidar, E., Reyes-Cadena, S., Molina-Jasso, D., Gallaga, J., & Silva-Miranda, A., et al., (2005). Genotoxic and cytotoxic studies of beta–sitosterol and pteropodine in mouse. *Journal of Biomedicine and Biotechnology, 2005*(3), 242–247.

Perrone, S., Tei, M., Longini, M., & Buonocore, G., (2016). The multiple facets of lutein: A call for further investigation in the perinatal period. *Oxidative Medicine and Cellular Longevity, 2016*, 1–8.

Pushpangadan, P., George, V., Ijinu, T., & Chithra, M., (2018). Ethnomedicine, health food and nutraceuticals–traditional wisdom of maternal and child health in India. *Edelweiss Applied Science and Technology,* 113–117. doi: 10.33805/2576.8484.124.

Raman, A., & Lau, C. (1996). Anti-diabetic properties and phytochemistry of *Momordica charantia* L. (Cucurbitaceae). *Phytomedicine, 2*(4), 349–362. doi:10.1016/s0944–7113(96)80080–8.

Rane, B. R., & Keservani, R., (2020). Introduction to nutraceuticals and dietary supplements. In: *Nutraceuticals and Dietary Supplements* (pp. 35–56). Apple Academic Press. ISBN: 9781771888738.

Rane, B. R., Bharath, M. S., Patil, R. R., Keservani, R. K., & Jain, A. S., (2020b). Novel approaches in nutraceuticals. In: Rajesh, K. K., Raj, K. K., & Anil, K. S., (eds.), *Enhancing the Therapeutic Efficacy of Herbal Formulations Through Novel Drug Delivery Systems* (pp. 241–266). IGI Global International Publisher, Pennsylvania, USA, Chapter 11. ISBN13: 9781799844532.

Rane, B. R., Patil, A. S., Keservani, R. K., & Jain, A. S., (2020a). Novel approaches in herbal formulation. In: Rajesh, K. K., Raj, K. K., & Anil, K. S., (eds.), *Enhancing the Therapeutic Efficacy of Herbal Formulations Through Novel Drug Delivery Systems* (pp. 43–68). IGI Global International Publisher, Pennsylvania, USA, Chapter 2. ISBN13: 9781799844532.

Reddy, N., Sathe, S., Pierson, M., & Salunkhe, D., (1982). Idli, an Indian fermented food: A review. *Journal Of Food Quality, 5*(2), 89–101. doi: 10.1111/j.1745-4557.1982.tb00736.x.

Santosh, K. J., Hare R. S., & Pragya, P., (2017). Chapter 1 – dietary fiber and human health: An introduction. *Dietary Fiber for the Prevention of Cardiovascular Disease*, 1–22. ISBN 9780128051306, https://doi.org/10.1016/B978-0-12-805130-6.00001-X.

Schneeman, B. O., (1999). Fiber, inulin and oligofructose: Similarities and differences. *Journal of Nutrition, 129*(7), 1424S–1427S.

Sharma, A. K., Keservani, R. K., & Gautam, S. P., (2020). *Herbal Product Development*. Apple Academic Press, CRC Press, Taylor & Francis Group. ISBN: 9781771888776.

Shay, K. P., Moreau, R. F., Smith, E. J., Smith, A. R., Hagen, T. M. Alpha-Lipoic Acid as a Dietary Supplement: Molecular Mechanisms and Therapeutic Potential. *Biochimica et Biophysica Acta (BBA) – General Subjects 2009, 1790*(10), 1149–1160. https://doi.org/10.1016/j.bbagen.2009.07.026 (accessed on 28 February 2023).

Shi, Y., Zhou, K., Li, D., Guyonnet, V., Hincke, M., & Mine, Y., (2021). Avian eggshell membrane as a novel biomaterial: A review. *Foods, 10*(9), 2178.

Singh, P., Kesharwani, R. K., & Keservani, R. K., (2017a). Antioxidants and vitamins: Roles in cellular function and metabolism. In: *Sustained Energy for Enhanced Human Functions and Activity* (pp. 385–407). Academic Press. ISBN:9780128054130.

Singh, S., Kesari, A., Rai, P., & Watal, G., (2007). Assessment of glycemic potential of *Musa paradisiaca* stem juice. *Indian Journal of Clinical Biochemistry, 22*(2), 48–52. doi: 10.1007/bf02913313.

Smith, A., Shenvi, S., Widlansky, M., Suh, J., & Hagen, T., (2004). Lipoic acid as a potential therapy for chronic diseases associated with oxidative stress. *Current Medicinal Chemistry, 11*(9), 1135–1146. doi: 10.2174/0929867043365387.

Srivastava, A., & Shivanandappa, T., (2010). Hepatoprotective effect of the root extract of *Decalepis hamiltonii* against carbon tetrachloride–induced oxidative stress in rats. *Food Chemistry, 118*(2), 411–417. doi: 10.1016/j.foodchem.2009.05.014.

Srivastava, A., Harish, S., & Shivanandappa, T., (2006). Antioxidant activity of the roots of *Decalepis hamiltonii* (Wight & Arn.). *LWT – Food Science and Technology, 39*(10), 1059–1065. doi: 10.1016/j.lwt.2005.07.005.

Swami, S., Thakor, N., Haldankar, P., & Kalse, S., (2012). Jackfruit and its many functional components as related to human health: A review. *Comprehensive Reviews in Food Science and Food Safety, 11*(6), 565–576. doi: 10.1111/j.1541-4337.2012.00210.x.

Tamang, J., (2015). Naturally fermented ethnic soybean foods of India. *Journal Of Ethnic Foods, 2*(1), 8–17. doi: 10.1016/j.jef.2015.02.003.

Trends, O., (2022). *Dietary Fiber Market: Global Industry Trends, Share, Size, Growth, Opportunity and Forecast 2022–2027 – GII.* Retrieved from: https://www.giiresearch.com/report/imarc1053370-dietary-fiber-market-global-industry-trends-share.html (accessed on 28 January 2023).

Uruakpa, F. O., Ismond, M. A. H., & Akobundu, E. N. T. (2002). Colostrum and Its Benefits: A Review. *Nutrition Research, 22*(6), 755–767. https://doi.org/10.1016/s0271–5317(02)00373–1 (accessed on 28 February 2023).

Vuong, T., Rønning, S., Suso, H., Schmidt, R., Prydz, K., Lundström, M., et al., (2017). The extracellular matrix of eggshell displays anti-inflammatory activities through NF-κB in LPS-triggered human immune cells. *Journal Of Inflammation Research, 10*, 83–96.

Wong, J. M. W., Comelli, E. M., Kendall, C. W. C., Sievenpiper, J. L., Noronha, J. C., & Jenkins, D. J. A., (2017). Dietary fiber, soluble and insoluble, carbohydrates, fructose, and lipids. *The Microbiota in Gastrointestinal Pathophysiology*, 187–200. doi: 10.1016/b978-0-12-804024-9.00022-7.

Yonzan, H., & Tamang, J., (2010). Microbiology and nutritional value of selroti, an ethnic fermented cereal food of the Himalayas. *Food Biotechnology, 24*(3), 227–247. doi: 10.1080/08905436.2010.507133.

Yoo, J., Park, K., Yoo, Y., Kim, J., Yang, H., & Shin, Y., (2014). Effects of egg shell membrane hydrolysates on anti-inflammatory, anti-wrinkle, anti-microbial activity and moisture–protection. *Korean Journal for Food Science of Animal Resources, 34*(1), 26–32.

CHAPTER 3

ROLE OF DIETARY FIBERS IN DIABETES

BHAWANA SHARMA,[1] AMUL MISHRA,[2] BHUSHAN R. RANE,[3] PIUSH SHARMA,[1] SHIV GARG,[1] and SAVITA RATHORE[1]

[1]*Maharishi Arvind College of Pharmacy, Ambabari Circle, Ambabari, Jaipur, Rajasthan, India*

[2]*B. N. University, Udaipur, Rajasthan, India*

[3]*Shri D. D. Vispute College of Pharmacy and Research Center, Panve, Maharashtra, India*

ABSTRACT

Diabetes is a chronic metabolic disease marked by elevated blood glucose (or blood sugar) levels. It can harm the heart, blood vessels, eyes, kidneys, and nerves. Around 422 million people worldwide suffer from diabetes. It is directly responsible for 1.6 million fatalities per year, the majority of whom live in low- and middle-income nations. In recent decades, both the number of cases and the incidence of diabetes have increased considerably. Preventing diabetes requires tight control of blood glucose and insulin levels, as well as systematic infection to retain insulin receptor and pancreatic cell function. This can be achieved by implementing early and long-term lifestyle changes, like changing dietary and physical activity habits to achieve better weight control, when possible, a preferred strategy to pharmacological therapy due to its safety, efficacy, and affordability. The goal of this chapter is to demonstrate how dietary fiber plays a role in diabetes. When dietary fiber is included in a meal, it reduces postprandial glycemic and insulinemic excursions, hence altering plasma lipid levels in patients with type 2 diabetes. In comparison to insoluble fiber, Soluble fiber has been demonstrated to be

Food Supplements and Dietary Fiber in Health and Disease. Bhushan R. Rane, Raj K. Keservani, Durgesh Singh, Nayan A. Gujarathi, and Ashish S. Jain, (Eds.)
© 2024 Apple Academic Press, Inc. Co-published with CRC Press (Taylor & Francis)

more effective at lowering postprandial blood glucose, insulin, and serum lipid levels. The viscosity of dietary fiber is also discovered to play an important role; the higher the viscosity, the bigger the effect. Longer glucose absorption, longer hepatic insulin extraction, enhanced insulin sensitivity at the mobile level, and bile acid binding are some of the probable pathways for metabolic benefits with dietary fiber. In the United Kingdom, Food and Drug Administration and The National Advisory Committee both have advised a daily dietary fiber consumption of 20–35 grams per person.

3.1 INTRODUCTION

In 1953 the term "dietary fiber" was coined by'Hipsley.'He described the non-digestible plant constituents which make up the cell wall (Potty, 1996). It refers to a broad range of compounds that are extensively but incompletely digested by symbiotic bacteria in the large intestine, resulting in fatty acid but without providing carbs to the host. Dietary fiber is described as "the edible sections of plant or comparable carbohydrates that are difficult to digest and absorb in the human small intestine, but ferment completely or partially in the large intestine" by the American Association of Cereal Chemists (AACC). Polysaccharide, oligosaccharides, lignin, and other plant components make up dietary fibers. Dietary fiber (Keservani et al., 2010a,b, 2020) has a number of physiological benefits, including laxation, blood cholesterol reduction, and blood glucose reduction. Depending on the structural components shown in Table 3.1, these unavailable carbohydrates are divided into two groups like structural and non-structural materials.

TABLE 3.1 Unavailable Carbohydrates in Food Classification

Principal Diet Sources	Description	Classical Nomenclature
Structural materials of plant cell wall	Structure polysaccharides	Hemicellulose, celluloses, and some pectins
	Noncarbohydrate constituents	Minor constituents, lignin
Non-structural materials, either found naturally or used as food additives	Different polysaccharides from a wide range of sources	Gums, mucilages, pectin, chemically modified polysaccharides, algal polysaccharides

The most popular way to classify DFs is by their water solubility, though grading based on gel-formation properties, viscosity, or the degree of fermentation by gut flora could also be useful (Russell et al., 2016). Gums, gels, mucillages, pectic compounds, and a fraction of hemicelluloses are among the soluble. The insoluble fiber is made up of noncarbohydrate fiber. The noncarbohydrate fiber component, lignin, cellulose, and some hemicelluloses, especially those coupled with lignin, make up the insoluble fibers. Soluble fibers, in particular, have already been shown to have an effect on glucose and lipid metabolism (Ienkins et al., 1978). It is fermented in the colon to produce gas and short-chain fatty acids, but because the acids are quickly removed, they add little to fecal weight. The effects of soluble fibers in the small intestinal lumen could be related to their ability to slow down nutrient absorption from the bulk phase. Several studies have already been conducted to see if the fiber effect may be predicted based on its physiochemical qualities. There is also proof that the particle size is important and that the milling process can produce coarse particles, which have been proven to regulate intestinal transit time (Payler et al., 1975), but fine bran may have a considerably smaller impact on fecal mass and potentially cause constipation (Wrick et al., 1976). A decrease in metabolic capacity with reduced postprandial insulin levels and glucose is observed because Cooking, drying, boiling, or pureeing cereals, lentils, or fruit may damage the fiber structure or other features of the food (Jenkins et al., 1982).

Dietary fibers are one of the natural constituents of fruits (Ramulu & Rao, 2003), vegetables (Escalada-Pla et al., 2007), legumes (Ancona et al., 2004), spices (Sowbhagya et al., 2007), cereals (Hamid & Luan, 2000), etc.

3.2 COMPONENTS OF DIETARY FIBER

Due to variation in dietary fiber content from source to source and the type of fiber, they play an important role in physiology. The fiber components of cellulose, pectin, etc., depending on the sources and varies greatly with cereals and vegetables (Nawirska & Kwasniewska, 2005).

1. **Celluloses:** This polysaccharide is a linear structure and made up of numerous glucose units connected together. Cellulose is a dietary fiber that is insoluble and forms the main wall of plant cells. Many animals can digest this fiber because they already have the enzyme cellulase in their bodies, but humans do not contain this enzyme; hence, it goes undigested. Despite the fact that cellulose is not digested by humans, its water-holding and roughage-forming properties bulk up the stool and facilitate defecation.

2. **Hemicellulose:** This contains slightly less in number of glucose and other sugar structures which are joint to each other in a branched structure, as compared to cellulose. In an alkaline media, these insoluble fibers become somewhat soluble and perform the same role as cellulose in our bodies.
3. **Lignin:** This polysaccharide is found in plant cells between the gaps of cellulose and hemicellulose and is a noncarbohydrate polysaccharide. Lignin is another insoluble dietary fiber that is difficult to digest.
4. **Beta Glucan:** These are the soluble fibers that our gut bacteria ferment. They function as prebiotics, allowing probiotics to feed on them and make short-chain fatty acids as a result. This soluble fiber is primarily responsible for blood sugar regulation, lipid balance, and immune enhancement.
5. **Pectin:** This is soluble fiber and is found in citrus fruits. Pectins are generally utilized in jams and jellies because when heated with sugar, they form a thick gel-like structure.
6. **Guar Gum:** It is a soluble fiber and is consists of two sugars, i.e., galactose and mannose. It comes from a legume called Guar. Because of its tendency to gel in water, this fiber is also employed as a thickener in various food processing sectors.
7. **Inulin:** This fiber is derived from chicory roots. Like other soluble fibers, it functions as a prebiotic in our bodies, promoting immunity and preserving intestinal health.

Given the therapeutic potential of dietary fiber, more fiber-rich food products may be beneficial to one's health. Natural and unprocessed sources of fiber include brans, separated sources such as cellulose and different gums, modified sources such as carboxy methyl cellulose (CMC), and non-plant sources such as xylans and polydextrose (Gordon, 1989). Many fibers, such as soybean-based fiber (Claye et al., 1996), rice bran (Chaudhary & Awasthi, 2009), commercial pectin (Potty, 1996), oat bran (Malkki & Virtanen, 2001), are now commercially accessible on the market for food enrichment. Dietary fiber has also gained importance as epidemiological studies related to the inadequate intake of dietary fiber leads to the incidence of a wide spectrum of diseases (Lue et al., 1991). These polymers have distinct functional properties that can be exploited to develop new food compositions. Carr et al. (2003) proposed the intestinal viscosity content in hamsters and rats, claiming that viscosity of dietary fiber lowers the cholesterol, and this effect is responsible for high elimination of cholesterol from the body. The health advantages, as well as functional qualities including hydration capacity, have also created a renewed interest in dietary fiber research. Many fiber supplements have also been studied, including those made from by-products of the processing of fruits, spices, legumes, vegetables, and other foods. Increased fiber supplementation not only boost the health benefits and functional qualities of many meals, but it might also help food producers in terms of the environment (Makee & Latner, 2000).

- Unconventional sources of fiber, such as sweet orange peel (Chau & Huang, 2003), passion fruit seed fiber (Chau & Huang, 2004), apple pomace (Sudha et al., 2007a), rice bran (Hamid & Luan, 2000), and coconut fiber, have recently been investigated for their potential applications and physiological benefits (Raghavendra et al., 2006). However, data on the content and usefulness of dietary fiber derived from vegetables is limited, with studies focusing on only a few plants such as carrots (Chau et al., 2007), potato peels (Arora & Camire, 1994), and cabbage (Chau et al., 2007; Jongaroontaprangsee et al., 2007).
- Dietary fibers are multifunctional substances that have a good impact on the activities of the human body. Cardiovascular illnesses, diverticulosis, diabetes mellitus, colon cancer, appendicitis, constipation, hemorrhoids, hernia, duodenal ulcer, gall stone, obesity, and other ailments of the gastrointestinal tract can all be helped by consuming enough dietary fiber (Slavin, 2005; Gomez et al., 2010). Increased usage of fiber supplements can thus improve not only the health benefits and functional qualities of food, but also bring environmental benefits to food producers and inspire food scientists to explore new sources of fibers as a functional ingredient (Makee & Latner, 2000).

3.3 RECOMMENDED DIETARY FIBER INTAKE

- Due to a lack of proper methodology, quantifying total dietary fibers has been difficult until recently. For measuring total dietary fiber in food, a standard method is adopted by The Association of Official Analytical Chemists (AOAC)(Southgate 1969 and Southgate 1985), which is based on gravimetric determination and enzymatic degradation of the residue after performing an extensive investigation (Deutsh et al., 1986). Physiologists, on the other hand, have different needs than analytical chemists. For quantitative determination of the content of the water soluble and insoluble components and for the identification of individual sugar polymers, polygalacturonic acids, galactomannans, 3-glucans, rhamnogalacturans, arabinogalactans. To measure these subfractions, the Southgate chemical fractionation procedure (Southgate, 1969) coupled with gas liquid chromatography (Southgate, 1985) which is the best available standard; it was used by Anderson (1986) to extract an extensive list of the fiber content of many foodstuffs in common usage.

- As per the American Diabetes Association, consumption of fiber in diabetic patients should be increased to 14 g fiber/1000 kcal daily, or roughly 25 g per day for women and 38 g per day for men, to match with the general population (Evert et al., 2014). Although it is advised that 50% of all grains consumed be whole grains, no precise recommendations have been provided regarding the optimal types of dietary fiber consumption (Evert et al., 2014). It is widely accepted that obtaining a fiber consumption of >50 g/d without the use of dietary fiber supplements is challenging. Soluble-fiber supplements, such as pectin, alginate, xanthan gum, guar gum, glucomannan, psyllium, glucan concentrates, and different fiber combinations, are the most often used dietary fiber supplements (Papathanasopoulos et al., 2010).
- According to the German Society for Nutrition (DGE), daily fiber consumption should be at least 30 g. If there are no contraindications and a high fluid intake is also required, a higher fiber intake was suggested for diabetic patients. The Diabetes and Nutrition Study Group of the European Association for the Study of Diabetes (EASD) has recently advised a daily fiber intake of more than 40 g or more than 20 g per 1000 calories (Toeller et al., 2005). Around 50% insoluble fiber and 50% water-soluble fiber should make up this amount of fiber (Parash Chettri et al., 2020).
- The US Food and Drug Administration and The National Advisory Committee in the United Kingdom have both advised a daily dietary fiber consumption of 20–35 grams per person (Prasad et al., 1995) due to the increasing importance of dietary fiber in human nutrition.

3.4 IMPORTANCE OF DIETARY FIBER

Dietary fiber has many benefits as flows (Healey et al., 2018; Wakai et al., 2007):

1. **Dietary Fiber and Colorectal Cancer:** The consumption of dietary fiber lowers the risk of colon cancer. Dietary fiber fermentation promotes the proliferation of probiotic bacteria in the colon, which outnumber harmful bacteria. During fermentation, organisms also create Butyrate, a chemical with anti-cancer potential. Bingham et al. (2003) studied people aged 25 to 70 years old from 10 European nations. It was discovered that by doubling fiber intake through food, the incidence of colorectal cancer was lowered by 40%. A study done by Wakai et al. (2007) proposed that increasing total dietary fiber consumption reduced the incidence of colorectal cancer.
2. **Dietary Fiber and Cardiovascular Disease:** Dietary fiber consumption has also been associated to a lower risk of cardiovascular disease. Their gel-forming ability is credited with preventing blood glucose and cholesterol spikes. After enzymatic activity on these soluble fiber gels, they slowly release energy, providing long-lasting fullness and preventing untimely cravings and, as a result, weight gain. Another aspect that helps to minimize bad cholesterol levels is that organisms make short-chain fatty acids when they ferment soluble fibers (SFA). SFA generation inhibits hepatic cholesterol synthesis, hence inhibiting LDL synthesis (Low-Density Lipoprotein). Burley et al. (2013) investigated a link between intake of dietary and low risk of heart diseases.
3. **Dietary Fiber and Diabetes:** Dietary fiber, as previously stated, forms a gel-like material that prevents immediate glucose release and offers long-term energy. It is good for diabetics because of its feature. The InterAct Consortium (2015) conducted research in which participants were given additional cereal and vegetable fiber-rich diets. Its findings indicated a reduced risk of type 2 diabetes with dietary fiber.
4. **Dietary Fiber and Gut Health:** Soluble fiber fermentation by bacteria enhances the body's ability to absorb nutrients. This also reduces the risk of infection and keeps our stomach in good shape. Nausea, acidity, bloating, abdominal cramps, indigestion, heartburn, and gastric pain are all symptoms that are prevented by a healthy gut, Healey et al. (2018) published a study with comparable results. It was discovered that those who consume a high amount of dietary fiber have a larger gut microbiota than those who consume a low amount of dietary fiber.

5. **Dietary Fiber and Constipation:** Constipation is a condition that many people face these days. To relieve constipation, many people take laxatives on a regular basis, but long-term use of the medications may have negative effects. This is where dietary fiber can help. Its propensity to hold water aids in constipation relief, as dietary fiber softens feces and makes them easier to pass. Irritable bowel syndrome (IBS) and diverticulosis show symptom of constipation, as well as stress, poor eating patterns, irregular meals, and a sedentary lifestyle. Nutritionists advise such persons to boost their dietary fiber intake because it can help with bowel motions. Cabre (2011) conducted a study that supported dietary fiber's capabilities.
6. **Dietary Fiber and Obesity:** Dietary fiber helps to keep blood sugar and lipid levels in check, as well as reducing the body's predisposition to gain weight. The slowly released glucose keeps us full for a long time, resulting in satiety and preventing unplanned snacking in between meals. It aids in avoiding excessive calorie intake, which is the primary cause of weight gain. Vijver et al. did a study in the Netherlands (2009). According to the findings, those who consume a high number of whole grains have a lower BMI and are less likely to gain weight than those who consume a low number of whole grains. Dietary fiber intake in both groups were carefully monitored, and the researchers recommended that people eat a fiber-rich diet.

3.5 DIABETES AND DIETARY FIBER

Diabetes is a long-term metabolic disorder characterized by excessive blood glucose (or sugar) levels. It can cause catastrophic damage to the heart, blood vessels, eyes, kidneys, and nerves. The most prevalent type of diabetes is type 2 diabetes, which affects largely adults and occurs when the body becomes resistant to insulin or does not make enough of it. During the previous three decades, type 2 diabetes has become much more common in countries of all income levels. Type 1 diabetes is characterized by the pancreas' inability to produce insulin on its own. It's also known as insulin-dependent diabetes or juvenile diabetes. Access to low-cost diabetes medications, such as insulin, is critical for patients' survival. By 2025, a global agreement has been achieved to halt the rise in diabetes and obesity.

Around 422 million people globally are affected by diabetes. Diabetes is directly responsible for 1.6 million deaths each year, the bulk of which occur in low- and middle-income nations. Both the number of cases and the frequency of diabetes have risen dramatically in recent decades.

Poor blood glucose management is a major contributor to the onset of vascular diabetes complications. Many new hypoglycemic medications and insulin formulations have been available for diabetic patients with a broad range of durations and peak action times, but none of them can completely supersede the importance of food in regulating postprandial hyperglycemia. Pharmacological approaches are unable to control daily plasma glucose fluctuations, whereas dietary treatment is effective in controlling hyperinsulinemia, dislipidemia, and other cardiovascular risk factors by avoiding the rapid rise and fall in plasma glucose levels caused by meal consumption.

Controlling blood glucose and insulin levels, as well as systematic infection to preserve insulin receptor and pancreatic cell function, are key to preventing diabetes. This can be achieved by implementing early and long-term lifestyle changes, like changing dietary and physical activity habits to achieve better weight control, a favored strategy to drug therapy, when possible, due to its safety, efficacy, and cost (Weisman et al., 2018, Williamson, 2018; Ibrahim et al., 2018).

Modifying one's lifestyle is an important aspect of managing diabetes. "Medical nutrition therapy" is the most common approaches to this. Medical nutrition therapy aims to improve blood glucose management, lipid profiles, and by controlling blood pressure in type 2 diabetic patients in order to reduce the risk of cardiovascular diseases (Bantle et al., 2008). Medical nutrition therapy has been proven to reduce glycosylated hemoglobin (HbA1c) levels by 1% to 2% in an individual with type 2 diabetes (Pastors et al., 2003). It's also been proven to lower low-density lipoprotein cholesterol, which is a key sign for reducing the risk of cardiovascular disease (Yu-Poth et al., 1999). In those with type 2 diabetes, the American Diabetes Association recommends a specific diet as part of medical nutrition therapy for secondary and tertiary prevention. Consumption of fiber-rich foods is a part of this diet (Bantle et al., 2008). Increased fiber content lowers the glycemic index of diets, which has also been investigated for many years in the treatment of diabetes (Anderson et al., 1979; Jenkins et al., 2002; Marangoni et al., 2008).

The hypothesis is that a lower glycemic index will result in smaller blood glucose rises, and consequently lower blood glucose and HbA1c levels. Despite the fact that increased fiber consumption has also been associated to a lower risk of diabetes (Meyer et al., 2000; Wannamethee et al., 2009), the research on fiber intake and diabetes control is conflicting. Many of the research on fiber intake and glycemic control, in particular, are tiny and have mixed results; some suggest an increase in diabetes control while others show no difference (Karhunen et al., 2010; Liese et al., 2003; Anderson et al., 1999; Pick et al., 1996; Priebe et al., 2008; Ostman et al., 2006).

3.6 PHYSIOLOGIC EFFECTS OF FIBER

High fiber intake has been linked to reduced postprandial increase in blood glucose concentration, as well as a lower baseline glucose concentration, improved insulin sensitivity, and lower cholesterol levels.

3.6.1 ALTERED TRANSIT TIME

Early research suggested that gelling fiber could slow down bulk-phase diffusion in a model of small intestine absorption (Jenkins et al., 1978). However, later research concentrated on the influence of viscous fiber on the time it takes for the stomach to empty (Holt et al., 1979). The slowing of stomach emptying was assumed to be the most essential process of fiber, which was supported by the fact that postprandial hyperglycemia was reduced, when fiber was added to meals, many studies on the effects of guar gum and pectin on gastric emptying employed hypertonic liquid test meals (Holt et al., 1979; Wilmshurst et al., 1980; Leeds et al., 1981), and the results may not be applicable to the emptying of solid dry matter meals (Jenkins et al., 1977; Jenkins et al., 1980). Harju et al. (Harju et al., 1983; Harju et al., 1984) employed pectin and guar gum to help individuals with dumping syndrome feel better. Guar gum was found to delay the stomach emptying time for solids in the latter research (Harju et al., 1984). In diabetic subjects, stomach emptying is delayed, and glucose levels are lower. Blackburn et al. (1984) found no association between the two, implying that this process may contribute but cannot be the only cause of the reduced postprandial reactions.

3.6.2 EFFECTS WITHIN SMALL INTESTINE

Soluble fibers, such as guar and pectin, showed increased intestinal transit time (Holt et al., 1979), whereas insoluble fibers, such as wheat bran and whole grains, shorten transit time and increase intestinal bulk. The glucose-lowering effects of D-xylose may be due to a reduced rate of carbohydrate absorption rather than increased overall glucose utilization or suppression of hepatic glucose synthesis, according to studies (Jenkins et al., 1978). By modifying mixing, motility, and convection; intraluminal digesting rates; unstirred layer thickness; inhibition of maximum transport capacity; altered pH profile; and, with long-term therapy, altered intestinal morphology is observed due to the presence of fiber in the small intestine. Small intestine perfusion investigations in healthy people showed, Blackburn et al. (1984) proposed that fiber slowed intestinal motility and hence decreased convection. *In vitro* experiments have also shown that the soluble fibers' inclination to form gels can enhance unstirred layer thickness, effectively with the gut creating a gel-filtration system (Wilmshurst et al., 1980). Human investigations, on the other hand, revealed that only pectin caused enhancement in the thickness of the unstirred water layer. Such case was not observed with guar, and the evidence suggests to a slower rate of bulk diffusion in this case (Blackburn et al., 1984). Fiber may also pack carbohydrate molecules, insulating them from digesting enzymes in the colon and reducing approach to the intestinal wall, according to some theories (Jenkins et al., 1980). Antienzyme activity may be present in certain high fiber foods (Jenkins et al., 1980). Pancreatic enzyme activity and secretion have both been demonstrated to be reduced by fiber (Sommer et al., 1980; Dunaif et al., 1981).

3.6.3 GUT HORMONE EFFECTS

Dietary fiber has also been demonstrated to affect the release of gut hormones, as one might predict given its potential to modify the pace and nutrient absorption place in the gut. After eating fiber-supplemented meals, gastric inhibitory polypeptide (GIP) response, an insulin secretion trigger, was lower in healthy diabetic people and patients with post gastrectomy dumping syndrome than after eating control food (Kay et al., 1981; Morgan et al., 1979). Levitt et al. reported no reduction in GIP responses to a mixed meal with reduced quantities of fiber, but did find much decreased plasma glucagon responses, which was replicated by others (Jenkins et al., 1979). Although this could have contributed to the lower hyperglycemia, it's also possible that the fiber-supplemented meal reduced amino acid absorption. The demonstration of increased plasma somatostatin release with fiber was a fascinating finding (Shimoyama et al., 1982).

Somatostatin slows carbohydrates and glucose absorption in the small intestine, possibly influencing the benefits of fiber. More research is certainly required.

3.6.4 PERIPHERAL METABOLIC EFFECTS

Several investigations have shown the decreased blood glucose levels observed following fiber eating are linked to either unaltered or lower insulin levels (Jenkins et al., 1977; Morgan et al., 1979). These acute effects are not due to enhanced insulin sensitivity, but rather to a reduced rate of intestinal transit and a diminished stimulus; however, some studies have found that chronic fiber ingestion is linked to reduced baseline glucose levels and lower C-peptide excretion in the urine (Jenkins et al., 1980; Mann et al., 1984), suggesting an increase in insulin sensitivity or a reduced demand for insufflation. Indeed, an increase in insulin binding to monocyte receptor for insulin has been shown in the studies that have looked into this (Pederson et al., 1982, Hjollund et al., 1983; Ward et al., 1982). This impact may be particularly important in obese patients. Changes in binding, on the other hand, must be distinguished from weight loss and improved diabetic control.

Christiansen et al. (1980) attempted to investigate the action of guar on requirement of insulin in seven individuals with insulin-dependent diabetes mellitus using an artificial pancreas (Biostator) (IDDM). They discovered that the average 24-hour requirements were lowered by 12.4%.

3.6.5 ABSORPTION OF ORGANIC SUBSTANCES

The presence of ionizable groups in fibers like uronic acid residues in pectins and hemicelluloses, affects their cation-exchange ability. Some fibers have this feature, which allows them to bind minerals (Ward et al., 1982) such as calcium, iron, and zinc, as well as organic compounds (Christiansen et al., 1980; James et al., 1078). Insoluble fibers like cellulose have been proven to bind Ca^{2+}, and phytin meals, which are high in insoluble fiber, have been linked to a low level of insufficiency. *In vitro* studies have suggested that fiber in the stomach may also bind cholesterol and bile salts, interfering with cholesterol's enterohepatic circulation (Harmuth-Hoene et al., 1983; Tuomilehto et al., 1983). Fiber can also show actions in the intestine that promote fiber's lipid- and cholesterol-lowering effects, according to changes in lipid metabolism (Simpson et al., 1981; Bosello et al., 1980). These include impacts on the production of low-density chylomicra and the site of lipid absorption (Bosello et al., 1980). Alterations in very low-density lipoprotein (VLDL) turnover provide an alternative pathway.

3.6.6 EFFECTS ON LARGE BOWEL

By bacterial fermentation of fiber in the colon, short-chain fatty acids are produced, which may restrict fatty acid mobilization and intestinal synthesis, as well as reduce gluconeogenesis (Blackburn et al., 1984). Short-chain fatty acids, including acetate, propionate, and butyrate are generated in the colon by bacterial fermentation of indigestible DF polysaccharides (Jenkins et al., 2000), with the percentage of different SCFAs varying dependent on the substrate and, in the end, the gut microbiota. Increased SCFA synthesis is thought to be advantageous because it lowers hepatic glucose output and improves lipid homeostasis. SCFA also acts as a direct target for G protein-coupled receptors GPR-41 and GPR-43. An intriguing observation was that oral treatment of the GPR41 ligand propionate nearly doubled plasma levels of anorexigenic leptin in mice, despite no effect on food intake (Covington et al., 2006).

In randomized controlled cross-over research in healthy women, measures of insulin sensitivity improved to a comparable level with all Dietary Fiber, independent of pace of colonic fermentation. Even while the poor accuracy of all the available methods to assess colonic rate of fermentation in humans must be considered, our findings suggest that a dose-dependent relationship between DF fermentability and enhanced indicators of insulin sensitivity is improbable.

Furthermore, SCFA may cause adipogenesis via GPR43 (Covington et al., 2006), and colonization of germfree mice (gnotobiotic) with a strong saccharolytic member of the normal human gut microbiota, as well as the dominant human methane-producing germ, evolved in significantly improved colonic fermentation efficacy, which was correlated with enhanced de novo lipogenesis and obesity in the host (Backhed et al., 2007).

The gut microbiota of obese persons differs from that of lean subjects, and modifications toward the "lean microbiome" can be seen in obese subject who loses weight (Backhed et al., 2007). Even though the recipients of the "obese microorganisms" had equivalent energy consumption, the recipients of the "obese microbes" showed a higher growth of fat mass when the gut microbiota from obese mice or lean mice was transplanted to germ-free mice (Backhed et al., 2007).

A four-week continuous subcutaneous infusion of LPS increased weight growth, liver fat, inflammatory indicators, and insulin resistance markers in the same way that a high-fat diet did (Cani et al., 2007). These results suggest that DF consumption may change the proportions of particular gut flora members, tying the ideas of bacterial colonization, inflammation, and insulin resistance together.

Diabetes risk may be reduced by eating a diet rich in insoluble cereal Dietary Fiber and whole grains, according to prospective cohort studies. There is no compelling evidence is available that soluble DF from fruits and vegetables plays a significant effect in this scenario. Many protective mechanisms proposed for DF ingestion are common in both soluble and insoluble DF (low energy density, moderate weight loss, effects on inflammatory markers, increased satiety, and gut hormones) or are relevant with soluble viscous DF consumption (low energy density, moderate weight loss, effects on inflammatory markers, increased satiety, and gut hormones) (nutritional absorption is hampered, stomach emptying is slowed, postprandial glucose responses are reduced, total and LDL cholesterol is lowered, and colonic fermentation is reduced). As a result, additional undiscovered processes appear to be at work in reducing diabetes risk in people eating a lot of insoluble cereal DF. Increased insulin sensitivity could be a hopeful element contributing to the favorable effects of insoluble DF intake, albeit the mechanisms behind this phenomenon need to be elucidated. A modification in the relationship of gut microbiotic ecosystems, as well as indirect and direct effects on yet unknown hormonal and molecular components in the host that may be changed in subjects eating high DF diets, are all hypothesized processes.

3.7 EFFECTS OF HIGH-FIBER DIETS ON PATIENTS WITH DIABETES

The benefits of fiber on carbohydrate metabolism in diabetes have been studied using two approaches: the first employs refined fibers such as guar and pectin, and the second enhances the fiber content of the diet with naturally occurring fibers. Diverse forms of fiber have been utilized in studies, which may have quite different effects. Dose of fiber used has varied from study to study. Combinations of soluble and insoluble fibers with potentially opposing effects have been employed. The effects of changing the macronutrient and fiber content of the diet have made it difficult to attribute them only to fiber. It's been difficult to separate the benefits of fiber from those of carbohydrate restriction, weight loss, calorie restriction, and the beginning level of diabetes control. Fiber's effects on plasma lipids and lipoproteins have been inconsistently studied.

Jenkins et al. in Oxford (Jenkins et al., 1977, Jenkins et al., 1976), Levitt et al. (1978) in South Africa and Goulder et al., (1978) in the United Kingdom were among the first to establish that the non-absorbable polysaccharides guar and pectin reduced postprandial glycemia in both diabetic and non-diabetic patients, often with less insulin secretion. The most efficient fibers had the highest viscosity (Jenkins et al., 1978), that might be linked to a slowdown of stomach emptying (Jenkins et al., 1978; Holt et al., 1979) or reduced diffusion of digestive products. Fiber that was provided in capsules (Hall et al., 1980), dusted on foo, or eaten before a meal (Jenkins et al., 1979) was shown to be ineffective, thus it had to be mixed into the food (Wilmshurst et al., 1980).

Fiber consumption with one meal was observed to reduce hyperglycemia with a subsequent meal. Nonviscous fibers, like those contained in wheat bran, had less of an impact than viscous fibers, which were proven to be effective (Wilmshurst et al., 1980). Fiber's immediate effects may be dose dependent. Test meals supplemented with a total of 26 g guar and pectin produced lower glucose and insulin responses in diabetic subjects. In IDDM, the glucose response decreased by 30%, while in noninsulin-dependent diabetic mellitus (NIDDM), the insulin response decreased by 42 to 60% (Jenkins et al., 1980; Vinik et al., 1988). Others' research indicated that the decrease in insulin response did not occur with 9–18 g but occurred with 26 g, implying a dose-dependent impact. Short-term metabolic tests followed the test-meal experiments, showing that 14–26 g guar given daily with meals, decreased urine glucose and 3-hydroxybutyrate losses by 40% compared to the control period. Longer-term studies with guar granulate confirmed these findings, which also showed decreased insulin responses and improved postprandial blood glucose levels. Urinary glucose levels and insulin needs were reduced for up to a year in investigations (Table 3.2 and Figure 3.1).

TABLE 3.2 Effect of Dietary Fiber on Cholesterol and Blood Glucose

Percent Reduction of Fasting Blood Glucose	Percent Reduction of Cholesterol
0	–2
5	–1
10	1
15	3
20	5
25	11
30	13

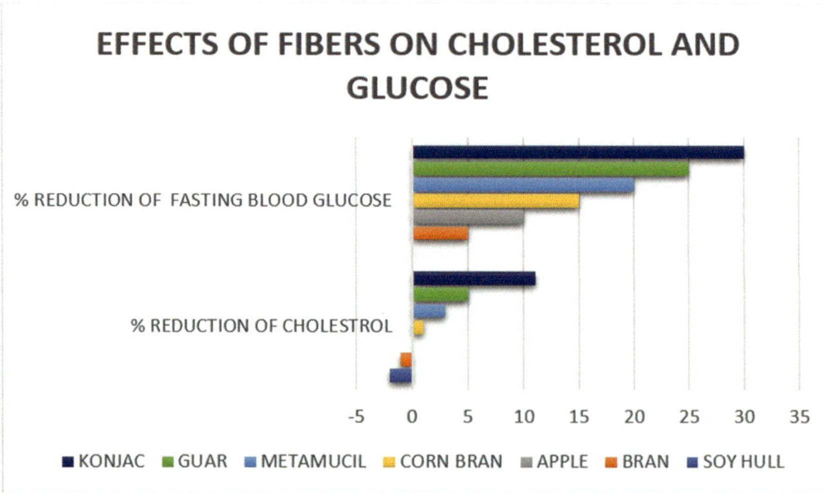

FIGURE 3.1 Compiled data from literature to show that soluble fibers have a positive influence on cholesterol and glucose levels while insoluble and fruit fibers had a weak or negative effect.

However, until recently, there was no commercially available pure fiber preparation that was suitable for clinical usage. At a Guar Symposium in London in December 1985, many new findings from Finland, England, and Ireland were presented. The majority of research found that adding varied quantity of guar to a regular meal plan had favorable effects, but they were short-term and poorly controlled (Fuessl et al., 1985).

3.8 ROLE OF DIETARY FIBER IN TREATMENT OF DIABETIC PATIENTS

Findings that compared a fat-modified diet to a low-fat/high carbohydrate diet found that the former was obviously superior. However, if a low-fat/high-carbohydrate diet is compared to a low-fat/high-carbohydrate diet in which fiber rich foods replace starch as the main carbohydrate source, the outcome does not have to be the same. Dietary fiber has been shown in studies to have significant impacts on blood glucose and lipoprotein metabolism (Vinik et al., 1988).

Dietary fiber has many definitions; however, the one that seems most relevant from a physiological and clinical standpoint was coined in the 1970s by Trowell (2005), who first claimed that dietary fiber may play a major role in diabetes. According to this definition, dietary fibers are made up of plant polysaccharides that are resistant to breakdown by human digestive enzymes. The pioneering studies of Kiehm et al. (1976) who showed a dramatic decrease in insulin dosage and good blood glucose control in insulin-treated diabetic patients by prescribing a high-carbohydrate/high-fiber diet, demonstrated the importance of dietary fiber in the treatment of diabetic patients. A dietary experiment was conducted to see how dietary fiber and carbohydrate affect blood glucose and lipoprotein metabolism separately (Leeds et al., 1981). They compared a fat-modified diet, in which olive oil was the main source of fat, to a low-fat/high-carbohydrate diet, in which the high-carbohydrate quota was achieved by increasing the consumption of fiber-rich foods, in six IDDM and eight NIDDM patients (legumes, fruit, vegetables).

Carbohydrate and fat accounted for 42 and 37% of total calorie consumption in the first diet, respectively, whereas these dietary elements accounted for 53 and 30% in the second diet. Both diets were low in cholesterol and saturated fat, with similar calorie, mono disaccharide, and protein contents. A third diet was included in the experiment to assess independently the effects of dietary fiber and carbohydrate on glucose and lipoprotein metabolism. This was similarly a low-fat/high-carbohydrate diet (53% carbohydrate, 30% fat), but the carbohydrate quota was mostly fiber-depleted starchy items in this case (bread, potatoes). The fat-modified diet had 20 grams of fiber per day, 54 grams per day in the fiber-enriched low-fat/high-carbohydrate diet, and 16 grams per day in the fiber-depleted low-fat/high-carbohydrate diet. The three diets, all of which were made up entirely of natural foods, were ingested in a random order for 10 days while the patients were in a metabolic ward. When comparing the fat-modified diet to the fiber-rich low-fat/high-carbohydrate diet, the latter came out on top. The fiber-rich low-fat/high-carbohydrate diet significantly reduced postprandial and daily average blood glucose concentrations in both IDDM and NIDDM patients. Fasting glucose levels were also reduced, but the difference did not reach statistical significance (Table 3.3).

TABLE 3.3 Effect on Blood Glucose Levels Obtained by Changing Diet to Low-Carbohydrate/High-Fiber

Fat-Modified Diet to Low-Carbohydrate/High-Fiber	Blood Glucose	
	Insulin-Dependent	Non-Insulin-Dependent
Fasting	–2.8	–0.2
2-h-postprandial	–3	–1
Average daily	–1	–1.2

In both categories of diabetic individuals, LDL cholesterol concentrations were significantly lower following the fiber-rich low-fat/high-carbohydrate diet compared to the fat-modified diet; however, VLDL triglyceride levels were not significantly changed. The fiber-rich high carbohydrate diet significantly reduced HDL-Chol values in both IDDM and NIDDM patients (Table 3.4).

TABLE 3.4 Effect on Serum Lipoprotein Composition by Changing Diet from Low-Carbohydrate/High-Fiber to High-Carbohydrate-Fiber

Serum Lipoprotein	Blood Glucose	
	Insulin-Dependent	Non-Insulin-Dependent
LDL cholesterol	–0.7	–0.8
HDL cholesterol	–0.3	–0.29
VLDL triglycerides	–0.35	0.4

The high-carbohydrate content of fiber-rich low-fat/high-carbohydrate diet has been attributed to their positive benefits rather than fiber. As a result, the effects of fiber on glucose and lipoprotein metabolism in general were investigated in this study. This was accomplished by contrasting the outcomes of two different diets with the same carbohydrate quota (53% of calories in both diets) and just the amount of fiber (16 vs. 54 g/day) that differed only in the amount of fiber (16 vs. 54 g/day). This study reveals that increasing dietary fiber in the diet can reduce postprandial and average daily blood glucose concentrations by 25 and 15%, respectively, and LDL-cholesterol and VLDL triglyceride levels by 25 and 10%, respectively, in both IDDM and NIDDM patients. On the other hand, dietary fiber had no influence on fasting blood glucose levels or HDL cholesterol concentrations. Other organizations have verified the findings of this investigation. Simpson et al. (1981) proposed that a high-carbohydrate/high-fiber diet can also be followed by diabetic patients in their usual home setting without major feasibility issues and with the same beneficial metabolic effects. Other diabetic youngsters, pregnant diabetic women, patients with secondary failure to oral hypoglycemic medications, and diabetic patients with chronic renal failure have all had similar outcomes (Kinmouth et al., 1982; Ney et al., 1982; Lousley et al., 1984; Parillo et al., 1988) (Table 3.5).

TABLE 3.5 Low-Fat, High-Carbohydrate Diets with Mostly Starch or Fiber-Rich Meals have Metabolic Consequences (Increase, Reduction, No Impact)

	Blood Glucose	Plasma Insulin	Insulin Sensitivity	Plasma Lipoproteins		
				VLDL	LDL	HDL
High starch	Increased	Increased	Decreased	Increased	Decreased	No effect/Decreased
High fiber	Decreased	No effect	Increased	Decreased	Decreased	No effect/Decreased

Abbreviations: VLDL: very-low-density lipoprotein; LDL: low-density lipoprotein; HDL: high-density lipoprotein.

Other studies, on the other hand, have not been able to replicate the improvement in blood glucose control in diabetic individuals by eating a high-carbohydrate/high-fiber diet (Hollenbeck et al., 1986; Beattie et al., 1988). In studies where whole-meal cereals were the primary sources of dietary fiber, however, no significant effects of a high-fiber diet were observed (Hollenbeck et al., 1986). This disparity can be explained in part by the differing characteristics of fiber found in cereals, legumes, fruits, and some vegetables, on the one hand, and legumes, fruits, and some vegetables, on the other. The latter food contains mostly water-soluble, gel-forming fiber that can delay the mixing of food with intestinal juice, delaying digestion and absorption of nutrients; cereal fiber, on the other hand, is mostly non-water-soluble and unable to affect the rate of food digestion in the small intestine (Vinik et al., 1988 and Leeds AR 1987). Few studies state that dietary fiber has no influence on blood glucose control, blood glucose concentrations were measured only when the subjects were fasting, whereas glucose metabolism occurs during the postprandial period (Hollenbeck et al., 1986).

Another factor to consider when evaluating the metabolic features of the high-carbohydrate/high-fiber diet is the influence of such a diet on insulin sensitivity. This has only been done in non-diabetic people, but the results appear to show that high-carbohydrate/high-fiber diets can enhance insulin sensitivity (Fugawa et al., 1990). According to whether fiber-depleted starchy foods or unprocessed vegetable foods (fiber-rich) are present in the high-carbohydrate diet, the findings of the comparison between a fat-modified diet and a low-fat/high carbohydrate diet travel in opposite ways (Table 3.4). In both IDDM and NIDDM patients, the low-fat/high-carbohydrate diet provides substantial metabolic advantages over the fat-modified diet (contrary to what was found in the previous section for the starch-rich diet).

It improves blood glucose control (especially in the postprandial period), lowers plasma and LDL cholesterol levels, and inhibits the rise in plasma triglyceride levels that occurs when dietary carbohydrates are increased. It may also help with peripheral insulin sensitivity. In terms of fiber-rich foods' impact on plasma lipoprotein metabolism, keep in mind that their potential to lower plasma cholesterol and LDL concentrations is independent of other dietary changes. Reduced dietary cholesterol and saturated fat, as well as increased fiber-rich food consumption, have an additive effect in decreasing plasma cholesterol and LDL levels. In NIDDM patients, the total impact of this combined dietary approach is a decrease in plasma cholesterol of up to 30% (Riccardi et al., 1984).

Improvements in blood glucose control have been linked to an increase in fiber consumption in various studies. Weight losses, a reduction in total food energy, variation in the total CHO content of the diet, variations in type of CHOs in the diet, and the incorporation of substantial amounts of legumes (peas and beans) all complicate interpretation of the data (Hollenbeck et al., 1986; Beattie et al., 1988; Leeds 1987; Fugawa et al., 1990). Starch digestibility is known to be influenced by the organization and structure of starch granules, as well as how starch-containing foods are processed (Keys, 1970) (Table 3.6).

TABLE 3.6 Food Fiber and Plasma Glucose Rise (Added to Glucose Solution or Mixed Meal)

Studies Conducted By	Fiber Used	Amount of Fiber (g)	Reduction in Glucose Rise	
			Yes	No
Jenkins et al.	Guar gum	12	+	–
Morgan et al.	Guar gum	10	+	–
Levitt et al	Guar gum	5	+	–
–	Pectin	5	–	–
Williams et al.	Guar gum	10	–	+
Blackburn et al.	Guar gum	9–14.5	+	–
Jarjis et al.	Guar gum	2.5–14.5	+	–
Jenkins et al.	Gum tragacanth	12	+	–
Jenkins et al.	Pectin	12	–	+
Holt et al.	Pectin	14.5	+	–
Williams et al.	Pectin	10	–	+
Sandhu et al.	Pectin	7.5–15	–	+

TABLE 3.6 *(Continued)*

Studies Conducted By	Fiber Used	Amount of Fiber (g)	Reduction in Glucose Rise	
			Yes	No
Jarjis et al.	Psyllium	7	–	+
Pastors et al.	Psyllium	6.8	+ (14%)	–
Thomas et al.	Soy polysaccharide	10	–	+
Williams et al.	Locust bean	10	–	+
Tredger et al.	Beet fiber*	20	–	+
Hagander et al.	Beet fiber*	11	+ (25%)	–
Braaten et al.	Oat gum	14.5	+	–

*Beet fiber is composed primarily of pectins, hemicelluloses, and cellulose (Liese et al., 2003). It has low viscosity (Karhunen et al., 2010). Oat gum used in Yu-Poth et al. (1999) had a high viscosity.

Several studies have found that adding more fiber to a diet has no effect (Parillo et al., 1988). It's still unclear whether consuming big amounts of fiber in the form they naturally come in foods has a beneficial effect on blood glucose levels in diabetics. It'll be a difficult task to fix. A drop-in serum cholesterol has also been observed in many of these investigations. This drop is most likely due to a reduction in total dietary fat and saturated fatty acid content, at least in part. A rise in plant-based mono- and polyunsaturated fatty acids could also have contributed. In maximum studies, an independent effect attributable to the fiber content of the diet cannot be determined (Tables 3.7 and 3.8).

TABLE 3.7 Effect of Dietary Fiber on Glucose Control (Guar Gum)

	Fiber Added (g)	Duration	CHO Content Changed	Result
Jenkins et al.	14–26	1 yr.	No	Urine glucose decreased
Aro et al.	21	3 mo (x-over)*	Unknown	Improved modestly
Ray et al.	30	8 wk	Unknown	Improved
Smith	14–20	3 mo	Unknown	Improved modestly
Najemnik et al.	15	2 wk (x-over)*	Unknown	Improved modestly
Holman et al.[±]	15	8 wk (x-over)*	No	Not improved

TABLE 3.7 *(Continued)*

	Fiber Added (g)	Duration	CHO Content Changed	Result
Beattie et al.±	15	20 wk (x-over)*	No	Not improved
Uusitupa et al.±	15	3 mo (x-over)*	No	Not improved
Lalor et al.	15	3 mo (x-over)*	No	Improved modestly

*x-over refers to a crossover design.
± GHb was used to assess effect on integrated glucose concentration.

Several studies have also been reported. Few of these are very well controlled, and a crossover design has also been used; in others, the design was less stringent. Guar gum, pectin, psyllium powder, soybeans, polysaccharides, oat bran, and others have been used (Tables 3.5 and 3.6) (Pyorala et al., 1987; Rosengren et al., 1989; Riccardi et al., 1987; Wolever et al., 1990).

TABLE 3.8 Effect of Dietary Fiber Addition on Glucose Control

	Fiber Added (g)	Duration	CHO Content Changed	Result
Pectin	36	6 wk	No	Not improved
Jenkins et al.	20	3 mo	No	Not improved
Gardner et al.*	26–52	4 wk	No	Not improved
Mahalko et al.	20	2 wk	No	Fasting glucose increased
Schwartz				
Cereal/bran fiber	22	3 wk (x-over)ᵗ	No	Improved modestly±
Karlstrom et al.	23–37	10–15 days	No	Improved modestly±
Monnier et al.	10–15	20 wk	No	Not improved
Beattie et al.*				
Beet fiber	16	6 wk (x-over)ᵗ	No	Not improved
Karlander et al.*				

*GHb used to assess the effect on integrated glucose concentration.
ᵗ x-over refers to a crossover design.
± Modest improvement, decrease of <1—1.5 mM in plasma glucose.

However, because of the study designs utilized and variability in the type and amount of fiber added, the data in several of these trials are difficult to interpret. Furthermore, in other research, the diet was not strictly supervised

(Tables 3.5 and 3.6). Several long-term studies have recently been published in which excellent, randomized, crossover designs were used and the food composition was controlled. In addition, rather than using isolated plasma or urine glucose measurements, GHbs was employed as an indicator of glucose control in this study. In these investigations, there was little or no improvement in glucose management (Pyorala et al., 1987; Riccardi et al., 1987; Jenkins et al., 1979, 1980).

3.9 CONCLUSION

Dietary guidelines for diabetic patients should focus on the overall increase in dietary fiber and encourage the intake of natural fiber-rich foods based on such experimental evidence. Diets rich in fiber are an important part of diabetes therapy. They improve glycemic management, blood lipids, body weight, and inflammation, among other things and also lowers the risk of premature death. These advantages were not limited to any fiber type or type of diabetes, and they were shown across the intake spectrum, while those going from low to moderate or high intakes saw greater improvements in glycemic control. Diabetes affects 537 million persons worldwide. Based on the above findings, increasing daily fiber intake by 15 g or 35 g should be a realistic aim for diabetics.

KEYWORDS

- **blood glucose control**
- **carboxy methyl cellulose**
- **diabetes care**
- **dietary fiber intake**
- **ferment soluble fibers**
- **plasma cholesterol levels**

REFERENCES

American Diabetes Association. (2007). Nutrition Recommendations and Interventions for Diabetes: A position statement of the American Diabetes Association. *Diabetes Care 1*

January 2007; 30 (suppl_1): S48–S65. https://doi.org/10.2337/dc07-S048 (accessed on 28 February 2023).

Anderson, J. W., (1986). *Plant Fiber in Foods*. Lexington, KY, HCF Diabetes Res. Found.

Anderson, J. W., Allgood, L. D., Turner, J., Oeltgen, P. R., & Daggy, B. P., (1999). Effects of psyllium on glucose and serum lipid responses in men with type 2 diabetes and hypercholesterolemia. *Am. J. Clin. Nutr., 70*, 466–473.

Anderson, J. W., Midgley, W. R., & Wedman, B., (1979). Fiber and diabetes. *Diabetes Care, 2*, 369–377.

Backhed, F., Manchester, J. K., Semenkovich, C. F., & Gordon, J. I., (2007). Mechanisms underlying the resistance to diet–induced obesity in germ–free mice. *Proc. Natl. Acad. Sci., USA., 104*, 979–984.

Bantle, J. P., Wylie-Rosett, J., Albright, A. L., et al., (2008). Nutrition recommendations and interventions for diabetes: A position statement of the American Diabetes Association. *Diabetes Care, 31*(Suppl1), S61–78. American Diabetes Association.

Beattie, V. A., Edwards, C. A., Hosker, J. P., Cullen, D. R., Ward, J. D., & Read, N. W., (1988). Does adding fiber to low energy, high carbohydrate, low fat diet confer any benefit to the management of newly diagnosed overweight type II diabetics*? Br. Med., 296*(11), 47–49.

Blackburn, N. A., Redfern, J. S., Jarjis, H., Holgate, A. M., Hanning, I., Scarpello, J. H. B., Johnson, I. T., & Read, N. W., (1984). The mechanism of action of guar gum in improving glucose tolerance in man. *Clin. Sci., 66*, 329–336.

Bosello, O., Ostuzzi, R., Armellini, F., Micciolo, R., & ScuroL, A., (1980). Glucose tolerance and blood lipids in bran–fed patients with impaired glucose tolerance. *Diabetes Care, 3*, 46–49.

Cani, P. D., Amar, J., Iglesias, M. A., Poggi, M., Knauf, C., Bastelica, D., Neyrinck, A. M., Fava, F., Tuohy, K. M., et al., (2007). Metabolic endotoxemia initiates obesity and insulin resistance. *Diabetes, 56*(17), 61–72.

Christiansen, J. S., Bonnevie-Nielsen, V., Svendsen, P. A., Rubin, P., Rønn, B., & Nerup, J. (1980). Effect of guar gum on 24-hour insulin requirements of insulin–dependent diabetic subjects as assessed by an artificial pancreas. *Diabetes Care, 3*(6), 59–62.

Covington, D. K., Briscoe, C. A., Brown, A. J., & Jayawickreme, C. K., (2006). The G-protein-coupled receptor 40 family (GPR40–GPR43) and its role in nutrient sensing. *Biochem. Soc. Trans., 34*, 770–773.

Deutsch, M. J., (1986). Vitamins and other nutrients. General referee reports, committee on foods II. */ Assoc Off Anal. Chem., 69*, 259.

Devinder, D., Mona, M., Hradesh, R., & Patil, R. T., (2012). Dietary fiber in food: A review. *J. Food Sci. Technol., 49*(3), 255–266. doi: 10.1007/s13197-011-0365-5PMCID: PMC3614039.

Diabetes Drafting Group, (1985). Prevalence of small vessel disease and large vessel disease in diabetic patients from 14 centers: The WHO multinational study of vascular disease in diabetics. *Diabetologia, 28*, 715–740.

Dunaif, G., & Schneeman, B. O., (1981). The effect of dietary fiber on human pancreatic enzyme activity *in vitro. Am. Clin. Nutr., 34*(10), 34, 35.

Evert, A. B., Boucher, J. L., Cypress, M., Dunbar, S. A., Franz, M. J., Mayer-Davis, E. J., Neumiller, J. J., Nwankwo, R., Verdi, C. L., Urbanski, P., et al., (2014). Nutrition therapy recommendations for the management of adults with diabetes. *Diabetes Care, 37*(Suppl 1), S120–143.

Fuessl, H., Adrian, T. E., Bacarese-Hamilton, A. J., & Bloom, S. R., (*1985*). *Effects of Guar on Plasma Glucose and Gut Hormone Response in Type II Diabetics* (p. 59). Br Diabetes Assoc Spring Meeting, Oxford, UK.

Fugawa, N. K., Anderson, J. W., Hageman, G., Young, V. R., & Minaker, K. L., (1990). High carbohydrate, high fiber diets increase peripheral insulin sensitivity in healthy young and old adults. *Am. J. Clin. Nutr., 52*, 524–528.

Gatti, E., Catenazzo, G., Camisasca, E., Torri, A., Denegri, E., & Sirtori, C. R., (1984). Effects of guar–enriched pasta in the treatment of diabetes and hyperlipidemia. *Ann. Nutr. Metab., 28*, 1–10.

Goulder, T. J., Alberti, K. G. M. M., & Jenkins, D. A., (1978). Effect of added fiber on the glucose and metabolic response to a mixed meal in normal and diabetic subjects. *Diabetes Care, 1*, 351–355.

Hall, S. E. H., Bolton, T. M., & Hetenyi, G. Jr., (1980). The effect of branon glucose kinetics and plasma insulin in non-insulin dependent insulin dependent diabetes mellitus. *Diabetes Care, 3*, 520–525.

Harju, E., & Larmi, T. K., (1983). Efficacy of guar gum in preventing the dumping syndrome. *Parenter. Enterol. Nutr., 7*, 470–472.

Harju, E., Heikkila, J., & Larmi, T. K., (1984). Effect of guar gum on gastric emptying after gastric resection. *Parenter. Enterol. Nutr., 8*, 18–20.

Harmuth-Hoene, A. E., (1983). The influence of guar on the nitrogen balance, the absorption of minerals and trace elements and the digestible energy in 6 female test subjects. Beitr Infusionther Klin Ernaehr Forsch Prax, *12*, 68–80.

Healey, G., Murphy, R., Butts, C., Brough, L., Whelan, K., & Coad, J., (2018). Habitual dietary fiber intake influences gut microbiota response to an insulin-type fructan prebiotic: A randomized, double-blind, placebo-controlled, cross-over, human intervention study. *British Journal of Nutrition, 119*(2), 176–189. doi: 10.1017/S0007114517003440.

Hjollund, E., Pedersen, O., Richelsen, B., Beck-Nielsen, H., & Sorensen, N. S., (1983). Increased insulin binding to adipocytes and monocytes and increased insulin sensitivity of glucose transport and metabolism in adipocytes from noninsulin–dependent diabetics after a low–fat/high–starch/high–fiber diet. *Metabolism, 32*(10), 67–75.

Hollenbeck, G. B., Coulston, A. M., & Reaven, G. M., (1986). To what extent does increased dietary fiber improve glucose and lipid metabolism in patients with non-insulin dependent diabetes mellitus (NIDDM). *Am. I Clin. Nutr., 43*, 16–24.

Holt, S., Heading, R. C., Carter, D. C., Prescott, L. F., & Tothill, P., (*1979*). Effect of gel fiber on gastric emptying and absorption of glucose and paracetamol. *Lancet, 1*(6), 36–39.

https://www.who.int/health-topics/diabetes#tab=tab_ (accessed on 28 January 2023).

Ibrahim, M., Tuomilehto, J., Aschner, P., Beseler, L., Cahn, A., Eckel, R. H., et al., (2018). Global status of diabetes prevention and prospects for action: A consensus statement. *Diabetes Metab. Res. Rev., 34*, e3021.

Inter Act Consortium, (2015). Dietary fiber and incidence of type 2 diabetes in eight European countries: The EPIC-inter act study and a meta-analysis of prospective studies. *Diabetologia, 58*(7), 1394–1408.

James, W. P. T., Branch, W. J., & Southgate, D. A., (1978). Calcium binding by dietary fiber. *Lancet, 1*, 638–639.

Jenkins, A. L., Jenkins, D. J., Zdravkovic, U., Wursch, P., & Vuksan, V., (2002). Depression of the glycemic index by high levels of beta-glucan fiber in two functional foods tested in type 2 diabetes. *Eur. J. Clin. Nutr., 56*, 622–628.

Jenkins, D. J. A., Goff, D. V., Leeds, A. R., Alberti, K. G. M. M., Wolever, T. M. S., Gassull, M. A., & Hockaday, T. D. R., (1976). Unabsorbable carbohydrates and diabetes: Decreased post–prandial hyperglycemia. *Lancet, 2*, 172–174.

Jenkins, D. J. A., Leeds, A. R., Gassull, M. A., Cochet, B., & AlbertiKGM, M., (1977). Decrease in postprandial insulin and glucose concentrations by guar and pectin. *Ann. Intern. Med., 86*, 20–23.

Jenkins, D. J. A., Leeds, A. R., Gassull, M. A., Cochet, B., & Alberti, K. G. M. M., (1977). Decrease in postprandial insulin and glucose concentrations for guar and pectin. *Ann. Intern. Med., 86*, 20–23.

Jenkins, D. J. A., Thorne, M. J., Camelon, K., Jenkins, A., Rao, A. V., Taylor, R. H., Thompson, L. U., et al., (1982). Effect of processing on digestibility and the blood glucose response: A study of lentils. *Clin. Nutr., 36*(10), 93–101.

Jenkins, D. J. A., Wolever, T. M. S., Leeds, A. R., Gassull, M. A., Haisman, P., Dilawarie, J. B., Goff, D. V., et al., (1978). Dietary fibers, fiber analogues and glucose tolerance: Importance of viscosity. *Br. Med. J., 1*(13), 92–94.

Jenkins, D. J. A., Wolever, T. M. S., Leeds, A. R., Gassull, M. A., Haisman, P., Dilawarie, J. B., Goff, D. V., et al., (1978). Dietary fibers, fiber analogues and glucose tolerance: Importance of viscosity. *Br. Med. J., 1*(13), 92–94.

Jenkins, D. J. A., Wolever, T. M. S., Nineham, R., Bacon, S., Smith, R., & Hockaday, T. D., (1979). Dietary fiber and diabetic therapy: A progressive effect with time. *Adv. Exp. Med. Biol., 119*, 275–279.

Jenkins, D. J. A., Wolever, T. M. S., Nineham, R., Sarson, D. L., Bloom, S. R., Ahern, J., Albert, K. G. M. M., & Hockaday, T. D. R., (1980). Improved glucose tolerance four hours after taking guar with glucose. *Diabetologia, 19*, 21–24.

Jenkins, D. J. A., Wolever, T. M. S., Taylor, R. H., Ghafari, H., Jenkins, A. L., Barker, H., & Jenkins, M. J., (1980). Rate of digestion of foods and postprandial glycaemia in normal and diabetic subjects. *Fir. Med. Jf., 281*, 14–17.

Jenkins, D. J., Kendall, C. W., Axelsen, M., Augustin, L. S., & Vuksan, V., (2000). Viscous and nonviscous fibers, nonabsorbable and low glycaemic index carbohydrates, blood lipids and coronary heart disease. *Curr. Opin. Lipidol., 11*, 49–56.

Karhunen, L. J., Juvonen, K. R., Flander, S. M., et al., (2010). A psyllium fiber-enriched meal strongly attenuates postprandial gastrointestinal peptide release in healthy young adults. *J. Nutr., 140*(7), 37–44.

Kay, R. M., Grobin, W., & Track, N. S., (1981). Diets rich in natural fiber improve carbohydrate tolerance in maturity–onset, noninsulin dependent diabetics. *Diabetologia, 20*, 18–21.

Keservani, R. K., Kesharwani, R. K., Sharma, A. K., Vyas, N., & Chadoker, A., (2010b). Nutritional supplements: An overview. *International Journal of Current Pharmaceutical Review and Research, 1*(1), 59–75.

Keservani, R. K., Kesharwani, R. K., Vyas, N., Jain, S., Raghuvanshi, R., & Sharma, A. K., (2010a). Nutraceutical and functional food as future food: A review. *Der Pharmacia Lettre, 2*(1), 106–116.

Keservani, R. K., Sharma, A. K., & Kesharwani, R. K., (2020). *Nutraceuticals and Dietary Supplements: Applications in Health Improvement and Disease Management*. CRC Press. ISBN: 9781771888738.

Keys, A., (1970). Coronary heart disease in seven countries. *Circulation, 41*(Suppl. 1), 1–211.

Kiehm, T. G., Anderson, J. W., & Word, K., (1976). Beneficial effects of a high–carbohydrate, high fiber diet on hyper glycemic diabetic men. *Am. Clin. Nutr., 29*, 895–899.

Kinmouth, A. L., Angus, R. M., Jenkins, P. H., Smith, M. A., & BaumJ, D., (1982). Whole foods and increased dietary fiber improve blood glucose control in diabetic children. *Arch Dis. Child, 57*, 187–194.

Leeds, A. R., (1987). Dietary fiber: Mechanisms of action. *Int IObes., 11*(Suppl. 1), 3–7.

Leeds, A. R., Ralphs, D. N. L., Ebied, F., Metz, G., & Dilawari, J. B., (1981). Pectin in the dumping syndrome: Reduction of symptoms and plasma volume changes. *Lancet, 1*(10), 75–78.

Levitt, N. S., Vinik, A. L., Sive, A. A., Child, P. T., & Jackson, W. P. U. (1980). The effect of dietary fiber on glucose and hormone responses to a mixed meal in normal subjects and in diabetic subjects with and without autonomic neuropathy. *Diabetes Care, 4*(5), 15–19.

Li, Y. O., & Komarek, A. R., (2017). Dietary fiber basics: Health, nutrition, analysis, and applications. *Food Quality and Safety, 1*(1), 47–59.

Liese, A. D., Roach, A. K., Sparks, K. C., Marquart, L., D'Agostino, R. B. J., & Mayer-Davis, E. J., (2003). Whole-grain intake and insulin sensitivity: The insulin resistance atherosclerosis study. *Am. J. Clin. Nutr., 78*, 965–971.

Lousley, S. E., Jones, D. B., & Slauyhter, P., (1984). High carbohydrate high fiber diets in poorly controlled diabetes. *Diabetic Med., 1*, 21–25.

Mann, J. I., (1984). Lines to legumes: Changing concepts of diabetic diets. *Diabetic Med., 1*, 191–198.

Marangoni, F., & Poli, A., (2008). The glycemic index of bread and biscuits is markedly reduced by the addition of a proprietary fiber mixture to the ingredients. *Nutr. Metab Cardiovasc Dis., 18*, 602–605.

Meyer, K. A., Kushi, L. H., Jacobs, D. R. Jr., Slavin, J., Sellers, T. A., & Folsom, A. R., (2000). Carbohydrates, dietary fiber, and incident type 2 diabetes in older women. *Am. J. Clin. Nutr., 71*, 921–930.

Morgan, L. M., Goulder, T. J., Tsiolakis, D., Marks, V., & AlbertiKGM, M., (1979). The effect of unabsorbable carbohydrate on gut hormones: Modification of post–prandial GIP secretion by guar. *Diabetologia, 17*, 85–89.

Ney, D., Hollingsworth, D. R., & Cousin, L., (1982). Decreased insulin requirement and improved control of diabetes in pregnant women given a high–carbohydrate, high–fiber, low fat diet. *Diabetes Care, 5*, 529–533.

Ostman, E. M., Frid, A. H., Groop, L. C., & Bjorck, I. M., (2006). A dietary exchange of common bread for tailored bread of low glycaemic index and rich in dietary fiber improved insulin economy in young women with impaired glucose tolerance. *Eur. J. Clin. Nutr., 60*, 334–341.

Papathanasopoulos, A., & Camilleri, M., (2010). Dietary fiber supplements: Effects in obesity and metabolic syndrome and relationship to gastrointestinal functions. *Gastroenterology, 138*(1), 65–72.

Parash, C., & Suriyakala, P. C., (2020). Role of dietary fibers in reducing the risk of type 2 diabetes. Int. *J. Phys. Educ. Sports Health, 7*(4), 71–77. doi: https://doi.org/10.22271/kheljournal.2020.v7.i4b.1772.

Parillo, M., Riccardi, G., Pacioni, D., Lovine, C., Contaldo, F., Isernia, C., De Marco, F., et al., (1988). Metabolic consequences of feeding a high–carbohydrate high fiber diet to diabetic patients with chronic kidney failure. *Am. Clin. Nutr., 48*, 265–269.

Pastors, J. G., Franz, M. J., Warshaw, H., Daly, A., & Arnold, M. S., (2003). How effective is medical nutrition therapy in diabetes care? *J. Am. Diet. Assoc., 103*(8), 27–31.

Payler, D. K., Pomare, E. W., Heaton, K. W., & Harvery, R. F., (1975). The effect of wheat bran on intestinal transit. *Gut, 16*, 209–213.

Pederson, O., Hjollund, E., Lindskov, H. O., Helms, P., Sorensen, N. S., & Ditzel, J., (1982). Increased insulin receptor binding to monocytes from insulin–dependent diabetic patients after a low–fat, high–starch, high–fiber diet. *Diabetes Care, 5*, 284–291.

Pick, M. E., Hawrysh, Z. J., Gee, M. I., Toth, E., Garg, M. L., & Hardin, R. T., (1996). Oat bran concentrate bread products improve long–term control of diabetes: A pilot study. *J. Am. Diet Assoc., 96*(12), 54–61.

Priebe, M. G., Van, B. J. J., De Vos, R., & Vonk, R. J., (2008). Whole grain foods for the prevention of type 2 diabetes mellitus. *Cochrane Database Syst. Rev*., (1), CD006061.

Pyorala, K., Loast, M., & Uusitupa, N., (1987). Diabetes and atherosclerosis: An epidemiological view. *Diabetes Metab. Rev., 3*, 463–524.

Riccardi, G., Rivellese, A. A., & Mancini, M., (1987). The use of diet to lower plasma cholesterol levels. *Eur. Heart, 8*(Suppl. E), 79–85.

Riccardi, G., Rivellese, A., Pacioni, D., Genovese, S., Mastranzo, P., & Mancini, M., (1984). Separate influence of dietary carbohydrate and fiber on the metabolic control in diabetes. *Diabetologia, 26*, 116–121.

Rosengren, A., Welin, L., Tsipogianni, A., & Wilhelmesen, L., (1989). Impact of cardiovascular risk factors on coronary heart disease and mortality among middle aged diabetic men: A general population study. *Br. Med. I., 299*(11), 27–31.

Russell, W. R., Baka, A., Bjorck, I., Delzenne, N., Gao, D., Griffiths, H. R., Hadjilucas, E., et al., (2016). Impact of diet composition on blood glucose regulation. *Crit. Rev. Food Sci. Nutr., 56*(4), 541–590.

Sarker, M., & Rahman, M., (2017). Dietary fiber and obesity management. *Adv. Obes. Weight Manag. Control., 7*(3), 295–297.

Shimoyama, R., Uehara, S., Itagaki, Y., Izumiyama, S., & Hirayama, A., (1982). Effects of guar intake on plasma somatostatin like immunoreactivity in diabetic patients. *HokkaidoIgaku Zasshi, 57*, 727–732.

Simpson, H. C. R., Simpson, R. W., Lousley, S., Carter, R. D., Geekie, M., Hockaday, T. D. R., & Mann, J., (1981). A high carbohydrate leguminous fiber diet improves all aspects of diabetic control. *Lancet, 1*, 1–5.

Sommer, H., & Kasper, H., (1980). The effect of dietary fiber on the pancreatic excretory function. *Hepato–Gastroenterology, 27*, 477–483.

Southgate, D. A. T., (1969). Determination of carbohydrates in foods. II. Unavailable carbohydrates. *J. Sci. Food Agric., 20*, 331–335.

Southgate, D. A. T., (1985). The measurement and characterization of cereal dietary fiber. In: *Proc Brood and Gezondheid,* (Vol. 10, p. 1727). Brussels.

The InterAct Consortium, (2015). *Diabetologia, 58*, 1394. https://doi.org/10.1007/s00125-015-3585-9.

Toeller, M., (2005). Evidence-based nutritional recommendations for the treatment and prevention of diabetes mellitus. *Diabetes und Stoffwechsel, 14*, 75–94.

Tuomilehto, J., Karttunen, P., Vinni, S., Kostiainen, E., & Uusitupa, M., (1983). A double–blind evaluation of guar gum in patients with dyslipidaemia. *Hum. Nutr. Appl. Nutr., 37*, 109–116.

Vinik, A., & Jenkins, D. J. A., (1988). Dietary fiber in management of diabetes. *Diabetes Care, 11*, 160–173.

Wakai, K., Date, C., Fukui, M., et al., (2007). Dietary fiber and risk of colorectal cancer in the Japan collaborative cohort study. *Cancer Epidemiology, Biomarkers & Prevention, 16*(4).

Wannamethee, S. G., Whincup, P. H., Thomas, M. C., & Sattar, N., (2009). Associations between dietary fiber and inflammation, hepatic function, and risk of type 2 diabetes in older men: Potential mechanisms for the benefits of fiber on diabetes risk. *Diabetes Care, 32*(18), 23–25.

Ward, G. M., Simpson, R. W., Simpson, H. C., Naylor, B. A., Mann, J. I., & Turner, R. C., (1982). Insulin receptor binding increased by high carbohydrate low fat diet in non-insulin–dependent diabetics. *Eur. Clin. Invest, 12*, 93–96.

Weisman, A., Fazli, G. S., Johns, A., & Booth, G. L., (2018). Evolving trends in the epidemiology, risk factors, and prevention of type 2 diabetes: A review. *Can. J. Cardiol. 34*, 552–564.

Williamson, D. A., (2018). Prevention of type 2 diabetes: What is the right target population? *Expert Rev. Endocrinol. Metab.,* 13.

Wilmshurst, P., & Crawley, J. C. W., (1980). The measurement of gastric transit time in obese subjects using 24Na and the effects of energy content and guar gum on gastric emptying and satiety. *Br. J. Nutr., 44*, 1–6.

Wolever, T. M. S., Jenkins, D. J. A., Vuksan, V., Josse, R. G., Wong, G. S., & Jenkins, A. L., (1990). Glycemic index of foods in individual subjects. *Diabetes Care, 13*, 126–132.

Wrick, K. L., (1976). The influence of dietary fiber source on human intestinal transit and stool output. *J. Nutr., 29*(14), 74–79.

Yu-Poth, S., Zhao, G., Etherton, T., Naglak, M., Jonnalagadda, S., & Kris-Etherton, P. M., (1999). Effects of the national cholesterol education program's step I and step II dietary intervention programs on cardiovascular disease risk factors: A meta-analysis. *Am. J. Clin. Nutr., 69*, 632–646.

CHAPTER 4

ROLE OF DIETARY FIBERS IN OBESITY

HEMANT P. SURYAWANSHI,[1] PRAMOD N. PATIL,[2]
RINA H. SURYAWANSHI,[3] and RAJESH A. AHIRRAO[4]

[1]*PG College of Pharmaceutical Science and Research, Chaupale, Maharashtra, India*

[2]*RCP, Institute of Technology, Shirpur, Maharashtra, India*

[3]*NTV'S Sharada Junior College, Joganipada, Maharashtra, India*

[4]*PG College of Pharmaceutical Science and Research, Nandurbar, Maharashtra, India*

ABSTRACT

Obesity is a multifaceted chronic disease having psychological, social, cultural, genetic, physiological, metabolic, and behavioral causes. Overweight and obesity are on the rise globally, in developing and developed nations. Obesity is primarily treated by calorie restriction and increased physical exercise. Despite eventual weight recovery, dieting as part of a lifestyle change results in long-term weight loss. Intensive behavioral therapy, including nutrition and activity changes, is recommended. Dietary fiber has a number of functions in the body, one of which is to aid in the control of energy intake and the prevention of obesity. Dietary fiber's distinctive physical and chemical features are linked to its importance in regulating energy intake and obesity development, which aid in early satiety signals and better or prolonged satiety signals. Early satiety signals may be induced by cephalic and gastric phase responses to the bulking effects of dietary fiber on energy density and palatability, whereas viscosity-producing effects of certain fibers may enhance satiety through intestinal phase events related to altered gastrointestinal function and subsequent fat absorption delay.

Food Supplements and Dietary Fiber in Health and Disease. Bhushan R. Rane, Raj K. Keservani, Durgesh Singh, Nayan A. Gujarathi, and Ashish S. Jain, (Eds.)
© 2024 Apple Academic Press, Inc. Co-published with CRC Press (Taylor & Francis)

Fiber-rich diets, whether obtained through fiber supplementation or high-fiber diets or diets that include high-fiber foods, have a lower calorie density than high-fat diets in general. There's also evidence that women respond better to dietary fiber changes than men. When dietary fiber is provided, obese persons are more inclined to eat less, according to the link between body weight and fiber's effect on energy consumption.

4.1 INTRODUCTION

Dietary fiber has a variety of purposes in the diet, one of which is to aid with energy intake control and reduce the risk of obesity (Jarouliya & Keservani, 2019). The significance of dietary fiber in controlling energy intake and obesity development is linked to its unique physical and chemical properties, which aid in early satiety signals and better or prolonged satiety signals. Early satiety signals may be induced by cephalic- and gastric-phase responses to dietary fiber's bulking effects on energy density and palatability; whereas the viscosity-producing actions of some fiber may increase satiety intestinal-phase events related to altered gastrointestinal function and subsequent fat absorption delay. Fiber-rich diets, whether obtained through fiber supplementation or the incorporation of high fiber foods into meals, have a lower calorie density than high fat diets in general. The ability of fiber to add bulk and weight to the diet contributes to this. There's also evidence that women respond better to dietary fiber changes than men. Obese people are more likely to eat less when dietary fiber is included, according to the link between body weight and fiber's effect on energy consumption (Britt Burton-Freeman).

4.1.1 OBESITY

Obesity is a multifaceted chronic illness with psychological, social, cultural, genetic, physiologic, metabolic, and behavioral causes and effects. Obesity and overweight persons are on the rise in both developing and developed countries at worrisome rates (Obesity, 2015; *Yazdi*, 2015).

Obesity is defined as a condition in which a person's excess body fat has accumulated to the point where it poses a health risk (Obesity, 2015). Obesity is characterized as having a BMI of higher than 30 kg/m^2, which is calculated by dividing a person's weight by their height squared. Overweight is defined as having a BMI between 25 and 30 kg/m^2 (Obesity, 2015). In several East

Asian countries, lower values are used (Kanazawa, 2005). Obesity has been associated with a variety of diseases and conditions, including cardiovascular disease, type-II diabetes, obstructive sleep apnea, cancer, osteoarthritis, and asthma (Haslam, 2005). Obesity, as a result, has been related to a shorter life expectancy. Although it has not been proven to be a direct cause of disease, a high BMI puts you at risk for diseases caused by diet, exercise, and the environment (Chiolero, 2018). Obesity increases the risk of clinical depression, and obesity is caused by melancholy (*Luppino, 2010)*.

On an individual, social, and environmental level, diet, physical activity, mechanization, urbanization, genetic susceptibility, medications, mental diseases, financial strategies, disorders related to endocrine glands, etc., are all contributing factors to obesity (Obesity, 2015; *Yazdi*, 2015; *Kassotis, 2020; Bleich, 2008)*.

Obesity prevention necessitates a multifaceted approach that includes community, family, and individual treatments (Obesity, 2015; Chiolero, 2018). Doctors propose dietary changes and exercise as the two major treatments (Haslam, 2005). Reduced energy-dense foods, such as high-fat or high-sugar foods, and increased dietary fiber (Keservani et al., 2010a, b, 2020) consumption can improve diet quality (Obesity, 2015). Medications can be used in conjunction with a healthy diet to control appetite or fat absorption (Yanovski, 2014). If diet, exercise, and medicine don't help, a gastric balloon or surgery to shrink the stomach or shorten the intestines may be utilized, increasing the time it takes for you to feel full and limiting your ability to absorb nutrients from meals (*Colquitt, 2014; Imaz, 2008*).

Obesity is a leading preventable cause of death in both adults and children around the world, and rates are rising (Obesity, 2015; Encyclopedia, 2015). In 195 nations, 600 million adults (12%) and 100 million children were obese in 2015 (Afshin, 2017). Obesity is more prevalent in women than it is in men (Obesity, 2015). Obesity is one of the most pressing public health issues of the 21st century (Dibaise, 2013). Obesity was classified as a condition by several medical organizations in 2013, including the American Medical Association and the American Heart Association (*Jensen, 2014; Pollack, 2013; Weinstock, 2013)*.

4.2 COMPLICATIONS OF OBESITY

CHD (*Lu, 2014*), angina pectoris and heart failure (*Haslam, 2005; Aune, 2016*), hypertension, improper cholesterol level, DM, birth defects, menstrual cycle disorders, infertility, increased complications during general anesthesia Stroke, depression in women, osteoarthritis (*Haslam, 2005*), pulmonary embolism (*Darvall, 2007*), complications during pregnancy (*Haslam, 2005; Arendas, 2008*), erectile dysfunction (*Corona, 2014*), migraines (*Bigal, 2008*), carpal tunnel syndrome (*Sharifi-Mollayousefi, 2008*), dementia (*Beydoun, 2008*), idiopathic intracranial hypertension (*Wall, 2008*), multiple sclerosis (*Munger, 2009*), fatty liver disease, cholelithiasis, Hepatocellular carcinoma (*Dibaise, 2013*), cancer of esophagus, colon rectum, pancreas, gallbladder, endometrium, kidney, Leukemia (*Basen, 2011*), obesity, asthma (*Haslam, 2005; Poulain, 2006*), Urinary incontinence (*Hunskaar, 2008*), chronic renal failure (*Ejerblad, 2006*), gout (*Aune, 2014*), poor mobility (*Tukker, 2009*), lower back pain (*Molenaar, 2008*).

4.3 RESPONSIBLE FACTORS FOR OBESITY

The carbohydrate-insulin hypothesis proposed that eating processed, high glycemic load carbohydrates produces hormonal changes in the body that enhance calorie deposition in adipose tissue, stimulate appetite, and decrease energy expenditure (Ludwig, 2018). The majority of cases of obesity, according to calorie hypothesis, calories are produced by a combination of excessive dietary energy intake and a lack of physical exercise (Lau, 2007). Genetics, medical factors, and psychological disorders account for a small number of cases (*Bleich, 2008*).

4.3.1 LIFESTYLE

Obesity is largely caused by a sedentary lifestyle (Seidell, 2005). There has been a significant movement toward less physically demanding jobs worldwide (Obesity, 2008; WHO, 2009; Ness-Abramof, 2006), moreover, at least 30% of the global population does not get enough exercise (WHO, 2009). This is owing to a rise in the use of vehicles and a rise in the use of labor-saving technology in the house (Obesity, 2008; WHO, 2009; Ness-Abramof, 2006). Physical activity levels in youngsters appear to be declining as a result of decreased walking and physical education (Salmon, 2007). In both children and adults, there is a relationship between television and mobile phone presentation time and the risk of obesity (*Gortmaker, 1996; Vioque, 2000; Tucker, 1991*).

4.3.2 HEREDITY

Obesity, like many other medical diseases, is the consequence of a complex interaction of hereditary and environmental variables (Albuquerque, 2017). Obesity is caused by polymorphisms in numerous genes that influence hunger and metabolism when there is enough dietary energy. When a favorable environment is available, more than 41 of these locations in the human genome have been related to the development of obesity as of 2006 (Poirier, 2006).

4.3.3 PRESENCE OF OTHER DISEASES

Obesity can be exacerbated by some physical and mental diseases, as well as the pharmaceuticals used to treat them. Several rare genetic syndromes, hypothyroidism, Cushing's syndrome, and growth hormone insufficiency are among the medical conditions that raise the risk of obesity (Rosén, 1993). Patients with psychotic diseases are more likely to be overweight or obese than people without mental illnesses (Chiles, 2010).

4.3.4 SOCIAL FACTORS

There have been numerous theories presented to explain the relationship between BMI and socioeconomic level. The wealthy in industrialized countries are said to be able to buy more nutritious food, are subjected to more societal pressure to maintain their weight and have more opportunities with higher physical fitness needs. Smoking has a significant impact on one's weight. Over the course of 10 years, those who stop smoking acquire an average of 4.4 kg for men and 5.0 kg for women (Flegal, 1995). Obesity rates are rising in developing countries as a result of urbanization. Obesity rates in China are normally under 5%, but in some cities, obesity rates exceed 20% (Obesity, 2009). Early-life malnutrition is likely to play a role in emerging countries' rising obesity rates (Caballero, 2001).

4.3.5 GUT BACTERIA

The study of infectious diseases' influence on metabolism is still in its early phases. The gut flora of lean and obese adults has been demonstrated to differ.

There is evidence that gut flora has an impact on metabolic capacity. This apparent change is thought to confer a larger capability for energy harvesting, which contributes to obesity. Obesity has yet to be definitively determined as the direct cause or outcome of these variations (DiBaise, 2008).

4.3.6 ANTIBIOTICS

Antibiotic use in children has been related to a higher risk of obesity later in life (Antibiotics, 2018; Cox, 2015).

4.3.7 VIRUSES

A relationship between viruses and obesity has been discovered in humans and a range of animal species. It's unclear how much these connections have contributed to the obesity epidemic's rise (Falagas, 2006).

4.4 PREVENTION AND MANAGEMENT OF OBESITY WITH DIETARY FIBERS

Plant components that are not broken down by human digestive enzymes are referred to as dietary fiber (Dietary Fiber, 2018). All polysaccharides and lignin that are not digested by the human digestive tract's endogenous secretion are considered dietary fiber. A physiological definition, such as "dietary components resistant to mammalian enzyme degradation," or a chemical definition, such as "the sum of non-starch polysaccharides and lignin," is currently used by the majority of animal nutritionists (Jha, 2021).

Lignin, a major source of dietary insoluble fiber, has been demonstrated to influence the rate at which soluble fibers are broken down (Dietary, 2005). Short-chain fatty acids are formed when insoluble fibers, such as resistant starch, are fermented, providing energy to colonocytes (Dietary Fiber, 2018; Keenan, 2015; Lockyer, 2017). Coronary heart disease, cancer of colon, and type II diabetes can all be prevented with a diet high in dietary fiber and whole grains (Reynolds, 2019).

Dietary fibers can alter the composition of the contents of the gastrointestinal tract, altering the absorption of other nutrients and substances (Eastwood, 2005). Soluble fiber becomes a gelatinous, viscous material when it absorbs water. Few kinds of insoluble fiber bulk up the feces but aren't fermented, but others, like wheat bran, can ferment slowly in the colon in addition to bulking up the feces (Anderson, 2009; De Paepe, 2020). In the colon, soluble fibers are fermented more than insoluble fibers (Rosin, 2002; Bach Knudsen, 2001; Phillips, 2013; Williams, 2000).

Soluble and insoluble fiber can be found in legumes, whole grains and cereals, vegetables, fruits, nuts, and seeds, among other foods (Fiber, 2019; Dietary, 2005). A diet rich in fiber is linked to improved health and a reduced risk of a variety of diseases (Fiber, 2019; Veronese, 2018).

Soluble and insoluble fiber sources are the two types of fiber found in the diet. Both forms of fiber are found in variable levels in plant diets, depending on the fiber's viscosity and fermentability (Dietary Fiber, 2018; Institute of Medicine, 2001). Fiber consumption has different health benefits based on the type of fiber consumed and the benefits that may occur in the gastrointestinal system (Gallaher, 2006). Bulking fibers including cellulose, hemicellulose, and psyllium absorb and hold water, which aids in consistency. Psyllium and beta-glucan are viscous fibers that thicken the feces (Institute of Medicine, 2001). Resistant starch and inulin are fermentable fibers that support the bacteria and microbiota of the large intestine and are digested to produce short-chain fatty acids, which have a range of functions in gut health (Bedford, 2018; Cummings, 2001).

1. **Soluble Fiber:** It's a type of fiber that dissolves in water and ferments in the colon, producing gases and physiologically active by-products including short-chain fatty acids made by gut bacteria. It is also known as fermentable fiber or prebiotic fiber. Two examples include beta-glucans and raw guar gum. Psyllium is a bulking fiber that absorbs water in the digestive system, making feces easier to pass. It's a non-fermented, soluble, viscous fiber. Because soluble fiber is viscous and inhibits stomach emptying, it gives humans a longer feeling of fullness (Fiber, 2019). Soluble non-viscous fibers found in legumes and bananas (Keenan, 2015; Fiber, 2019). Soluble fibers, such as beta-glucans from oats or barley, have been found to lower LDL cholesterol levels in the blood, which is a risk factor for cardiovascular disease (Fiber, 2019; Veronese, 2018; FDA, 2008).
2. **Insoluble Fiber:** It does not dissolve in water and is not digested by digestive enzymes in the upper GI tract. Examples include wheat bran, cellulose, and lignin. Coarsely powdered insoluble fiber increases mucus secretion in the large intestine, which adds weight. Insoluble fiber that has been finely milled has the opposite effect and

can even promote constipation (Fiber, 2019). Resistant starches and other insoluble fibers can be fermented in the colon (Lockyer, 2017).

Non-starch polysaccharides, as well as other plant components like cellulose, resistant starch, resistant dextrins, inulin, lignins, chitins (in fungi), pectins, beta-glucans, and oligosaccharides, make up dietary fiber (Fiber, 2019; Dietary Fiber, 2018; Dietary, 2005) (Table 4.1).

TABLE 4.1 Types and Sources of Fibers

SL. No.	Nutrient	Source
A.	**Water Insoluble Dietary Fibers**	
1.	Cellulose	Cereals, fruit, vegetables
2.	Chitin	In fungi and insects
3.	Hemicellulose	Cereals, bran, timber, legumes
4.	Hexoses	Wheat, barley
5.	Pentose	Rye, oat
6.	Lignin	Stones of fruits, vegetables, cereals
7.	Xanthan gum	Production with Xanthomonas-bacteria from sugar substrates
8.	Resistant starch	Corn, barley, wheat, legumes, raw bananas, and potatoes (Lockyer, 2017)
B.	**Water Soluble Dietary Fibers**	
1.	Arabinoxylan	Psyllium (Fischer, 2004)
2.	Fructans	In some plant taxa, starch can be used to replace or augment starch as a storage carbohydrate.
3.	Inulin	Topinambour, chicory, etc.
4.	Pectin	In the fruit skin (apples), vegetables
5.	Alginic acids	In algae
6.	Carrageen	Red algae
7.	Raffinose	Legumes
8.	Polydextrose	Synthetic polymer

4.4.1 FOOD CONTAINS DIETARY FIBERS

Dietary fibers can be found in fruits, vegetables, and entire grains. Fiber is abundant in fruits, dark green vegetables, orange vegetables, cooked dry beans (legumes), starchy vegetables, other vegetables, entire grains, and meat.

Dietary fiber is found in plants and is commonly consumed whole, raw, or cooked, but it can also be obtained in nutritional supplements and fiber-rich processed meals. The highest fiber grain bran products, such as crude corn bran (79 g per 100 g) and crude wheat bran (43 g per 100 g), are used as components in processed meals (Search, 2015).

4.4.2 PLANT SOURCES

Several plants have a lot of fiber, both soluble and insoluble. Plums and prunes, for example, have a thick skin that shields the juicy flesh inside. The peel contains insoluble fiber, whereas the pulp contains soluble fiber. Grapes are also high in fiber (Stacewicz-Sapuntzakis, 2001) (Table 4.2).

TABLE 4.2 Plant Sources of Fibers

SL. No.	Source of Soluble Fiber	Source of Insoluble Fiber
1.	Legumes like peas, soybeans, and other beans	Whole grain foods
2.	Oats, rye, chia, and barley	Wheat and corn bran
3.	Fruits like avocados, plums, prunes, berries, figs, ripe bananas, and the upper of apples	Beans and peas
4.	Vegetables – broccoli and carrots	Nuts and seeds
5.	Root tubers and root vegetables such as sweet potatoes and onions	Potato and onion skins
6.	Psyllium seed and flax seeds	Lignans
7.	Almonds	Vegetables such as green beans, cauliflower, celery, and nopal
8.	Legumes	Avocado and unripe bananas
9.	Oats, rye, chia, and barley	The upper part of kiwi fruit, grapes, and tomatoes (Alvarado, 2001)

4.4.3 FIBER SUPPLEMENTS

These are just a few examples of fiber supplements and food additives that have been on the market. These could be sold to consumers for nutritional purposes, the treatment of gastrointestinal issues, and health benefits like cholesterol reduction, colon cancer risk reduction, and weight loss.

Irritable bowel syndrome symptoms like diarrhea or constipation, as well as stomach discomfort, may benefit from soluble fiber supplements (Friedman, 1989). Irritable bowel disease (Ewaschuk, 2006), such as Crohn's disease (Guarner, 2005), ulcerative colitis (Seidner, 2005; Seidner, 2003), and Clostridium difficile colitis (Ward, 1997), may be helped by prebiotic soluble fiber products containing inulin or oligosaccharides, leading to the making of fatty acids with short chain, which have anti-inflammatory properties in the bowel. So, by adjusting meal choices as part of a comprehensive dietary plan, fiber supplements may help control irritable bowel syndrome (MacDermott, 2007).

As a supplement, high-amylose maize resistant starch has been employed and has been shown to improve insulin sensitivity and glycemic control (Robertson, 2012; Maki, 2012; Johnston, 2010), as well as promote regularity (Phillips, 1995) and possibly relieve diarrhea (Ramakrishna, 2000; Raghupathy, 2006; Ramakrishna, 2008). According to one preliminary finding, resistant maize starch may aid in the treatment of ulcerative colitis symptoms (James, 2012).

4.4.3.1 INULIN

Most plants include inulins, which are oligosaccharides with nutritional value as carbohydrates or, more specifically, as fructans, a polymer of fructose, a natural plant sugar. For usage in cooked foods, manufacturers extract inulin from enhanced plant sources such as chicory roots or Jerusalem artichokes (Kaur, 2002). It can be used to substitute sugar, oil, and flour in powdered nutritional supplements to improve flow and mixing capabilities. It could also be beneficial to your health as a prebiotic fermentable fiber (Roberfroid, 2007).

Inulin is a fermentable prebiotic fiber that is digested by gut bacteria to form short-chain fatty acids that help with calcium, magnesium, and iron absorption (Abrams, 2005; Tako, 2008).

The principal downside of inulin is that it ferments in the intestine, potentially producing gas and digestive pain in most people at doses greater than 15 gm/day (Grabitske, 2009). People with digestive issues have found that eliminating fructose and inulin from the diet has helped them (Shepherd, 2006). While lower inulin intake levels have been shown to cause changes in the microbiota in clinical studies, higher inulin intake levels may be necessary to achieve body weight improvements (Liber, 2013).

4.4.3.2 VEGETABLE GUMS

Supplements made from vegetable gum fiber are a relatively recent product on the market. Vegetable gum fibers, which are commonly offered as a powder, dissolve quickly and have no aftertaste. They have shown to be useful in treating irritable bowel syndrome in preliminary clinical trials (Parisi, 2002). Vegetable gum fibers include guar gum and gum Arabic.

4.5 FUNCTIONING IN THE INTESTINE

Bulking, viscosity, and fermentation are three ways dietary fibers help (Gallaher, 2006). Various fibers have different effects, emphasizing that a varied diet is beneficial to overall health. Some fibers predominantly contribute through a single method. Cellulose and wheat bran, for example, have good bulking properties but are only lightly fermented. Many dietary fibers, on the other hand, for example, can help you in more than one of these ways. Psyllium, for example, provides both bulk and viscosity.

Bulking fibers (e.g., psyllium) can be soluble or insoluble. They absorb water and can increase stool weight and regularity greatly. In the intestine, the majority of bulking fibers are not fermented or are just moderately fermented (Gallaher, 2006).

The contents of the digestive tract are thickened by viscous fibers, potentially lowering sugar absorption, post-meal glycemic response, and fat absorption. Because of their viscosity and thickening qualities, they are commonly used in small amounts in food formulations. Some viscous fibers are partially or completely fermented in the intestine, while others are only moderately fermented or not fermented at all (Gallaher, 2006).

The bacteria in the large intestine consume fermentable fibers, moderately increasing fecal volume and generating short chain fatty acids as by-products by a wide range of physiological functions. Fully fermented dietary fibers include resistant starch, inulin, fructo-oligosaccharide, and galacto-oligosaccharide. Fibers, both insoluble and soluble, are included. Dietary fibers can alter the nature of the contents of the gastrointestinal tract by adding bulk and viscosity, as well as how other nutrients and chemicals are absorbed (Keenan, 2012; Dietary, 2005; Eastwood, 2005). Certain soluble fibers attach to bile acids in the small intestine as a result of cytochrome P450-mediated cholesterol oxidation, making them less likely to re-enter the body and reducing blood cholesterol levels (Anderson, 2009).

The consumption of insoluble fiber has been associated with a reduced risk of diabetes (Foods, 2005), however, the exact mechanism is unknown (Weickert, 2008). Resistant starch, a form of insoluble dietary fiber, has been shown to improve insulin sensitivity in healthy persons (Robertson, 2003; Robertson, 2005), type 2 diabetics (Zhang, 2007), and people with insulin resistance (Zhang, 2007), Type 2 diabetes may be less common as a result of this research (Robertson, 2012; Maki, 2012; Johnston, 2010).

4.6 COLON

The colon can be divided into two parts:

- On the right, a fermenter (cecum and ascending colon) (Hellendoorn, 1983). Microorganisms use dietary fiber, resistant starch, fat, and protein to salvage nutrients on the right side of the colon, and the end-products are absorbed for utilization by the body (Jarouliya & Keservani, 2019a).
- The left colon (transverse, descending, and sigmoid) has an impact on continence. The presence of bacteria in the colon leads the colon to have a high metabolic activity, which is predominantly reductive, whereas the liver is oxidative. The substrates of the cecum are either biliary excretion products or materials that have passed through the whole gut. Dietary fiber has an effect on the colon are:
    - o Fermentation of some food fibers by bacteria;
    - o As a result, bacterial bulk increases;
    - o An increase in the activity of bacterial enzymes;
    - o After fermentation, changes in the fiber residue's water retaining capacity.

The cecum swells when some dietary fibers are ingested, and this is now regarded to be a normal physiological reaction. This rise could be the result of a variety of things, including as the fiber's longer cecal stay, greater bacterial mass, or higher bacterial end products. Pectin, gum Arabic, oligosaccharides, and resistant starch are fermented to yield short-chain fatty acids (mainly acetic, propionic, and n-butyric), as well as carbon dioxide, hydrogen, and methane. Almost all of these short chain fatty acids will be absorbed by the intestines. This means that fecal short-chain fatty acid estimates ignore cecal or colonic fermentation in favor of absorption efficiency, fiber residue's potential to sequester short-chain fatty acids, and fiber fermentation throughout the colon, which will likely continue until the substrate is depleted. The gut mucosa is affected by short chain fatty acid production in a variety of ways.

4.7 METABOLISM OF CHOLESTEROL

Dietary fiber can alter cholesterol metabolism by regulating digestion, absorption, and excretion at each stage (Brown, 1999), including:

- The caloric energy of foods via a bulking effect;
- Reduced time it takes for the stomach to empty;
- Absorption activity based on the glycemic index;
- The ileum slows bile acid absorption, allowing bile acids to pass through to the cecum;
- The cecum's bile acid metabolism is changed or increased;
- Short-chain fatty acids obtained by fiber fermentation, notably propionic acid, have an indirect effect on cholesterol metabolism in the liver;
- Bile acid binding to fiber or bacteria in the cecum causes increased fecal loss from the enterohepatic circulation.

4.8 EFFECTS OF FIBER CONSUMPTION

Fiber may boost health through a variety of mechanisms, according to preliminary study (Boerjan, 2003):

1. **Soluble and Insoluble Fiber:** Increases dietary volume without boosting caloric content as much as digestible carbohydrates, resulting in satiety and possibly a reduction in appetite.
2. **Soluble Fiber Only:** During digestion, it attracts water and creates a thick gel, slowing stomach emptying, reducing intestinal transit time, shielding carbohydrates from enzymes, and delaying glucose absorption (Dietary fiber, 2018; Gropper, 2008), reducing blood sugar fluctuation (Dietary fiber, 2018; Gropper, 2008). Lowers total and LDL cholesterol levels, potentially lowering heart disease risk (Dietary fiber, 2018).
3. **Insoluble Fiber Only:** Reduces the risk of diabetes in diabetics by regulating blood sugar levels and lowering glucose and insulin levels (Dietary fiber, 2018; Food, 2005). Food moves more quickly through

the digestive system, making regular defecation simpler. Constipation can be alleviated by bulking up the stool.

Because fiber does not bind to minerals or vitamins, it does not hinder their absorption. On the other hand, fermentable fiber sources appear to improve mineral absorption, notably calcium absorption (Greger, 1999; Raschka, 2005; Scholz-Ahrens, 2007).

4.9 DIETARY RECOMMENDATIONS

4.9.1 UNITED KINGDOM

In 2018, the British Nutrition Foundation released a statement that clarified the description of dietary fiber and outlined the possible health benefits that have been demonstrated to far, as well as raising the recommended daily minimum consumption for healthy people to 30 gm (Dietary fiber, 2018; Hooper, 2015).

4.9.2 UNITED STATES

Adult men ages 19 to 50 should consume 38 gm of dietary fiber per day, men 51 and older 30 gm, and adult women ages 19 to 50 should consume 25 gm per day, women 51 and older 21 gm, according to current recommendations from the United States National Academy of Medicine (NAM) of the National Academy of Sciences. Three studies found that persons who consumed the most fiber had a median of 14 gm of fiber per 1,000 calories and had the lowest risk of coronary heart disease, especially those who ate more cereal fiber (Fiber, 2019; Dietary, 2005; Institute of Medicine, 2005).

North Americans consume less than half of the dietary fiber required for optimum health on average. This percentage could be as low as 20% in today's youth's preferred food choices, a fact that experts feel leads to the high levels of obesity seen in many industrialized countries (Suter, 2005). Food goods with fiber health claims have been approved by regulatory bodies such as the FDA of the United States, acknowledging the growing body of scientific data that greater fiber intake has physiological benefits. The FDA defines which ingredients are considered "fiber," and product labels must state that adding the fiber ingredient has a physiological benefit (Aubrey, 2017). The FDA has allowed approved fiber products to make health claims, such as claiming that frequent use can lower blood cholesterol levels, which can reduce the risk of coronary heart disease (Health claims, 2008) and several kinds of cancer (Health claims, 2008).

The FDA has approved the following viscous fiber sources (Fiber, 2019):

- Seed husk of Psyllium (7 gm/day);
- Oat bran, whole oats, or rolled oats; or whole grain or dry milled barley (3 gm/day).

Consumption of fermentable fiber on a regular basis may lower the risk of chronic diseases (Tungland, 2002; Lee, 2008; Theuwissen, 2008). A lack of fiber in the diet can cause constipation (What, 2015).

4.9.3 EUROPEAN UNION

Dietary fiber intakes of 25 gm/day are acceptable for normal laxation in adults, according to the European Food Safety Authority's (EFSA) Panel on Nutrition, Novel Foods, and Food Allergens (NDA), which is in responsibility of establishing Dietary Reference Values for carbohydrates and dietary fiber (Scientific, 2010; Maragkoudakis, 2017).

4.9.4 FERMENTATION

Edible plant parts or similar carbohydrates resistant to digestion and absorption in the human small intestine with total or partial fermentation in the large intestine, according to the American Association of Cereal Chemists (AACC International, 2007).

The fiber containing sections of a plant that we consume, such as the skin, pulp, seeds, stems, leaves, and roots, are referred to as "edible components of plants." There are insoluble and soluble sources for certain plant components.

Soluble fermentable fiber is found in complex carbohydrates including starch, oligosaccharides, and poly-saccharides.

Fermentation in the large intestine can be complete or partial. The colon is a section of the large intestine where extra nutrient absorption occurs through the fermentation process. Fermentation occurs when colonic bacteria work on the food material, resulting in the generation of gases and short-chain fatty acids. Butyric, acetic, and propionic are short-chain fatty acids with important health impacts, according to scientific evidence (Wong, 2006).

Shorter-chain carbohydrates cannot be digested, but they are converted to short-chain fatty acids and gases through fermentation in the colon. Fiber molecules with partial or low fermentability, according to a 2002 journal publication (Tungland, 2002), include:

- Cellulose;
- Methylcellulose;
- Hemicellulose;
- Lignans;
- Plant waxes.

Compounds in fibers with a high fermentability include:

- Resistant starch;
- Betaglucans;
- Pectins;
- Natural gums;
- Inulins;
- Oligosaccharides.

4.9.5 SHORT-CHAIN FATTY ACIDS (SCFA)

Short-chain fatty acids are formed when fermentable fiber is fermented (Jha, 2021). SCFAs play a role in a variety of physiological processes that promote health, including (Wong, 2006):

- Act on pancreatic insulin secretion and hepatic glycogen breakdown regulation to stabilize blood glucose levels.
- Regulate glucose absorption by inducing glucose transporter gene expression in the intestinal mucosa (Drozdowski, 2002).
- Provide colonocyte nutrition, primarily through the SCFA butyrate.
- Reduce LDL cholesterol and triglyceride levels in the blood, which are associated to atherosclerosis, by suppressing cholesterol synthesis in the liver.
- A lower colonic pH (i.e., a higher level of acidity in the colon) protects the lining from colonic polyp formation and improves mineral absorption from the food.
- Boost the production of T helper cells, antibodies, leukocytes, cytokines, and lymph systems, all of which contribute to immune defense.

- Improve the colonic mucosal layer's barrier properties, minimizing inflammatory and adhesion irritants while also boosting immunological function.

The colonic mucosa absorbs SCFAs, which pass through the intestinal wall and into the portal circulation, where the liver transports them to the general circulatory system.

SCFAs have a wide range of effects on major regulatory systems, including blood glucose and cholesterol levels, the environment in the colon, and intestinal immune activity (Roy, 2006; Scholz-Ahrens, 2007).

Butyrate, propionate, and acetate are the most common SCFAs in humans, with butyrate serving as the primary source of energy for colonocytes, propionate intended for liver absorption, and acetate entering the peripheral circulation to be processed by peripheral organs.

4.9.6 FDA-APPROVED PRODUCTS AND HEALTH CLAIM

The FDA allows food makers in the United States to claim that consuming meals containing 1.7 g of psyllium husk soluble fiber or 0.75 g of oat or barley soluble fiber as betaglucans on a daily basis may reduce the risk of heart disease (FDA, 2008).

Beta-glucan can be found in soluble fiber from the following sources:

- Oat bran;
- Rolled oats;
- Whole oat flour;
- Oatrim;
- Barley, both whole grain and dry milled;
- Psyllium husk soluble fiber with a purity level of at least 95%.

Diets low in saturated fat and cholesterol, as well as soluble fiber from select of the following foods, may minimize the risk of heart disease, according to the official label. According to FDA regulation 21 CFR 101.81, daily dietary intake amounts of soluble fiber from the sources listed above are linked to a lower risk of coronary heart disease, are:

- About 3 gm soluble beta-glucan fiber per day from whole oats, barley, or a mixture of entire oats and barley.
- Psyllium seed husk provides 7 gm or more soluble fiber per day (Soluble Fiber, 2008).

Soluble fiber from grains is another approved health claim for lowering the risk of some types of cancer and heart disease by eating fruits and vegetables (FDA, 2008). According to a qualified health claim granted by the FDA in December 2016, resistant starch from high-amylose maize may lower the incidence of type 2 diabetes by enhancing insulin sensitivity. The FDA issued new labeling advice for isolated or synthesized dietary fiber in 2018, outlining how different forms of dietary fiber should be labeled (Elaine, 2018).

4.10 INVESTIGATION

As of 2019, a clinical investigation on the possible health advantages of a high-fiber diet indicated wide patterns of lower risk of various cancers, cardiovascular diseases (Keservani et al., 2016a), and type 2 diabetes (Fiber, 2019; Veronese, 2018). According to a nine-year study of 3,88,000 adults aged 50 to 71, those who consumed the highest fiber had a 22% decreased risk of dying during that time (Park, 2011). In addition to a lower risk of death from heart disease, fiber-rich diets, particularly grains, have been associated with a lower risk of infectious and respiratory illnesses and cancer (Keservani et al., 2015).

4.11 CONCLUSION

The shift in lifestyle has resulted in a major decline in the consumption of fruits (Keservani et al., 2016b), vegetables, and legumes. This is because the amount of fiber in the diet pattern in any modern society has been demonstrated to be far below the required threshold. A diet high in dietary fiber is a good way to maintain a healthy weight because it has a favorable impact throughout the gastrointestinal tract, starting with the release and management of satiety hormones and regulating metabolite levels such as HDL, LDL, and triglycerides. Dietary fiber promotes rapid evacuation and serves as a carbon source for numerous lactic bacteria, which ferment the fiber and produce a variety of useful metabolites, such as short-chain fatty acids.

Obesity is a risk factor for cardiovascular, diabetes, and metabolic problems consequently the bulk of studies looked at the multiple effects of fiber intake on weight loss and obesity management. Given the benefits of fiber intake, researchers are interested in developing fiber-enriched food products by incorporating fruits, vegetables, or extracted fiber from other sources into the meal. More fruits and vegetables, as well as fiber-rich meals, should be included in the diet chart to help with obesity management.

KEYWORDS

- **diabetes**
- **fibers**
- **heredity**
- **obesity**
- **satiety**
- **short-chain fatty acids**
- **weight loss**

REFERENCES

Abrams, S. A., Griffin, I. J., Hawthorne, K. M., Liang, L., Gunn, S. K., Darlington, G., & Ellis, K. J., (2005). A combination of prebiotic short- and long-chain inulin-type fructans enhances calcium absorption and bone mineralization in young adolescents. *The American Journal of Clinical Nutrition, 82*(2), 471–476. doi: 10.1093/ajcn.82.2.471. PMID 16087995.

Afshin, A., Forouzanfar, M. H., Reitsma, M. B., Sur, P., Estep, K., & Lee, A., (2017). Health effects of overweight and obesity in 195 countries over 25 years. *The New England Journal of Medicine, 377*(1), 13–27. doi: 10.1056/NEJMoa1614362. PMC 5477817. PMID 28604169.

Albuquerque, D., Nóbrega, C., Manco, L., & Padez, C., (2017). The contribution of genetics and environment to obesity. *British Medical Bulletin, 123*(1), 159–173. doi: 10.1093/bmb/ldx022. PMID 28910990.

Alvarado, A., Pacheco-Delahaye, E., & Hevia, P., (2001). Value of a tomato byproduct as a source of dietary fiber in rats (PDF). *Plant Foods for Human Nutrition, 56*(4), 335–348. doi: 10.1023/A:1011855316778. PMID 11678439. S2CID 21835355.

Anderson, J. W., Baird, P., Davis, R. H., Ferreri, S., Knudtson, M., Koraym, A., et al., (2009). Health benefits of dietary fiber (PDF). *Nutrition Reviews, 67*(4), 188–205. doi: 10.1111/j.1753-4887.2009.00189.x. PMID 19335713.

Arendas, K., Qiu, Q., & Gruslin, A., (2008). Obesity in pregnancy: Pre-conceptional to postpartum consequences. *Journal of Obstetrics and Gynaecology Canada, 30*(6), 477–488. doi: 10.1016/s1701-2163(16)32863-8. PMID 18611299.

Aubrey, A., (2017). *The FDA Will Decide Whether 26 Ingredients Count as Fiber*. National Public Radio.

Aune, D., Norat, T., & Vatten, L. J., (2014). Body mass index and the risk of gout: A systematic review and dose-response meta-analysis of prospective studies. *European Journal of*

Nutrition, 53(8), 1591–1601. doi: 10.1007/s00394-014-0766-0. PMID 25209031. S2CID 38095938.

Bach, K. K. E., (2001). The nutritional significance of "dietary fiber" analysis. Animal feed science and technology. *The Role of Dietary Fiber in Pig Production, 90*(1), 3–20. doi: 10.1016/S0377-8401(01)00193-6. ISSN 0377-8401.

Basen-Engquist, K., & Chang, M., (2011). Obesity and cancer risk: Recent review and evidence. *Current Oncology Reports, 13*(1), 71–76. doi: 10.1007/s11912-010-0139-7. PMC 3786180. PMID 21080117.

Bedford, A., & Gong, J., (2018). Implications of butyrate and its derivatives for gut health and animal production. *Animal Nutrition, 4*(2), 151–159. doi: 10.1016/j.aninu.2017.08.010. PMC 6104520. PMID 30140754.

Beydoun, M. A., Beydoun, H. A., & Wang, Y., (2008). Obesity and central obesity as risk factors for incident dementia and its subtypes: A systematic review and meta-analysis. *Obesity Reviews (Meta-Analysis), 9*(3), 204–218. doi: 10.1111/j.1467-789X.2008.00473.x. PMC 4887143. PMID 18331422.

Bigal, M. E., & Lipton, R. B., (2008). Obesity and chronic daily headache. *Current Pain and Headache Reports (Review), 12*(1), 56–61. doi: 10.1007/s11916-008-0011-8. PMID 18417025. S2CID 23729708.

Bleich, S., Cutler, D., Murray, C., & Adams, A., (2008). Why is the developed world obese? *Annual Review of Public Health (Research Support), 29*, 273–295. doi: 10.1146/annurev.publhealth.29.020907.090954. PMID 18173389.

Boerjan, W., Ralph, J., & Baucher, M., (2003). Lignin biosynthesis. *Annual Review of Plant Biology, 54,* 519–546. doi: 10.1146/annurev.arplant.54.031902.134938. PMID 14503002.

Brown, L., Rosner, B., Willett, W. W., & Sacks, F. M., (1999). Cholesterol–lowering effects of dietary fiber: A meta–analysis. *The American Journal of Clinical Nutrition, 69*(1), 30–42. doi: 10.1093/ajcn/69.1.30. PMID 9925120.

Burton-Freeman, B. (2000). Amgen, incorporated, thousand oaks, CA. *Symposium: Dietary Composition and Obesity: Do We Need to Look Beyond Dietary Fat?*

Caballero, B., (2001). Introduction. Symposium: Obesity in developing countries: Biological and ecological factors. *The Journal of Nutrition (Review), 131*(3), 866S–870S. doi: 10.1093/jn/131.3.866s. PMID 11238776.

Cavaglieri, C. R., Nishiyama, A., Fernandes, L. C., Curi, R., Miles, E. A., & Calder, P. C., (2003). Differential effects of short–chain fatty acids on proliferation and production of pro–and anti-inflammatory cytokines by cultured lymphocytes. *Life Sciences, 73*(13), 1683–1690. doi: 10.1016/S0024-3205(03)00490-9. PMID 12875900.

Chiles, C., & Van, W. P. J., (2010). Psychiatric aspects of the obesity crisis. *Psychiatr. Times. 27*(4), 47–51.

Chiolero, A., (2018). Why causality, and not prediction, should guide obesity prevention policy. *The Lancet Public Health, 3*(10), e461, e462. doi: 10.1016/S2468-2667(18)30158-0. ISSN 2468-2667. PMID 30177480.

Colquitt, J. L., Pickett, K., Loveman, E., & Frampton, G. K., (2014). Surgery for weight loss in adults. *The Cochrane Database of Systematic Reviews (Meta-Analysis, Review), 8*(8), CD003641. doi: 10.1002/14651858.CD003641.pub4. PMID 25105982.

Corona, G., Rastrelli, G., Filippi, S., Vignozzi, L., Mannucci, E., & Maggi, M., (2014). Erectile dysfunction and central obesity: An Italian perspective. *Asian Journal of Andrology, 16*(4), 581–591. doi: 10.4103/1008 82X.126386. PMC 4104087. PMID 24713832.

Coudray, C., Demigné, C., & Rayssiguier, Y., (2003). Effects of dietary fibers on magnesium absorption in animals and humans. *The Journal of Nutrition, 133*(1), 1–4. doi: 10.1093/jn/133.1.1. PMID 12514257.

Cox, L. M., & Blaser, M. J., (2015). Antibiotics in early life and obesity. *Nature Reviews Endocrinology, 11*(3), 182–190. doi: 10.1038/nrendo.2014.210. PMC 4487629. PMID 25488483.

Cummings, J. H., (2001). *The Effect of Dietary Fiber on Fecal Weight and Composition* (3rd edn., p. 184). Boca Raton, Florida: CRC Press. ISBN 978-0-8493-2387.

Darvall, K. A., Sam, R. C., Silverman, S. H., Bradbury, A. W., & Adam, D. J., (2007). Obesity and thrombosis. *European Journal of Vascular and Endovascular Surgery, 33*(2), 223–233. doi: 10.1016/j.ejvs.2006.10.006. PMID 17185009.

De Paepe, K., Verspreet, J., Courtin, C. M., & Van De, W. T., (2020). Microbial succession during wheat bran fermentation and colonization by human faecal microbiota as a result of niche diversification. *The ISME Journal, 14*(2), 584–596. doi: 10.1038/s41396-019-0550-5. PMC 6976558. PMID 31712738.

Dibaise, J. K., & Foxx-Orenstein, A. E., (2013). Role of the gastroenterologist in managing obesity. *Expert Review of Gastroenterology & Hepatology (Review), 7*(5), 439–451. doi: 10.1586/17474124.2013.811061. PMID 23899283. S2CID 26275773.

DiBaise, J. K., Zhang, H., Crowell, M. D., Krajmalnik-Brown, R., Decker, G. A., & Rittmann, B. E., (2008). Gut microbiota and its possible relationship with obesity. Mayo *Clinic Proceedings (Review), 83*(4), 460–469. doi: 10.4065/83.4.460. PMID 18380992.

Dietary Fiber: British Nutrition Foundation, (2018). Archived from the original.

Drozdowski, L. A., Dixon, W. T., McBurney, M. I., & Thomson, A. B., (2002). Short–chain fatty acids and total parenteral nutrition affect intestinal gene expression. *Journal of Parenteral and Enteral Nutrition, 26*(3), 145–150. doi: 10.1177/0148607102026003145. PMID 12005453.

Eastwood, M., & Kritchevsky, D., (2005). Dietary fiber: How did we get where we are? *Annual Review of Nutrition, 25*, 1–8. doi: 10.1146/annurev.nutr.25.121304.131658. PMID 16011456.

EFSA Panel on Dietetic Products, Nutrition, and Allergies (NDA); Scientific Opinion on Dietary Reference Values for carbohydrates and dietary fibre. EFSA Journal 2010; 8(3):1462 [77 pp.]. doi:10.2903/j.efsa.2010.1462. Available online: www.efsa.europa.eu.

Elaine, W., (2018). *FDA Unveils Dietary Fibers Guidance: Good News for Inulin, Polydextrose, Some Gray Areas Remaining*. FoodNavigatorUSA.com.

Ewaschuk, J. B., & Dieleman, L. A., (2006). Probiotics and prebiotics in chronic inflammatory bowel diseases. *World Journal of Gastroenterology, 12*(37), 5941–5950. doi: 10.3748/wjg.v12.i37.5941. PMC 4124400. PMID 17009391.

Falagas M. E., & Kompoti, M. (2006). Obesity and infection. *Lancet Infect Dis. 6*(7), 438–46. doi: 10.1016/S1473–3099(06)70523–0. PMID: 16790384.

Falagas, M. E., & Kompoti, M., (2006). Obesity and infection. *The Lancet*.

FDA/CFSAN: A Food Labeling Guide: Appendix C Health Claims, (2008). Wayb ack Machine.

Fiber, (2019). Linus Pauling Institute, Oregon State University.

Fischer, M. H., Yu, N., Gray, G. R., Ralph, J., Anderson, L., & Marlett, J. A., (2004). The gel–forming polysaccharide of psyllium husk (*Plantago ovata* Forsk). *Carbohydrate Research, 339*(11), 2009–2017. doi: 10.1016/j.carres.2004.05.023. PMID 15261594.

Flegal, K. M., Troiano, R. P., Pamuk, E. R., Kuczmarski, R. J., & Campbell, S. M., (1995). The influence of smoking cessation on the prevalence of overweight in the United States. *The New England Journal of Medicine, 333*(18), 1165–1170. doi: 10.1056/NEJM199511023331801. PMID 7565970.

Food and Nutrition Board, Institute of Medicine of the National Academies, (2005). *Dietary Reference Intakes for Energy, Carbohydrate, Fiber, Fat, Fatty Acids, Cholesterol, Protein, and Amino Acids (Macronutrients)* (pp. 380–382). National Academies Press.

Friedman, G., (1989). Nutritional therapy of irritable bowel syndrome. *Gastroenterology Clinics of North America, 18*(3), 513–524. PMID 2553606.

Gallaher, D. D., (2006). *Dietary Fiber* (pp. 102–110). Washington, D.C.: ILSI Press. ISBN 978-1-57881-199-1.

Gallaher, D. D., (2006). *Present Knowledge in Nutrition* (9 edn., pp. 102–110). Washington, D.C.: ILSI Press. ISBN 978-1-57881-199-1.

Gortmaker, S. L., Must, A., Sobol, A. M., Peterson, K., Colditz, G. A., & Dietz, W. H., (1996). Television viewing as a cause of increasing obesity among children in the United States, 1986–1990. *Archives of Pediatrics & Adolescent Medicine (Review), 150*(4), 356–362. doi: 10.1001/archpedi.1996.02170290022003. PMID 8634729.

Grabitske, H. A., & Slavin, J. L., (2009). Gastrointestinal effects of low–digestible carbohydrates. *Critical Reviews in Food Science and Nutrition, 49*(4), 327–360. doi: 10.1080/10408390802067126. PMID 19234944. S2CID 205689161.

Greger, J. L., (1999). Nondigestible carbohydrates and mineral bioavailability. *The Journal of Nutrition, 129*(7 Suppl), 1434S, 1435S. doi: 10.1093/jn/129.7.1434S. PMID 10395614.

Gropper, S. S., Smith, J. L., & Groff, J. L., (2008). *Advanced Nutrition and Human Metabolism* (5th edn., p. 114). Cengage Learning. ISBN 978-0-495-11657-8.

Guarner, F., (2005). Inulin and oligofructose: Impact on intestinal diseases and disorders. *The British Journal of Nutrition, 93*(1), S61–65. doi: 10.1079/BJN20041345. PMID 15877897.

Haslam, D. W., & James, W. P., (2005). Obesity. *Lancet (Review), 366*(9492), 1197–1209. doi: 10.1016/S0140-6736(05)67483-1. PMID 16198769. S2CID 208791491.

Health Claims: Fiber-Containing Grain Products, Fruits, and Vegetables and Cancer. Electronic Code of Federal Regulations: US Government Printing Office, current as of 20 October 2008.

Hellendoorn, E. W., (1983). Fermentation as the principal cause of the physiological activity of indigestible food residue. In: Spiller, G. A., (ed.), *Topics in Dietary Fiber Research* (pp. 127–168). Plenum Press, New York.

Hooper, B., Spiro, A., & Stanner, S., (2015). 30 g of fiber a day: An achievable recommendation?. *Nutrition Bulletin, 40*(2), 118–129. doi: 10.1111/nbu.12141.

Hunskaar, S., (2008). A systematic review of overweight and obesity as risk factors and targets for clinical intervention for urinary incontinence in women. *Neurourology and Urodynamics (Review), 27*(8), 749–757. doi: 10.1002/nau.20635. PMID 18951445. S2CID 20378183.

Imaz, I., Martínez-Cervell, C., García-Alvarez, E. E., Sendra-Gutiérrez, J. M., & González-Enríquez, J., (2008). Safety and effectiveness of the intragastric balloon for obesity. A meta–analysis. *Obesity Surgery, 18*(7), 841–846. doi: 10.1007/s11695-007-9331-8. PMID 18459025. S2CID 10220216.

Institute of Medicine, (2001). *Dietary Reference Intakes, Proposed Definition of Dietary Fiber* (p. 25). Washington, D.C.: Institute of Medicine Press. ISBN 978-0-309-07564-0.

Institute of Medicine, (2005). *Dietary Reference Intakes for Energy, Carbohydrate, Fiber, Fat, Fatty Acids, Cholesterol, Protein, and Amino Acids* (pp. 387, 388). Washington, DC: The National Academies Press. Retrieved 8 June 2021.

Institute of Medicine. 2005. Dietary Reference Intakes for Energy, Carbohydrate, Fiber, Fat, Fatty Acids, Cholesterol, Protein, and Amino Acids. Washington, DC: The National Academies Press. https://doi.org/10.17226/10490.

Jacob C. Seidell (2005). *Epidemiology of Obesity, 5*(1), 3–14. doi: 10.1055/s-2005–871737.

James, S., (2012). *P208 Abnormal Fiber Utilization and Gut Transit in Ulcerative Colitis in Remission: A Potential New Target for Dietary Intervention*. Presentation at European Crohn's & Colitis Organization meeting, Feb. 16–18, 2012 in Barcelona, Spain. European Crohn's & Colitis Organization.

Jarouliya, U., & Keservani, R. K., (2019). Pathways leading to child obesity. In: Debasis, B., (ed.), *Global Perspectives on Childhood Obesity: Current Status, Consequences and Prevention* (2nd edn., pp. 137–146). Academic Press, Elsevier, Chapter 12. ISBN: 9780128128404.

Jarouliya, U., & Keservani, R. K., (2019a). Protein function as cell surface and nuclear receptor in human diseases. In: Sanjay, B., & Debarshi, K. M., (eds.), *Medicinal Chemistry with Pharmaceutical Product Development* (pp. 1–32). Apple Academic Press, CRC Press, Taylor & Francis Group. Chapter 1. ISBN: 9781771887106.

Jensen, M. D., Ryan, D. H., Apovian, C. M., Ard, J. D., Comuzzie, A. G., Donato K. A., et al., (2023). American College of Cardiology/American Heart Association Task Force on Practice Guidelines; Obesity Society. 2013 AHA/ACC/TOS guideline for the management of overweight and obesity in adults: a report of the American College of Cardiology/American Heart Association Task Force on Practice Guidelines and The Obesity Society. Circulation. 2014 Jun 24; *129*(25 Suppl 2), S102–38. doi: 10.1161/01.cir.0000437739.71477.ee. Epub 2013 Nov 12. Erratum in: Circulation. 2014 Jun 24;*129*(25 Suppl 2), S139–40. PMID: 24222017; PMCID: PMC5819889.

Jha, R., & Mishra, P., (2021). Dietary fiber in poultry nutrition and their effects on nutrient utilization, performance, gut health, and on the environment: A review. *Journal of Animal Science and Biotechnology, 12*(1), 51. doi: 10.1186/s40104-021-00576-0. PMC 8054369. PMID 33866972.

Johnston, K. L., Thomas, E. L., Bell, J. D., Frost, G. S., & Robertson, M. D., (2010). Resistant starch improves insulin sensitivity in metabolic syndrome. *Diabetic Medicine, 27*(4), 391–397. doi: 10.1111/j.1464-5491.2010.02923.x. PMID 20536509. S2CID 27570039.

Kanazawa, M., Yoshiike, N., Osaka, T., Numba, Y., Zimmet, P., & Inoue, S., (2005). Criteria and classification of obesity in Japan and Asia-Oceania. Nutrition and fitness: Obesity, the metabolic syndrome, cardiovascular disease, and cancer. *World Review of Nutrition and Dietetics, 94,* 1–12. doi: 10.1159/000088200. ISBN 978-3-8055-7944-5. PMID 16145245. S2CID 19963495.

Kassotis, C. D., Vandenberg, L. N., Demeneix, B. A., Porta, M., Slama, R., & Trasande, L., (2020). Endocrine-disrupting chemicals: Economic, regulatory, and policy implications. *The Lancet Diabetes & Endocrinology, 8*(8), 719–730. doi: 10.1016/S2213-8587(20)30128-5. ISSN 2213-8587. PMC 7437819. PMID 32707119.

Kaur, N., & Gupta, A. K., (2002). Applications of inulin and oligofructose in health and nutrition (PDF). *Journal of Biosciences, 27*(7), 703–714.

Keenan, M. J., Martin, R. J., Raggio, A. M., McCutcheon, K. L., Brown, I. L., Birkett, A., et al., (2012). High-amylose resistant starch increases hormones and improves structure and function of the gastrointestinal tract: A microarray study. *Journal of Nutrigenetics and Nutrigenomics, 5*(1), 26–44. doi: 10.1159/000335319. PMC 4030412. PMID 22516953.

Keenan, M. J., Zhou, J., Hegsted, M., Pelkman, C., Durham, H. A., Coulon, D. B., & Martin, R. J., (2015). Role of resistant starch in improving gut health, adiposity, and insulin resistance. *Advances in Nutrition, 6*(2), 198–205. doi: 10.3945/an.114.007419. PMC 4352178. PMID 25770258.

Keservani, R. K., Kesharwani, R. K., & Sharma, A. K. (2015). Pulmonary and respiratory health: Antioxidants and nutraceuticals. In: Debasis, B., Harry, G. P., & Anand, S., (eds.), *Nutraceutical and Functional Foods in Human Life and Disease Prevention* (pp. 279–295). Boca Raton, Fl. CRC Press, Taylor and Francis, Chapter 17.

Keservani, R. K., Kesharwani, R. K., Sharma, A. K., Vyas, N., & Chadoker, A., (2010b). Nutritional supplements: An overview. *International Journal of Current Pharmaceutical Review and Research, 1*(1), 59–75.

Keservani, R. K., Kesharwani, R. K., Vyas, N., Jain, S., Raghuvanshi, R., & Sharma, A. K., (2010a). Nutraceutical and functional food as future food: A review. *Der Pharmacia Letter, 2*(1), 106–116.

Keservani, R. K., Sharma, A. K., & Kesharwani, R. K., (2016a). Nutraceutical and functional foods for cardiovascular health. In: *Food Process Engineering* (pp. 257–278, 291–312). Apple Academic Press, CRC Press. ISBN: 9781771884020.

Keservani, R. K., Sharma, A. K., & Kesharwani, R. K., (2016b). Medicinal effect of nutraceutical fruits for the cognition and brain health. *Scientifica,* 10. Article ID 3109254. doi: 10.1155/2016/3109254.

Keservani, R. K., Sharma, A. K., & Kesharwani, R. K., (2020). *Nutraceuticals and Dietary Supplements: Applications in Health Improvement and Disease Management*. CRC Press. ISBN: 9781771888738.

Lau, D. C., Douketis, J. D., Morrison, K. M., Hramiak, I. M., Sharma, A. M., & Ur, E., (2007). 2006 Canadian clinical practice guidelines on the management and prevention of obesity in adults and children [summary]. *CMAJ (Practice Guideline, Review), 176*(8), S1–13. doi: 10.1503/cmaj.061409. PMC 1839777. PMID 17420481.

Lee, Y. P., Puddey, I. B., & Hodgson, J. M., (2008). Protein, fiber and blood pressure: Potential benefit of legumes. *Clinical and Experimental Pharmacology & Physiology, 35*(4), 473–476. doi: 10.1111/j.1440-1681.2008.04899.x. PMID 18307744. S2CID 25086200.

Liber, A., & Szajewska, H., (2013). Effects of inulin-type fructans on appetite, energy intake, and body weight in children and adults: Systematic review of randomized controlled trials. *Annals of Nutrition & Metabolism, 63*(1, 2), 42–54. doi: 10.1159/000350312. PMID 23887189.

Lockyer, S., & Nugent, A. P., (2017). Health effects of resistant starch. *Nutrition Bulletin, 42*, 10–41. doi: 10.1111/nbu.12244.

Lu, Y., Hajifathalian, K., Ezzati, M., Woodward, M., Rimm, E. B., & Danaei, G., (2014). Metabolic mediators of the effects of body-mass index, overweight, and obesity on coronary heart disease and stroke: A pooled analysis of 97 prospective cohorts with 1·8 million participants. *Lancet, 383*(9921), 970–983. doi: 10.1016/S0140-6736(13)61836-X. PMC 3959199. PMID 24269108.

Ludwig, D. S., & Ebbeling, C. B., (2018). The carbohydrate-insulin model of obesity: Beyond calories in, calories out. *JAMA Internal Medicine, 178*(8), 1098. doi: 10.1001/jamainternmed.2018.2933. PMC 6082688.

Luppino, F. S., De Wit, L. M., Bouvy, P. F., Stijnen, T., Cuijpers, P., Penninx, B. W., & Zitman, F. G., (2010). Overweight, obesity, and depression: A systematic review and meta-analysis of longitudinal studies. *Archives of General Psychiatry, 67*(3), 220–229. doi: 10.1001/archgenpsychiatry.2010.2. PMID 20194822.

MacDermott, R. P., (2007). Treatment of irritable bowel syndrome in outpatients with inflammatory bowel disease using a food and beverage intolerance, food and beverage avoidance diet. *Inflammatory Bowel Diseases, 13*(1), 91–96. doi: 10.1002/ibd.20048. PMID 17206644. S2CID 24307163.

Maki, K. C., Pelkman, C. L., Finocchiaro, E. T., Kelley, K. M., Lawless, A. L., Schild, A. L., & Rains, T. M., (2012). Resistant starch from high-amylose maize increases insulin sensitivity in overweight and obese men. *The Journal of Nutrition, 142*(4), 717–723. doi: 10.3945/jn.111.152975. PMC 3301990. PMID 22357745.

Maragkoudakis, P., (2017). *Dietary Fiber*. EU Science Hub. Joint Research Center.

Matthew Weinstock (2013). *The Facts About Obesity*. H & HN. American Hospital Association.

Molenaar, E. A., Numans, M. E., Van, A. E. J., & Grobbee, D. E., (2008). [Considerable comorbidity in overweight adults: Results from the Utrecht Health Project]. *Nederlands Tijdschrift Voor Geneeskunde (English abstract) (in Dutch), 152*(45), 2457–2463. PMID 19051798.

Munger, K. L., Chitnis, T., & Ascherio, A., (2009). Body size and risk of MS in two cohorts of US women. *Neurology (Comparative Study), 73*(19), 1543–1550. doi: 10.1212/WNL.0b013e3181c0d6e0. PMC 2777074. PMID 19901245.

Ness-Abramof, R., & Apovian, C. M., (2006). Diet modification for treatment and prevention of obesity. *Endocrine (Review), 29*(1), 5–9. doi: 10.1385/ENDO:29:1:135. PMID 16622287. S2CID 31964889.

Obesity and Overweight, (2008). World Health Organization. Archived from the original on 18 December 2008.

Obesity and Overweight, (2009). World Health Organization.

Parisi, G. C., Zilli, M., Miani, M. P., Carrara, M., Bottona, E., Verdianelli, G., et al., (2002). High-fiber diet supplementation in patients with irritable bowel syndrome (IBS): A multicenter, randomized, open trial comparison between wheat bran diet and partially hydrolyzed guar gum (PHGG). *Digestive Diseases and Sciences, 47*(8), 1697–1704. doi: 10.1023/A:1016419906546. PMID 12184518. S2CID 27545330.

Park, Y., Subar, A. F., Hollenbeck, A., & Schatzkin, A., (2011). Dietary fiber intake and mortality in the NIH-AARP diet and health study. *Archives of Internal Medicine, 171*(12), 1061–1068. doi: 10.1001/archinternmed.2011.18. PMC 3513325. PMID 21321288.

Phillips, G. O., (2013). Dietary fiber: A chemical category or a health ingredient? *Bioactive Carbohydrates and Dietary Fiber, 1*(1), 3–9. doi: 10.1016/j.bcdf.2012.12.001. ISSN 2212-6198.

Phillips, J., Muir, J. G., Birkett, A., Lu, Z. X., Jones, G. P., O'Dea, K., & Young, G. P., (1995). Effect of resistant starch on fecal bulk and fermentation-dependent events in humans. *The American Journal of Clinical Nutrition, 62*(1), 121–130. doi: 10.1093/ajcn/62.1.121. PMID 7598054.

Poirier, P., Giles, T. D., Bray, G. A., Hong, Y., Stern, J. S., Pi-Sunyer, F. X., & Eckel, R. H., (2006). Obesity and cardiovascular disease: Pathophysiology, evaluation, and effect of weight loss. *Arteriosclerosis, Thrombosis, and Vascular Biology (Review), 26*(5), 968–976.

CiteSeerX 10.1.1.508.7066. doi: 10.1161/01.ATV.0000216787.85457.f3. PMID 16627822. S2CID 6052584.

Pollack, A., (2013). A.M.A. *Recognizes Obesity as a Disease*. The New York Times. Archived from the original on 24 June 2013.

Prescrire.org (2018). Antibiotics during infancy: a risk factor for obesity? *Prescrire Int., 27*(194), 155–157.

Raghupathy, P., Ramakrishna, B. S., Oommen, S. P., Ahmed, M. S., Priyaa, G., Dziura, J., et al., (2006). Amylase-resistant starch as adjunct to oral rehydration therapy in children with diarrhea. *Journal of Pediatric Gastroenterology and Nutrition, 42*(4), 362–368. doi: 10.1097/01.mpg.0000214163.83316.41. PMID 16641573. S2CID 4647366.

Ramakrishna, B. S., Subramanian, V., Mohan, V., Sebastian, B. K., Young, G. P., Farthing, M. J., & Binder, H. J., (2008). A randomized controlled trial of glucose versus amylase resistant starch hypo-osmolar oral rehydration solution for adult acute dehydrating diarrhea. *PLOS One, 3*(2), e1587. Bibcode:2008PLoSO.3.1587R. doi: 10.1371/journal.pone.0001587. PMC 2217593. PMID 18270575.

Ramakrishna, B. S., Venkataraman, S., Srinivasan, P., Dash, P., Young, G. P., & Binder, H. J., (2000). Amylase-resistant starch plus oral rehydration solution for cholera. *The New England Journal of Medicine, 342*(5), 308–313. doi: 10.1056/NEJM200002033420502. PMID 10655529.

Raschka, L., & Daniel, H., (2005). Mechanisms underlying the effects of inulin-type fructans on calcium absorption in the large intestine of rats. *Bone, 37*(5), 728–735. doi: 10.1016/j.bone.2005.05.015. PMID 16126464.

Reynolds, A., Mann, J., Cummings, J., Winter, N., Mete, E., & Te Morenga, L., (2019). Carbohydrate quality and human health: A series of systematic reviews and meta-analyses. *Lancet, 393*(10170), 434–445. doi: 10.1016/S0140-6736(18)31809-9. PMID 30638909. S2CID 58632705.

Roberfroid, M. B., (2007). Inulin-type fructans: Functional food ingredients. *The Journal of Nutrition, 137*(11 Suppl), 2493S–2502S. doi: 10.1093/jn/137.11.2493S. PMID 17951492.

Robertson, M. D., Bickerton, A. S., Dennis, A. L., Vidal, H., & Frayn, K. N., (2005). Insulin-sensitizing effects of dietary resistant starch and effects on skeletal muscle and adipose tissue metabolism. *The American Journal of Clinical Nutrition, 82*(3), 559–567. doi: 10.1093/ajcn.82.3.559. PMID 16155268.

Robertson, M. D., Currie, J. M., Morgan, L. M., Jewell, D. P., & Frayn, K. N., (2003). Prior short-term consumption of resistant starch enhances postprandial insulin sensitivity in healthy subjects. *Diabetologia, 46*(5), 659–665. doi: 10.1007/s00125-003-1081-0. PMID 12712245.

Robertson, M. D., Wright, J. W., Loizon, E., Debard, C., Vidal, H., Shojaee-Moradie, F., et al., (2012). Insulin-sensitizing effects on muscle and adipose tissue after dietary fiber intake in men and women with metabolic syndrome. *The Journal of Clinical Endocrinology and Metabolism, 97*(9), 3326–3332. doi: 10.1210/jc.2012-1513. PMID 22745235.

Rodríguez-Cabezas, M. E., Gálvez, J., Camuesco, D., Lorente, M. D., Concha, A., Martinez-Augustin, O., et al., (2003). Intestinal anti-inflammatory activity of dietary fiber (*Plantago ovata* seeds) in HLA-B27 transgenic rats. *Clinical Nutrition, 22*(5), 463–471. doi: 10.1016/S0261-5614(03)00045-1. PMID 14512034.

Rosén, T., Bosaeus, I., Tölli, J., Lindstedt, G., & Bengtsson, B. A., (1993). Increased body fat mass and decreased extracellular fluid volume in adults with growth hormone deficiency.

Clinical Endocrinology, 38(1), 63–71. doi: 10.1111/j.1365-2265.1993.tb00974.x. PMID 8435887. S2CID 25725625.

Rosin, P. M., Lajolo, F. M., & Menezes, E. W., (2002). Measurement and characterization of dietary starches. *Journal of Food Composition and Analysis, 15*(4), 367–377. doi: 10.1006/jfca.2002.1084. ISSN 0889–1575.

Saemann, M. D., Bohmig, G. A., & Zlabinger, G. J., (2002). Short-chain fatty acids: Bacterial mediators of a balanced host-microbial relationship in the human gut. *Wiener Klinische Wochenschrift, 114*(8, 9), 289–300. PMID 12212362.

Salmon, J., & Timperio, A., (2007). Prevalence, trends and environmental influences on child and youth physical activity. Pediatric fitness (review). *Medicine and Sport Science, 50,* 183–199. doi: 10.1159/000101391. ISBN 978-3-318-01396-2. PMID 17387258.

Sara Berg, M. S., (2023). *Foods That Spike a Patient's Blood Glucose are Not What You Think.* American Medical Association.

Scholz-Ahrens, K. E., & Schrezenmeir, J., (2007). Inulin and oligofructose and mineral metabolism: The evidence from animal trials. *The Journal of Nutrition, 137*(11 Suppl), 2513S–2523S. doi: 10.1093/jn/137.11.2513S. PMID 17951495.

Search, USDA Food Composition Databases, (2015). Nutrient Data Laboratory. USDA National Nutrient Database, US Department of Agriculture, Standard Release 28.

Seidner, D. L., Lashner, B. A., Brzezinski, A., Banks, P. L., Goldblum, J., Fiocchi, C., et al., (2005). An oral supplement enriched with fish oil, soluble fiber, and antioxidants for corticosteroid sparing in ulcerative colitis: A randomized, controlled trial. *Clinical Gastroenterology and Hepatology, 3*(4), 358–369. doi: 10.1016/S1542-3565(04)00672-X. PMID 15822041.

Sharifi-Mollayousefi, A., Yazdchi-Marandi, M., Ayramlou, H., Heidari, P., Salavati, A., Zarrintan, S., & Sharifi-Mollayousefi, A., (2008). Assessment of body mass index and hand anthropometric measurements as independent risk factors for carpal tunnel syndrome. *Folia Morphologica, 67*(1), 36–42. PMID 18335412.

Shepherd, S. J., & Gibson, P. R., (2006). Fructose malabsorption and symptoms of irritable bowel syndrome: Guidelines for effective dietary management. *Journal of the American Dietetic Association, 106*(10), 1631–1639. doi: 10.1016/j.jada.2006.07.010. PMID 17000196.

Soluble Fiber from Certain Foods and Risk of Coronary Heart Disease, U.S. Government Printing Office, Electronic Code of Federal Regulations, Title 21: Food and Drugs, Part 101: Food Labeling, Subpart E, Specific Requirements for Health Claims, 101.81 [1] June 2008.

Stacewicz-Sapuntzakis, M., Bowen, P. E., Hussain, E. A., Damayanti-Wood, B. I., & Farnsworth, N. R., (2001). Chemical composition and potential health effects of prunes: A functional food?. *Critical Reviews in Food Science and Nutrition, 41*(4), 251–286. doi: 10.1080/20014091091814. PMID 11401245. S2CID 31159565.

Suter, P. M., (2005). Carbohydrates and dietary fiber. Atherosclerosis: Diet and drugs. *Handbook of Experimental Pharmacology, 170*, 231–261. doi: 10.1007/3-540-27661-0_8. ISBN 978-3-540-22569-0. PMID 16596802.

Tako, E., Glahn, R. P., Welch, R. M., Lei, X., Yasuda, K., & Miller, D. D., (2008). Dietary inulin affects the expression of intestinal enterocyte iron transporters, receptors and storage protein and alters the microbiota in the pig intestine. *The British Journal of Nutrition, 99*(3), 472–480. doi: 10.1017/S0007114507825128. PMID 17868492.

Theuwissen, E., & Mensink, R. P., (2008). Water-soluble dietary fibers and cardiovascular disease. *Physiology & Behavior, 94*(2), 285–292. doi: 10.1016/j.physbeh.2008.01.001. PMID 18302966. S2CID 30898446.

Tucker, L. A., & Bagwell, M., (1991). Television viewing and obesity in adult females. *American Journal of Public Health, 81*(7), 908–911. doi: 10.2105/AJPH.81.7.908. PMC 1405200. PMID 2053671.

Tukker, A., Visscher, T. L., & Picavet, H. S., (2009). Overweight and health problems of the lower extremities: Osteoarthritis, pain and disability. Public Health Nutrition (Research Support), *12*(3), 359–368. doi: 10.1017/S1368980008002103. PMID 18426630.

Tungland, B. C., & Meyer, D., (2002). Nondigestible oligo- and polysaccharides (dietary fiber): Their physiology and role in human health and food. *Comprehensive Reviews in Food Science and Food Safety, 1*(3), 73–92. doi: 10.1111/j.1541-4337.2002.tb00009.x. PMID 33451232.

Veronese, N., Solmi, M., Caruso, M. G., Giannelli, G., Osella, A. R., Evangelou, E., et al., (2018). Dietary fiber and health outcomes: An umbrella review of systematic reviews and meta-analyses. *The American Journal of Clinical Nutrition, 107*(3), 436–444. doi: 10.1093/ajcn/nqx082. PMID 29566200.

Vioque, J., Torres, A., & Quiles, J., (2000). Time spent watching television, sleep duration and obesity in adults living in Valencia, Spain. *International Journal of Obesity and Related Metabolic Disorders (Research Support), 24*(12), 1683–1688. doi: 10.1038/sj.ijo.0801434. PMID 11126224.

Wall, M., (2008). Idiopathic intracranial hypertension (pseudotumor cerebri). *Current Neurology and Neuroscience Reports (Review), 8*(2), 87–93. doi: 10.1007/s11910-008-0015-0. PMID 18460275. S2CID 17285706.

Ward, P. B., & Young, G. P., (1997). Dynamics of Clostridium difficile infection. Control using diet. *Advances in Experimental Medicine and Biology, 412*, 63–75. doi: 10.1007/978-1-4899-1828-4_8. ISBN 978-1-4899-1830-7. PMID 9191992.

Weickert, M. O., & Pfeiffer, A. F., (2008). Metabolic effects of dietary fiber consumption and prevention of diabetes. *The Journal of Nutrition, 138*(3), 439–442. doi: 10.1093/jn/138.3.439. PMID 18287346.

WHO. *Physical Inactivity: A Global Public Health Problem.* World Health Organization.

Williams, B. A., Oostdam, A. J., Groot, J. C., Boer, H., & Tamminga, S., (2000). Effects of ageing on the *in vitro* fermentation of cell walls and cell contents of entire, fractionated and composite leaves of Italian ryegrass. *Journal of the Science of Food and Agriculture, 80*(4), 484–490. doi: 10.1002/(SICI)1097-0010(200003)80:4<484::AID-JSFA554>3.0.CO;2-Y. ISSN 1097-0010.

Wong, J. M., De Souza, R., Kendall, C. W., Emam, A., & Jenkins, D. J., (2006). Colonic health: Fermentation and short chain fatty acids. *Journal of Clinical Gastroenterology, 40*(3), 235–243. doi: 10.1097/00004836-200603000-00015. PMID 16633129. S2CID 46228892.

World Health Organization (2014). Obesity and Overweight. Fact Sheet No. 311. http://www.who.int/mediacentre/factsheets/fs311/en/.

Yanovski, S. Z., & Yanovski, J. A., (2014). Long-term drug treatment for obesity: A systematic and clinical review. *JAMA (Review), 311*(1), 74–86. doi: 10.1001/jama.2013.281361. PMC 3928674. PMID 24231879.

Yazdi, F. T., Clee, S. M., & Meyre, D., (2015). Obesity genetics in mouse and human: Back and forth, and back again. *PeerJ., 3*, e856. doi: 10.7717/peerj.856. PMC 4375971. PMID 25825681.

Zhang, W. Q., Wang, H. W., Zhang, Y. M., & Yang, Y. X., (2007). [Effects of resistant starch on insulin resistance of type 2 diabetes mellitus patients]. *Zhonghua Yu Fang Yi Xue Za Zhi [Chinese Journal of Preventive Medicine] (in Chinese), 41*(2), 101–104. PMID 17605234.

CHAPTER 5

ROLE OF DIETARY FIBER IN CORONARY HEART DISEASE (CHD)

ASHISH A. KARLE,[1] BHUSHAN R. RANE,[1] JAYVADAN K. PATEL,[2] NAYAN A. GUJARATHI,[3] HITENDRA S. MAHAJAN,[4] RAJ K. KESERVANI,[5] and RAMSANEH RAGHUWANSHI[6]

[1]*Shri D.D. Vispute College of Pharmacy and Research Center, Panvel, Maharashtra, India*

[2]*Department of Pharmaceutics, Nootan College of Pharmacy, Visnagar, Gujarat, India*

[3]*Department of Pharmaceutics, Shri Vile Parle Kelvani Mandal's Institute of Pharmacy, Dhule, Maharashtra, India*

[4]*Department of Pharmaceutics, R. C. Patel, Institute of Pharmaceutical Education and Research, Shirpur, Maharashtra, India*

[5]*Faculty of B. Pharmacy, CSM Group of Institutions, Prayagraj, Uttar Pradesh, India*

[6]*Professor, Department of Pharmaceutical Chemistry, Corporate Institute of Pharmacy, Bhopal, Madhya Pradesh, India*

ABSTRACT

The purpose of this review is to study the role of dietary fiber in coronary heart disease (CHD). Excessive LDL cholesterol, low HDL cholesterol, high blood pressure, family records, diabetes, smoking are the chance

Food Supplements and Dietary Fiber in Health and Disease. Bhushan R. Rane, Raj K. Keservani, Durgesh Singh, Nayan A. Gujarathi, and Ashish S. Jain, (Eds.)
© 2024 Apple Academic Press, Inc. Co-published with CRC Press (Taylor & Francis)

factors for CHD. Nutritional fibers are not digested by humans however they have a sequence of metabolic health advantages. Soluble and Insoluble are two major kinds of nutritional fiber. From these kinds of soluble dietary fiber is beneficial in the control of Coronary heart ailment. Soluble fiber assists lower general blood cholesterol levels by using lowering low-density lipoprotein, or "bad," levels of cholesterol. Studies additionally have proven that excessive-fiber meals may additionally produce other coronary heart health advantages, such as decreasing blood strain and irritation. Diverse mechanisms suggested with the aid of scientists which depends at the metabolic stage, dietary fiber, slows down gastric emptying and intestinal transit, decreases the price of intestinal carbohydrate absorption, and increases fecal bile acid excretion. Observational epidemiological evidence consistently demonstrates lower incidence of CHD and other long-term diseases among those with the highest intake of fruits, vegetables, and grains. Such a dietary pattern appears to offer protective effects that transcend lipid lowering and overall is typically lower in total fat, saturated fat, and cholesterol.

5.1 INTRODUCTION

5.1.1 CORONARY HEART DISEASE AND DIETARY FIBER

CHD is a type of heart disease in which coronary arteries, which are involved in supplying blood to the heart, get blocked due to the deposition of fatty material. CHD or coronary arteries disease, develops when the coronary arteries grow to be too slender that is narrow in size. It is due to low density lipoprotein (LDH) cholesterol blockages broadening withinside of the walls. The coronary arteries are the type of blood vessels that deliver oxygen and blood to the heart. CHD tends to increase the LDL cholesterol builds up at the artery partitions, developing plaques. These plaques reason the arteries to narrow, decreasing blood flow to the coronary artery or can reason infection in and hardening of the partitions of the blood vessel. A clot can occasionally impede blood flow, inflicting severe fitness problems. Coronary arteries are the main source which provides blood to the heart that feeds it oxygen. If those arteries narrow, the heart might not acquire sufficient oxygen-rich blood, specifically all through bodily activity (Figure 5.1).

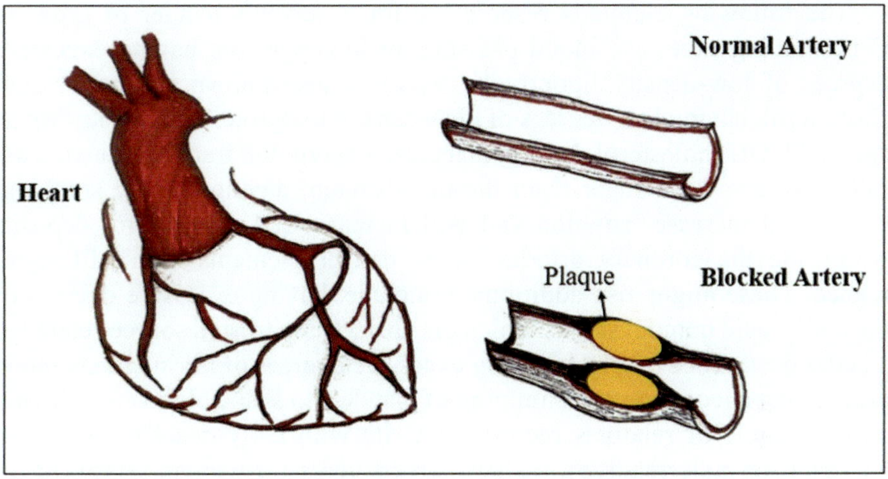

FIGURE 5.1 Diagrammatic representation of normal and blocked artery.

CHD develops due to the damage or harm to the internal layer of a coronary artery. This harm reasons fatty deposits of plaque to accumulate on the damaged site. These deposits encompass LDL cholesterol and different inflammatory merchandise from cells. This buildup is referred to as atherosclerosis. If portions of plaque spoil off or rupture, platelets will cluster withinside the region in an artery and restore the blood vessel. This cluster can block the artery and decrease or block blood flow, which can also additionally cause a coronary heart attack (Bingham et al., 2009) (Figure 5.2).

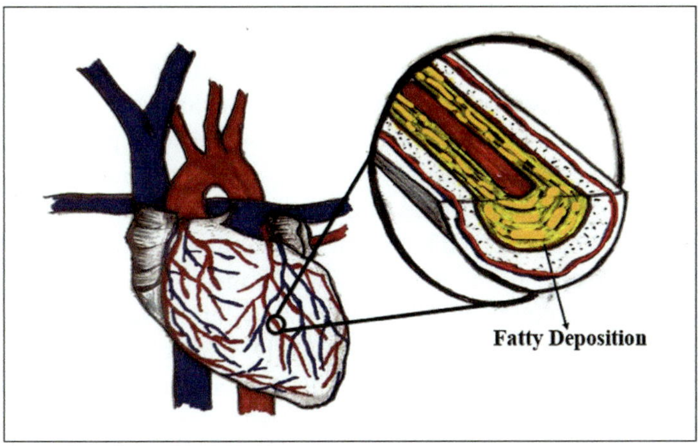

FIGURE 5.2 Fatty deposition narrowing the coronary artery.

The following elements responsible for a person's danger of growing CHD; having excessive blood pressure, or hypertension, having excessive degrees of low-density lipoprotein, which is also known as "bad," LDL cholesterol, having low degrees of high-density lipoprotein, which known as "good," HDL cholesterol, having diabetes, wherein the frame can't successfully take away the sugar from the bloodstream, having obesity smoking, which will increase irritation and will increase LDL cholesterol deposits withinside the coronary arteries Some danger elements aren't lifestyle-related. These might also additionally include: having excessive degrees of the amino acid homocysteine, which one 2015 study trusted source related to a better occurrence of CHD, having excessive degrees of fibrinogen, a blood protein that encourages the clumping of platelets to shape blood clots having an own circle of relatives records of CHD with early-onset (earlier than 55 years for male relatives, earlier than 65 years for woman relatives) for women, having been via untimely menopause. For men, being over 45 years of age having excessive degrees of lipoprotein mainly is likewise related to a better danger of cardiovascular disease. Trusted Source and CHD is a study of how the food regimen can lessen the danger of CHD.

Dietary fiber (Keservani et al., 2010a, b, 2020) which is found in particular in fruits, vegetables, whole grains, and legumes might be well recognized for its cap potential to save you or relieve constipation. But meals containing fiber can offer different fitness advantages as well, which include supporting to keep a healthful weight and reducing your danger of diabetes, coronary heart disorder, and risk of cancer. Selecting meals that have fiber isn't always difficult. It is necessary to find out how nutritional fiber you need, the meals that incorporate it, and a way to upload them to food and snacks. Additionally, dietary fiber referred to as roughage or bulk consists of the elements of plants that cannot digest or absorb by a human. Unlike different meals components, which include fats, proteins, or carbohydrates which your break down and absorb fiber isn't always digested by the body. Instead, it passes particularly intact through your stomach, small intestine, and colon and from your body.

CHD is one of the main causes of mortality yearly around 610,000 deaths in the U.S. are because of CHD. Now it's becoming one of the major causes of mortality across the globe which shows 78 million deaths in a year. This disease is mainly related to existence lifestyle. Many researchers studied and concluded that dietary fiber is useful in CHD. Dietary fiber is not digested through the human digestive system but its metabolic characteristic assists in decreasing LDL cholesterol, increasing suitable HDL cholesterol, lowering blood pressure (Crowe et al., 2012).

5.1.2 HUMAN DIETS' FIBER CONTENT

On the indication of very general, records on the distribution of fiber consumption are one of a kind establishments, the idea that dietary fiber can be a protective thing in human health. There is still a lack of correct information, and to be had estimates will nearly in reality alternate as technologies for figuring out meals consumption and fiber content material enhance. On average fiber intake in Western nations, current facts are available. Kay, Sabry, and Cosima observed that suggest nutritional fiber consumption changed into 19 gm/day in a pattern of 200 Canadian guys, with cereal-derived fiber accounting for nearly half of it. Bingham, Cummings, and McNeil, as well as Southgate, Bingham, and Robertson, located that normal nutritional fiber consumption for both women and men in round 20 gm/day in special investigations in England. Similar results were discovered in American facts primarily based on items on hand for intake, indicating a popular drop-in available nutritional fiber, particularly cereal-derived fiber. In evaluation to folks who ate numerous weight-reduction plans, vegetarians in the United Kingdom fed on two times as much fiber (Bingham et al., 2009).

5.1.3 CLASSIFICATION AND DIFFERENT TYPES OF DIETARY FIBER

- **Plant:**
  - Cellulose;
  - Non-cellulose(*example:* hemicellulosepectingumnon-carbohydrate). *Example:* Lignin.
- **Animal and Microbial Origin:**
  Example: Xanthan gum chitin.
  Structure and solubility are two characteristics that can be used to classify dietary fibers. Polysaccharides are classified as linear or nonlinear molecules based on their structure. They can also be classified as soluble or insoluble based on their solubility in water (Table 5.1).

TABLE 5.1 Examples of Water Soluble and Water Insoluble of Dietary Fibers

Water Soluble Dietary Fibers	Water Insoluble Dietary Fibers
Mucilages	Cutin
Gums	Lignin
Hemi cellulose	Cutin cellulose
Pectins	–

- **Dietary Fiber Soluble:** It is a dietary substance that is not digested by the enzymes and is soluble in warm (or) hot water but precipitates when combined with 4 parts ethyl alcohol. Gums are polysaccharides with complicated structures. Because they are largely indigestible, they are not part of the cell wall structure. Although a tiny proportion may be insoluble, it is present in soluble form. Unbranched-1,4 connected D-glucose units are interspersed with beta-1,3-linkages in these glucose polymers. Barley, rye, and oats have the largest concentrations.
  Pectins are polymer compounds made up of D-glucuronic acid polymers connected by 1,4 links. Sugars like galactose, arabinose, and glucose make up the side chains of the primary polymer. Pectins are mostly water-soluble, with solubility varying depending on the degree of esterification of galacturonic acid and the composition of component side chains. The inclusion of calcium salts increases gelling capability while reducing reliance on pH and sugar concentration. Because of its ion exchange and gelling properties due to the presence of galacturonic acid units, pectin is an important component of dietary fiber.
- **Dietary Fiber (Insoluble):**
- **Cellulose:** It is very less soluble in all-fiber; it is insoluble not only in cold or hot water but also in hot dilute acid and alkaline solutions, also cellulose, the principal cell wall structural linear conformation with a high grade of inter molecule H-bonding. Only powerful mineral acids and cellulose enzymes are capable of breaking the glycosidic bond between 1,4-linkages of glucose units. The human digestive system does not hydrate cellulose, which makes it a genuinely accessible carbohydrate. Microcrystalline cellulose is produced by acid hydrolysis of the amorphous portion. Cellulose is used as a bulky agent in food due to its water-absorbing ability and less solubility.
- **Hemicellulose:** It is a type of polysaccharide that contains branching and liner pentose and Hexose. It may be found in both soluble and insoluble forms. Pentosons are soluble hemicelluloses found in wheat grains. Hemicellulose is a weak alkaline solution. Xylose, arabinose, galactose, glucose, mannose, glucuronic acid, and galacturonic acid are examples of component monosaccharide units. In food items, both soluble and insoluble hemicelluloses play a vital role, with the former operating as SDF and IDF. Their capacity to bind water and function as a bulking agent distinguishes them. In the colon, hemicellulose is fermented to a larger extent than cellulose.

- **Lignin:** It is an amorphous, extremely water-insoluble polymeric substance made up of phenyl propane residues arranged in a matrix by condensation of phenolic alcohols such coniferyl, sinapyl, and p-coumaric. Lignin can bind bile salts and other organic matter, which can slow or prevent the absorption of nutrients in the small intestine.
- **Cutin and Plant Waxes:** These are hydrophobic lipid compounds present in the structure of plants and are closely related to structural polysaccharides. These are often present in very modest amounts.

5.1.4 DIETARY FIBER ADVANTAGES

1. **Digestion:** As insoluble fiber moves through the digestive tract, it binds to water, making feces softer and bulkier. Constipation, hemorrhoids, and diverticulosis may additionally all be handled and prevented with fiber, which may be observed in whole grain.
2. **LDL Cholesterol:** Low blood cholesterol levels have been related to a decreased hazard of coronary artery disease. Cholesterol is used by the body to make bile acids, that are removed on an ordinary basis. Due to the fact water-soluble fiber binds to bile acids, an excessive fiber diet can also bring about improved cholesterol excretion. Few fibers seem to have a more potent impact than others. The fiber in rolled oats is extra effective than the fiber in wheat at lowering blood levels of cholesterol.
3. **Reduce the Risk of Cancer:** Excessive-fiber diets may additionally lower the risk of a few cancers, consisting of colon cancer. Insoluble fiber complements the pace at which wastes are removed from the body, in accordance to analyze this could suggest that the body is much less explosive to risky compounds launched throughout digestion. Fiber ingestion might also decrease most cancers risk, although the mechanism is uncertain (Fahey et al., 2002).
4. **Weight Loss:** Individuals who need to shed pounds may discover that high-fiber diets are useful. Because of its propensity to take in water, fiber has no energy however produces a full sensation (Bingham et al., 2009).
5. **Diabetes and Weight Problems:** Recent research shows that consuming a high-fiber, whole-grain weight loss plan lowers the danger of obtaining type 2 diabetes and weight problems. Expanded

intake of fiber present in complete grains, rather than delicate grains, has been tested to lower the glycemic index and enhance insulin sensitivity, decreasing the chance of kind 2 diabetes and weight problems (Evans et al., 2017).

5.2 FOOD REGIMEN AND CORONARY HEART DISEASE

CHD can fade over the years, emphasizing the necessity of keeping a balanced diet. Plaque improvement in the arteries can restrict blood glide to the coronary heart symptoms like chest soreness and shortness of breath are due to a decline in blood flow. If CHD, left untreated, can result in a coronary heart attack or surprising cardiac arrest. Each of those disorders can be fatal. Medicine assists us to keep away from widespread issues. A beta-blocker may be prescribed to lower blood pressure, in addition to a medicinal drug to open arteries and allow blood to go with the flow. Plant-based totally diets can help lessen coronary heart disorder, coronary heart attacks, and unexpected cardiac arrest by way of increasing your intake of those foods which are excessive in nutrients and minerals, which assist to keep our heart risk free from disease also, that food which has low energy, which might useful resource with weight management. Fruits and greens lower cholesterol and protect the heart from CHD due to the fact they are high in fiber (Evans et al., 2017).

5.2.1 WHOLE GRAINS

Whole grains also can help to improve heart health and minimize the effects of CHD. Whole grains, like fruits and vegetables, are nutrient-dense and a great source of fiber as a result, they can resource inside the reduction of cholesterol and blood strain (Basu et al., 2007).

5.2.2 HEALTHY FATS

When a patient has CHD, he could consider that everyone fat is awful for him but, not all fats are harmful. Consuming healthful fats sparsely is probably beneficial to heart fitness. Healthful fats can assist to lower cholesterol and decrease the risk of heart assaults and strokes (Jiao et al., 2015).

5.2.3 PROTEIN THAT IS LOW IN FATS

Protein intake is also beneficial for your well-known health. Select proteins that are low in fats, however, be selective that kinds of fish excessive in omega-three fatty acids, which help lower LDL cholesterol and triglyceride levels, are wholesome choices. Salmon, herring, and different cold-water fish fall beneath this category.

5.3 DIETARY FIBER IN CORONARY HEART DISEASE

In some of the most important studies that tracked people for many years, excessive dietary fiber intake was related to a decreased risk of heart disorder. Researchers found that a high total dietary fiber consumption became associated with a 40% decreased danger of coronary heart disorder which was studied in Harvard on nearly 40,000 miles. The consequences of a Harvard research had been very comparable. Fiber intake has additionally been related to a reduced incidence of metabolic syndrome, a set of characteristics that raises the hazard of heart disease and diabetes, high blood pressure, excess weight (especially across the stomach), high triglyceride tiers, and LDL cholesterol are a number of those danger elements. A good fiber consumption, in line with numerous research, may additionally provide safety in opposition to this infection (Weickert et al., 2011).

5.3.1 VEGETABLES AND FRUITS

Although the botanic period "fruit" refers to a plant's seeds and surrounding tissues, the pulpy seeded tissues which have a sweet (oranges, apples, pears, blueberries) or bitter (lemons, limes, cranberries) flavor are frequently known as "fruits" for culinary purposes. Vegetables are useful for human consumption. Plant components together with stems and stalks (celery), roots (carrots), tubers (potatoes), bulbs (onions), leaves (spinach, lettuce), blossoms (artichokes), a few fruits (cucumbers, pumpkin, tomatoes), and seeds, in keeping with culinary terminology (beans, peas).

There was no interventional research that explicitly checked out the impact of greens and culmination on the risk of CHD danger reduction changed into installed in interventional trials when vegetable and fruit-eating became a part of the nutritional tips. Consumption of vegetables and culmination turned into connected to reduced blood strain, but the hyperlink to other CHD risk factors changed into unclear. Notwithstanding the absence of intervention trials, the yank coronary heart association (AHA) recommends that you eat at least eight culmination and veggies every day (Wada et al., 2015).

5.3.2 NUTS

Nuts (tree nuts and peanuts) have complex matrices wealthy in unsaturated fatty acids and other useful substances, including vegetable protein, fiber, minerals, tocopherols, phytosterols, and phenolic compounds. Tree nuts are defined as dry fruits with one seed whose ovary wall hardens as they mature. Almonds, hazelnuts, walnuts, pistachios, pine nuts, cashews, pecans, macadamias, and Brazil nuts are all part of this category.

Peanuts, which might be botanically groundnuts or legumes but are popularly categorized as part of the nut's meals category, are included in the client definition. Peanuts even have a nutritional profile that is comparable to that of tree nuts. Regardless of the truth that chestnuts are tree nuts, they fluctuate from all different not unusual nuts in that they're starchier and have a distinct dietary profile. Nut consumption is connected to a decreased incidence of coronary heart disorder, in line with epidemiological research. A dose-response pattern of courting turned into found in several of the investigations. In line with an evaluation of four studies from America, greater nut consumption is linked to a 35% lower threat of cardiovascular diseases (Fay et al., 2019).

5.3.3 SOYA

Soya protein is a protein (Keservani et al., 2015; Singh et al., 2017b) determined in soybeans that are often used as alternative animal protein in humans' diets. The soybean is a cholesterol-free, saturated-fats-free legume that is the best vegetable food that includes all necessary amino acids. Fiber, iron, calcium, zinc, and vitamin B (Singh et al., 2017a) nutrients are all discovered in soybeans. Phytoestrogen (isoflavones) (Keservani & Sharma, 2014) are plant components that have interaction with mammalian endocrine structures, and soybeans are the maximum and normally ingested source.

Minerals (calcium, potassium, and magnesium), protein (casein and whey), and vitamins (riboflavin and nutrition B12) blanketed in dairy merchandise can help save you CVD (Keservani et al., 2016a). Conversely, the quantity of saturated fat in dairy products raises worries approximately feasible dangerous cardiovascular effects.

5.4 MECHANISMS OF DIETARY FIBER IN CORONARY HEART DISEASE

The high potassium, magnesium, and calcium minerals content in dietary fiber products is the concept to be one of the causes for their blood pressure reducing advantages. The food plan, which includes an aggregate of culmination, vegetable servings in line with a day of dietary fiber (frequently low-fats), significantly reduced blood pressure. A link has been shown between calcium intake and a reduction in body weight and fats mass is positive effect has been shown to have a moderately reducing impact on hypertension, maximum likely because of bioactive peptides. The precise fatty acid composition, which is composed mostly of short-chain fatty acids and stearic acid, is liable for the lack of effect of high saturated fat content material on LDL-C ranges (Salman et al., 2016) (Figure 5.3).

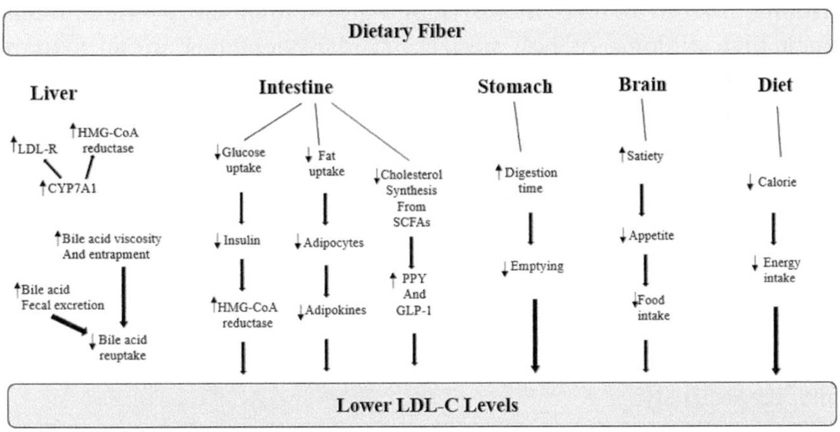

FIGURE 5.3 Mechanism of dietary fiber in lowering the risk of coronary heart disease.

5.4.1 *HYPOCHOLESTEROLEMIC RESULTS OF SOLUBLE NUTRITIONAL FIBERS*

The potential of soluble dietary fiber to lower blood general cholesterol and LDL-C in people is one of the first diagnosed and nicely-studied capabilities of the fiber. Psyllium, glucan, pectin, and guar gum are 4 important types of soluble dietary fiber that have been validated to decrease blood LDL-C in experimental trials of those fibers have additionally been permitted for health claims by using America food and Drug management (FDA): psyllium and glucan from whole oats and barley. Recent research at the outcomes of those and other soluble fibers on blood cholesterol has endured providing light on their viable involvement in reducing the chance of cardiovascular disease (Keservani et al., 2017). The latest research has checked out the effect of concentrated glucan derived from oat and barley sources on blood cholesterol levels (Villarini et al., 2018).

5.4.2 SOLUBLE FIBER FROM LEGUMES

Inside the common Western food regimen, whole grains, fruits (Keservani et al., 2016b), and vegetables are the maximum critical sources of soluble fiber; amongst greens, legumes are an excessive supply of both general and soluble dietary fiber. Chickpeas, for instance, consist of roughly 17.4 gm of total nutritional fiber in a 100 g, inclusive of 5 g of soluble dietary fiber. Because of their high diploma of polymerization, many legumes are an extremely good supply of resistant starch, providing a greater substrate for colonic fermentation and possibly extra SCFAs.

Non-soy legumes, including chickpeas, pinto beans, and navy beans, have been proven to reduce cholesterol levels in randomized managed research, and their excessive soluble fiber content is thought to be chargeable for this gain. Several researchers have checked out the cholesterol-decreasing blessings of non-soy legumes, that are automatically eaten up in Western diets, in the ultimate 12 months. Pinto and military beans are the most customarily eaten legumes inside the united states, with 3.6 lbs and 1.3 lbs in step with capita, respectively.

Fiber interacts with several areas of the digestive gadget, which include the mouth, belly, small intestine, and huge gut, and has an influence on fitness through many distinct pathways (colon). (i) Colonic feature with decreased transit time, improved stool size, and colonic fermentation (generation of SCFA); (ii) blood LDL cholesterol discounts; and (iii) blood glucose reductions are the three maximum widely documented fitness advantages. Different tactics, in line with published research, include stronger intestine plant life and decrease blood strain.

5.4.3 MECHANISMS OF FIBER INSIDE THE INTESTINE

Insoluble fibers along with cellulose and hemicellulose, in addition to psyllium, play a first-rate role in reducing transit time and growing stool size. Diets rich in legumes and whole grains are particularly useful at speeding up gut transit. Fibers are cholesterol-lowering are properly documented. The maximum thorough research into the consequences of glucans has been performed, and minimal consumption of 3 g is advised for health. The glucans enhance viscosity and limit bile acid reabsorption within the small gut, decreasing levels of cholesterol inside the bloodstream. Pectin, psyllium, and guar gum have also been shown to lower LDL cholesterol, soluble fibers like glucans affect glucose and insulin responses. Soluble fiber binds to carbohydrates in the small gut.

Soluble fiber's accelerated viscosity acts as a barrier, slowing glucose absorption at the same time as additionally inhibiting amylase, resulting in less starch digestion and more insulin sensitivity. Some fibers aid in weight reduction with the aid of increasing satiety. Soluble fibers, for example, in the belly integrate with partially digested food, slowing stomach emptying. β-glucans may produce an urge for food suppressants such as cholecystokinin, which can also make contributions to a feeling of fullness. Some varieties of soluble fiber were proven to lessen blood stress. This might appear within the equal way that sugar absorption is decreased, due to the fact insulinemia can cause endothelial dysfunction and hypertension. It's also feasible that it has whatever to do with satiety and weight reduction. Expanded fiber weight-reduction plan can also lower anti-inflammatory indicators like reactive protein while additionally growing additives, yet studies show that big increases are required to lessen C reactive protein to a proper stage. Although the modern-day paper specializes in CVD, it's miles important to word that fecal plant life fermentation to SCFA dilutes cancer agents, which is the mechanism maximum probable to be concerned in decreasing the risk of colon cancer, and some fibers might also affect estrogen metabolism through inhibiting reabsorption and synthesis, which could explain the link between nutritional fiber and decreased breast most cancers threat. The impact of various types of fiber on the intestine microbiota, of which bacteria represent the most essential aspect, is much less well understood. Growing useful microorganisms and regulating gene expression are two possibilities that have been proposed (Boshuizen et al., 2010).

5.4.4 FIBER AND CHOLESTEROL METABOLISM

Although the molecular tactics behind the results of nutritional fiber on cholesterol metabolism had been broadly explored, the molecular mechanisms concerned are nevertheless unfamous. Vegetarians and semi-vegetarians have lower cholesterol and LDL cholesterol levels, as well as decreased LDL cholesterol and LDL to HDL cholesterol/HDL levels kept at optimum level. According to Keys et al., some forms of dietary fiber can lower plasma general LDL cholesterol in human beings a long time in the past. Because then, several studies have proven that high consumption of nutritional fiber, specifically fermentable fiber, lowers serum overall cholesterol and LDL levels of cholesterol substantially.

Most effective pectins changed into beneficial in lowering plasma LDL cholesterol in hypercholesterolemic casein rabbits after partial substitution of noticed dust, citrus pectin, cellulose, and wheat bran. In pectin-fed rabbits, impartial steroid excretions were more.

Dietary fibers partially hinder the enterohepatic cycle, preventing bile acid re-use within the liver and raising hepatic manufacturing of the proscribing enzyme 7-cholesterol hydroxylase (CYP7A1), which converts LDL cholesterol to cholic acid. As a result, more bile acids are produced whilst the quantity of LDL cholesterol to be had for inclusion in lipoproteins decreases (e.g., VLDL). LDL cholesterol may be used in lipoproteins (e.g., VLDL) (Martinez de Prado et al., 2014).

Fiber compounds have a fermentability ranging from 10% to 90%. Lignin and cellulose are the least fermentable of these materials, whereas pectin, gums, resistant starch, mucilage, and positive oligosaccharides are highly fermentable. CO_2, CH_4, H_2, and quick-chain fatty acids are produced in the course of anaerobic fermentation (butyric, propionic, and acetic acids). Intestinal fitness is stepped forward through the manufacturing of butyric acid, which is connected to the regeneration of microbiota and colonocytes, as well as the decrease of intestinal inflammation and the danger of neoplasia. Due to their excessive P content, algal fibers are much less fermentable than the ones of other plant meals (HVT et al., 2018).

5.4.5 EFFECT OF FIBERS ON BLOOD PRESSURE

Information on the effects of dietary fibers on blood strain is scarcer than information on their effects on cholesterol levels, and much less is thought about the processes concerned at the moment. It has been proposed that nutritional fiber (and hence LDL and HDL concentrations) impact arterial endothelial and smooth muscle, thereby changing arterial contraction tone. However, it's viable that fiber impacts cardiac input/output and total peripheral resistance through regulating the sympathetic and parasympathetic neural structures or converting the concentrations of a ramification of nearby or systemic regulators (e.g., K^+, CO_2, H^+, prostaglandins, thromboxanes, NO) dietary fibers may additionally impact the pastime of the angiotensin-changing enzyme (ACE) within the kidneys, that's vital for blood pressure control.

5.5 MARKETED PRODUCT OF DIETARY FIBER

- Daily fiber caps;
- Activated fiber powder;
- NutriFiber;
- Psyllium husk powder;
- Boven ingredient dietary fiber;
- Daily multifiber;
- Oat fiber powder;
- Fabulicious high fiber gummies;
- Mits pro fiber powder;
- Active fiber complex.

5.6 CONCLUSION

Medicines help to maintain risk associated with CHD but they have temporary benefits with many side effects. Dietary fiber is the edible part of the plant which is not digested by our body, but it will help to reduce the risk of CHD. CHD is associated with various risk factors like high cholesterol, high lipoprotein. Dietary fiber, particularly soluble dietary fiber reduces the bad cholesterol LDL level, reduces glucose absorption also lowers blood pressure. In this way, dietary fiber helps to reduce the risk of CHD. CHD is a major problem in the world and it is due to improper diet and poor lifestyle. Proper intake of dietary fiber reduces the risk of CHD. Dietary fiber shows this effect by reducing the LDL cholesterol level, maintaining blood pressure, proper mineral balance, and decreasing gastric transit time. Dietary fiber not only reduces the risk of CHD but also help to maintain blood glucose level, and reduce the risk of cancer.

5.7 FURTHER REMARKS

Based on the positive effects of dietary fibers on CHD risk factors, new studies are needed to further our understanding of the benefits of dietary fibers. In western, Mediterranean, or hypocaloric diets on emerging CHD risk factors like postprandial lipemia, thrombogenesis, blood coagulation factors, inflammation, antioxidant markers, lipoprotein lipase (LDL), and postprandial lipemia. Additionally, further research is needed on the probable interactions between other dietary compounds, medicines, and dietary fiber, as fiber compounds are known to interact with dietary macro- and micro-nutrients. Also, as there exists hypo and hyper responders to diet and drug treatment, more information regarding the fiber-gene interaction is needed to personalize and individualize die to therapy and pharmacotherapy.

KEYWORDS

- **angiotensin-changing enzyme**
- **coronary heart disease**
- **dietary fiber**
- **food and drug management**
- **heart disease**
- **lipoprotein lipase**
- **soluble fiber**

REFERENCES

Afshin, A., Sur, P. J., Fay, K. A., et al., (2007). Health effects of dietary risks in 195 countries, 1990–2017: A systematic analysis for the global burden of disease. *Lancet, 393*, 1958–1972.

Andersson, A., Tengblad, S., Karlstrom, B., Kamal-Eldin, A., Landberg, R., Basu, S., et al., (2007). Whole-grain foods do not affect insulin sensitivity or markers of lipid peroxidation and inflammation in healthy, moderately overweight subjects. *J. Nutr., 137*, 1401–1407.

Aune, D., Norat, T., Romundstad, P., et al., (2013). Whole grain and refined grain consumption and the risk of type 2 diabetes: A systematic review and dose-response meta-analysis of cohort studies. *Eur. J. Epidemiol., 28*, 845–858.

Bazzano, L. A., Ogden, L. G., Loria, C. M., & Whelton, P. K., (2003). Dietary fiber intake and reduced risk of coronary heart disease in US men and women: The national health and nutrition examination survey I epidemiologic follow-up study. *Arch. Intern. Med., 163*, 1897–1904.

Begg, C. B., & Mazumdar, M., (1994). Operating characteristics of a rank correlation test for publication bias. *Biometrics, 50*, 1088.

Berlin, J. A., Longnecker, M. P., & Greenland, S., (1993). Meta-analysis of epidemiologic dose-response data. *Epidemiology, 4*, 218–228.

Bingham, S. A., Gill, C., Welch, A., Cassidy, A., Runswick, S. A., Oakes, S., et al., (1997). Validation of dietary assessment methods in the UK arm of EPIC using weighed records, and 24-h urinary nitrogen and potassium and serum vitamin C and carotenoids as biomarkers. *Int. J. Epidemiol., 26*, S137–S151.

Bohlscheid-Thomas, S., Hoting, I., Boeing, H., & Wahrendorf, J., (1997). Reproducibility and relative validity of energy and macronutrient intake of a food frequency questionnaire developed for the German part of the EPIC project. *Int. J. Epidemiol., 26*, S71–S81.

Brown, L., Rosner, B., Willett, W. W., & Sacks, F. M., (1999). Cholesterol-lowering effects of dietary fiber: A meta-analysis. *Am. J. Clin. Nutr.,* 69.

Brown, L.,Rosner, B., Willett, W. W., & Sacks, F. M., (1999). Cholesterol-lowering effects of dietary fiber: A meta-analysis. *Am. J. Clin. Nutr.,* 69.

Burkitt, D. P., Walker, A. R. P., & Painter, N. S., (1974). Dietary fiber and disease. *JAMA, 229*, 1068–1074.

Burr, M. L., Fehily, A. M., Gilbert, J. F., Rogers, S., Holliday, R. M., Sweetnam, P. M., et al., (2008). Effects of changes in fat, fish, and fiber intakes on death and myocardial reinfarction: Diet and reinfarction trial (DART). *Eur. J. Clin. Nutr., 2*, 757–761.

Burr, M. L., Fehily, A. M., Gilbert, J. F., Rogers, S., Holliday, R. M., Sweetnam, P. M., et al., (1989). Effects of changes in fat, fish, and fiber intakes on death and myocardial reinfarction: Diet and reinfarction trial (DART). *Lancet, 2*, 757–761.

Cochran, W. G., (1954). The combination of estimates from different experiments. *Biometrics, 10*, 101.

Crowe, F. L., Key, T. J., Appleby, P. N., et al., (2012). Dietary fiber intake and ischaemic heart disease mortality: The European prospective investigation into cancer and nutrition-heart study. *Eur. J. Clin. Nutr., 66*, 950.

Crowe, F. L., Roddam, A. W., Key, T. J., Appleby, P. N., Overvad, K., Jakobsen, M. U., et al., (2011). Fruit and vegetable intake and mortality from ischaemic heart disease: Results from the European prospective investigation into cancer and nutrition (EPIC)-heart study. *Eur. Heart J., 32*, 1235–1243.

Danesh, J., Saracci, R., Berglund, G., Feskens, E., Overvad, K., Panico, S., et al., (2007). EPIC-Heart: The cardiovascular component of a prospective study of nutritional, lifestyle and biological factors in 520 middle-aged participants from 10 European countries. *Eur. J. Epidemiol., 22*, 129–141.

Dong, J. Y., He, K., Wang, P., & Qin, L. Q., (2011). Dietary fiber intake and risk of breast cancer: A meta-analysis of prospective cohort studies. *Am. J. Clin. Nutr., 94*, 900.

Dong, J. Y., Zhang, Y. H., Wang, P., et al., (2012). Meta-analysis of dietary glycemic load and glycemic index in relation to risk of coronary heart disease. *Am. J. Cardiol., 109*, 1608–1613.

Du, H., Van, D. A. D., Boshuizen, H. C., et al., (2010). Dietary fiber and subsequent changes in body weight and waist circumference in European men and women. *Am. J. Clin. Nutr., 91*, 329.

Egger, M., Davey, S. G., Schneider, M., & Minder, C., (1997). Bias in meta-analysis detected by a simple, graphical test. *BMJ, 315*, 629.

Eshak, E. S., Iso, H., Date, C., et al., (2010). Dietary fiber intake is associated with reduced risk of mortality from cardiovascular disease among Japanese men and women. *J. Nutr., 140*, 1445–1453.

Eshak, E. S., Iso, H., Date, C., Kikuchi, S., Watanabe, Y., Wada, Y., et al., (2010). Dietary fiber intake is associated with reduced risk of mortality from cardiovascular disease among Japanese men and women. *J. Nutr., 140*, 1445–1453.

Evans, C. E., Greenwood, D. C., Threapleton, D. E., et al., (2015). Effects of dietary fiber type on blood pressure: A systematic review and meta-analysis of randomized controlled trials of healthy individuals. *J. Hypertens., 33*, 897–911.

Evans, C. E., Greenwood, D. C., Threapleton, D. E., et al., (2017). Glycemic index, glycemic load, and blood pressure: A systematic review and meta-analysis of randomized controlled trials. *Am. J. Clin. Nutr., 105*, 1176–1190.

Ferrari, P., Day, N. E., Boshuizen, H. C., Roddam, A., Hoffmann, K., Thiebaut, A., et al., (2008). The evaluation of the diet/disease relation in the EPIC study: Considerations for the calibration and the disease models. *Int. J. Epidemiol., 37*, 368–378.

Fuller, S., Beck, E., Salman, H., et al., (2016). New horizons for the study of dietary fiber and health: A review. *Plant Foods Hum. Nutr., 71*, 1–12.

Gianfredi, V., Salvatori, T., Villarini, M., et al., (2018). Is dietary fiber truly protective against colon cancer a systematic review and meta-analysis. *Int. J. Food Sci. Nutr., 69*, 904–915. 15.

Greenland, S., & Longnecker, M. P., (1992). Methods for trend estimation from summarized dose-response data, with applications to meta-analysis. *Am. J. Epidemiol., 135*, 1301–1309.

Greenwood, D. C., Threapleton, D. E., Evans, C. E., et al., (2013). Glycemic index, glycemic load, carbohydrates, and type 2 diabetes: Systematic review and dose-response meta-analysis of prospective studies. *Diabetes Care. Br. J. Nutr., 36*, 4166–4171.

Higgins, J. P., Thompson, S. G., Deeks, J. J., & Altman, D. G., (2003). Measuring inconsistency in meta-analyses. *BMJ, 327*, 557–560.

Hipsley, E. H., (1953). Dietary "fiber" and pregnancy toxaemia. *Brit. Med. J., 2*, 420.

Holbrook, A., Wright, M., Sung, M., Ribic, C., & Baker, S., (2011). Statin-associated rhabdomyolysis: Is there a dose-response relationship *Can. J. Cardiol., 27*, 146–151.

Howard, B. V., Van, H. L., Hsia, J., Manson, J. E., Stefanick, M. L., Wassertheil-Smoller, S., et al., (2006). Low-fat dietary pattern and risk of cardiovascular disease: The women's health initiative randomized controlled dietary modification trial. *JAMA, 295*, 655–666.

Jansen, M. C., Bueno-De-Mesquita, H. B., Buzina, R., et al., (1999). Dietary fiber and plant foods in relation to colorectal cancer mortality: The seven countries study. *Int. J. Cancer, 81*, 174.

Jaya, K. S. R., & Gordan, D. T., (1989). Functional properties vs. physiological action of total dietary fiber. *Cereal Food Worl., 34*, 517–523.

Jha, S. K., (2005). *Dietary Fiber for the Prevention of Cardiovascular Disease || Dietary Fiber and Human Health: An Introduction, 2*, 13–17.

Jiao, J., Xu, J. Y., Zhang, W., et al., (2015). Effect of dietary fiber on circulating C-reactive protein in overweight and obese adults: A meta-analysis of randomized controlled trials. *Int. J. Food Sci. Nutr., 66*, 114–119.

Katsouyanni, K., Rimm, E. B., Gnardellis, C., Trichopoulos, D., Polychronopoulos, E., & Trichopoulou, A., (1997). Reproducibility and relative validity of an extensive semi-quantitative food frequency questionnaire using dietary records and biochemical markers among Greek schoolteachers. *Int. J. Epidemiol., 26*, S118–S127.

Kaushik, S., Wang, J. J., Wong, T. Y., et al., (2009). *Glycemic Index, Retinal Vascular Caliber, and Stroke Mortality, 40*, 206–212.

Keservani, R. K., & Sharma, A. K., (2014). Flavonoids: Emerging trends and potential health benefits. *Journal of Chinese Pharmaceutical Sciences, 23*(12), 815.

Keservani, R. K., Kesharwani, R. K., Sharma, A. K., Vyas, N., & Chadoker, A., (2010b). Nutritional supplements: An overview. *International Journal of Current Pharmaceutical Review and Research, 1*(1), 59–75.

Keservani, R. K., Kesharwani, R. K., Vyas, N., Jain, S., Raghuvanshi, R., & Sharma, A. K., (2010a). Nutraceutical and functional food as future food: A review. *Der Pharmacia Lettre, 2*(1), 106–116.

Keservani, R. K., Sharma, A. K., & Jarouliya, U., (2015). Protein and peptide in drug targeting and its therapeutic approach. *Ars Pharmaceutica (Internet), 56*(3), 165–177.

Keservani, R. K., Sharma, A. K., & Kesharwani, R. K., (2016a). Nutraceutical and functional foods for cardiovascular health. In: *Food Process Engineering* (pp. 257–278, 291–312). Apple Academic Press, CRC Press. ISBN: 9781771884020.

Keservani, R. K., Sharma, A. K., & Kesharwani, R. K., (2016b). Medicinal effect of nutraceutical fruits for the cognition and brain health. *Scientifica,* 10. Article ID 3109254. doi: 10.1155/2016/3109254.

Keservani, R. K., Sharma, A. K., & Kesharwani, R. K., (2017). An overview and therapeutic applications of nutraceutical and functional foods. *Recent Advances in Drug Delivery Technology,* 160–201. ISBN:9781522507543.

Khan, K., Jovanovski, E., Ho, H. V. T., et al., (2017). The effect of viscous soluble fiber on blood pressure: A systematic review and meta-analysis of randomized controlled trials. *Nutrition, Metabolism, and Cardiovascular Diseases: NMCD, 28*, 3–13.

Khaw, K. T., & Barrett-Connor, E., (1987). Dietary fiber and reduced ischemic heart disease mortality rates in men and women: A 12-year prospective study. *Am. J. Epidemiol., 126*, 1093–1102.

Lia, A., Hallmans, G., Sandberg, A. S., Sundberg, B., Aman, P., & Andersson, H., (1995). Oat beta-glucan increases bile acid excretion and a fiber-rich barley fraction increases cholesterol excretion in ileostomy subjects. *Am. J. Clin. Nutr., 62*, 1245–1251.

Ma, Y., Hebert, J. R., Li, W., et al., (2008). Association between dietary fiber and markers of systemic inflammation in the women's health initiative observational study. *Nutrition. Arch. Intern. Med., 24*, 9419.

Margret, C. R., Mona, M., Hradesh, R., & Patil, R. T., (2012). *Dietary Fiber in Food, Food Sci. Technol., 49*, 255–266.

McEligot, A. J., Largent, J., Ziogas, A., Peel, D., & Anton-Culver, H., (2006). Dietary fat, fiber, vegetable, and micronutrients are associated with overall survival in post-menopausal women diagnosed with breast cancer. *Nutr. Cancer, 55*, 132.

Mente, A., DeKoning, L., Shannon, H. S., & Anand, S. S., (2009). A systematic review of the evidence supporting a causal link between dietary factors and coronary heart disease. *Arch. Intern. Med., 169*, 659–669.

Mozaffarian, D., Kumanyika, S. K., Lemaitre, R. N., Olson, J. L., Burke, G. L., & Siscovick, D. S., (2003). Cereal, fruit, and vegetable fiber intake and the risk of cardiovascular disease in elderly individuals. *JAMA, 289*, 1659–1666.

Ness, A. R., Hughes, J., Elwood, P. C., Whitley, E., Smith, G. D., & Burr, M. L., (2002). The long-term effect of dietary advice in men with coronary disease: Follow-up of the diet and reinfarction trial (DART*). Eur. J. Clin. Nutr., 56*, 512–518.

Niranjan, B. M., (2019). *Research Journal of Pharmacognosy and Phytochemistry, 11*(3).
Ocke, M. C., Bueno-De-Mesquita, H. B., Pols, M. A., Smit, H. A., Van, S. W. A., & Kromhout, D., (1997). The Dutch EPIC food frequency questionnaire. II. Relative validity and reproducibility for nutrients. *Int. J. Epidemiol.,* 26, S49–S58.
Olendzki, B. C., Ma, Y., Schneider, K. L., Merriam, P., Culver, A. L., Ockene, I. S., et al., (2009). A simple dietary message to improve dietary quality: Results from a pilot investigation. *Nutrition, 25*, 736–744.
Orsini, N., Bellocco, R., & Greenland, S., (2006). Generalized least squares for trend estimation of summarized dose-response data. *Stata J., 6*, 40–57.
Papathanasopoulos, A., & Camilleri, M., (2010). Dietary fiber supplements: Effects in obesity and metabolic syndrome and relationship to gastro-intestinal functions. *Gastroenterology, 138,* 65–72.
Park, Y., Subar, A. F., Hollenbeck, A., & Schatzkin, A., (2011). Dietary fiber intake and mortality in the NIH-AARP diet and health study. *Arch Intern. Med., 171*, 1061–1068.
Pereira, M. A., Reilly, E., Augustsson, K., et al., (2004). Dietary fiber and risk of coronary heart disease: A pooled analysis of cohort studies. *Arch. Intern. Med., 164*, 370.
Pereira, M. A., Reilly, E., Augustsson, K., Fraser, G. E., Goldbourt, U., Heitmann, B. L., et al., (2004). Dietary fiber and risk of coronary heart disease: A pooled analysis of cohort studies. *Arch. Intern. Med., 164*, 370–376.
Pietinen, P., Rimm, E. B., Korhonen, P., et al., (1996). Intake of dietary fiber and risk of coronary heart disease in a cohort of Finnish men. *Circulation J. Nutr., 94*, 2720–2727.
Pisani, P., Faggiano, F., Krogh, V., Palli, D., Vineis, P., & Berrino, F., (1997). Relative validity and reproducibility of a food frequency dietary questionnaire for use in the Italian EPIC centers. *Int. J. Epidemiol.,* 26, S152–S160.
Riboli, E., Elmståhl, S., Saracci, R., Gullberg, B., & Lindgarde, F., (1997). The Malmo food study: Validity of two dietary assessment methods for measuring nutrient intake. *Int. J. Epidemiol., 26*, S161–S173.
Riboli, E., Hunt, K. J., Slimani, N., Ferrari, P., Norat, T., Fahey, M., et al., (2002). *European Prospective Investigation into Heart Disease and Nutrition (EPIC), 5*, 1113–1124.
Richardson, D. P., (2003). Wholegrain health claims in Europe. *Proc. Nutr. Soc., 62*, 161–169.
Sánchez-Muniz, F. J., Bastida, S., Gutiérrez-García, O., & Carbajal, A., (2009). Olive oil-diet improves the simvastatin effects with respect to sunflower oil-diet in men with increased cardiovascular risk: A preliminary study. *Nutr. Hosp., 24*, 333–339.
Saravanya, K. S., & Kavitha, S., (2017). A study on properties of palmyra sprout. *International Journal of Current Research, 9*, 54299–54301.
Seal, C. J., Nugent, A. P., Tee, E. S., et al., (2016). Whole-grain dietary recommendations: The need for a unified global approach. *Br. J. Nutr., 115*, 2031–2038.
Singh, P., Kesharwani, R. K., & Keservani, R. K., (2017a). Antioxidants and vitamins: Roles in cellular function and metabolism. In: *Sustained Energy for Enhanced Human Functions and Activity* (pp. 385–407). Academic Press. ISBN:9780128054130.
Singh, P., Kesharwani, R. K., & Keservani, R. K., (2017b). Protein, carbohydrates, and fats: Energy metabolism. In: *Sustained Energy for Enhanced Human Functions and Activity* (pp. 103–115). Academic Press. ISBN:9780128054130.
Slimani, N., Deharveng, G., Unwin, I., Southgate, D. A. T., Vignat, J., Skeie, G., et al., (2007). The EPIC nutrient database project (ENDB): A first attempt to standardize nutrient databases across the 10 European countries participating in the EPIC study. *Eur. J. Clin. Nutr., 61*, 1037–1056.

Slimani, N., Ferrari, P., Ocke, M., Welch, A., Boeing, H., Van, L. M., et al., (2000). Standardization of the 24-h diet recall calibration method used in the European prospective investigation into cancer and nutrition (EPIC): General concepts and preliminary results. *Eur. J. Clin. Nutr., 54*, 900–917.

Slimani, N., Kaaks, R., Ferrari, P., Casagrande, C., Clavel-Chapelon, F., Lotze, G., et al., (2002). European prospective investigation into cancer and nutrition (EPIC) calibration study: Rationale, design and population characteristics. *Public Health Nutr., 5*, 1125–1145.

Streppel, M. T., Arends, L. R., Van't, V. P., Grobbee, D. E., & Geleijnse, J. M., (2005). Dietary fiber and blood pressure: A meta-analysis of randomized placebo-controlled trials. *Arch. Intern. Med., 165*, 150.

Streppel, M. T., Arends, L. R., Vant, V. P., Grobbee, D. E., & Geleijnse, J. M., (2005). Dietary fiber and blood pressure: A meta-analysis of randomized placebo-controlled trials. *Arch. Intern. Med., 165*, 150–156.

Streppel, M. T., Ocke, M. C., Boshuizen, H. C., Kok, F. J., & Kromhout, D., (2008). Dietary fiber intake in relation to coronary heart disease and all-cause mortality over 40 years: The Zutphen study. *Am. J. Clin. Nutr., 88*, 1119–1125.

Streppel, M. T., Ocke, M. C., Boshuizen, H. C., Kok, F. J., & Kromhout, D., (2008). Dietary fiber intake in relation to coronary heart disease and all-cause mortality over 40 y: The zutphen study. *Am. J. Clin. Nutr., 88*, 1119–1125.

Stroup, D. F., Berlin, J. A., Morton, S. C., et al., (2000). Meta-analysis of observational studies in epidemiology: A proposal for reporting. *JAMA, 283*, 2008–2012.

Subhashis, D., Jawahar, S., Muntaj, H., Purushotham, V., Sharmila, G., & Sireesha, K., (2002). Effect of fibers on heart disease. *IJP*, 6–14.

Thompson, W. G., Holdman, N. R., Janzow, D. J., Slezuk, J. M., Morris, K. L., & Zemel, M. B., (2011). Effect of energy-reduced diets high in dairy products and fiber on weight loss in obese adults. *Am. J. Clin. Nutr., 13*, 1344–1353.

Threapleton, D. E., Greenwood, D. C., Burley, V. J., Aldwairji, M., & Cade, J. E., (2013). Dietary fiber and cardiovascular disease mortality in the UK women's Cohort study. *Eur. J. Epidemiol., 28*, 335.

Threapleton, D. E., Greenwood, D. C., Evans, C. E., et al., (2013). Dietary fiber intake and risk of cardiovascular disease: Systematic review and meta-analysis. *BMJ, 347*, f6879.

Torre, L. A., Bray, F., Siegel, R. L., Ferlay, J., Lortet-Tieulent, J., & Jemal, A., (2015). Global cancer statistics. *CA Cancer J. Clin., 65*, 87.

Trowell, H., (1972). Ischemic heart disease and dietary fiber. *Am. J. Clin. Nutr., 25*, 926–932.

Trowell, H., (1972). Ischemic heart disease and dietary fiber. *Am. J. Clin. Nutr., 25*, 926–932.

Vaquero, M. P., Sanchez, M. F. J., Jiménez, R. S., Prats, O. P., Higueras, F. J., & Bastida, S., (2010). Major diet-drug interactions affecting the kinetic characteristics and hypolipidaemic properties of statins. *Nutr. Hosp., 25*, 193–206.

Vatanasuchart, N., Niyomwit, B., & Wongkrajang, K., (2009). Resistant starch contents and the *in vitro* starch digestibility of Thai starchy foods. *Kasetsart J. Nat. Sci., 43*, 178–186.

Wang, C. H., Qiao, C., Wang, R. C., & Zhou, W. P., (2015). Dietary fiber intake and pancreatic cancer risk: A meta-analysis of epidemiologic studies. *Sci. Rep., 5*, 10834.

Weickert, M. O., Mohlig, M., Schofl, C., et al., (2006). Cereal fiber improves whole-body insulin sensitivity in overweight and obese women. *Diabetes Care, 29*, 775.

Weickert, M. O., Roden, M., Isken, F., Hoffmann, D., Nowotny, P., Osterhoff, M., et al., (2011). Effects of supplemented isoenergetic diets differing in cereal fiber and protein content on insulin sensitivity in overweight humans. *Am. J. Clin. Nutr., 94*, 459–471.

Whelton, S. P., Hyre, A. D., Pedersen, B., Yi, Y., Whelton, P. K., & He, J., (2005). Effect of dietary fiber intake on blood pressure: A meta-analysis of randomized, controlled clinical trials. *J. Hypertens., 23*, 475–481.

Wu, Y., Qian, Y., Pan, Y., et al., (2015). Association between dietary fiber intake and risk of coronary heart disease: A meta-analysis. *Clin. Nutr., 34*, 603.

Yao, O. L., & Andrew, R. K., (2017). Dietary fiber basics: Health, nutrition, analysis and application. *Food Quality and Safety, 1*, 47–59.

Yue-Yue, Y., Sen, M., Xiao-Xi, W., & Xue-Ling, Z., (2017). Modification and application of dietary fiber in foods. *Hindawi Journal of Chemistry, 8*, 1–8.

Zhang, Z., Xu, G., Ma Yang, J., & Liu, X., (2013). Dietary fiber intake reduces risk for gastric cancer: A meta-analysis. *Gastroenterology, 145*, 113–120.

CHAPTER 6

ROLE OF DIETARY FIBER IN GUT HEALTH

SANKET DHARASHIVKAR,[1] MADHURI GAIKWAD,[2] GAUTAMI WARGHADE,[1] and TRUNALI GHUDE[1]

[1]*Dr. L. H. Hiranandani College of Pharmacy, Ulhasnagar, Maharashtra, India*

[2]*AIKTC School of Pharmacy, Panvel, Maharashtra, India*

ABSTRACT

Dietary fiber comprise of indigestible forms of carbohydrate, generally as polysaccharides that derives from plant-based products. Many studies have reported that people on high fiber diet have reduced risks of certain diseases such as cancers, cardiovascular disease, weight gain, and possibly diabetes. The gut microflora functions as a principal mediator of the advantageous effects of dietary fiber, such as the appetite regulation, processes of metabolism and persistent inflammatory pathways. The fiber rich diet such as vegetable, cereals, nuts, and fruits have a positive impact on health because consumption of fiber leads to reduced occurrence of several diseases. This chapter covers in detail the review about beneficial effect of dietary fibers in different diseases like constipation, loose motion, inflammatory bowel diseases, hiatal hernias, gastroesophageal reflux disease, Barrett's esophagus, diverticular disease, hemorrhoids, peptic ulcer, gastritis, celiac disease, irritable bowel syndrome, gallstone, and colon cancer. It also covers in detail about additional benefits of a high-fiber diet, *how to increase* high fiber diet, disadvantages of high fiber diet care to be taken after side effects and marketed products like Nutrova functional fiber, Organic whole husk

Food Supplements and Dietary Fiber in Health and Disease. Bhushan R. Rane, Raj K. Keservani, Durgesh Singh, Nayan A. Gujarathi, and Ashish S. Jain, (Eds.)
© 2024 Apple Academic Press, Inc. Co-published with CRC Press (Taylor & Francis)

psyllium, Actifiber, Celevida, Prohance D, D-Protin, Nimbose, Tummycool powder, Pro360 NutriFiber, Rohn Fiber supplement, Vidaslim, Nutricology Dietary Fiber Cellulose Powder, Urban Platter Oats Fiber Powder, Inulin dietary fiber, Naturolax-A, 1 mg high fiber, AcuraglobeFiber-S for Gastrointestinal Health, Activated Fiber 90 Tablets, Benefiber Prebiotic Fiber Supplement, Pro360 NutriFiber, Water Soluble Fiber, Health Drink Powder.

6.1 INTRODUCTION

Dietary fibers are the product of plant parts that our body can't absorb or digest. They are also called roughage or bulk and unlike other food components, which includes fats, carbohydrates or proteins that our body can metabolize and absorb, fiber passes through our body undigested (Pereira et al., 2004; Rimm et al., 1996). The daily need of dietary fiber for an adult is shown in Table 6.1.

TABLE 6.1 Daily Recommendations of Fiber for an Adult

	Age 50 or Less	Age 51 or More
Male	38 grams	30 grams
Female	25 grams	21 grams

Fiber is a kind of carbohydrate that the body is not able to break down. Most of the carbohydrates are metabolized into sugar molecules, but fibers cannot be digested into sugar molecules, instead they pass through the body un-metabolized. Most of us get about 15 g per day of fiber but the daily requirement for Children and adults is at least 20 to 30 g of fiber per day for good health. The fruits and vegetables, beans, and whole grains are great sources of fiber. Fiber comprise of polysaccharides that are non-starch, includes dextrins, inulin, lignin, cellulose chitins, pectin, beta-glucans, waxes, and oligosaccharides (Brown et al., 1999; McKeown et al., 2002). The two types of dietary fiber are soluble and insoluble fibers. People don't require to concentrate much about this difference since most of the high fiber containing foods contain both insoluble and soluble fiber. So that, they can focus on overall fiber intake. After coming in contact with water soluble fiber forms a solid gel mass in the stomach. Later that gel is broken down by bacteria in the large intestine. Some calories are provided to the individual by soluble fibers. Soluble fiber provides various benefit like reducing the blood

LDL cholesterol level by changing the body's absorption of dietary fat and cholesterol, reducing absorption of carbohydrates through digestion, which helps in regulating body's sugar levels helping to keep hunger and blood sugar in check. Beans, fruits, oats, nuts, and vegetables are good sources of soluble fiber (McKeown et al., 2004; Fung et al., 2002). Insoluble fiber is beneficial to the people who having problem of constipation or irregular bowels because they do not dissolve in water and pass mostly as it is through the gastrointestinal tract. It cannot supply calories. Insoluble fiber helps a people for easy passage of stool by building bulk in the stool. The good sources of insoluble fiber are fruits (Keservani et al., 2016b), nuts, vegetables, whole grain foods. Different plant foods contain different amounts of soluble and insoluble fiber. A wide variety of fiber rich foods should be there in our diet to receive the greatest gut health benefit (Liu et al., 2000).

6.2 BENEFITS OF A HIGH-FIBER DIET IN GUT HEALTH

Dietary fiber is a crucial part of a healthy diet. This is essential for keeping the gut healthy and to avoid the possibility of persistent health conditions. Many people do not get enough fiber from their diets, as stated by some impression, only 5% of the people meet the adequate intake requirements. It states that most people could get health benefits by increasing their daily fiber intake (Schulze et al., 2004; Krishnan et al., 2007). Eating fiber has many health benefits as mentioned below. Dietary fiber (Keservani et al., 2010a, b, 2017, 2020) has a useful effect on gastrointestinal disorders, such as constipation, loose motion, inflammatory bowel diseases, hiatal hernias, gastroesophageal reflux disease, Barrett's esophagus, diverticular disease, hemorrhoids, peptic ulcer, gastritis, celiac disease, irritable bowel syndrome, gallstone, and even colon cancer.

6.2.1 CONSTIPATION

Fiber is important to maintain the gut healthy and constipation can be prevented or relieved by eating enough fiber, which in turn helps waste to excrete easily out of the body. It as well boosts healthy gut microbial flora. Dietary fiber encourages regular bowel movements, increases the bulk of stool, and minimize the period that waste remains inside the intestines. Dietary fiber softens the stool and also increases its weight and size. The chances of constipation can be decreased by increasing the bulk of stool which makes it easier to pass (Aldoori et al., 1998; Fuchs et al., 1999).

6.2.2 LOOSE MOTION

Because of diarrhea, undigested food moves too fast, due to this intestine cannot absorb water, this in turn results in loose stools. Fiber will help you to thicken the stool since it adds bulk to stool and absorbs water and by slowing down the transit time, fiber gives the large intestines an opportunity to absorb additional water (Farvid et al., 2016; Backhed et al., 2007).

6.2.3 INFLAMMATORY BOWEL DISEASES

The cause of inflammatory bowel diseases (IBD), such as Crohn's disease and ulcerative colitis, still remains uncertain. In industrialized countries, the incidence of IBD is continuously increasing. Several trials are carried out on animal models of IBD and human studies, in which they have reported that the addition of some types of dietary fiber can delay and reduce lesions of the intestinal mucosa throughout the course of the disease. The outlined effects are primarily observed because of increased luminal building of short chain fatty acids which are produced due to bacterial fermentation of un-digestible dietary fiber. Immunomodulatory properties of short chain fatty acids accelerate healing and regeneration processes of the intestinal epithelium, and they decrease colonic pH thereby stimulating growth of the healthy microflora and reducing growth of the pathogens (Basu et al., 2012; Bindels et al., 2017).

6.2.4 HIATAL HERNIAS

When the upper part of your stomach gets inside the chest cavity through a hole in the diaphragm hiatal hernia occurs. In patients suffering from hiatal hernia, the stomach acids can easily enter into the esophagus, the tube which carries food from our throat to our stomach. This may result in a condition called gastroesophageal reflux disease which causes a burning feeling in our throat and chest. The best way to reduce or prevent symptoms of hiatal hernia is to make dietary and lifestyle changes. Low acid producing food fibers are less likely to aggravate your hiatal hernia symptoms (Bouskra et al., 2008; Brooks et al., 2017).

6.2.5 *GASTROESOPHAGEAL REFLUX DISEASE*

Gastroesophageal reflux disease (GERD) is a gastric disorder which influence the lower esophageal sphincter, the valve that regulates the flow of food and drinks from your esophagus to your stomach. The movement of lower esophageal sphincter helps to block the stomach acids from traveling back up, but its failure to close properly contributes to the outflow of gastric contents back into the esophagus. When food stays in the gastric region for longer periods of time due to delayed gastric emptying, it can loosen the lower esophageal sphincter which permits gastric acid to come back up the esophagus. This affects the entire digestive tract, resulting in heartburn and esophagitis, ulcers, and cancer. A person who suffers from gastroesophageal reflux disease can make a few deliberate dietary changes to help lessen these effects. Making a few intentional dietary changes is one of the simpler steps which can help a person who suffers from gastroesophageal reflux disease to lessen these effects. The foods include fruits, vegetables, and grains have high fiber content which reduces acid reflux due to fiber's qualities as a digestive aid. Fiber absorbs liquid in the digestive system, which blocks the movement of stomach acid (Chassaing et al., 2014, 2015a).

6.2.6 *BARRETT'S ESOPHAGUS*

In Barrett's esophagus, the lining of the esophagus, the tube that connects your mouth and stomach gets injured by acid reflux. This means that the tissue in the esophagus has transformed to a type of tissue that is found in the intestine. Barrett's esophagus is thought to be caused by long-term acid reflux or heartburn in gastroesophageal reflux disease. Over time, the acid can irritate and change the tissues lining the esophagus. There is a risk of getting cancer in the esophagus due to chronic Barrett's esophagus. Consuming a great amount of fiber in your daily diet is adequate for your overall health. Medical research reported that this can also help prevent Barrett's esophagus from worsening and decrease the risk of cancer in the esophagus (Chassaing et al., 2015b, 2017).

6.2.7 DIVERTICULAR DISEASE

Diverticulosis occurs when small, bulging pouches (diverticuli) develop in the lower part of the intestine, usually in the colon. Contraction and stretching during bowel movements can intensify the condition. Not eating enough fiber place, you at a much higher risk of developing diverticulitis. Fibers might give benefits by enlarging fecal mass and regulating bowel movements, as well as acting as prebiotics in the colon and favoring health-promoting species of the intestinal microflora. Around 25 to 30 grams of fiber should be consumed daily (Etienne-Mesmin et al., 2016; Dewulf et al., 2011).

6.2.8 HEMORRHOIDS

Hemorrhoids are normal features of anatomy. They become a problem when hemorrhoids start to generate pain, itchiness or bleed. The people who have irregular bowel movements are more likely to suffer from hemorrhoids. Consumption of more high fiber, low fat, whole foods can often lessen or prevent the symptoms of hemorrhoids. Fiber increase stool weight, reducing the colon transit time, increase water retention in the colon, which results in softer stools that can pass more easily. Fiber in our diet work better when they are taken along with water and other liquids, such as fruit juices and clear soups (Flythe et al., 2010; Everard et al., 2013).

6.2.9 PEPTIC ULCER

Peptic ulcer progresses due to variability between the factors that damage the mucosa and those for its protection, resulting in a lesion of the lining of the upper digestive tract. It is one of the most common diseases in the world, having some complications which are major causes of morbidity and mortality. For individuals with peptic ulcer it is advisable to take 20 to 30 g/day fibers since it can act as buffers, reduce the concentrations of bile acids in the stomach and the intestinal transit time, resulting in decreased abdominal bloating, thus less discomfort and pain in the gastrointestinal tract (Gulhane et al., 2016; Gibson et al., 1999).

6.2.10 GASTRITIS

The term gastritis is a general term that refers to any condition that involves inflammation of the lining of the stomach. Gastritis can be acute or chronic, acute gastritis is unexpected and severe, while chronic gastritis is long-lasting. Symptoms include indigestion, abdominal pain, nausea, and bloating. Eating certain foods and avoiding others can help people manage their gastritis symptoms. Foods like whole grains, fruits, vegetables, and beans that are high in fiber can help (Harlow et al., 2014; Hamilton et al., 2017).

6.2.11 CELIAC DISEASE

Celiac disease is a digestive and serious autoimmune disease that occurs in genetically predisposed people where the small intestine is damaged due to the consumption of gluten. It is predicted to affect roughly 1 in 100 people worldwide. Having enough fiber in the diet is very important for people with celiac disease. Some with celiac disease suffer with diarrhea, but the intestinal damage heals after they are placed on a gluten-free diet. The diarrhea stops, but sometimes, constipation develops. Gluten-free whole grains like amaranth, millet, quinoa, sorghum, and teff should be tried. Of course, gluten-free foods such as brown or wild rice and baked potatoes with their skins can also be eaten (Lee et al., 2011; Kinnebrew et al., 2010).

6.2.12 IRRITABLE BOWEL SYNDROME

Irritable bowel syndrome is one of the most common and severe conditions for which patients seek medical attention. Certain food practices may contribute to symptoms of constipation, diarrhea, bloating, gas, and abdominal pain. Addition of fiber to your diet might help to improve bowel function and reduce symptom severity. For improving irritable bowel syndrome, fiber supplementation, particularly psyllium, is both safe and effective. Fiber treatment is most beneficial to the patients who are susceptible to constipation (Liu et al., 2016; Lindemans et al., 2015).

6.2.13 GALLSTONE

The gallbladder is an organ located directly under the liver. It works with the liver to store and release bile, which helps in the digestion of fats in food. Gallstones are the hardened deposits of digestive fluid formed in the gallbladder. Gallstones, can lead to abdominal pain, mostly after meals, anorexia, vomiting, and sickness. The recommended amounts of dietary fiber should be including diet to keep your gallbladder healthy. Insoluble dietary fiber may help to speed intestinal transit time, reduce the production of bile acids and serve in decreasing bile cholesterol levels (Rabot et al., 2010; Miles et al., 2017).

6.2.14 COLON CANCER

In a handful of studies, it is reported that fibers are linked to lowering the risk of colon cancer, and now new research suggests that fiber can also help colon cancer survivors to live longer. People who had deliberately added fiber to their diet noticed improvement in their risk of dying due to cancer. A 20% reduction was seen in patients dying from colon cancer was seen by the addition of fiber rich food in their diet. Taking high-fiber cereals and whole grains had a great influence on survival, followed by fiber-rich vegetables and then fruits. Fiber helps to move food through the digestive system at a greater rate and limiting the time potential carcinogens sit in the intestines. Fiber can also show anti-inflammatory properties (Salazar et al., 2015; Rankin et al., 2016).

6.3 ADDITIONAL BENEFITS OF A HIGH-FIBER DIET

6.3.1 REDUCED RISK OF DIABETES

Adding more fiber to your diet can also have benefits for diabetes. Fiber slows down the absorption of sugar in the body and prevents blood sugar from rising after meals. Type 2 diabetes. Soluble fiber may slow the absorption of sugar and help improve blood sugar levels in people with diabetes (Smith et al., 2013).

6.3.2 MANAGEMENT OF WEIGHT

Weight loss is regulated by the addition of a high amount of dietary fiber in your diet. After eating high-fiber foods, a person feels full longer, which can help people stick to a diet. High fiber intake increased weight loss and adherence to a calorie restriction diet. They fill you up, so people are likely to eat less and stay full longer, and high-fiber foods tend to take longer to eat and have less energy, meaning they have fewer calories for you (Sonnenburg et al., 2016).

6.3.3 REDUCED CHOLESTEROL LEVELS

Beans, oats, flaxseed, and oat bran containing soluble Fiber helps lower total blood cholesterol levels by lowering levels of "bad," or low-density lipoprotein cholesterol. Studies have also shown that high-fiber foods may have other heart health benefits, like lowering blood pressure and inflammation (Sonnenburg & Sonnenburg 2014).

6.3.4 PROTECTION AGAINST HEART DISEASE

Consuming high fiber diets can lower the incidence of cardiovascular disease (Keservani et al., 2016a), reduce blood pressure and reduction in mortality rate from these conditions. Cardioprotective effects may be due to fiber lowering total cholesterol and low-density lipoprotein (LDL) cholesterol, also known as "bad cholesterol" and a major complication of heart disease (Ashkan et al., 2017; Sugimoto et al., 2008).

6.4 HOW TO INCREASE HIGH FIBER DIET?

1. **Jump-Start Your Day:** A high-fiber breakfast cereal containing— 5 or more grams of fiber a serving should be chosen for breakfast. Add some tablespoons of wheat bran without being able to handle your favorite cereal.
2. **Switch to Whole Grains:** Eat at least half of all grains as whole grains. Breads should be chosen that list whole grain, whole wheat flour, or another whole grain as the first ingredient on their label and contain at least 2 grams of fiber per serving. Try to include brown rice, wild rice, barley, whole wheat pasta, and bulgur wheat.
3. **Bulk Up Baked Goods:** Replace whole-grain flour for half or all of the white flour when baking. Try to add crushed bran cereal, unprocessed wheat bran or uncooked oatmeal to muffins, cakes, and cookies.

4. **Lean on Legumes:** The excellent sources of fiber are beans, peas, and lentils. Try adding beans to a canned soup or green salad. Or make nachos with chilled black beans, lots of fresh veggies, whole grain chips, and salsa.
5. **Eat More Fruit and Vegetables:** Eat five or more portions daily. Fruits and vegetables contain great amount of fiber, as well as vitamins (Singh et al., 2017a) and minerals.
6. **Make Snacks Count:** Fresh fruit, raw vegetables, low-fat popcorn, and whole grain crackers are good snack choices. Nuts or dried fruits are also a healthy option, and they do contain high-fiber. However, keep in mind that nuts and dried fruits are very high in calories.

Dietary fiber content of some food products are given in Table 6.2 (Turnbaugh et al., 2006).

TABLE 6.2 Dietary Fiber Content of Some Food Products

Food	Serving Size	Dietary Fiber (g)	Calories
Wheat bran flakes (ready-to-eat cereal)	3/4 of a cup	4.9–5.5	90–98
High fiber bran (ready-to-eat cereal)	½–3/4 of a cup	9.1–14.3	60–81
Canned, chickpeas	half a cup	8.1	176
Cooked, lentils	half a cup	7.8	115
Cooked, pinto beans	half a cup	7.7	122
Cooked, black beans	half a cup	7.5	114
Cooked, lima beans	half a cup	6.6	108
Canned, white beans	half a cup	6.3	149
Kidney beans	half a cup	5.7	112
Raw pear	1 medium fruit	5.5	101
Canned, plain, cooked beans	half a cup	5.2	119
Avocados	half a cup	5	120
Mixed vegetables, cooked from frozen	half a cup	4	59
Blackberries	half a cup	3.8	31
Collards, cooked	half a cup	3.8	32
Cooked, sweet potato	1 medium vegetable	3.8	103
Popcorn, without oil	3 cups	3.5	93
Almonds	1 ounce (oz)	3.5	164
Cooked, whole wheat spaghetti	1/2 a cup	3.2	87

TABLE 6.2 *(Continued)*

Food	Serving Size	Dietary Fiber (g)	Calories
Orange	1 medium fruit	3.1	69
Banana	1 medium fruit	3.1	105
Oat bran muffins	1 small muffin	3	178
Dry roasted, pistachios	1 oz	2.8	161
Oil roasted, pecans	1 oz	2.7	203
Cooked, quinoa	half a cup	2.6	111

6.5 DISADVANTAGES OF HIGH FIBER DIET

Eating too much fiber results in bloating, gas, and constipation. These side effects can occur when a person consumes more than 70 g of fiber per day. This is uncommon but can occur when someone is following a vegan, raw, or whole-food diet. High-fiber foods are good for your health. Adding too much fiber too quickly can encourage gas, bloating, and cramping. Increase the fiber in your diet moderately for a few weeks. This gives the natural bacteria in your digestive system time to adjust to the change. Fiber works best when it absorbs water, making stool soft and bulky so drink plenty of water. People who are allergic to high-fiber foods have a hard time consuming enough fiber. They should check with their doctor and try to find alternative sources of fiber that do not cause allergic reactions.

Some of the most common symptoms of too much fiber are:

- Bloating;
- Gas;
- Feeling full;
- Abdominal pain;
- Constipation or diarrhea;
- Dehydration;
- Malabsorption of some essential nutrients;
- Increase or decrease in weight;
- Nausea;
- Intestinal obstruction in very few cases.

Bowel movements become easier due to fiber. It also encourages fermentation and formation of gas. Therefore, intake of excessive fiber frequently affects the digestive system. Consumption of too much fiber can interfere with the body's ability to absorb important nutrients, resulting in nutrient insufficiency. This happens because the fiber binds with minerals like calcium, magnesium, zinc, and iron (Verdam et al., 2013).

6.6 CARE TO BE TAKEN AFTER SIDE EFFECTS

The symptoms of taking too much fiber (Wang et al., 2014) can be decreased by:

- Reduction in fiber consumption;
- Increasing fluid intake;
- Regular exercise;
- Avoiding food that increases swelling, like chewing gum.

An individual with serious symptoms can select to acquire a low-fiber diet that is taking 10 g of fiber till their signs and symptoms may be higher managed. For individuals with serious digestive conditions, this type of diet is mostly prescribed.

A low-fiber diet comprises:

- Bread and grain products containing less than 2 g of fiber per serving;
- Canned and cooked fruits and vegetables;
- Perfectly cooked meats.

6.7 MARKETED PRODUCTS

Many products are available in market few of them are discussed below:

1. **Nutrova Functional Fiber:** It consists of fenugreek galactomannan' from fenugreek (methi) seeds: exceptionally soluble fiber that passes material across the digestive system, helps to absorb fats & sugars, and nourish our good gut bacteria. It also consists of gluten-free wheat fiber extract: excellent non-soluble fiber which helps to add bulk to stool and stimulate bowel movements. Mix 1 measuring spoon of nutrova functional fiber are to be mixed with 1 glass of water before consumption (Weitkunat et al., 2015). It feeds our appropriate intestine bacteria (as a prebiotic), for higher intestine health, improves bowel movements, lipid tiers and trendy well-being Ideal for low-carbohydrate diets/diets missing in high-fiber foods.

2. **Organic Whole Husk Psyllium:** Dietary fiber organic whole husk psyllium, which is certified by Organic India, is derived from the seeds of the herb Plantago ovata, which is a bulk-forming dietary fiber. It consists of both soluble and insoluble fiber and naturally supports the entire digestive system. Healthy elimination and regularity is promoted by adding psyllium to the diet. The soluble fiber from psyllium, as well as a healthy diet, can decrease the possibility of health disease. This product contains Organic husk Psyllium and Gluten Free-Kosher. It contains no sugar, sodium, cholesterol, fat or additives and is of pharmacopeia grade. Mix it (1 tablespoon) with at least 200 ml of juice, other beverage or water. Stir well and drink immediately. If it is too viscous, add more liquid and stir. It is recommended to drink an additional glass of water afterwards to ensure hydration (Weitkunat et al., 2015).
3. **Actifiber:** It is 100% organic, soluble fiber nutrition that helps manage blood sugar level naturally and it is clinically proven. It also helps to regulate blood sugar fluctuations usually seen after having food. It helps to take control and manage diabetes better on prolonged use. Actifiber Natural Sugar Control is recommended by doctors and should be part of the daily diet of diabetics. Ideally, start by mixing 1 sachet with a glass of water with your morning meal. Additional servings can be added with subsequent meals, salads, coffee, tea, etc. (Kesharwani et al., 2016). It is effective in controlling carbohydrates. When Actifiber is added to your food, it dissolves and combines with your food into a gel. Controls post-meal sugar fluctuations because mealtime carbohydrates are digested more slowly, and sugars are slowly released with fewer spikes right after a meal. Helps better control diabetes during long-term use. Regularly improves insulin resistance in 8 weeks and glucose metabolism in 12 weeks. It's also easy to consume. Leaves no taste, odor or color when dissolved. You won't even know if you've added it to food, so you can even cook or bake with it (Winner et al., 2016).
4. **Celevida:** The Dr. Reddy Celevida polygenic disease powder is sugar-free and safe for consumption for diabetics. The powder has been clinically evidenced to regulate glucose spikes within the body, whereas it continues to supply essential nutrients. It's high in supermolecule (Keservani et al., 2015; Singh et al., 2017b) and fiber. About 100 g of the powder contains 30 g protein and 12 g fiber. It conjointly contains a low glycemic index of concerning 36,

that slows down digestion and also the rate at which carbohydrates (Singh et al., 2017b) are absorbed by the body, so supporting weight management. Patient must drink the Celevida powder frequently for a healthy and active lifestyle. It comprise of defatted soya bean flour, cocoa powder, gram flour, milk powder, high oleic flower oil, soya oil, fructo-oligosaccharide powder, corn dextrin, ragi flour, mineral concoction, emulsifier, sodium chloride, bulking agent, sweetener, vitamin premix and anti-caking agent (Winer et al., 2016).

5. **Prohance D:** This powder has soluble fibers that provide a feeling of fullness and additionally help management sterol levels. The special formula of Prohance D is dead suited to Diabetic patients to assist them keep their glucose levels low. Moreover, the ingredient during this concoction helps to stop the spike in blood sugar right when meals, therefore serving to in diabetic care management. This health supplement also helps in delaying hunger and at identical time provides the daily supermolecule demand of diabetic patients. This biological process health drink also contains a healthy mixture of Fats and 27 essential Vitamins and Minerals that facilitate enhance the system of diabetic individuals. Furthermore, this health supplement is freed from trans-fats, milk sugar and gluten, creating it fully eater and gluten-free so even people with disorder will simply consume it. Patient ought to pour a 175 cubic centimeter of either heat or cold water into a glass and blend 50 grams or half-dozen leveled scoops of the Prohance D powder into this glass. Stir well making certain that no lumps are remaining. Once employing a shaker rather than a glass, shake smartly before overwhelming this drink (Zhang et al., 2014).
6. **D-Protin:** It is enriched with fiber for easy and smooth digestion, which also helps improve your digestive health. D-Protin contains no added sugars or trans fats and is gluten free. Contains antioxidants and promotes heart health with heart-friendly soy proteins. Deficiency symptoms, especially in diabetics due to an adequate combination of macro- and micro-nutrients. Macronutrients provide a slow and sustained release of energy throughout the day and improve lean body mass. Micronutrients improve glucose metabolism, with zinc and chromium being essential for the formation and use of insulin. It consists of skimmed milk powder, maltodextrin, soy protein isolate, inulin (fiber), sunflower oil, evening primrose oil, algae oil powder, sucralose (sugar-free sweetener), vitamins, minerals, and flavor. The

patient should add 2 tablespoons of D-Protin to 1/3 glass of warm milk or water and stir until dissolved. Add the remaining milk or water to prepare 1 glass of nutritious drink. Enjoy twice daily, morning and evening, or as recommended by your healthcare practitioner (Zhang et al., 2014).

7. **Nimbose:** It is a completely unique fiber method made from decided on herbal soluble & insoluble for typical intestine and digestive fitness (belly fitness dietary supplements). This intestine fitness powder additionally possesses anti-inflammatory benefits. This prebiotic fiber complement may be quite simply jumbled in water/juices and fed on immediately. Product has been formulated with perfect flavor and smooth dispersibility. Nimbose is the proprietary intestine fitness dietary supplements addressing decrease gastric fitness issues. This patent implemented digestion complement method improves bowel movements, relieves constipation, boosts immunity, and allows in pressure management. It is the Best digestive resource for a couple of intestine fitness/digestive fitness issues. This superior prebiotics for intestine fitness includes best herbal ingredients. This clinically tested intestine cleanse powder is flawlessly secure to apply and not using a damaging events. It is without problems dispersible and geared up to apply product (Zheng et al., 2013).
8. **Tummycool Powder:** It is enriched with 100% herbal lively elements like sanaya, harad, bael, isabgol, amla, kaladana, gulab, saunf, bahera, black salt, sendha salt, and ajwain. Effective and fiber wealthy elements upload bulk in stool that facilitates relieve constipation and raise wholesome digestion. Tummycool powder has herbal elements like isabgol and amla that stimulates intestinal contractions and peristaltic actions that offer alleviation from constipation. Tummy cool is non-dependency forming and sugar-unfastened that's why it may be utilized by diabetic sufferers too. Tummycool powder is enriched with fiber rich elements like saunf, amla, and ajwain that facilitates in right digestion. Patient need to take 1–2 tablespoons (5–10 g) of tummy cool powder with a pitcher of lukewarm water at mattress time or as endorsed with the aid of using physician (Zheng et al., 2013).
9. **Pro360 NutriFiber:** It is 100% herbal origin, plant primarily based totally wheat dextrin water soluble fiber without a brought preservatives and its sugar unfastened system that allows to control your blood glucose, helps weight control and digestive bowel mechanism.

Pro360 NutriFiber dissolves absolutely in water and does now no longer have any color, flavor or smell. Just upload 1 scoop (approx. 5 g) two times a day, in water or in your preferred meals to make Pro360 NutriFiber for each day intake. Pro360 NutriFiber may be brought to any meal or drinks which makes you to experience much less hungry. This allows to hold the load and to control the diabetes withinside the lengthy term. The advantages of this product encompass low caloric value, low glycemic index, low insulinemic index, prebiotic effects. It is imported from France and carries 100% wheat dextrin powder (Zheng et al., 2008).

10. **RohnFiber Supplement:** It is one of the dietary supplements with the best ratio of insoluble and soluble fiber with delivered advantages of prebiotic to decorate intestine fitness, lessen constipation and regularize bowel movements. It may also be useful for coronary heart and diabetic care. This fiber complement includes inulin which acts as a prebiotic. Inulin keeps the fitness of useful intestine bacteria, which complements the technique of digestion. This complement may be used for normal bowel movement, for treating constipation for piles and fissures, for lowering LDL cholesterol and to controls diabetes. It is crafted from excessive nice oat and inulin fibers and impartial in taste, so it is able to be combined with chapati dough, juices, milk shakes, or may be sprinkled on any meals item (Zindl et al., 2013).
11. **Vidaslim:** This coffee weight management powder jar of 400 g is an excessive fiber dietary complement that facilitates in weight loss. Vidaslim consists of 38 vitamins that assist growth lean muscle boom which aids in weight loss. Vidaslim products also boost metabolism. It is a meal replacer that makes one slim in a healthy way. It is trans-fat free and gluten-free, made with natural ingredients and contains no harmful chemicals. Vidaslim Coffee Management Powder contains: Energy, Fat, Carbohydrates, Dietary fiber, Protein, White kidney bean extract, L-Carnitine, Green tea extract, Ginseng. It helps lower bad cholesterol in your body. It allows in weight reduction and development of general fitness as its miles wealthy in critical vitamins. This boosts immune machine and power levels. Vidaslim Coffee Weight-control powder allows to enhance metabolism. It includes in experienced tea and coffee, each of that have caffeine. Therefore, it will increase the fats burning process.

    Direction of use: Mix 4 scoops of Vidaslim Coffee Weight Management Powder in 100 ml of water and eat at lunch or dinner.

12. **NutriCology Dietary Fiber Cellulose Powder:** It is an excellent source of insoluble fiber to support bowel function. It supports healthy elimination and digestive regularity. It is free of wheat and gluten, dairy, eggs, soy, fish, shellfish, peanuts, tree nuts, corn, and yeast.
    Direction of Use: Drink 1 teaspoon blended with water two or three instances each day earlier than meals, or as directed.
13. **Urban Platter Oats Fiber Powder:** Urban oats platter fiber is a handy technique of including useful insoluble fiber on each day diet. It is a light, barely yellowish, satisfactory grained nutritional fiber listen extracted from oat spelt bran. Fiber enables adjust digestive health. Due to its impartial and inert character, it could be utilized in drinks, pasta, and different programs without affecting flavor or smell.
    Direction of use: Add this fiber to smoothies, chapatis, breads, soups or snacks for brought fiber consumption and simplicity of digestion.
14. **Inulin Dietary Fiber:** Inulin is a soluble dietary fiber extracted from Chicory root as it's far complete of inulin. It is a non-digestible oligosaccharide. It is used as sugar and fat alternative and as fiber enrichment. It is utilized in gut fitness, calorie reduction, and blood sugar management. Especially it's far advanced for sugar alternative. It is a nicely tolerated, natural bulking agent, easy to disperse, white colored, tasteless, and odorless. Especially it's far advanced for fats mimetic effect. Inulin helps the increase of useful intestine microorganism. This maintains the intestine microorganism balanced and can have numerous fitness benefits. Inulin can help relieve constipation by causing more frequent bowel movements and better stool consistency.
    Direction of use: Take 1 teaspoon 1 to a few instances daily.
15. **Naturolax-A:** It includes isabgol fiber from herbal sources, a method which has effervescence upon blending with water. It enables in bowel movement: Adds soluble fiber to stool making it tender and massive thereby triggering the bowel to settlement and flow the stool out. Direction of use: Add one heaped teaspoon (approx. 5.6 gm) of Naturolax-a in an empty glass, fill the glass with water Stir the aggregate such that the contents need to get combined with water and drink it at once.
16. **1 mg High Fiber:** It includes pre- and probiotics unflavored with resistant maltodextrin, inulin, and guar gum. It supports

gastrointestinal fitness and lowers the glycemic index of food. Prebiotics and probiotics help the frame in constructing and retaining up a wholesome network of microorganism and diverse microorganisms. It helps the intestine and aids withinside the digestion process. It helps in supplying wholesome microorganism and in addition rowing a surroundings where in specific microorganisms can flourish.

17. **AcuraglobeFiber-S for Gastrointestinal Health:** Prebiotic soluble fiber maintain healthier gut flora help in weight management helps in intestinal protection bowel regularity and aid gut fitness fiber-S is a specialized method containing combo of particular prebiotic soluble nutritional fibers that allows to fulfill the day by day requirement for the Dietary Fiber and aid gastrointestinal fitness. Fiber-S stimulates "Good" Bacteria withinside the gut which allows in keep intestine fitness. It is an smooth to mix, with clean flavor powder. prebiotic soluble Fiber, Maintain more healthy gut flora, help in weight management, helps in intestinal protection, bowel regularity and aid gut fitness.
18. **Activated Fiber 90 Tablets:** Activated fiber pills, a mix of nutritional fiber's such as citrus pea and oat fiber, are a handy manner to growth your consumption of wholesome fiber daily. It is an aggregate of soluble and insoluble nutritional fiber's that allows cut back Appetite via way of means of presenting a sense of fullness and lowering the indulgence to overeat. Directions to use: One to 2 pills with meal, 3 instances consistent with day.

    It helps to improve digestion key benefits:

    i. It includes pea and oat fiber to increase your fiber intake;
    ii. Helps improve digestion.
19. **Benefiber Prebiotic Fiber Supplement:** Soluble fiber supplement for digestive health bene fiber daily prebiotic fiber powder provides the daily fiber helps to maintain good digestive health in a sugar and gluten free unflavored fiber powder form. This fiber supplement nourishes the good bacterium in the intestines with a dextrin and supports an environment for good digestive health.

    i. It helps maintain digestive health & prevents constipation;
    ii. This sugar-free supplement aims to control sugar levels & lowers cholesterol levels;
    iii. It helps raise energy levels by meeting fiber requirements.

    Directions for use: For a while 12 and older, stir teaspoons of Benefiber prebiotic fiber complement powder into 4 to 8 oz. of a non-carbonated beverage or smooth meals 3 instances daily. For kids a while 6 to 11, use one teaspoon of this powder 3 instances daily.

20. **Pro360 NutriFiber Water Soluble Fiber Health Drink Powder:** Pro360 NutriFiber – water soluble nutritional fiber nutrients supplement – to manipulate diabetic, weight control, digestive health. It is plant primarily based totally wheat dextrin water soluble fiber without a delivered preservatives and its sugar unfastened components that enables to manipulate the sugar level, helps your weight control and digestive bowel mechanism.
    Directions for use: Just add 1 scoop (approx. 5 g) twice a day, in water or in food to make Pro360 NutriFiber in daily intake.

6.8 CONCLUSION

Dietary fiber is a crucial component of a healthy diet, with research which links a high fiber diet with lowered risks of many health disorders, such as cardiovascular disorder, type 2 diabetes, and specific cancers. Fiber is also essential for keeping the bowels healthy. Fiber helps to control bowel movements so they are not too loose or too hard and may lower the risk of diverticulosis, diverticulitis, and colorectal cancer. Fiber is good for the gastrointestinal tract because it gives bulk to the stool, helping in colonic lubrication and transit. The bulk or quantity of cloth within side the gastrointestinal tract is extra due to the fact fiber isn't digestible, and for this reason, it stays for the duration of the transit through the small intestine. Most human beings do now no longer meet their needful everyday requirement of fiber. People can grow this degree through intake of excessive fiber foods, end result and veggies with the skins on, or through taking fiber dietary supplements if this isn't feasible. The current review suggests that dietary fiber has the prospect of altering the gut microflora and change metabolic regulation in humans. Most high-fiber foods are considered generally healthy since they are low in calories, sugar, and fat. After eating high-fiber foods one may feel fuller and thereby less tendency to overeat. Additionally, high-fiber diets are often part of a low-cholesterol, heart-healthy diet. A high-fiber diet can contribute greatly to keep the gastrointestinal tract healthy as well as to a general healthy lifestyle. For best results, people are always advised to follow a healthful diet alongside an active lifestyle.

KEYWORDS

- **constipation**
- **dietary fiber**
- **gastroesophageal reflux disease**
- **gastrointestinal disorders**
- **gut microflora**
- **prebiotic effect**
- **weight management**

REFERENCES

Aldoori, W. H., Giovannucci, E. L., Rockett, H. R., Sampson, L., Rimm, E. B., & Willett, W. C., (1998). A prospective study of dietary fiber types and symptomatic diverticular disease in men. J. Nutr., 128, 714–719.

Ang, Z., & Ding, J. L., (2016). GPR41 and GPR43 in obesity and inflammation – protective or causative. *Front. Immunol., 7*, 1–5.

Ashkan, A., Mohammad, H. F., Marissa, B. R., Patrick, S., Kara, E., Alex, L., et al., (2017). Health effects of overweight and obesity in 195 countries over 25 years. *N. Engl. J. Med., 377*, 13–27.

Backhed, F., Manchester, J. K., Semenkovich, C. F., & Gordon, J. I., (2007). Mechanisms underlying the resistance to diet-induced obesity in germ-free mice. *Proc. Natl. Acad. Sci. USA., 104*, 979–984.

Basu, R., O'Quinn, D. B., Silberger, D. J., Schoeb, T. R., Fouser, L., Ouyang, W., Hatton, R. D., & Weaver, C. T., (2012). Th22 cells are an important source of IL-22 for host protection against enteropathogenic bacteria. *Immunity., 37*, 1061–1075.

Bindels, L. B., Segura, M. R. R., Gomes-Neto, J. C., Mutemberezi, V., Martinez, I., Salazar, N., Cody, E. A., Quintero-Villegas, M. I., Kittana, H., De Los Reyes-Gavilan, C. G., et al., (2017). Resistant starch can improve insulin sensitivity independently of the gut microbiota. *Microbiome, 5*, 12.

Bouskra, D., Brezillon, C., Berard, M., Werts, C., Varona, R., Boneca, I. G., & Eberl, G., (2008). Lymphoid tissue genesis induced by commensals through NOD1 regulates intestinal homeostasis. *Nature, 456*, 507–510.

Brooks, L., Viardot, A., Tsakmaki, A., Stolarczyk, E., Howard, J. K., Cani, P. D., Everard, A., Sleeth, M. L., Psichas, A., Anastasovskaj, J., et al., (2017). Fermentable carbohydrate stimulates FFAR2-dependent colonic PYY cell expansion to increase satiety. *Mol. Metab., 6*, 48–60.

Brown, L., Rosner, B., Willett, W. W., & Sacks, F. M., (1999). Cholesterol-lowering effects of dietary fiber: A meta-analysis. Am. J. Clin. Nutr., 69, 30–42.

Chassaing, B., Koren, O., Goodrich, J. K., Poole, A. C., Srinivasan, S., Ley, R. E., & Gewirtz, A. T., (2015). Dietary emulsifiers impact the mouse gut microbiota promoting colitis and metabolic syndrome. *Nature, 519*, 92–96.

Chassaing, B., Ley, R. E., & Gewirtz, A. T., (2014a). Intestinal epithelial cell toll-like receptor 5 regulates the intestinal microbiota to prevent low-grade inflammation and metabolic syndrome in mice. *Gastroenterology, 147*, 1363–1377.

Chassaing, B., Miles-Brown, J., Pellizzon, M., Ulman, E., Ricci, M., Zhang, L., Patterson, A. D., et al., (2015b). Lack of soluble fiber drives diet-induced adiposity in mice. *Am. J. Physiol. Gastrointest. Liver Physiol., 309*, G528–G541.

Chassaing, B., Shreya, M. R., Lewis, J. D., Srinivasan, S., & Gewirtz, A. T., (2017). Colonic microbiota encroachment correlates with dysglycemia in humans. *Cell Mol. Gastroenterol. Hepatol., 4*, 205–221.

Dewulf, E. M., Cani, P. D., Neyrinck, A. M., Possemiers, S., Van, H. A., Muccioli, G. G., Deldicque, L., Bindels, L. B., Pachikian, B. D., Sohet, F. M., et al., (2011). Inulin-type fructans with prebiotic properties counteract GPR43overexpression and PPARgamma-related adipogenesis in the white adipose tissue of high-fat diet-fed mice. *J. Nutr. Biochem., 22*, 712–722.

Etienne-Mesmin, L., Vijay-Kumar, M., Gewirtz, A. T., & Chassaing, B., (2016). Hepatocyte toll-like receptor 5 promotes bacterial clearance and protects mice against high-fat diet-induced liver disease. *Cell Mol. Gastroenterol. Hepatol., 2*, 584–604.

Everard, A., & Cani, P. D., (2013). Diabetes, obesity and gut microbiota. *Best Pract. Res. Clin. Gastroenterol., 27*, 73–83.

Farvid, *M. S.*, Eliassen, *A. H.*, Cho, E., Liao, X., Chen, W. Y., & Willett, *W. C.*, (*2016*). *Dietary fiber intake in young adults and breast cancer risk. Pediatrics, 137(3), 1–9.*

Flythe, M. D., & Aiken, G. E., (2010). Effects of hops (*Humulus lupulus* L.) extract on volatile fatty acid production by rumen bacteria. *J. Appl. Microbiol., 109*, 1169–1176.

Fuchs, C. S., Giovannucci, E. L., Colditz, G. A., et al., (1999). Dietary fiber and the risk of colorectal cancer and adenoma in women. N. Engl. J. Med., 340, 169–176.

Fung, T. T., Hu, F. B., Pereira, M. A., et al., (2002). Whole-grain intake and the risk of type 2 diabetes: A prospective study in men. Am. J. Clin. Nutr., 76, 535–540.

Gibson, G. R., (1999). Dietary modulation of the human gut microflora using the prebiotics oligofructose and inulin. *J. Nutr., 129*, 1438S–1441S.

Gulhane, M., Murray, L., Lourie, R., Tong, H., Sheng, Y. H., Wang, R., Kang, A., Schreiber, V., Wong, K. Y., Magor, G., et al., (2016). High fat diets induce colonic epithelial cell stress and inflammation that is reversed by IL-22. *Sci. Rep., 6*, 1–17.

Hamilton, M. K., Ronveaux, C. C., Rust, B. M., Newman, J. W., Hawley, M., Barile, D., Mills, D. A., & Raybould, H. E., (2017). Prebiotic milk oligosaccharides prevent development of obese phenotype, impairment of gut permeability, and microbial dysbiosis in high fat-fed mice. *Am. J. Physiol. Gastrointest. Liver Physiol., 312*, G474–G487.

Harlow, B. E., Lawrence, L. M., Kagan, I. A., & Flythe, M. D., (2014). Inhibition of fructan-fermenting equine faecal bacteria and *Streptococcus bovis* by hops (*Humulus lupulus* L.) beta-acid. *J. Appl. Microbiol., 117*, 329–339.

Keservani, R. K., Kesharwani, R. K., Sharma, A. K., Vyas, N., & Chadoker, A., (2010b). Nutritional supplements: An overview. *International Journal of Current Pharmaceutical Review and Research, 1*(1), 59–75.

Keservani, R. K., Kesharwani, R. K., Vyas, N., Jain, S., Raghuvanshi, R., & Sharma, A. K., (2010a). Nutraceutical and functional food as future food: A review. *Der Pharmacia Lettre, 2*(1), 106–116.

Keservani, R. K., Sharma, A. K., & Jarouliya, U., (2015). Protein and peptide in drug targeting and its therapeutic approach. *ARS Pharmaceutica (Internet), 56*(3), 165–177.

Keservani, R. K., Sharma, A. K., & Kesharwani, R. K., (2016a). Nutraceutical and functional foods for cardiovascular health. In: *Food Process Engineering* (pp. 257–278, 291–312). Apple Academic Press, CRC Press. ISBN: 9781771884020.

Keservani, R. K., Sharma, A. K., & Kesharwani, R. K., (2016b). Medicinal effect of nutraceutical fruits for the cognition and brain health. *Scientifica,* 10. Article ID 3109254, doi: 10.1155/2016/3109254.

Keservani, R. K., Sharma, A. K., & Kesharwani, R. K., (2017). An overview and therapeutic applications of nutraceutical and functional foods. *Recent Advances in Drug Delivery Technology,* 160–201. ISBN:9781522507543.

Keservani, R. K., Sharma, A. K., & Kesharwani, R. K., (2020). *Nutraceuticals and Dietary Supplements: Applications in Health Improvement and Disease Management*. CRC Press. ISBN: 9781771888738.

Kesharwani, R. K., Singh, P., & Keservani, R. K., (2016). Green coffee bean extract and chlorogenic acids: Chemistry and novel antioxidant benefits. In: Bagchi, D., Moriyama, H., & Swaroop, A., (eds.), *Green Coffee Bean Extract in Human Health* (pp. 1–17). Boca Raton, Taylor and Francis, USA. Chapter 1. ISBN: 9781498716376.

Kinnebrew, M. A., Ubeda, C., Zenewicz, L. A., Smith, N., Flavell, R. A., & Pamer, E. G., (2010). Bacterial flagellin stimulates toll-like receptor 5-dependent defense against vancomycin-resistant *Enterococcus* infection. *J. Infect. Dis., 201*, 534–543.

Krishnan, S., Rosenberg, L., Singer, M., et al., (2007). Glycemic index, glycemic load, and cereal fiber intake and risk of type 2 diabetes in US black women. Arch. Intern. Med., 167, 2304–2309.

Lee, Y. S., Li, P., Huh, J. Y., Hwang, I. J., Lu, M., Kim, J. I., Ham, M., Talukdar, S., Chen, A., Lu, W. J., et al., (2011). Inflammation is necessary for long-term but not short-term high-fat diet-induced insulin resistance. *Diabetes, 60*, 2474–2483.

Lindemans, C. A., Calafiore, M., Mertelsmann, A. M., O'Connor, M. H., Dudakov, J. A., Jenq, R. R., Velardi, E., Young, L. F., Smith, O. M., Lawrence, G., et al., (2015). Interleukin-22 promotes intestinal-stem-cell-mediated epithelial regeneration. *Nature, 528*, 560–564.

Liu, S., Willett, W. C., Stampfer, M. J., et al., (2000). A prospective study of dietary glycemic load, carbohydrate intake, and risk of coronary heart disease in US women. Am. J. Clin. Nutr., 71, 1455–1461.

Liu, T. W., Cephas, K. D., Holscher, H. D., Kerr, K. R., Mangian, H. F., Tappenden, K. A., & Swanson, K. S., (2016). Nondigestible fructans alter gastrointestinal barrier function, gene expression, histomorphology, and the microbiota profiles of diet-induced obese C57BL/6J mice. *J. Nutr., 146*, 949–956.

McKeown, N. M., Meigs, J. B., Liu, S., Saltzman, E., Wilson, P. W., & Jacques, P. F., (2004). Carbohydrate nutrition, insulin resistance, and the prevalence of the metabolic syndrome in the Framingham offspring cohort. Diabetes Care, 27, 538–546.

McKeown, N. M., Meigs, J. B., Liu, S., Wilson, P. W., & Jacques, P. F., (2002). Whole-grain intake is favorably associated with metabolic risk factors for type 2 diabetes and cardiovascular disease in the Framingham offspring study. Am. J. Clin. Nutr., 76, 390–398.

Miles, J. P., Zou, J., Kumar, M. V., Pellizzon, M., Ulman, E., Ricci, M., Gewirtz, A. T., & Chassaing, B., (2017). Supplementation of low- and high-fat diets with fermentable fiber exacerbates the severity of DSS-induced acute colitis. *Inflamm. Bowel Dis., 23*, 1133–1143.

Pereira, M. A., O'Reilly, E., Augustsson, K., et al., (2004). Dietary fiber and risk of coronary heart disease: A pooled analysis of cohort studies. Arch. Intern. Med., 164, 370–376.

Rabot, S., Membrez, M., Bruneau, A., Gerard, P., Harach, T., Moser, M., Raymond, F., et al., (2010). Germ-free C57BL/6J mice are resistant to high-fat-diet-induced insulin resistance and have altered cholesterol metabolism. *FASEB J., 24*, 4948–4959.

Rankin, L. C., Girard-Madoux, M. J., Seillet, C., Mielke, L. A., Kerdiles, Y., Fenis, A., Wieduwild, E., Putoczki, T., Mondot, S., Lantz, O., et al., (2016). Complementarity and redundancy of IL-22-producing innate lymphoid cells. *Nat Immunol., 17*(2), 179–186.

Rimm, E. B., Ascherio, A., Giovannucci, E., Spiegelman, D., Stampfer, M. J., & Willett, W. C., (1996). Vegetable, fruit, and cereal fiber intake and risk of coronary heart disease among men. JAMA, 275, 447–451.

Salazar, N., Dewulf, E. M., Neyrinck, A. M., Bindels, L. B., Cani, P. D., Mahillon, J., De Vos, W. M., Thissen, J. P., Gueimonde, M., De Los Reyes-Gavilan, C. G., et al., (2015). Inulin-type fructans modulate intestinal *Bifidobacterium* species populations and decrease fecal short-chain fatty acids in obese women. *Clin. Nutr., 34*, 501–507.

Schulze, M. B., Liu, S., Rimm, E. B., Manson, J. E., Willett, W. C., & Hu, F. B., (2004). Glycemic index, glycemic load, and dietary fiber intake and incidence of type 2 diabetes in younger and middle-aged women. Am. J. Clin. Nutr., 80, 348–356.

Singh, P., Kesharwani, R. K., & Keservani, R. K., (2017a). Antioxidants and vitamins: Roles in cellular function and metabolism. In: *Sustained Energy for Enhanced Human Functions and Activity* (pp. 385–407). Academic Press. ISBN:9780128054130.

Singh, P., Kesharwani, R. K., & Keservani, R. K., (2017b). Protein, carbohydrates, and fats: Energy metabolism. In: *Sustained Energy for Enhanced Human Functions and Activity* (pp. 103–115). Academic Press. ISBN:9780128054130.

Smith, P. M., Howitt, M. R., Panikov, N., Michaud, M., Gallini, C. A., Bohlooly, Y. M., Glickman, J. N., & Garrett, W. S., (2013). The microbial metabolites, short-chain fatty acids, regulate colonic Treg cell homeostasis. *Science, 341*, 569–573.

Sonnenburg, E. D., & Sonnenburg, J. L., (2014). Starving our microbial self: The deleterious consequences of a diet deficient in microbiota-accessible carbohydrates. *Cell Metab., 20*, 779–786.

Sonnenburg, E. D., Smits, S. A., Tikhonov, M., Higginbottom, S. K., Wingreen, N. S., & Sonnenburg, J. L., (2016). Diet-induced extinctions in the gut microbiota compound over generations. *Nature, 529*, 212–215.

Sugimoto, K., Ogawa, A., Mizoguchi, E., Shimomura, Y., Andoh, A., Bhan, A. K., Blumberg, R. S., et al., (2008). IL-22 ameliorates intestinal inflammation in a mouse model of ulcerative colitis. *J. Clin. Invest., 118*, 534–544.

Turnbaugh, P. J., Ley, R. E., Mahowald, M. A., Magrini, V., Mardis, E. R., & Gordon, J. I., (2006). An obesity-associated gut microbiome with increased capacity for energy harvest. *Nature, 444*, 1027–1031.

Verdam, F. J., Fuentes, S., De Jonge, C., Zoetendal, E. G., Erbil, R., Greve, J. W., Buurman, W. A., et al., (2013). Human intestinal microbiota composition is associated with local and systemic inflammation in obesity. *Obesity (Silver Spring), 21*, E607–E615.

Wang, X., Ota, N., Manzanillo, P., Kates, L., Zavala-Solorio, J., Eidenschenk, C., Zhang, J., Lesch, J., Lee, W. P., Ross, J., et al., (2014). Interleukin-22 alleviates metabolic disorders and restores mucosal immunity in diabetes. *Nature, 514*, 237–241.

Weitkunat, K., Schumann, S., Petzke, K. J., Blaut, M., Loh, G., & Klaus, S., (2015). Effects of dietary inulin on bacterial growth, short-chain fatty acid production and hepatic lipid metabolism in gnotobiotic mice. *J. Nutr. Biochem., 26*, 929–937.

Winer, D. A., Luck, H., Tsai, S., & Winer, S., (2016). The intestinal immune system in obesity and insulin resistance. *Cell Metab., 23*, 413–426.

Woting, A., & Blaut, M., (2016). The intestinal microbiota in metabolic disease. *Nutrients, 8*(4), 202.

Zhang, B., Chassaing, B., Shi, Z., Uchiyama, R., Zhang, Z., Denning, T. L., Crawford, S. E., Pruijssers, A. J., Iskarpatyoti, J. A., Estes, M. K., et al., (2014). Viral infection. Prevention and cure of rotavirus infection via TLR5/NLRC4- mediated production of IL-22 and IL-18. *Science, 346*, 861–865.

Zheng, X., Qiu, Y., Zhong, W., Baxter, S., Su, M., Li, Q., Xie, G., Ore, B. M., Qiao, S., Spencer, M. D., et al., (2013). A targeted metabolomic protocol for short chain fatty acids and branched-chain amino acids. *Metabolomics, 9*, 818–827.

Zheng, Y., Valdez, P. A., Danilenko, D. M., Hu, Y., Sa, S. M., Gong, Q., Abbas, A. R., Modrusan, Z., Ghilardi, N., De Sauvage, F. J., et al., (2008). Interleukin- 22 mediates early host defense against attaching and effacing bacterial pathogens. *Nat. Med., 14*, 282–289.

Zindl, C. L., Lai, J. F., Lee, Y. K., Maynard, C. L., Harbour, S. N., Ouyang, W., Chaplin, D. D., & Weaver, C. T., (2013). IL-22-producing neutrophils contribute to antimicrobial defense and restitution of colonic epithelial integrity during colitis. *Proc. Natl. Acad. Sci. USA, 110*, 12768–12773.

PART II
Food Supplements

CHAPTER 7

INTRODUCTION AND OVERVIEW OF FOOD SUPPLEMENTS

DILIP O. MORANI,[1] MANGESH S. BANSOD,[1] BHUSHAN R. RANE,[1] ASHISH S. JAIN,[1] and PRAVIN O. PATIL[2]

[1]*Shri D.D. Vispute College of Pharmacy and Research Center, Panvel, Maharashtra, India*

[2]*H.R. Patel Institute of Pharmaceutical Education and Research, Shirpur, Maharashtra, India*

ABSTRACT

The nutrients that may not be consumed in sufficient amounts are delivered by food supplements, often referred to as dietary supplements. Food supplements are available in different dosage forms like tablets, capsules, liquid, etc., and mainly contain minerals, vitamins, amino acids, and other components. The market for healthy food supplements was approximated to be worth USD 310.4 billion in 2020 and is predicted to further grow at a rate of 6.2% per year. Additionally, the COVID-19 pandemic has developed awareness among consumers regarding the importance of health. Thus, customers are purchasing nutrition supplements to boost their overall health. The World Health Organization (WHO) states that taking dietary supplements and eating a nutritious diet is very much important for boosting the immune system and key approach for a successful recovery from various illnesses, including COVID-19 infection.

Food Supplements and Dietary Fiber in Health and Disease. Bhushan R. Rane, Raj K. Keservani, Durgesh Singh, Nayan A. Gujarathi, and Ashish S. Jain, (Eds.)
© 2024 Apple Academic Press, Inc. Co-published with CRC Press (Taylor & Francis)

7.1 INTRODUCTION TO FOOD SUPPLEMENTS

The development of food habits is a very complex phenomenon that is influenced by a number of factors like income, prices, religion, region, family structure and habits, technological advancements, and stress levels. Various epidemiologic studies over the past 50 years have shown that diets dominated by vegetables, fruits, and dietary fibers reduce and prevent the chances of various diseases like obesity, diabetes, cardiovascular diseases as well as also enhance human health. High dietary intake of vegetables, fruits, and whole grains is mainly associated with decreased chances of developing various chronic diseases that are the highest causes of death in most industrialized countries, including the United States and Europe (Efsa, 2008; Liu, 2004). It is stated that one-third of all cancer deaths in industrialized countries may be minimized through appropriate dietary formulations. The type of fruit or vegetables that seems to be protective against cancer includes raw vegetables followed by alliums, vegetable, tomatoes, and carrots, green, and cruciferous vegetables (Denny & Buttriss, 2005).

According to 1994 Act of United state Dietary Supplement Health and Education (DHSEA), the dietary supplement may be defined by using various criteria; namely:

- A product planned to complement the diet that carries one or more dietary components like vitamin, mineral, dietary substance, amino acid, herb or other botanical for use by human to complete the diet by increasing total daily intake or metabolite, extract, concentrate, constituent or combination of such components (Zeisel, 1999);
- A product meant for administration in the form of capsule, tablet, liquid or pill form;
- A product not meant for use as the single item of meal or diet or as conventional food;
- Anything named as dietary supplement; and
- Products like newly approved drug, licensed biologic or certified antibiotic which was marketed as dietary food or supplement before approval certification or license (Kalra, 2003).

Due to their potential nutritional benefits, food supplements are considered demanding sources of nutrients which have nutritional or physiological results. As a result, their primary intention is to enrich a person's regular diet. Food supplements are becoming increasingly popular around the world, with plant extracts and botanicals particularly well-liked as they are supposed to be safer and healthier than manufactured medications. They are also expected to have no harmful side effects. The rise in sales also increases awareness of dietary supplements. The concentration of vitamins and minerals are limited in food supplements as reported in the European Union (EU), which is controlled by food laws and current legislation (Directive, 2002). While in the United States (US), the Food and Drug Administration (FDA) specifies the phrase "dietary supplement" as a certified one (FDA).

According to FDA, dietary supplements are products which contain one or more dietary ingredients that are taken up by mouth. Food supplements are available in various combinations and in a wide range of doses. But a certain amount of nutrient is required for our body to function and higher doses may not be necessarily better. Some substances may be harmful or may produce adverse effects in higher doses. Therefore, food supplements can be legally sold with warning 'not to exceed the dose' and appropriate dose recommendation for safeguarding the consumer's health. In general, women use more food supplements than men (Rovira et al., 2013).

7.2 BENEFITS OF FOOD SUPPLEMENTS

There are many advantages of taking the food supplements. Some of the important benefits are:

- Food supplements can treat digestive disorder such as lactose intolerant by taking lactase supplement on or particular deficiency.
- Benefits of dietary supplements are associated with acquiring specific nutrients from whole food.
- Further, food supplements can raise macronutrients like protein which is absorbed in the form of the whole food. For example, high protein supplement can help children of delayed growth to increase their height and weight and strengthen the immune system.

7.3 LIMITATIONS OF FOOD SUPPLEMENTS

The following are the drawbacks of taking food supplements:

- There is potential harm of regularly taking the food supplements in the diet which can outweigh the advantages they offer.
- Food supplements are not regulated by US FDA and also the contents of the container may not be similar with contents on label. Therefore,

the food supplements are usually taken under the guidance of health care personnel for the purpose of maximum safety.

- Furthermore, some food supplement may also be toxic at high doses. For instance, excessive intake of vitamin D can damage kidney and vitamin A may cause birth defects and liver damage.

7.4 CLASSIFICATION OF FOOD SUPPLEMENTS

Depending on the origin (natural or synthetic), food supplements may be distinguished. According to the form or texture in which they available, food supplements are classified as:

- Mineral and vitamin supplements either in the form of multi-minerals or multivitamins or not;
- Protein supplements either in the form of tablet or liquid in combination;
- Amino acids of every composition and form;
- Meal surrogates in the form of wafers, biscuits or powder;
- Supplements for increasing weight;
- Carbohydrate supplements with or without vitamins and electrolytes;
- Activator supplements for growth and other hormones;
- Supplements having natural anabolic effect and not included in banned substances list;
- Food ingredients like garlic, royal jelly, yeast;
- Herbs;
- Supplements of basic fatty acids.

The some of the classes, their examples and contents of food supplements are given in Table 7.1.

TABLE 7.1 Classification of Food Supplements Along with Examples and Contents

SL. No.	Class	Content	Examples
1.	Activator	Growth hormone and other hormones	Amino acids
2.	Carbohydrate	Vitamins and electrolytes	Dextrose
3.	Food and foodstuff	Yeast, royal jelly, garlic	Fish oil, vitamins, and minerals

TABLE 7.1 *(Continued)*

SL. No.	Class	Content	Examples
4.	Herbs	Other plant source and amino acid	Fiber, ginseng
5.	Minerals	Oily minerals	Selenium, multi-mineral tablets
6.	Multi-minerals and multivitamins	Both vitamin and mineral	Calcium supplement, vitamin D
7.	Oil supplements	Oily base with minerals and vitamins	Primrose oil, cod liver oil
8.	Vitamins	Oily vitamins	Vitamin B, vitamin C

7.5 NEED OF DIETARY SUPPLEMENTS

A healthy balance diet cannot be substituted by Food supplements (European Commission). The diet that contains plenty of whole grains, vegetables, fruits, healthy fats and adequate protein must provide all the essential nutrients necessary for good health. Many European countries confirmed that public information should concentrate dietary guidelines on based food (Eufic, 2009). Nowadays, everyone unable to take a healthy diet due to today's modern lifestyle. Dietary survey of Europe shows that micronutrients intake is below optimum (Troesch, 2012). The Eurreca project of Europe has found insufficient intakes of vitamin D, vitamin C, folic acid, iodine, calcium, and selenium (Eu, Eurreca). According to a national survey, recent comparisons have shown more concern on vitamin D intake, whereas some specific age groups have lesser intake of minerals (Mensink, 2012). For example, there is more concern on iron intake in teenage girls in Denmark, France, Germany, Poland, and the United Kingdom (UK). Further, in young women, poor iron content may lead to increase the risk of infants being born with less birth weight, deficiency of iron and delayed in brain development (Radlowski & Johnson, 2013). Moreover, in pregnant women, folate status is important and critical. Therefore, they are required to take folic acid before conception and used up to 12 weeks of pregnancy. However, the risk of having a baby with neural tube defect like spina bifida will be minimized by the optimum status of folate. Specific group of people requiring advice about food supplements are given in Table 7.2.

TABLE 7.2 Specific Group of People Requiring Advice about Food Supplements

SL. No.	Specific Group	Supplements
1.	Breastfeeding individuals	Vitamin D
2.	Children under five years age	Vitamin D, vitamin C, vitamin A
		Children having good appetite who eat a wide variety of food may not require them.
3.	People of age above 50	Folate, Vitamin B12, Vitamin D
		Frail elderly may be benefited by low dose multivitamin supplement
4.	People with darker skin or insufficient sun exposure	Vitamin D
5.	Vegans	Vitamin D, vitamin B12
6.	Women of childbearing age	Folic acid and vitamin D, specifically iron

7.6 SAMPLE PREPARATION AND EXTRACTION PROCEDURES FOR FOOD SUPPLEMENTS

Most of the producers have stated that their products contain some amount of plant extract, but the information does not confirm about the content of bioactive substances. The composition and content of bioactive substances depends on climate, season, soil, temperature, and other factors. However, a contradiction exists between active substance content in one dose and the amount of extract used and may have on dosing which can lead to either inefficient preparation or overdose. It should be acknowledged that most of the extracts are in solid form while considering methods of sample preparation for food supplements. Hence, the first step is pulverizing and homogenizing several dosage forms in sample handling procedures. Solid liquid extraction with ultrasound followed by filtration, centrifugation or both are common methods for the detection of bioactive substances in food supplements.

7.6.1 SOLID-LIQUID EXTRACTION (SLE)

Solid-liquid extraction (SLE) with ultrasound is the most commonly used method for determination of bioactive substances or adulterants of plant extract. This is due to extracted substance soluble in the solvent used for extraction. Moreover, the solvent used require no reconstitution and compatible with the method of instrumentation. The fastest and complete solid extraction can be achieved by using solvents of large exchange surfaces and short diffusion paths and by pulverizing and homogenizing solid samples. After sonification, filtration is (Brabcová et al., 2013; Šatínský et al., 2013; Omar et al., 2014; Fibigr et al., 2016) and then centrifugation (Fibigr et al., 2016) is required to remove undissolved material. In order to obtain high yield of analyzed substance and promote extraction, shaking (Cerezo et al., 2013), stirring (Lorenzo et al., 2014), and vortex mixing (Austin et al., 2014) of samples in extraction solvent have been reported before conducting sonification, filtration, and centrifugation. Different aqueous and acidified mixtures of methanol are as extraction solvent apart from methanol which is the common solvent for extraction.

7.6.2 SOLID PHASE EXTRACTION (SPE)

In mass spectrometry (MS), HRMS (high resolution mass spectrometry), and tandem mass spectrometry (MS/MS) analysis that required a high purity of analyzed samples, various forms of SPE are used as cleaning step. Thus, before analysis, extracts from the soft gels subjected to dispersive solid phase extraction (DSPE) for reducing the presence of co-separated from lipid substances in the oily matrix in the final sample; (Vaclavik et al., 2014). In food supplements, for the determination of phenolic compounds by ultra-high performance liquid chromatography-quadrupole time-of-flight mass spectrometry (UHPLC-Q-TOF-MS) (Hu et al., 2015), graphene oxide was used as sorbent for dispersive micro-solid phase extraction (DMSPE). SPE dependent molecularly imprinted polymers (MIPs) were used and reported in order to reduce effects of matrix in MS. The suitability of MIPs-UHPLC-MS/MS methods was checked by lovastatin detection in food supplements dependent on red yeast rice (Svoboda et al., 2017) for analyzing real samples. MIPs offer high selectivity and thus, used for the preparation of samples for complex plant matrix. However, for the extraction of biologically active substances from plant extracts, available MIP sorbents are less.

7.6.3 LIQUID-LIQUID EXTRACTION (LLE) AND MICRO-EXTRACTION METHODS

In dietary supplements, for the determination of anorectic drugs, phosphodiesterase 5 inhibitors and stimulants, LLE was commonly utilized for liquid chromatography-high resolution mass spectrometry (LC-HRMS). For the substances dispersed in 1M sodium hydroxide solution, a combination of ethyl ether/pentane (1:9) used as acceptor liquid (Shi et al., 2014). Before analysis of plant sterols and stanols, saponification of esterified forms is required. LLE of free sterols and stanols was done after 80°C saponification with ethanolic solution of 2M KOH when liquid chromatography (LC) or gas chromatography (GC) was used. Vortex mixing of sample solution was performed with LLE by diluted aqueous hydrochloric acid (HCl) and n-hexane in liquid chromatography method with charged aerosol detection (LC-CAD). Then, filtration of the organic part was performed and injection into the chromatographic system was done (Fibigr et al., 2017). This type of method of preparation of sample is rapid in contrast to method used in gas chromatography with flame ionization detector and mass spectrometry analysis in which before sample injected into GC system, reconstitution, and derivatization were performed (Srigley & Haile, 2015). After extraction of desired analytes, LLE used as cleaning step in all mentioned works. In all mentioned works, internal standards had to be used for correction in loss of analyte in sample preparation procedure including LLE which can introduce a margin of error due to its varying nature while measuring target analytes. However, this method is not environment friendly as per its standard design. Hence, old approach of LLE has been replaced by new methods such as dispersive liquid-liquid micro-extraction (DLLME), liquid-liquid micro-extraction (LLME) and single drop micro-extraction (SDME) (Ocaña-González et al., 2016; Hashemi et al., 2017; Spietelun et al., 2014). For analyzing food supplements, these methods are rarely used because of sufficient sample amounts and no necessity to reach detection limits.

7.6.4 OTHER PROCEDURES

Ground and dried food supplements samples were mixed with (65%) concentrated nitric acid and subjected to mineralization by microwave digestion for the inductively coupled plasma-mass-spectrometry (ICP-MS). Then, clear solutions transferred to volumetric flasks and finally, volume was makeup with deionized water (Filipiak-Szok et al., 2015). Using microwave digester equipped with temperature and pressure sensors was performed for simple and faster microwave assisted extraction (MAE) method in two works involving ICP-MS (Hsieh & Jiang, 2013; Yang et al., 2014).

7.7 ANALYTICAL METHODS

7.7.1 LIQUID CHROMATOGRAPHY (LC) METHODS

For analyzing bioactive substances in food supplements based on plant extracts, Reverse phase liquid chromatography (RP-LC) coupled with photodiode array (PDA) or ultraviolet-visible (UV-vis) is common method (Magiera et al., 2015; Wang et al., 2015; Fibigr et al., 2017; Fibigr et al., 2017). Fluorescence detector can also be used in order to obtain better selectivity and sensitivity (Moretón-Lamas et al., 2017). Other types of detectors like evaporative light scattering detectors (ELSD) (Avula et al., 2014) and charged aerosol detectors (CAD) had to be used in UV in case of low response of analytes. Though these detectors have a universal response to all semi-volatile or non-volatile analytes that do not contain fluorophore or chromophore in their molecules, they do not require derivatization and their sensitivity is quite good, but they are not widely used because of lack of spectral data and limited linear range.

The absence of real requirements is the main drawback of the PDA approach for studying compounds with comparable spectral homes and might result in misidentification of analytes. Thus, by using liquid chromatography tandem mass spectrometry (LC-MS/MS), this drawback can be reduced. Further, by using this instrumentation, low detection limits can be achieved. New ionization techniques in addition to sensitivity and selectivity have appreciated the use of LC-MS/MS for soft ionization of compounds. The most ionization techniques are performed by electrospray (ESI) (Avula et al., 2012; Hu et al., 2015; Cerezo et al., 2016; Svoboda et al., 2017; Paíga et al., 2017; Nantia et al., 2017; Shi et al., 2017; Filipiak-Szok et al., 2015).

ICP-MS has been employed in work dealing with metal analysis like toxic adulterants and bioactive compounds in plant extracts. Further, ICP-MS enables rapid analysis with good accuracy and precision for the determination of trace elements in plants. However, results obtained from reported works state that food supplements and medicinal plants contain elements in the range of μg/g and that concentration of elements varies widely. In studies samples, the content of toxic elements significantly differed from one another. This variation is described by agronomic and environmental conditions, growing in contaminated areas, differential exposure to pollution, bad purchasing sources and poor storage conditions (Yang et al., 2014). Furthermore, ICP-MS equipped with high performance liquid chromatography (HPLC) was used for the determination of cobalt (Hsieh & Jiang, 2013) and selenium (Havlíková et al., 2014) in dietary supplements.

Recently, alternative separation and determination techniques are useful for the analysis of plant extracts and assays of bioactive substances due to current advancement in accessories and equipment has increased their quality and reliability. Separation efficiency and elution speed was increased with satisfactory sensitivity and resolution by columns of core shell technology (Wong et al., 2014) and smaller particles. Elution speed can also be increased by using Monolithic column. In contrast to conventional C18 stationary phase, alternative stationary phases such as cyanopropyl, pentafluoro phenyl (Srigley & Haile, 2015) and phenyl-hexyl are used for different selectivity. These alternative stationary phases have many advantages like better selectivity, higher separation efficiency and shorter retention times.

7.7.2 GAS CHROMATOGRAPHY (GC) METHODS

Gas chromatography (GC) was used to determine adulterants and bioactive compounds in plant extracts which because of their way of detection and physic-chemical properties are not easily analyzed by LC method. Flame Ionization detector (FID) becomes used for the dedication of plant stanols and sterols and assay of methyl sulfonyl methane (MSM) in multicomponent meals supplements (Šatínský et al., 2014). For analysis of low concentrations of adulterants in plant extracts need sensitive and selective detection technique like MS triple quadruple coupled with GC (GC-MS/MS) (Hayward et al., 2013; Páleníková et al., 2015). In case of unavailability of reference standards or peak co-elution, identification of analytes could be based on MS spectra (Caligiani et al., 2013). Around 5% phenyl methyl polysiloxane capillary column of 30 meters length is the most common separation column.

The derivatization step required is the main disadvantage of GC when moderate polar or non-polar substances are analyzed to achieve symmetric peaks, enhance separation and detection of these compounds and ensure satisfactory precision. Thus, for analysis of bioactive substances and detection of adulterants in plant extracts, LC is a common method as compared with GC.

7.7.3 SUPERCRITICAL FLUID CHROMATOGRAPHY (SFC) METHODS

For determination of bioactive substances having similar structures and for the separation of isomers, an important alternative method is SFC (Ganzera,

2015; Sánchez-Hernández, 2016; Wang et al., 2016). Also, it acts as a substitute to normal phase liquid chromatography (NPLC) used to analyze plant extracts. In SFC, Carbon dioxide (CO_2) is mostly used as mobile phase as it is used eco-friendly. In comparison to conventional gases, SFC offer lower viscosity, higher dissolving capacity, diffusivity, and density above its critical pressure and temperature. Thus, because of these unique characteristics, SFC is considered as effective tool for analyzing thermally unstable and non-volatile compounds. Further, as compared with HPLC, SFC gives higher flow rates and shorter run times. For separating hydrophobic compounds such as carotenoids which are difficult to separate by conventional LC or with long run times, SFC is more effective due to low polarity of CO_2 (Li et al., 2015). Also, for increasing the polarity, co-solvent like methanol can be utilized. The recent advancements in technology, particularly in the use of particles having a size smaller than 2 μm in ultra-high-performance liquid chromatography (UHPLC) may be applied to the ultra-high performance supercritical fluid chromatography (UHPSFC).

7.7.4 OTHER TECHNIQUES

Various other techniques are also used for assay determination and testing purity of plant extract as compared with other methods. These methods include Fourier transform infrared spectroscopy (FTIR), nuclear magnetic resonance (NMR) and thin layer chromatography (TLC).

For detection of regulated plants and herbs in plant dietary supplements (Deconinck et al., 2017), illegally added drugs in dietary supplements (Zhang et al., 2014) and quantitative determination of coenzyme Q10 from food supplements (Racz et al., 2015), the use of near infrared spectral imaging technology has been utilized. Detection limit of FTIR could not reach to the level of HPLC and high performance liquid chromatography mass spectrometry (HPLC-MS) techniques due to its properties. Wherein, for complex plant material, near infrared spectral imaging require only minutes while HPLC require time up to hours. Further, before using techniques which are time consuming and more precise, spectral imaging gives screening for illegally added drugs and adulterants in food supplements.

NMR is an important tool for quantification of bioactive substance in food supplement. Proton nuclear magnetic resonance (^1H NMR) spectroscopy is a strong tool which gives reliable results quantitatively in a short period of time. This method is more important as it minimizes sample preparation and enables analysis of a large number of samples without human intervention. To determine the total content of statin in red yeast rice (Lachenmeier et al., 2012) and coenzyme Q10 (Monakhova et al., 2013) in dietary supplements, simple, and direct ^{1}H NMR was employed. Detection, identification, and quantification of adulterants in dietary food supplements marketed for increasing sexual performance (Gilard et al., 2015) and weight loss (Hachem et al., 2016), was done by using this instrumentation.

To automate different steps, increase resolution and allow for accurate quantitative measurement, several modifications have been done in the fundamental method of TLC. Due to instability of TLC, the advanced form, i.e., high performance thin layer chromatography (HPTLC) can be a more important tool for qualitative and quantitative analysis of problematic compounds. To detect antidiabetic chemicals in dietary supplements from adulterated diabetic plants, rapid *in situ* method was developed. Surface enhance Raman spectroscopy (SERS) was utilized for qualitative identification of trace substances on HPTLC plate after separating analytes and pharmaceutical matrix components by HPTLC (Zhu et al., 2014). To confirm structure elucidation or identification of carotenoids resolved on TLC plate, new camag thin layer chromatography-mass spectrometry (TLC-MS) interface is considered as useful technique (Rodić et al., 2012). For qualitative comparison of barley juice extracts obtained from different origins, HPTLC can be used. For analyzing plant extracts, HPTLC gives simple and rapid solution as HPTLC fingerprint analysis have shown chemical uniformity accompanied by some qualitative differences (Havlíková et al., 2014). The suitability of analytical methods for the detection of specific group of bioactive substances in dietary supplements are given in Figure 7.1.

Storage and distribution of medicinal plants and their improper handling may result in fungi contamination which can further lead to mycotoxin production. Due to lack of surveillance, increased consumption of contaminated plant extracts may create health problems. Food supplement may become contaminated with mycotoxins and lead to health and hazardous problems (Ashiq et al., 2014). In the analysis of 50 commercial products, ultra-performance liquid chromatography – tandem mass spectrometer (UHPLC-MS/MS) method was developed, evaluated, and used for detection of 34 mycotoxins in dietary supplements containing coffee bean extracts. Presence of fumonisin B1, mycophenolic acid, ochratoxin A and B, and 10 to 36% contaminated preparations was confirmed (Vaclavik et al., 2013). LC-MS/MS method can also be used in other works. Alternaria mycotoxins, enniatins, zearalenone, and fusarium trichothecenes were the main contaminating mycotoxins.

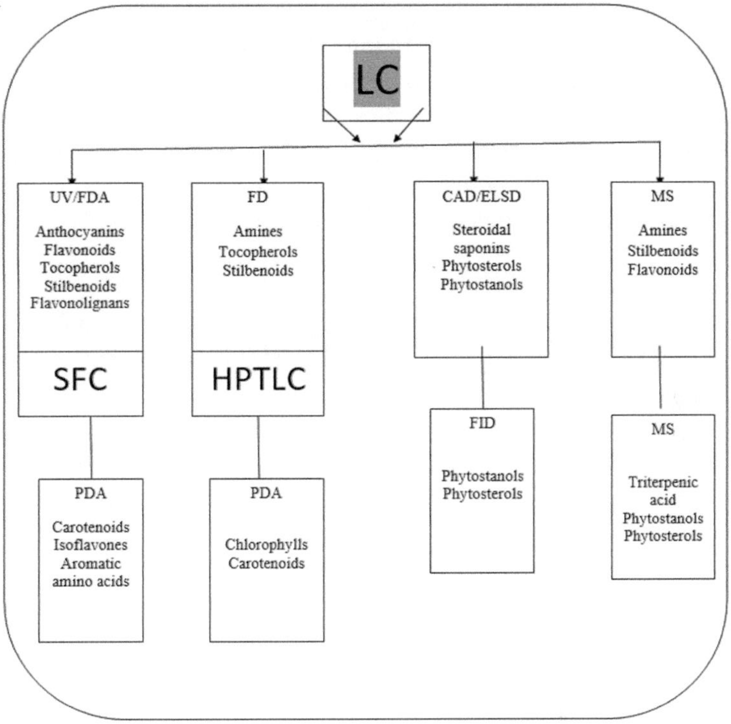

FIGURE 7.1 Suitability of analytical methods for detection of specific group of bioactive substances in dietary supplements.

7.7.5 ANALYSIS OF ENDOCRINE DISRUPTORS (EDS) IN PLANT EXTRACTS OF DIETARY SUPPLEMENTS

EDs interact with human or animal endocrine system is synthetic compounds and affects its function. In food supplements, EDs may have different origins based on plant extracts, for instance, from bioaccumulation in the food chain or plant contaminated by industrial pollution. Bio-accumulate and persistent compounds include polychlorinated biphenyl, alkylphenols, dioxins, and dichlorodiphenyltrichloroethane that can cause risk in livestock and plant manufacturing. Marketed herbal preparations are formulated as capsule that contains ethanolic extract of active compounds or dried enriched plant material (Veprikova et al., 2015). While producing dietary supplements based on plant extract, the common practice is not to avoid co-isolation of potential contaminants. Therefore, due to their similar physic-chemical properties of biologically active compounds, they may be present in raw materials and co-extracted. Thus, their enrichment may vary from trace levels to exceeding limits and cause a health hazard to consumers.

For instance, 8% of tested samples of organophosphorus pesticide residues in conventional Chinese medicine meals supplements (Li et al., 2017) were positive for contamination, but the pesticide content was lower than the limit set by the United States environmental protection agency.

7.7.6 DETERMINATION OF ADULTERANTS, CONTAMINANTS, AND PHARMACEUTICALS IN DIETARY SUPPLEMENTS

To increase the stated claims on the labels, anorectic, and antidiabetic drugs are added illegally to the food supplements and chemical substances like phosphodiesterase-5 (PDE-5) inhibitors and undeclared pharmaceuticals are considered as serious issues regarding purity of dietary supplements. Hence, it may create a challenge for analysts and lead to serious health problems to consumers. One special case is adulterant detection of high glucose levels based on *Stevia rabaudiana* extracts. But the findings were confusing for consumers who are suffering from diabetes and trying to maintain their sugar level.

In the last few years, advanced detection technique like high-resolution MS (HRMS) has enabled non-targeted and complex analysis of tested dietary supplements. Ultra-high-performance liquid chromatography-HRMS (UHPLC-HRMS) is used for the determination of anorectic drugs (Shi et al., 2014; Strano-Rossi et al., 2015), PDE-5 inhibitors, pharmaceuticals (Vaclavik et al., 2014), and secondary metabolites in plant extracts. For analyzing alkaloids, anti-hypertensive drugs, multiple pharmaceuticals and steroidal hormones occurring in supplement preparations, MS has been used (Martínez-Domínguez et al., 2015). Some work on assessing the purity of plant extracts and food supplements have been reported for additional analytical techniques like Fourier transform near infra-red spectroscopy (FT-NIR) for pharmaceutical drugs (Zhang et al., 2014), NMR for PDE-5 inhibitors and thin layer chromatography-surface enhance Raman spectroscopy (TLC-SERS) for antidiabetics (Zhu et al., 2014).

7.8 QUALITY ASSURANCE/QUALITY CONTROL (QA/QC)

Quality assurance/quality control (QA/QC) control must be established in order to guarantee reliable and precise results. Different validation guidelines are available for reference, such as European pharmacopeia recommendations international conference on harmonization (ICH), US FDA guidelines on bioanalytical method validation, US pharmacopeial convention, and others. No complete validation method is available for analyzing bioactive substances and contaminants in food supplements which includes accuracy and precision, carryover, linearity, matrix effect, recovery, robustness, stability of samples, selectivity, and sensitivity of proposed methods in reported works. The control of all these parameters were declared by the above-mentioned guidelines and recommendations. For LC, GC, and SFC methods, system suitability test is an essential part of the validation procedure. For identification of bioactive substances, retention, and spectra times were commonly employed. Due to complexity of plant extracts, method cannot give guarantee of analyzed substance in reference and sample solutions and therefore, verification of analyzed substance has to be carried out. Such verification can be easily done by HRMS, MS, and MS/MS. For adulterants, such types of validation parameters are present in FDA guidelines, official medicines control laboratory (OMCL) and audited under International standard organization (ISO) 17025.

7.9 SCOPE OF FOOD SUPPLEMENTS

There is limited information available regarding the use of dietary supplements among athletes. In 2001, the global market of food supplements was 46 billion US dollars, and in 2000, the US supplement market was 16.7 billion US dollars. Athletes make up a certain portion of the overall food supplements market, and wide ranges of products are targeted for both the active population and those who are engaged in competitive sports. A meta-analysis of 51 published surveys involving 10,274 female and male athletes showed 46% overall prevalence of food supplement use (Sobal & Marquart, 1994). However, the prevalence of use depends on sport, athletes of different age groups, cultural background and standards of performance. In some cases where strength and power are important in sports, the use of food supplements is usual.

Only a few studies have tried to quantify the frequency or amount of supplement use, but it appears that athletes frequently exceed the dosage recommendations of food supplements. This is due to many reasons like feeling of "more is better" or because of opponents or team mates are using higher doses or due to competition. In some preparations, the amount of food supplement may be very less as compared with the amount essential for efficacy, particularly when expensive ingredients are involved, whereas in some preparations, the dose of food supplements may be higher than the effective dose, e.g., creatine. Individual athlete estimates prove that some may consume a larger number of different food supplements on a regular basis and the amounts consumed are higher than those proven to be safe. Most people assume that 'natural' dietary supplements are safe, but long-term high doses of many of these supplements can be harmful. Iron, zinc, and other metals are most commonly consumed by many people in quantities that are known to be harmful. Athletes and often those who advise them to take food supplements were appeared to be completely unaware of the dangers. Various reasons for use of food supplements include:

- To meet demands of high competition;
- To get benefited for performance;
- To make up the inadequate diet;
- To match with team-mates;
- Advised by coach or supervisor.

7.10 CONCLUSION

In this chapter, we tried to give a recapitulation of different analytical and sample preparation methods for assessing the purity of plant extracts and determination of bioactive substances in food supplements based on plant extract. HPLC coupled with Photodiode Array Ultraviolet (PDA/UV) detectors is the preferred technique for bioactive substances. This is because this method is already established in many laboratories which perform regular analysis of various samples, not just in dietary supplements. SFC gives high selectivity for separations of isomeric compounds whereas GC method is used for determination of bioactive substances. For determination of specific groups of bioactive substances, suitable analytical techniques and their detection methods are given in Figure 7.1.

For testing the purity of plant extracts, UHPLC coupled with HRMS, MS, MS/MS methods are used. Due to low concentration of target compound, advance instrumentation is needed to cover a wide range of analytes and complexity of sample matrices. For the protection of consumers, quality control test should be performed beginning from raw material to finished product. However, no analytical method can give assurity about quality control of all the parameters of food supplements. This indicates the necessity of advanced methods for making purity assessments of plant extracts and advance techniques for assuring quality control of food supplements based on plant extracts. Therefore, health safety of consumers will be improved.

KEYWORDS

- **dietary supplements**
- **dispersive solid phase extraction**
- **Food Drug Administration**
- **food supplements**
- **high resolution mass spectrometry**
- **mass spectrometry**
- **nutraceuticals**
- **nutritional supplements**

REFERENCES

Ashiq, S., Hussain, M., & Ahmad, B., (2014). Natural occurrence of mycotoxins in medicinal plants: A review. *Fungal Genet. Biol., 66*, 1–10.

Austin, K. G., Travis, J., Pace, G., & Lieberman, H. R., (2014). Analysis of 1,3 dimethylamylamine concentrations in *Geraniaceae*, geranium oil and dietary supplements. *Drug Test. Anal., 6*, 797–804.

Avula, B., Wang, Y. H., Ali, Z., Smillie, T. J., & Khan, I. A., (2014). Chemical fingerprint analysis and quantitative determination of steroidal compounds from *Dioscorea villosa*, Dioscorea species and dietary supplements using UHPLC-ELSD. *Biomed. Chromatogr., 28*, 281–294.

Avula, B., Wang, Y. H., Wang, M., Smillie, T. J., & Khan, I. A., (2012). Simultaneous determination of sesquiterpenes and pyrrolizidine alkaloids from the rhizomes of *Petasites hybridus* (L.) G.M. et Sch. and dietary supplements using UPLC-UV and HPLC-TOF-MS methods. *J. Pharm. Biomed. Anal., 70*, 53–63.

Brabcová, I., Kovářová, L., Šatínský, D., Havlíková, L., & Solich, P., (2013). A fast HPLC method for determination of vitamin E acetate in dietary supplements using monolithic column. *Food Anal. Methods, 6*, 380–385.

Caligiani, A., Malavasi, G., Palla, G., Marseglia, A., Tognolini, M., & Bruni, R., (2013). A simple GC–MS method for the screening of betulinic, corosolic, maslinic, oleanolic and ursolic acid contents in commercial botanicals used as food supplement ingredients. *Food Chem., 136,* 735–741.

Cerezo, A. B., Leal, Á., Álvarez-Fernández, M. A., Hornedo-Ortega, R., Troncoso, A. M., & García-Parrilla, M. C., (2016). Quality control and determination of melatonin in food supplements. *J. Food Compos. Anal., 45*, 80–86.

Deconinck, E., Djiogo, C. A. S., Bothy, J. L., & Courselle, P., (2017). Detection of regulated herbs and plants in plant food supplements and traditional medicines using infrared spectroscopy. *J. Pharm. Biomed. Anal., 142*, 210–217.

Denny, A., & Buttriss, J. (2005). Synthesis Report No 4: Plant Foods and Health: Focus on Plant Bioactives, British Nutrition Foundation. https://www.bezpecnostpotravin.cz/UserFiles/File/Kvasnickova2/EuroFIR_4.pdf (accessed on 12 February 2023).

Di Lorenzo, C., Dos Santos, A., Colombo, F., Moro, E., Dell'Agli, M., & Restani, P., (2014). Development and validation of HPLC method to measure active amines in plant food supplements containing *Citrus aurantium* L. *Food Control, 46*, 136–142.

Directive2002/46/EC, http://eur-lex.europa.eu/legal-content/EN/TXT/?uri=CELEX:32002L0046 (accessed on 28 January 2023).

EFSA (European Food Safety Authority), (2008). Scientific opinion of the panel on dietetic products, nutrition and allergies on a request from the EC on food-based dietary guidelines. *The EFSA J.,* 1–44.

EU project EURRECA. https://eurreca.net (accessed on 28 February 2023).

Fibigr, J., Šatínský, D., & Solich, P., (2016). A study of retention characteristics and quality control of nutraceuticals containing resveratrol and polydatin using fused-core column chromatography. *J. Pharm. Biomed. Anal., 120*, 112–119.

Fibigr, J., Šatínský, D., & Solich, P., (2017). A new approach to the rapid separation of isomeric compounds in a *Silybum marianum* extract using UHPLC core-shell column with F5 stationary phase. *J. Pharm. Biomed. Anal., 134*, 203–213.

Fibigr, J., Šatínský, D., & Solich, P., (2017). A UHPLC method for the rapid separation and quantification of phytosterols using tandem UV/charged aerosol detection – A comparison of both detection techniques. *J. Pharm. Biomed. Anal., 140*, 274–280.

Fibigr, J., Šatínský, D., & Solich, P., (2017). A UHPLC method for the rapid separation and quantification of anthocyanins in acai berry and dry blueberry extracts. *J. Pharm. Biomed. Anal., 143*, 204–213.

Fibigr, J., Šatínský, D., Havlíková, L., & Solich, P., (2016). A new method for rapid determination of indole-3-carbinol and its condensation products in nutraceuticals using core–shell column chromatography method. *J. Pharm. Biomed. Anal., 120*, 383–390.

Filipiak-Szok, A., Kurzawa, M., & Szłyk, E., (2015). Determination of toxic metals by ICP-MS in Asiatic and European medicinal plants and dietary supplements. *J. Trace Elem. Med. Bio., 30*, 54–58.

Ganzera, M., (2015). Supercritical fluid chromatography for the separation of isoflavones. *J. Pharm. Biomed. Anal., 107*, 364–369.

Gilard, V., Balayssac, S., Tinaugus, A., Martins, N., Martino, R., & Malet-Martino, M., (2015). Detection identification and quantification by 1H NMR of adulterants in 150 herbal dietary supplements marketed for improving sexual performance. *J. Pharm. Biomed. Anal., 102*, 476–493.

Hachem, R., Assemat, G., Martins, N., Balayssac, S., Martino, V., Gilard, R., et al., (2016). Proton NMR for detection, identification and quantification of adulterants in 160 herbal food supplements marketed for weight loss. *J. Pharm. Biomed. Anal., 124*, 34–47.

Hashemi, B., Zohrabi, P., Kim, K. H., Shamsipur, M., Deep, A., & Hong, J., (2017). Recent advances in liquid-phase microextraction techniques for the analysis of environmental pollutants. *Trac-Trend. Anal. Chem., 97*, 83–95.

Havlíková, L., Šatínský, D., Opletal, L., & Solich, P., (2014). A fast determination of chlorophylls in barley grass juice powder using HPLC fused-core column technology and HPTLC. *Food Anal. Methods, 7*, 629–635.

Hayward, D. G., Wong, J. W., Shi, F., Zhang, K., Lee, N. S., DiBenedetto, A. L., & Hengel, M. J., (2013). Multiresidue pesticide analysis of botanical dietary supplements using salt-out acetonitrile extraction, solid-phase extraction cleanup column, and gas chromatography–triple quadrupole mass spectrometry. *Anal. Chem., 85*, 4686–4693.

Hsieh, Y., & Jiang, S., (2013). Determination of selenium compounds in food supplements using reversed-phase liquid chromatography–inductively coupled plasma mass spectrometry. *Microchem. J., 110*, 1–7.

https://food.ec.europa.eu/safety/labelling-and-nutrition/food-supplements_en (accessed on 12 February 2023).

https://www.eufic.org/en/healthy-living/article/food-based-dietary-guidelines-in-europe (accessed on 12 February 2023).

Hu, S. S., Cao, W., Da, J. H., Dai, H. B., Cao, J., Ye, L. H., Li, X. Y., & Chu, C., (2015). Dispersive micro solid-phase extraction with graphene oxide for the determination of phenolic compounds in dietary supplements by ultra-high-performance liquid chromatography coupled with quadrupole time-of-flight tandem mass spectrometry. *Food Anal. Methods, 8,* 833–840.

Kalra, E. K., (2003). Nutraceutical–definition and introduction. *AAPS Pharm. Sci., 5*, 25. Available online: http://www.aapsj.org/view.asp?art=ps050325 (accessed on 28 January 2023).

Lachenmeier, D. W., Monakhova, Y. B., Kuballa, T., Löbell-Behrends, S., Maixner, S., Kohl-Himmelseher, M., Waldner, A., & Steffen, C., (2012). NMR evaluation of total statin content and HMG-CoA reductase inhibition in red yeast rice (*Monascus* spp.) food supplements. *Chin. Med-UK, 7*, 1–7.

Li, B., Zhao, H., Liu, J., Liu, W., Fan, S., Wu, G., et al., (2015). Application of ultra-high performance supercritical fluid chromatography for the determination of carotenoids in dietary supplements. *J. Chromatogr. A, 1425*, 287–292.

Li, J., Li, D., Wu, J., Qin, J., Hu, J., Huang, W., Wang, Z., Xiao, W., & Wang, Y., (2017). Simultaneous determination of 35 ultra-trace level organophosphorus pesticide residues in Sanjie Zhentong capsules of traditional Chinese medicine using ultra high performance liquid chromatography with tandem mass spectrometry. *J. Sep. Sci., 40*, 999–1009.

Liu, R. H., (2004). Potential synergy of phytochemicals in cancer prevention: Mechanism of action. *J. Nutr., 134*, 3479S–3485S.

Magiera, S., Baranowska, I., & Lautenszleger, A., (2015). UHPLC–UV method for the determination of flavonoids in dietary supplements and for evaluation of their antioxidant activities. *J. Pharm. Biomed. Anal. 102*, 468–475.

Martínez-Domínguez, G., Romero-González, R., & Frenich, A. G., (2015). Determination of toxic substances, pesticides and mycotoxins, in ginkgo biloba nutraceutical products by liquid chromatography orbitrap mass spectrometry. *Microchem. J., 118*, 124–130.

Mensink, G. B., Fletcher, R., Gurinovic, M., et al., (2012). Mapping low intake of micronutrients across Europe. *British Journal of Nutrition, 14*, 1–19.

Monakhova, Y. B., Ruge, I., Kuballa, T., Lerch, C., & Lachenmeier, D. W., (2013). Rapid determination of coenzyme Q10 in food supplements using 1 H NMR spectroscopy. *Int. J. Vitam. Nutr. Res., 83*, 67–72.

Moretón-Lamas, E., Lago-Crespo, M., Lage-Yusty, M. A., & López-Hernández, J., (2017). Comparison of methods for analysis of resveratrol in dietary vegetable supplements. *Food Chem., 224*, 219–223.

Nantia, E. A., Moreno-González, D., García-Campaña, A. M., & Gámiz-Gracia., L., (2017). High-throughput methodology for the determination of carbamates in food supplements by UHPLC–MS/MS. *Chromatographia., 80*, 63–70.

Ocaña-González, J. A., Fernández-Torres, R., Bello-López, M. Á., & Ramos-Payán, M., (2016). New developments in microextraction techniques in bioanalysis. A review. *Anal. Chim. Acta, 905*, 8–23.

Omar, J. M., Yang, H., Li, S., Marquardt, R. R., & Jones, P. J. H., (2014). Development of an improved reverse-phase high-performance liquid chromatography method for the simultaneous analyses of trans-/cis resveratrol, quercetin, and emodin in commercial resveratrol supplements. *J. Agric. Food Chem., 62*, 5812–5817.

Paíga, P., Rodrigues, M. J. E., Correia, M., Amaral, J. S., Oliveira, M. B. P. P., & Delerue-Matos, C., (2017). Analysis of pharmaceutical adulterants in plant food supplements by UHPLC-MS/MS. *Eur. J. Pharm. Sci., 99*, 219–227.

Páleníková, A., Martínez-Domínguez, G., Arrebola, F. J., Romero-González, R., Hrouzková, S., & Frenich, A. G., (2015). Multifamily determination of pesticide residues in soya-based nutraceutical products by GC/MS–MS. *Food Chem., 173*, 796–807.

Racz, A., Vass, A., Heberger, K., & Fodor, M., (2015). Quantitative determination of coenzyme Q10 from dietary supplements by FT-NIR spectroscopy and statistical analysis. *Anal. Bioanal. Chem., 407*, 2887–2898.

Radlowski, E. C., & Johnson, R. W., (2013). Perinatal iron deficiency and neurocognitive development. *Frontiers in Human Neuroscience, 7*, 585.

Rodić, Z., Simonovska, B., Albreht, A., & Vovk, I., (2012). Determination of lutein by high-performance thin-layer chromatography using densitometry and screening of major dietary carotenoids in food supplements. *J. Chromatogr. A, 1231*, 59–65.

Rovira, M. A., Grau, M., Castañer, O., et al., (2013). Dietary supplement use and health-related behaviors in a Mediterranean population. *Journal of Nutrition Education and Behavior, 45*(5), 386–391.

Sánchez-Hernández, L., Bernal, J. L., Del Nozal, M. J., & Toribio, L., (2016). Chiral analysis of aromatic amino acids in food supplements using subcritical fluid chromatography and chirobiotic T2 column. *J. Supercrit. Fluid, 107*, 519–525.

Šatínský, D., Jägerová, K., Havlíková, L., & Solich, P., (2013). A new and fast HPLC method for determination of rutin, troxerutin, diosmin and hesperidin in food supplements using fused-core column technology. *Food Anal. Methods, 6*, 1353–1360.

Šatínský, D., Pospíšilová, M., & Sladkovský, R., (2014). A new gas chromatography method for quality control of methylsulfonylmethane content in multicomponent dietary supplements. *Food Anal. Methods, 7*, 1118–1122.

Shi, F., Guo, C., Gong, L., Li, J., Dong, P., Zhang, J., Cui, P., Jiang, S., Zhao, Y., & Zeng, S., (2014). Application of a high-resolution benchtop quadrupole-Orbitrap mass spectrometry for the rapid screening, confirmation and quantification of illegal adulterated phosphodiesterase-5 inhibitors in herbal medicines and dietary supplements. *J. Chromatogr. A, 1344*, 91–98.

Shi, H., Zhao, Y., Sun, J., Yu, L. L., & Chen, P., (2017). Chemical profiling of glucosinolates in cruciferous vegetables based dietary supplements using ultra-high performance liquid chromatography coupled to tandem high resolution mass spectrometry. *J. Food Compos. Anal., 61*, 67–72.

Sobal, J., & Marquart, L. F., (1994). Vitamin/mineral supplement use among athletes: A review of the literature. *International Journal of Sport Nutrition, 4*, 320–324.

Spietelun, A., Marcinkowski, Ł., De La Guardia, M., & Namieśnik, J., (2014). Green aspects, developments and perspectives of liquid phase microextraction techniques. *Talanta, 119*, 34–45.

Srigley, C. T., & Haile, E. A., (2015). Quantification of plant sterols/stanols in foods and dietary supplements containing added phytosterols. *J. Food Compos. Anal., 40*, 163–176.

Strano-Rossi, S., Odoardi, S., Castrignanò, E., Serpelloni, G., & Chiarotti, M., (2015). Liquid chromatography–high resolution mass spectrometry (LC–HRMS) determination of stimulants, anorectic drugs and phosphodiesterase 5 inhibitors (PDE5I) in food supplements. *J. Pharm. Biomed. Anal., 106*, 144–152.

Svoboda, P., Sander, D., Plachká, K., & Nováková, L., (2017). Development of matrix effect-free MISPE-UHPLC– MS/MS method for determination of lovastatin in Pu-erh tea, oyster mushroom, and red yeast rice. *J. Pharm. Biomed. Anal., 140*, 367–376.

Troesch, B., (2012). Dietary surveys indicate vitamin intakes below recommendations are common in representative Western countries. *British Journal of Nutrition, 108*(4), 692–698.

Vaclavik, L., Krynitsky, A. J., & Rader, J. I., (2014). Targeted analysis of multiple pharmaceuticals, plant toxins and other secondary metabolites in herbal dietary supplements by ultra-high performance liquid chromatography–quadrupole-orbital ion trap mass spectrometry. *Anal. Chim. Acta, 810*, 45–60.

Vaclavik, L., Vaclavikova, M., Begley, T. H., Krynitsky, A. J., & Rader, J. I., (2013). Determination of multiple mycotoxins in dietary supplements containing green coffee bean extracts using ultrahigh-performance liquid chromatography−tandem mass spectrometry (UHPLC-MS/MS). *J. Agric. Food Chem., 61*, 4822−4830.

Veprikova, Z., Zachariasova, M., Dzuman, Z., Zachariasova, A., Fenclova, M., Slavikova, P., Vaclavikova, M., et al., (2015). Mycotoxins in plant-based dietary supplements: Hidden health risk for consumers. *J. Agric. Food Chem., 63*, 6633−6643.

Wang, M., Carrell, E. J., Chittiboyina, A. G., Avula, B., Wang, Y. H., Zhao, J., et al., (2016). Concurrent supercritical fluid chromatographic analysis of terpene lactones and ginkgolic acids in ginkgo biloba extracts and dietary supplements. *Anal. Bioanal. Chem., 408*, 4649–4660.

Wang, Y., Avula, B., Tang, W., Wang, M., Elsohly, M. A., & Khan, I. A., (2015). Ultra-HPLC method for quality and adulterant assessment of steviol glycosides sweeteners – *Stevia rebaudiana* and stevia products. *Food Addit. Contam. A, 32*, 674–685.

Wong, Y. F., Makahleh, A., Saad, B., Ibrahim, M. N. M., Rahim, A. A., & Brosse, N., (2014). UPLC method for the determination of vitamin E homologues and derivatives in vegetable oils, margarines and supplement capsules using pentafluorophenyl column. *Talanta, 130*, 299–306.

Yang, F., Jiang, S., & Sahayam, A. C., (2014). Combined use of HPLC–ICP-MS and microwave-assisted extraction for the determination of cobalt compounds in nutritive supplements. *Food Chem., 147*, 215–219.

Zhang, R., Yin, L., & Jin, S., (2014). Detection of illegally added drugs in dietary supplements by near-infrared spectral imaging. *J. Innov. Opt. Heal. Sci., 7*, 1–7.

Zhu, Q., Cao, Y., Cao, Y., Chai, Y., & Lu, F., (2014). Rapid on-site TLC–SERS detection of four anti-diabetes drugs used as adulterants in botanical dietary supplements. *Anal. Bioanal. Chem., 406*, 1877–1884.

CHAPTER 8

ROLE OF FOOD SUPPLEMENTS IN DIABETES

JAVESH KASHINATH PATIL,[1] Y. HASNI SAYYED HAMID,[1] and MUKESH R. PATEL[2]

[1]*Poojya Sane Guruji Vidya Prasarak Mandal's College of Pharmacy, Shahada, Nandurbar, Maharashtra, India*

[2]*Assistant Registrar, Shri Govind Guru University, Godhra, Gujarat, India*

ABSTRACT

Diabetes mellitus is one of the prevailing metabolic disorders affecting globally. The current data says around 422 million people are affected with diabetes globally and this fact of global spreading is very well understood by the recognized institutions such as WHO, USDA, IDF, and CDA. Prediabetes, type 1, type 2, gestational diabetes, and other specific etiologic types are a few important classes of diabetes with urbanization, lifestyle, and genetic susceptibility as the main cause. Diet and supplements had a great role in prevention as well as management of diabetes, even the long-term complications of diabetes can be prevented or delayed. The common dietary supplements recommended in diabetes are micronutrients, antioxidants, dietary fibers, vitamins, and phyto foods. The details of all these dietary materials beneficial in diabetes along with examples, source, role, mechanism, and other recent research are explained in the chapter.

Food Supplements and Dietary Fiber in Health and Disease. Bhushan R. Rane, Raj K. Keservani, Durgesh Singh, Nayan A. Gujarathi, and Ashish S. Jain, (Eds.)
© 2024 Apple Academic Press, Inc. Co-published with CRC Press (Taylor & Francis)

8.1 INTRODUCTION

Diabetes mellitus (DM) is a heterogeneous set of metabolic disorders of fat and protein characterized by elevated blood sugar/glucose levels for a longer period that result in various health issues to many important organs of the body (Bai et al., 2019; NCCIH, 2021). The DM can be diagnosed using blood glucose level testing and associated with some common symptoms such as more hunger and fatigue, increased thrust (polydipsia), frequent urination (polyuria), itchy and dry skin, pain, and numbness in feet and legs, and blurred vision (Terri, 2021).

The current statistic of World Health Organization (WHO) had reported that DM is rapidly spreading globally. The prevalence of the disorder among the adult population of the world was 4.7% in 1980 that had risen to 8.5% in 2014 and presently accounting for around 422 million people affected with DM (WHO, 2021). On the other hand, as per the latest data of 2019 of the International Diabetes Federation (IDF), the burden of DM globally is around 463 million adults which growing fast estimated to be double by 2030 (IDF, 2020). Even after community healthcare initiatives to reduce the prevalence of this chronic illness, it is predicted that about 414 million individuals globally suffer from T2DM, with the number expected to climb to over 640 million by 2040 (Itsiopoulos et al., 2018). The top five countries having the maximum dominance of DM are India, China, the United States, Indonesia, and Japan. In India alone, more than 65 million adults are linked with diabetes it accounts for around 6.5 to 7.2% of the adult population (Harsh, 2015; Chandraguptala et al., 2020). While in China as per the 2010 study around 92 million cases were registered and around 150 million cases of early symptoms were found (BBC, 2010). The developed countries of Europe and America, namely the United Kingdom, Canada, and the United States are also showed a significant number of cases viz. 3.8 million, 2.4 million, and 29.1 million, respectively (WHO, 2021).

Diabetes mellitus is not a life-threatening condition, but surely reduces the quality of life and life expectancy hence considered as one of the primary reasons of morbidity and mortality globally. Around 5% augmentations in untimely mortality cases from DM are observed all over the globe. Around 1.5 million Fatalities are caused only by diabetes in 2019. The expected major health-related complications are microvascular and macrovascular complications that result in end-stage renal disease, ischemic heart diseases (IHD), stroke, gangrene of the lower extremities, and loss of sight in adults (WHO, 2021; Harsh Mohan, 2015; Jenny & Karin, 2016). Apart from the impact of DM on health, it impacted socially too; its high prevalence especially in association with micro- and macrovascular complications implied a high social and financial cost and had resulted in high co-morbidity and mortality rates in the affected population globally (Alberto, 2018).

8.1.1 CAUSES OF DIABETES MELLITUS

Looking to the context of causes of diabetes mellitus, it was very evident that developed countries of Asia, Europe, and America are having high prevalence while underdeveloped countries such as African countries showed low incidence. These facts now directly linking the DM as a condition associated with urbanization, lifestyle, and genetic susceptibility. People with obesity, low levels of physical activity and high caloric diet are easily susceptible to DM especially type 2 than type 1. In addition to this people with clinical conditions such as hypertension, dyslipidemia, systemic inflammation, metabolic complications, smokers, and age are also susceptible to DM and very prone to vascular complications of DM (Harsh, 2015; Jenny & Karin, 2016). Genetics do have a vital play in the progression of DM, especially in type 1 diabetes (T1D) and few atypical types of DM are straightforwardly inherited like maturity – onset diabetes in the young (MODY), and diabetes because of mitochondrial DNA mutations (WHO, 2021).

8.1.2 TYPES OF DIABETES MELLITUS

Diabetes mellitus for the convenience of understanding had been classified in a different way like primary (idiopathic) and secondary types, juvenile-onset, and maturity-onset types, insulin-dependent (IDDM) and non-insulin-dependent (NIDDM) types, and likewise much more, but all these classifications now outdated and underwent key revisions in recent times due to improved knowledge of etiology and pathogenesis of DM (Harsh, 2015). The very recent classification of DM is depicted in Table 8.1 (Rebecca, 2019).

8.1.2.1 PREDIABETES

It's a clinical condition where blood sugar level is over normal but it is not sufficient which can be used to diagnose DM. Prediabetes does not show any clinical symptoms but it is understood that a person with prediabetes will convert to type 2 DM over some time which is approximately 10 years. The conversion from prediabetes to type to DM can be reversed by doing lifestyle changes, dietary changes, and exercise (Rebecca, 2019; Mayo Clinic, 2021).

8.1.2.2 TYPE 1 DM

Previously it was called insulin-dependent diabetes or juvenile-onset diabetes and nearly constitutes 10% of cases of DM. It was understood that Type 1 DM occurs at a young age and the patient was dependent on Insulin for treatment hence the nomenclature was there, but the recent understanding of etiology had changed the concept. Based on the etiology, type 1 DM can be of two subtypes; Subtype 1A (immune-mediated) DM or deficiency or Subtype 1B (idiopathic) DM (Harsh, 2015; Rebecca, 2019).

8.1.2.2.1 Subtype 1A (Immune-Mediated) DM

This subtype is an autoimmune condition; the self-antibodies of a person destroy the β-cells of the pancreas leading to a deficiency of insulin.

8.1.2.2.2 Subtype 1B (Idiopathic) DM

This subtype is not an autoimmune condition but exemplifies insulin deficiency. The reason for deficiency of insulin is not clear hence also called idiopathically but here the patient is having a tendency to develop ketosis.

8.1.2.3 TYPE 2 DM

This type of DM is a little milder compared to type 1 DM but still holds major health complications. Type 2 DM contributes around 80% of cases of DM usually affects people of age above 30 years. Type 2 DM was formerly named maturity-onset diabetes, or non-insulin-dependent diabetes mellitus (NIDDM). The type 2 DM etiology is not clear but the pancreas was not able to synthesize a sufficient quantity of insulin results in hyperglycemia or the recent advancement says that sufficient insulin was created but patient develops the insulin resistance due to this developed insulin is ineffective and could not control blood sugar level in its normal range leading to type 2 DM (Harsh, 2015; Rebecca, 2019).

8.1.2.4 OTHER SPECIFIC ETIOLOGIC TYPES OF DM

In addition to the two key forms explain above, around 10% of cases of DM appear due to different etiological reasons such as family history, obesity, routine bodily sluggishness, race, and traditions, impaired glucose tolerance, hyper-tension, vascular diseases, and many more.

8.1.2.5 GESTATIONAL DIABETES

This is a type of DM associated with pregnancy, around 1 to 10% of pregnant women show the development of insulin resistance in middle or late pregnancy, which results in elevated blood glucose levels called gestational diabetes. Even though their blood sugar levels return to normal subsequent to delivery, such ladies are more likely to acquire diabetes later in life.

TABLE 8.1 Types and Subtypes of Diabetes Mellitus

SL. No.	Types	Subtypes
1.	Prediabetes	–
2.	Type 1 DM	• Subtype 1A (immune-mediated) DM • Subtype 1B (idiopathic) DM
3.	Type 2 DM	–
4.	Other specific types	• The genetic defect of β-cell • Endocrinopathies • Diseases of the exocrine pancreas • The genetic defect of insulin • Drug- or chemical-induced • Immune-mediated DM • Infections • Genetic syndrome
5.	Gestational DM	–

8.1.3 PATHOPHYSIOLOGY OF DIABETES MELLITUS

Diabetes has a complicated etiology that involves multiple hormones namely insulin, glucagons, and growth hormone and the interplay of these hormones and there direct connection with liver and kidney makes it more complex. Based on the etiology DM may be considered as the result of either reduced insulin secretion within the body or decreased capacity of the body to utilize glucose. In the case of Type 1 DM, there is a complete lack of insulin due to the destruction of β-cells of the pancreas either due to autoimmune or some idiopathic reasons. The three important interlinked mechanisms can be considered as key for the pathogenesis of Type 1 DM, and these include genetic susceptibility at the time of birth, autoimmunity, and activity of CD4+ T lymphocytes or infections or environmental factors that triggers the action of destruction of β-cells of the pancreas. In Type 2 DM body losses its ability to utilize glucose due to a low level of insulin or resistance to insulin by peripheral tissue ends up with a high plasma glucose level. Type 2 DM affects a larger segment of people despite this fact of high rates of incidence of DM we know very less about its pathogenesis and etiology. The fact is the deficiency of insulin is not the result of the destruction of the pancreatic cell but the inability of pancreatic cells to meet the requirement of the body for insulin. The identification of exact underline factors is not possible but can be summarized as the existence of multiple diseases, hereditary or genetic defects, obesity, increased glucose production, or resistance to insulin at the receptor level (Jahangir, 2019; Harsh, 2015). Hyperglycemia irrespective of type and etiology can harm nerves and blood vessels, primarily those in the eyes, heart, and kidneys, if treatment is delayed. Diabetic neuropathy, retinopathy, cardiovascular disease (Keservani et al., 2016a), and nephropathy are all possible consequences. Without correct intervention, blindness, renal failure, and a higher incidence of heart attack or stroke may occur (Sharon et al., 2018; Diabetes.org, 2017; Gillespie, 2006; Weinstock et al., 2021).

8.2 ROLE OF FOOD SUPPLEMENTS IN DIABETES

The basis of diabetic prevention and cure, in combination with medicine, is a commitment to a diet and eating patterns. Alternative treatments include supplemental insulin, a specific food, and/or medicines which alter blood glucose levels, based on the kind and severity of the diabetes. Patients may also need to take biological and active/nutritional supplements, which are pharmaceuticals made from natural ingredients. In diabetes patients, dietary restrictions combined with metabolic disturbances might lead to impaired absorption of certain vital nutrients. As an outcome, mineral, and vitamin shortages are common among these individuals (Vladimir et al., 2017).

Food intake is the most adjustable of the different risk variables that add to the inception and advancement of type 2 diabetes mellitus. A substantial increase in the prevalence suggests that a meal richer in more phytochemicals, antioxidant potential, and polyphenolic (Keservani & Sharma, 2014) substances is linked to a reduced incidence of diabetes and its contributing variables. Diverse pharmacological and non-pharmacological therapies have been developed according to the etiology of insulin resistance and type 2 diabetes mellitus with the goal of enhancing control of blood sugar and preventing diabetic complications (Nimesh & Ashwlayan, 2018). Non-pharmacological therapies include many important food supplements.

In the United States and across the globe, food supplements are a booming business. According to trade statistics, the revenue of these merchandises for all indications in the U.S. total is greater than $30 billion, with worldwide sales exceeding $100 billion. Despite the absence of proof for several famous supplements on the market, supplement consumption remains popular among buyers. Supplements (Keservani et al., 2010a, b) may be used by consumers to maintain or improve their health, to rectify a nutritional shortfall, or to treat a specific health issue. The regulatory system for food supplements in the United States differs significantly from that for medicines. Before a novel drug may be used on the market, its manufacturers must produce proof of its safety and efficacy to the US-FDA for assessment and approval. Dietary supplements are not held to similar standards. Dietary supplements are not designed to diagnose, cure, avoid, or treat any ailment, according to federal law. As a result, before to product introduction on the market, FDA approved proof of supplement's effectiveness and safety also isn't necessary. Similarly, there are no rules governing the legality of product claims, except that claiming a supplement helps to avoid, cure or treat an illness is prohibited. Promotion of manufactured supplementary product as an anti-diabetic product cannot be done, but the maker can mention that it is helpful in balancing the sugar level needed to remain healthy. Actually, customers may find it challenging to distinguish these distinctions when interpreting the possible effects of a supplement (Hannon et al., 2020; Shahbandeh, 2019; Mikulic, 2018; Starr, 2015).

When compared with the general population, those with diabetes were 1.6 times more likely to take complementary alternative medicine (CAM), according to a study that looked at the Medical Expenditure Panel Survey. As per the data mentioned in a nationally representative telephone poll, 57% of diabetic respondents used complementary and alternative medicine in the year 2017. CAM includes spiritual healing, acupuncture, massages, along with dietary supplements, which play a vital role in CAM. Because so many patients are eager to attempt complementary and alternative medicine, it's crucial to look into nutritional supplements that could help with prevention (Sharon et al., 2018; Gloria Yeh et al., 2002).

According to dietary pattern studies, a high consumption of whole grains, vegetables, and fruits may protect against type 2 diabetes. A low-glycemic-index diet has also been associated to a decreased occurrence of type 2 diabetes. It is ambiguous; however, which minerals or dietary components are responsible for this impact. Dairy foods, which are high in calcium and magnesium, have also been linked to a lowered incidence of type 2 diabetes mellitus, however the benefit was shown in two trials for dairy products having low-fat values (Raquel et al., 2009).

Medical nutrition therapy (MNT) is advantageous to circumvent diabetes, controlling diabetes, and delaying or prevent the development of diabetic complications. As a result, it is crucial at all three stages of diabetes prevention. To primarily prevent diabetes, adopt MNT and public health interventions in those who are obese or have pre-diabetes. Adopt MNT for diabetes, metabolic management as a secondary preventive to avoid complications. Adopt MNT to postpone and control diabetic complications as a tertiary preventive to avoid morbidity and death (ADA, 2008).

8.3 FOOD SUPPLEMENTS BENEFICIAL IN DIABETES

8.3.1 MICRONUTRIENTS

A growing amount of research suggests that certain micronutrients like Vanadium, Magnesium, Chromium, and Selenium are associated to the risk of Type 2 diabetes. The detailed description of mentioned micronutrients sources, significance, and mechanism in the management of diabetes is explained in subsections.

8.3.1.1 Vanadium

Although vanadium is just a trace mineral in the biosphere, it is the earth's surface's 21st most prevalent element. It can be found as a mere salt or as a polyoxovanadate in a variety of minerals. Vanadium is a trace element that is present in human food as well as iron and some other transition metal supplements. The usual diet provides around 2 mg of vanadium per day, while the body contains 20 to 25 mg of vanadium under normal conditions. Vanadium is present in a variety of cereals, as well as in dill seed, carrot, peas, maize, radish, tomato, black pepper, and pear, since it is typically taken up by crops cultivated in soils with high vanadium. Eggs, meat, fish (liver), vegetable oils, buckwheat, and oats are also abundant in vanadium. These natural sources are believed to be harmless than over the counter (OTC) medications due to their organic state (Crans et al., 2019; Walsh, 2021).

According to research, vanadium works similarly to insulin in moving glucose into cells, making it beneficial in both type 1 and type 2 diabetes. Supplementing with vanadium further reduced fasting blood sugar, cholesterol, and hemoglobin A1c levels. Fasting glucose levels (the amount of sugar in the blood when you wake up in the morning) can be improved with doses ranging from 45 to 150 mg per day. These dose levels have been found to be safe and well-tolerated by the majority of persons in toxicity tests. During the first week of usage or at higher dose levels (up to 400 mg per day), some people suffer minor gastrointestinal discomfort (Saurabh & Vrish, 2018).

The inhibitory impact of Vanadium on the action of protein tyrosine phosphatases (PTP) is one of the mechanisms proposed for the insulin like result of this element. This action is caused by antagonism between vanadate anions (VO_4^{3-}) and phosphate anions (PO_4^{3-}). Vanadium contributes significantly to receptor activation by inhibiting PTP-1B. Further, which inactivates the insulin-receptor (INS-IR) that performs a vital function in the metabolism of glucose, probably through prevention of detachment of phosphates from the residues of tyrosine phosphates of the beta subunit of INS-IR. The insulin induced signal transduction is the outcome of the stimulation of the PI3K-Akt pathway, which is engaged in the metabolism of lipids and carbohydrates. As an outcome, the transportation of glucose into cells becomes more efficient. The influence of reactive oxygen species (ROS) (produced by Vanadium compounds) on PTP-1B activity has also been postulated. Furthermore, vanadium also inhibits gluconeogenesis and glycogenolysis, and stimulates glycogenogenesis. Vanadium compounds or complexes are reported to have insulin-mimetic characteristics, implying that they play a role in glucose metabolism (Scibior et al., 2020; Trevino et al., 2019).

8.3.1.2 MAGNESIUM

Magnesium (Mg) is an element which the person needs for good health. Magnesium is needed for a range of body activities, involving muscular and neuronal performance, cardiac output, and blood glucose levels, along with protein, DNA, and bone synthesis. Magnesium is present naturally in a range of foodstuffs, with high concentrations in leguminous fruits, bran cereal, whole grains, spinach, some seeds, and nuts. A good amount of magnesium is present in milk, yogurt, and milk products. Additionally, it is also included in a few fortified foodstuffs. Magnesium can be found in multivitamin and mineral supplements, as well as numerous food supplements. Magnesium chloride, magnesium lactate, magnesium aspartate, and magnesium citrate, are more readily absorbed forms of magnesium in dietary supplements. Magnesium is also found in certain heartburn and laxatives and indigestion relief medications.

Consumption of so less magnesium doesn't quite cause noticeable symptoms in the short term. The kidneys assist retain magnesium by reducing the quantity lost in urine whenever healthy persons have low intakes. Low magnesium intake prolonged time, on the other hand, might result in magnesium insufficiency. Furthermore, some medical disorders and medicines might impair the body's capacity to absorb magnesium or increase the quantity of magnesium excreted, resulting in magnesium shortage. Nausea, vomiting, loss of appetite, tiredness, and weakness are symptoms of magnesium deficit. Muscular cramps, numbness, tingling, seizures, behavioral changes, and an irregular heart rhythm are all symptoms of severe magnesium deficiency. The per-day requirement of Magnesium recommended is about 400–420 mg and 310–320 mg for men and women, respectively. Magnesium supplements in high amounts can induce diarrhea and abdominal cramps. Extremely high dosages (more than 5,000 mg daily) can be fatal (NIH, 2021; NCCIH, 2021).

A vital role of Magnesium is observed in balancing insulin and glucose metabolism, and Mg insufficiency is frequent among adults having Type 2 diabetes. Although hypomagnesemia is a widespread symptom in people with type 2 diabetes, it has also been associated to an augmented risk of acquiring the disease. Magnesium, the most common intracellular divalent cation, is engaged in the enzymatic process of glucose metabolic pathways, high-energy phosphate, and energetic metabolism as an important co-factor. One meta-analysis of probable research suggests a dose-response relationship between diets magnesium consumption and the risk of type-2 diabetes (Yingting et al., 2018; Barbagallo et al., 2015; Dong et al., 2011; Rodriguez et al., 2011). The intracellular magnesium translocation is one suggested process. Insulin has a role in intracellular magnesium shifts, and intracellular magnesium appears to control insulin function in oxidative glucose metabolism. The insulin mediated glucose uptake and sensitivity to insulin is decreased as a result of impairment of tyrosine kinase action at the level of insulin receptor and that occurs due to less intracellular concentration of magnesium (Yeung et al., 2018). Several researchers have examined whether consuming magnesium supplements might benefit persons with diabetes or individuals who are at possibility of getting it. However, the results of the studies aren't conclusive. Additional research is needed to discover whether magnesium can help with diabetes management (NIH, 2021).

8.3.1.3 CHROMIUM

Chromium, among the most abundant minerals in the earth's surface and ocean, may be found in a variety of oxidation states in our ecosystem, including metallic (Cr^0), trivalent (+3), and hexavalent (+6) chromium. The last one is very hazardous and is primarily produced by oxidation of its more widespread and naturally existing trivalent chromium. Chromium is an important trace mineral that may be found in a variety of foods in trivalent form (William & Frank, 2004). Your body can't utilize glucose efficiently if you don't get enough chromium in your diet. According to an analysis, using chromium supplements along with standard treatment improved blood sugar control in patients with diabetes (mainly type 2) who had impaired glycemic control.

Large dosages of chromium supplements have been reported to induce stomach pain and bloating, as well as renal damage, muscle issues, liver failure, thrombocytopenia, hemolysis, mood swings and skin reactions. Hypoglycemia may be more prevalent among patients who take insulin or insulin secretagogues with chromium. The protracted implications of chromium supplementation haven't been well investigated (NCCIH, 2021; Campbell, 2010).

By potentiating insulin activity, chromium may have a function in carbohydrate, protein, and lipid metabolism. Even though the underlying mechanism for this action has yet to be discovered, researchers believe that chromium links to an oligopeptide that produces a low molecular weight chromium-binding fragment called chromodulin that attaches to the insulin receptor and activating it to increase insulin function. Chromium may have antioxidant properties as well. Meats, grains, vegetables, fruits (grapes, oranges, apples, and bananas), brewer's yeast, spices, nuts, wine, and beer all contain chromium. The quantity of chromium in these meals, on the other hand, varies greatly relying on regional soil and water variables, as well as the farming and manufacturing techniques utilized to make these. The absorption of chromium from food is modest, ranging from 0.4 to 2.5%. Around 35 μg and 25 μg are the advised daily intakes of chromium for males and females, respectively. According to some studies, those with more severe insulin resistance and weaker glycemic control may benefit better from chromium supplementation.

The American Diabetes Association determined in its 2010 diabetes recommendations that since research has not conclusively demonstrated that chromium supplementation improves patients with diabetes or obesity, the association cannot endorse it. This decision was made based on contradictory information from trials that were either poorly controlled or uncontrolled. In a 2015 policy statement, the association determined that there is inadequate proof to justify the regular usage of chromium and other micronutrient supplements for sugar management in diabetic patient. More investigation is necessary to see if some individuals (medication usage, ethnicity, baseline insulin sensitivity, and obesity, for example) are more likely to benefit from chromium supplementation over others (NIH, 2021).

8.3.1.4 SELENIUM

Selenium may be found in both inorganic and organic forms in nature. In its organic state, Selenium is linked to proteins known as selenoproteins. Selenocysteine and selenomethionine are the two most common organic forms. Eggs, chicken, meat, seafood (fish), dairy foods (yogurt, milk, cheese, condensed milk, ice-cream, butter), fruits (apple, kiwi, grapes, mango, orange), grains, cereals, garlic, celery, lettuce, onion, green peas, pepper, and Brazilian nuts are all high in Selenium. Many enzymes, including glutathione hyperoxidase, deiodinase-Iodothyronine, selenoprotein P, and Thioredoxin-reductase include selenium. Glutathione hyperoxidase, which also contains selenocysteine, is an important antioxidant because it catalyzes the elimination of organic hydrogen peroxide and hyper-oxides from tissues. When these compounds are withdrawn from the human, compounds become toxic to biomembranes, causing them to break down (Karalis, 2019; Navarro-Alarcon and Cabrera-Vique, 2008).

Glutathione peroxidase, an enzyme that guards cell membranes from oxidative degradation, contains selenium. Glutathione peroxidase reduces the risk of oxidative damage caused by free radicals by metabolizing hydrogen peroxide. The presence of selenium in the diet affects the effectiveness of glutathione peroxidase. The protein complex Nuclear Factor-kappa B (NF-κB) is a transcription factor. It is found in cells and is engaged in cellular responses to stress, UV irradiation, free radicals, oxidized low-density lipoprotein, and viral or bacterial antigens, among other things. When cells are exposed to stressful stimuli, they produce NF-κB, which then moves to the cell's nucleus. Over the course of three months, everyday supplementation with 960 μg substantially decreased selenium NF-κB activity, according to a randomized study. Another research revealed a substantial decrease in serum urine albumin discharge rates and plasma Thio-barbituric acid reactive substances (TBARS) after using 100 μg per day for three months (Hannah & Frank, 2008).

Quantification of glucose, blood lipids, insulin, insulin resistance, and inflammatory indicators are observed to be improved in human clinical studies. Antioxidant enzyme action, blood sugar, and insulin sensitivity all improved in animal studies. Nevertheless, one review points to a link between selenium and diabetes incidence, as well as the hyperglycemic outcomes of selenium in rats (Panchal et al., 2017).

Selenium is a mineral that may be found in both plants and soil. Selenium is a trace element that is needed by the humans in tiny levels. Too much selenium can lead to gastrointestinal issues, nail snags, hair loss, and nerve damage, among other things (Miranda, 2007).

Food is the primary source of Selenium, and based on the kind of meal ingested, around 80% of the total of dietary Selenium is absorbed. Bioavailability of Selenium differs depending on the Selenium source and the subject's nutritional state, with organic forms of Selenium being considerably larger.

Because Selenium may replace sulfur in amino acids such as selenocystathionine, selenocysteine, and selenomethionine owing to their physicochemical resemblances, dietary protein concentration is another significant factor determining Selenium present in food. Seleno-compounds would also be utilized to make Se-amino acids (primarily selenomethionine and selenocysteine), which would then be integrated into vegetable proteins. As a result, the Selenium forms found in animal feed vegetable proteins are eventually used in the production of the animal's own proteins, promoting their accumulation in cattle. Several plant species have been identified as Selenium accumulators, including *Allium sativum* (Garlic), *Brassica napus* (Canola), *Brassica juncea* (Indian mustard), and certain mushrooms. They have the capacity to absorb huge quantities of Selenium (above 1000 mg Se/kg) without experiencing any harmful consequences (Navarro-Alarcon and

Cabrera-Vique, 2008). The daily requirement of Selenium recommended is about 55 μg for both men and women (NIH, 2021).

8.3.2 ANTIOXIDANTS

Antioxidants are natural or artificial compounds which is used to prevent or slowdown the cell damages of many kinds. They are commonly exist in foods like vegetables and fruits and available even as food supplement products. The common examples beneficial in diabetes are omega fatty acid, alpha-Lipoic acid, and carotenes.

8.3.2.1 OMEGA-3 FATTY ACID

Omega-3 fatty acids are a kind of polyunsaturated fatty acid (PUFAs). Omega-3 fatty acids (omega-3s), often known as "n-3s." Vitamin F is another term for omega-3 fatty acids, which comes from the word "fatty acids." Even though there are numerous distinct omega-3s, most systematic study focuses on three: alpha-linolenic acid, eicosapentaenoic acid (EPA), and docosahexaenoic acid (DHA). Alpha-linolenic acid has 18 C-atoms, but EPA and DHA have 20 and 22 carbon atoms, correspondingly, and are entitled "long-chain" omega-3s as well. Seafood possesses the omega-3s DHA as well as EPA (fish, mackerel, herring, tuna, sardines, shellfish, salmon, and nutritional supplements like fish oil, and krill oil). Alpha linolenic acid is present in vegetable oils including soybean, flaxseed, pumpkin seed, and canola oils, as well as several other plant-based foods, such as black walnuts and Chia seeds. These healthy fats increase muscular activity, reduce blood clotting, aid digestion, and facilitate cell division and development, which are all necessary for the proper functioning of numerous organs. The average daily intake recommended is about 2.06 gm and 1.59 gm for males and females, respectively (Sandoiu, 2017; Gammone et al., 2019; NCCIH, 2021; NIH, 2021).

In diabetic individuals, omega-3 was linked to a substantial decrease in Apolipoprotein AII (Natto et al., 2019). Proteinuria was decreased in those with type 2 diabetes mellitus as well as type 1 diabetic mellitus who took omega-3s. Only type 2 diabetes persons had this association considerably (Chewcharat et al., 2021).

The major reason of morbidity and mortality in type 2 diabetes is cardiovascular disease (CVD). Plant-derived alpha-linolenic acid has also been found to lower CVD mortality, although it has distinct effects on CVD risk variables than EPA and DHA, as revealed by a previous meta-analysis comprising 12 studies with 744 individuals, 120 of whom had type 2 diabetes. One research validates omega-3 PUFAs' triglyceride-lowering benefits, reveals possible dose-response effects, and suggests thrombogenesis improvements. LDL levels are raised by omega-3 PUFAs without a change in lipid particle size. Modification in traditional jeopardy variables is inadequate to clarify the decreases in CVD threat associated with omega-3 PUFAs (Hartweg et al., 2009). A huge populace-based case control research found that taking a cod-liver oil plus vitamin D supplement in the first year of life dramatically decreased the danger of childhood-onset type-1 diabetes (Li, 2019).

8.3.2.2 ALPHA LIPOIC ACID (ALA)

Antioxidant alpha-lipoic acid is a vitamin-like molecule. ALA is a sulfur-containing molecule found in human cells and is needed for energy generation in the mitochondria. Alpha-lipoic acid is found in small quantities in many foods. Brussels sprouts, broccoli, spinach, beets, tomatoes, carrots, yams, potatoes, yeast, and rice bran are among the vegetables. Alpha-lipoic acid can also be found in red meat, particularly organ meat (kidney and liver).

The most prevalent usage of alpha-lipoic acid in diabetics is to relieve nerve discomfort (diabetic neuropathy). ALA has garnered a lot of interest as a prospective therapy for diabetic peripheral neuropathy because of its antioxidant qualities and capacity to enhance blood vessel circulation to the nerves. Germany has approved ALA in high doses for the cure of these nerve-related indications. It's also used to treat obesity and excessive blood cholesterol or other fats (lipids).

Alpha-lipoic acid appears to assist the body in resisting some types of cell damage while also restoring vitamin E and vitamin C levels. Alpha-lipoic acid has additionally been shown to enhance the functioning and conduction of neurons in diabetics. The body uses alpha-lipoic acid to break down carbohydrates and provide energy for the other organs. Alpha-lipoic acid exerts its effects as an antioxidant, which implies it may protect the brain from injury or damage. The antioxidant properties may also be beneficial in the treatment of some liver disorders (WebMD, 2021; Bradley & Walter, 2012).

It is frequently referred to be a universal antioxidant since it can rejuvenate several antioxidants such as Coenzyme Q10, vitamin C, vitamin E, and glutathione. Because of hyperglycemia provoked activation of the polyol pathway and production of advanced glycation end products (AGE) and reactive oxygen species (ROS), antioxidants have a role in diabetes therapy.

ALA protects diabetic cardiomyopathy (DCM) patients by inhibiting NF-κB activation, lowering matrix metalloproteinase-2, and lowering fas-ligand (Jeffrey et al., 2021).

Oxidation in diabetes causes hyperglycemia to worsen, and hyperglycemia causes additional oxidation, leading to cycle pathophysiology. Because ALA can interrupt this cycle by inhibiting oxidation, it's a promising treatment option for prediabetes and diabetes (Kaczor, 2020).

There is no set dosage for alpha-lipoic acid because it is an investigational therapy. However, for diabetes and neuropathy, studies have utilized 600–1,800 mg per day (Griffin, 2020). If you take alpha-lipoic acid with diabetic medicines, your blood glucose may drop excessively low. However, additional data is required to determine whether or not this relationship is of major significance (WebMD, 2021; Bradley & Walter, 2012).

8.3.3 DIETARY FIBERS

Every one of us had listened to this word have more fiber in our diet that make a good impact on human health, yes, it is true. The food containing dietary fibers are very perfectly alleviating conditions of digestion, constipation, heart diseases, and diabetes too. These dietary fibers obtained from plant and used as food by humans are bulky carbohydrates material that can't be get digested and can't be get absorb hence comes out undigested from the human body. High consumption of plant-based dietary fiber offers diminished or no absorption of cholesterol and easy evacuation of the content of the intestine, relieving constipation. The plant-based fibers recommended in the human diet are of two type's water-soluble and water-insoluble fibers and both are important and offer health benefits.

In the diet of patients with prediabetes or diabetes dietary fibers are especially recommended as it offers several benefits that help to combat with complications of diabetes. The first and foremost claim of fiber is that it is bulky, sticky, and non-digestible material when consumed shows a very slow rise in blood glucose following meals. Furthermore, as mention above it facilitate easy removal of intestinal content and interferes with absorption of cholesterol rendering lower chances of cardiac ailment and stroke, and in the case of diabetes, it is a double benefit because as per the notes of the Centers for Disease Control and Prevention (CDC) diabetics are more susceptible above-mentioned conditions (Diana & Kristeen, 2021; Mayo Clinic, 2021).

The common dietary fibers obtained from different sources as food for humans can be categorized into two broad groups based on it solubility and as soluble dietary fibers and insoluble dietary fibers.

8.3.3.1 SOLUBLE DIETARY FIBERS

This type of fiber is quite common and found in different plant sources the few common examples are oat, pea, beans, apple, citrus fruit, carrot, barley, and psyllium. The soluble fiber normally works by forming a gel-like material with water, and this gel-like consistency offers all the benefits including reduced incidence of developing Type 2 DM. As per the study published in Experimental and Therapeutic Medicine, in 2016 established the fact that; the soluble fibers offer help to increase insulin sensitivity, lowers blood sugar, and reduces cholesterol in patients with DM, and pronounced effect was observed in people with Type 2 DM. Additionally, weight reduction has been recorded. The human clinical investigation in the present research established the fact that around 20 gm of fiber per day in collaboration with a low-fat diet had significantly improved fasting blood sugar, low density lipoproteins levels, and insulin resistance index (Chunye et al., 2016).

8.3.3.2 INSOLUBLE DIETARY FIBERS

Insoluble fibers are non-digestible insoluble carbohydrates present in a range of foodstuff like cauliflower, nuts, celery, cucumbers, courgettes, edible seeds, fruit skins, green beans and potatoes, Whole-wheat flour, and wheat bran. These foods containing insoluble fiber promote the movement of GIT content by creating bulk facilitating the easy removal content any by this serve the role of laxative (Chunye et al., 2016; McKenzie, 2012). Eating extra insoluble dietary fiber has regularly been found to assist persons with type 2 diabetes manage their blood sugar levels. Insoluble fiber cannot be absorbed or broken down by the human body. As a result, unlike other carbohydrates does not induce an increase in postprandial blood glucose. On the other hand, due to increase bulk and bowel movement reduces the transit time of other food leading to lower absorption of glucose from the consumed diet. The indirect contribution of insoluble dietary fiber in the management of diabetes is that it helps in controlling the factors such as weight gain, high cholesterol, and free circulating low-density lipoproteins, and many more like those considered as diabetes inducers (Elizabeth et al., 2021).

8.3.3.3 IMPORTANT DIETARY FIBERS

Few important sources that provide both soluble and insoluble dietary fibers are explained below in detail:

1. **Cereals:** Or lentils are one of the important sources of soluble fibers. These cereals are usually composed of a high amount of carbohydrates, and around 50% of total carbohydrates present in cereals are fiber. As per the U.S. Department of Agriculture (USDA), 1 cup serving of cooked lentils provides around 15 gm of fiber and 230 calories hence can help in keeping blood sugar level stable (Diana & Kristeen, 2021) and also offers a lesser danger of CVD, obesity, and other chronic diseases related with metabolism (Caren & Katherine, 2011).
2. **Beans:** These are one of the important sources of soluble fiber and offer the best outcome if used in combination rather than single. The mixture of red kidney beans, black beans, and white beans in its cooked form offers the best quantity of soluble dietary fiber. One serving of all the above-mentioned beans was estimated to provide around 21 gm of Carbohydrates as dietary fiber, and that concentration of fiber is good enough to control blood sugar level and insulin sensitivity. In addition to soluble fibers beans also provide few insoluble fibers and a good sum of starch. Both these additional components help to improve insulin sensitivity and intestinal health (Diana & Kristeen, 2021).
3. **Whole Grains:** The inclusion of whole grains and products made of them is already established to have several health benefits due to their fiber composition. The benefits offered are reduced threat of non-communicable diseases (NCD), such as cancer, cardiac and vascular diseases, GIT disorders and diabetes more accurately type 2 diabetes. The composition of whole grains reveals the presence of both soluble and insoluble dietary fiber comprised of cellulose, fructan, arabinoxylan, xyloglucan, and β-glucan. The soluble fiber of a few whole grains offers an effective reduction in postprandial blood

glucose level by reducing glucose absorption through increased stomach viscosity as well as a better insulin response. There are some other whole grains like amaranth that are reported to offer benefit raised insulin levels and reduction in serum glucose levels (Nirmala & Iris, 2020).

4. **Artichokes (*Helianthus tuberosus*):** This tender, flavorful botanical material is an excellent supplier of both soluble as well as insoluble fiber. Artichoke is normally consumed as a steam-cooked or fermented meal and is now available as hydrolyzed cellulose extract. It was estimated that half a cup of artichoke offers around 4.8 gm fiber and additionally folate, vitamin C magnesium, and potassium according to USD. Health benefit offered by artichoke includes modulation of glucose metabolism, but the mechanism was not very well established. The findings suggest that it increases hepatic insulin sensitivity, mass, and function of β-cell and lovers the apoptosis of β-cell and reveres the insulin resistance (Diana & Kristeen, 2021; Hye et al., 2012; Lopez et al., 1996).
5. **Avocados (*Persea americana*):** The Hass avocado is a native edible fruit of Mexico covered with thick, bumpy skin of dark green, purplish-black color contributes 33% of the total weight of the fruit. The fruit provides rich nutrients, important phytochemicals such as mono and polyunsaturated fatty acids, omega 3 fatty acid, vitamin A, vitamin C, vitamin K, vitamin B6, folate, niacin, choline, and soluble and insoluble dietary fibers. The approximate composition of avocado was presented by USDA says that A ¼ cup serves more than 2 g of fiber and 3 gm of carbohydrates. The diverse chemical composition of fruit offers several benefits like a healthy blood lipid profile, enhanced bioavailability of fat-soluble vitamins, good cardiovascular health, weight management, and controlled diabetes (Diana & Kristeen, 2021; Mark & Adrienne, 2013). Learning available in the *Journal of the American College of Nutrition (JACN)* suggests avocados help to control blood sugar and insulin levels. It is further mentioned that fatty acid-rich avocados improve fasting pro-insulin levels in insulin-resistant animals, reduced the amount of post-prandial glucose and insulin, and increased the concentrations of High-density lipoprotein-C (HDL-C). In addition to this, it protects chances of cardiac issues which is normally twice in cases of the diabetic patient compared to normal people (Juan et al., 2007).

8.3.4 VITAMINS

Vitamins and minerals are recognized as vital nutritional components as they assist the body perform hundreds of processes, including bone and cellular restoration, wound healing, food transformation to energy, and immune system strengthening. To do all the above functions body takes the help of at least 30 vitamins, minerals, and dietary components that need to be taken through diet as the body is unable to produce it (Harvard, 2021). In people that have a history of prediabetes or diabetes, the inclusion of vitamins in the diet offers more benefits compared to normal people, the type of vitamin and quantity does have a significant role in diabetes management. The important vitamins that had a direct role in the management of diabetes are vitamin A, vitamin D, Vitamin E, vitamin C, vitamin K and B complex. The detailed explanation is in subsections.

8.3.4.1 VITAMIN D

Vitamin D is an oil-soluble vitamin had a very much proved role in bone health, but deficiency of vitamin D is considered a potential risk factor for Type 2 DM and even Type 1 DM. The β-cells of the pancreas and immune cells had the receptors for the active form of vitamin D (1-alpha, 25-dihydroxy vitamin D) hence it is understood that vitamin D had an active function in the synthesis of insulin and secretion in humans and animals. Therefore, vitamin D insufficiency might have a function in the etiology of both types of diabetes, and a greater understanding of the mechanisms at work could lead to the development of preventive measures (Mathieu et al., 2005). According to the data reported in the study around 72% of patients affected with type 2 DM were deficient in vitamin D and supplementation of Vitamin D at the doses of 4500 IU for two months had demonstrated a positive effect. The above findings hence clearly showed better glycemic control by Vitamin D supplementation. The mechanism through which Vitamin D works is that it improves the functioning of β-cells of the pancreas leads to the improved secretion of insulin and is also reported to show the increased response of insulin towards the body (Magda et al., 2016; Healthline, 2021).

8.3.4.2 VITAMIN C

Vitamin C, a water-soluble vitamin chemically also called ascorbic acid, is a potent antioxidant material and had a clear role in growth, repair, and immunity in humans. The vitamin supplement is frequently connected to offer protection from the common cold, immune-related ailments, cardiovascular disease, eye and skin diseases, and prenatal problems (Kathleen, 2021). In the context of protection offered by vitamin C in management or prevention of Type 2 DM was not very evident, but few emerging facts predominantly based on limited short term randomized trials thought to show the result for better glycemic control and reduced risk of Cardiovascular risk especially in cases of Type 2 DM (Shaun, 2021). To be very precise we can say that role of vitamin C supplement in glycemic control was published in Deakin University research on a very small Australian people group of 31 participants demonstrated that people with type 2 diabetes on a vitamin C supplement at 500 mg dose twice a day had a lowered blood glucose levels after eating of food by 36% (Kathleen, 2021).

8.3.4.3 VITAMIN A

Vitamin A and its active chemical form retinol are vital for humans and animals and execute several metabolic processes such as growth, cellular differentiation, and genetic expression and maintain normal homeostasis in humans under stress conditions via antioxidant properties. In addition to this, vitamin A had a crucial role in fetal development, sight, taste, hearing, appetite, spermatogenesis, and immune system. In connection with the liver, pancreas, and their metabolism it is not proved strongly but postulated that vitamin A and its active form retinal had involvement. It is believed that in hepatic lipid metabolism, adipogenesis, functioning of β-cell of the pancreas, and in raising insulin sensitivity, vitamin A is having a role, but the mechanism is not yet established (Brun et al., 2013). There is limited finding exist that claims deficiency of Vitamin A is found in chronic cases of Diabetes, prevention had offered by a high level of carotenoids and nephropathy complication of diabetes associated with urinal excretion of retinal (Roxana et al., 2015). The proposed mechanism for insulin sensitivity by vitamin A is that Retinol binding protein (RBP), specifically RBP4, transports retinol from the liver to peripheral tissues via attaching to appropriate cell receptors and has been associated with insulin sensitivity and lipid metabolism (Gavrilov et al., 2012; Kotnik et al., 2011; Pullakhandam et al., 2012).

8.3.4.4 VITAMIN E

Vitamin E is a fat-soluble vitamin that comes in numerous forms, but the human body exclusively uses alpha-tocopherol. Its primary function is in reproduction and popularly functions as an antioxidant, scavenging loose electrons (also known as "free radicals") which can cause cell injury. Prevention of blood clots in arteries very particularly in the heart and immunity-boosting are also associated with vitamin E supplements. The common food items rich in vitamin E are plant-based oils, nuts, seeds, fruits, and vegetables. Wheat germ oil, Sunflower, safflowers, and soybean oil, Almond, Peanut, peanut butter, Beet green, collard green, spinach, Pumpkins, Avocados, Asparagus, Mangos, and red bell peppers (The Nutrition source, 2020). The role of vitamin E and its associated chemical form had a direct relation with the onset and progression of diabetes, especially Type 2 DM. The biochemical investigation also revealed that people affected with DM show a lower level of vitamin E. Furthermore, it is established that it delays the inception of the diabetic complications as well as slows down the progression of the complications only middle-aged smokers are the exception (Jain & Jain, 2012). The underlined mechanism behind its role in the slow progression of DM is antioxidant (Brun et al., 2013). This antioxidant potential of vitamin E enhances insulin signaling and glycemic control in people having type 2 diabetes. Though, it is uncertain if supplementing with vitamin E improves insulin sensitivity and/or more metabolic factors linked to insulin resistance in overweight people (Patrick et al., 2004).

8.3.4.5 VITAMIN K

Vitamin K a fat-soluble vitamin (Singh et al., 2017a) very frequently found in vegetables and many animal foods, is complex comprised of two-component namely Phylloquinone and menaquinone. The most frequent type of Phylloquinone is the proximal, that is present in green leafy veggies, notably spinach, kale, and collard greens. Another form, Menaquinones, can be seen in certain fermented foodstuffs and animal meals. Some bacteria of the human body can also create menaquinones. The primary role of vitamin K is in the blood coagulation process and it is very well established that the important seven proteins involved in process of coagulation and additional proteins rely on vitamin K are γ-carboxyl-glutamate acid, and γ-glutamyl-carboxylase which are involved in metabolism of bones (Brun et al., 2013; The Nutrition Source, 2020). Vitamin k supplementation along with its due role also shows improved insulin sensitivity, glucose tolerance, and lower insulin resistance in cases of type 2 DM in humans (Manna & Kalita, 2016). The mechanism that operates by vitamin K for control of sugar, insulin sensitivity, and complication minimization is through multiple mechanisms namely increase in the insulinogenic index, insulinotropic effect, modulation of vitamin K dependent proteins, and prevention of inflammation (Hsing-Jung et al., 2020).

8.3.4.6 VITAMIN B COMPLEX

It is simply called vitamin B and is a complex group of eight water-soluble vitamins which are chemically diverse but put together as one group and offering an important function in cell metabolism and RBC production. The eight individual amino acid includes B12 (Cobalamin), B9 (Folic acid), B7 (Biotin), B6 (Pyridoxine), B5 (Pantothenic acid), B3 (Niacin), B2 (Riboflavin), and B1 (Thiamine) each one of these indispensable vitamins give to you on the whole bodily function including control of DM especially Type 2 DM (Emily, 2019).

Both vegetables and animals can provide B-complex vitamins, dietary ingredients like dairy products, egg, and meat are the best sources of vitamin B complex from the animal source while whole grains, potatoes pulses, legumes, beans, banana, chili peppers, etc., are few important sources of b-complex. Microbial sources do provide B-complex vitamin, and few important examples are nutritional yeast, brewer's yeast, and molasses (Winkler, 2006).

The role of B-complex concerning diabetes or in the functioning of the pancreas or insulin sensitivity was not very well understood, but all of these eight vitamins and especially riboflavin and pantothenic acid are linked with DM (Kamrul Hasan, 2017; Roxana, 2015). The role and mechanism of few important members of B-complex in support of care offered to DM are explained here in the next part of the discussion.

Vitamin B1 (thiamin) and B6 (Pyridoxine) were reported to have a beneficial role in lowering diabetic complications namely nephropathy and retinopathy (Kamrul, 2017). The Vitamin B1 may manipulate the development of neuropathic complications as it works as a coenzyme. The conductivity and transmission of neurons, glycation, and aldehyde groups transport is done by vitamin B1 as a coenzyme. Vitamin B6 actively contributes to the metabolism of glucose as it works as a coenzyme for glucose-phosphorylase for the consumption of glycogen in muscles and the liver. Over and above, the above discussion of mechanism the clinical study published had revealed the reversal of nephropathy associated with DNA-glycation in leukocytes after administration of thiamin and pyridoxine for five-month (Roxana, 2015).

The other two important members of the B complex namely Folate and B12 (cyanocobalamin) are recommended as a supplement for people suffering from DM. These supplementation via food or by any means became a must for DM cases that are on therapy with antidiabetic drugs metformin as this drug is reported to produce deficiency of folate and B12 (Kamrul Hasan, 2017; Roxana, 2015). The folic acid and vitamin B12 deficiency was reported in several places for the pathogenesis of Type 2 DM and studies had also reported its role in managing oxidative stress protection, better glycemic control via better serum insulin level, and sensitivity by folic acid and vitamin B12 supplementation.

Niacin is a candidate of vitamin B complex group that could reduce adhesion of monocyte to endothelial cells in diabetic patients. In amalgamation with additional B-complex vitamins like thiamin and riboflavin niacin offers protection from oxidative stress, insulin resistance and too exerts a negative result on the development of diabetic complications in DM cases (Roxana, 2015).

8.3.5 PLANT SUPPLEMENTS IN DIABETES MELLITUS

The use of contemporary medications for blood sugar control has resulted in several negative side effects, leading to a growing desire for safe and cost-effective alternatives. Phytoconstituents are found in medicinal plants, and some of them have modest to strong antihyperglycemic properties. Alkaloids, for example, have been shown to interact with proteins engaged in glucose homeostasis, resulting in a strong anti-diabetic benefit. Alkaloids have been shown to be strong α-glucosidase inhibitors and might be utilized as an option to insulin in the treatment of diabetes, however further research is needed to confirm their usefulness. By enhancing β-cell function, increasing glucose reabsorption, minimizing insulin resistance, or maintaining glucagon-like peptide-1 homeostasis, bioactive chemicals extracted from plants may reduce blood glucose levels. One of the primary reasons herbal medications are frequently utilized in the treatment of diabetes, particularly in rural areas, is their accessibility. As a result, the anti-diabetic potential of a diverse range of medicinal plants has been extensively studied in recent decades (Zulcafli et al., 2020). Some of the medicinal plants which are also consumed as essential dietary supplements are *Syzygium cumini, Momordica charantia,*

Trigonella foenum-graecum, Camellia sinensis, Terminalia chebula, Tinospora cordifoila, Benincasa hispida, etc. (Moradi et al., 2018; Patil & Patel, 2012).

8.3.5.1 SYZYGIUM CUMINI

Vernacular names of *S. cumini* (L.) are Jamun, Jambolan, Indian blackberry, Purple plum, Malabar plum, and Jamaica plum. The synonyms of *S. cumini* are *Eugenia jambolana, Eugenia cumini, and Syzygium jambolana* and it belongs to the Myrtaceae family. Traditional, as well as research finding, recommends the consumption of fruits, seeds, and leaves of Jamun to prevent and treat type 2 diabetes (Zulcafli et al., 2020).

Researchers have discovered the following mechanisms of action of Jambolan in diabetes: inhibition of carbohydrate cleaving enzymes, stimulation of insulin from remaining beta cells, increase in cathepsin-B activity, reduced oxidative stress, up-regulation of the glucose transporter Glut-4, increased glycogen content in liver and muscle cells, inhibition of the human peroxisome, development of insulin-positive cells from the pancreatic duct epithelial cells, proliferator-activated receptor gamma, and inhibition of insulinase in liver and kidney (Helmstadter, 2008).

8.3.5.2 MOMORDICA CHARANTIA

Vernacular names of *Momordica charantia* are Karela, Bitter melon, and Bitter gourd. The synonyms of *M. charantia* are *Momordica zeylanica* and *Momordica muricata* and it belongs to the Cucurbitaceae family. The parts of Karela used in diabetes are fruits, seeds, and leaves.

The mechanisms behind bitter melon's glucose-lowering actions have been studied in a number of research. Pancreatic secretion is stimulated, hepatic gluconeogenesis is reduced, and hepatic glycogen synthesis is increased, according to the stated processes. It also increases skeletal muscle glucose uptake. The insulin resistance index improved after consuming bitter melon, which might explain the lower fasting glucose level. The extract of Bitter melon shown the inhibitory action of α-glucosidase, α-amylase, and pancreatic lipase hence delays the absorption of glucose. The glucose uptake, utilization, and consumption are enhanced, thereby improves insulin resistance. According to one research, it's due to an augmention in glucagon-like peptide-1 production that may aid pancreatic β-cell proliferation and insulin secretion. Because of their antioxidant (Singh et al., 2017a) properties, the fruit extracts are able to inhibit the deposition of cross-linked advanced glycation end products and carboxymethyl lysine. Furthermore, three insulin-like active chemicals from bitter gourd have been revealed in the literature to inhibit the active site of glycogen synthase kinase 3 by interacting with it, decreasing glycogen synthase inactivation, and restoring glycogen levels (Liu et al., 2021; Kim et al., 2020).

8.3.5.3 TRIGONELLA FOENUM-GRAECUM

Vernacular names of *Trigonella foenum-graecum* are Fenugreek, Methi, Bahuparni. The synonym of *T. foenum-graecum* is *Trigonella tibetana* (Alef.) Vassilcz. and it belongs to the Fabaceae (Leguminosae) family (Nagulapalli et al., 2017; Biodiversity India, 2021).

Providing functional medicinal qualities to staple indigenous foods (e.g., Chapatis made of *Nigella sativa* flour) through phyto-pharmaceutical supplements like fenugreek can help in smoothly changing the diet to meet metabolic objectives while maintaining current dietary patterns for diabetic persons (Rao et al., 2020).

In type 2 diabetes patients, fenugreek reduces serum insulin and HOMA-IR (homeostatic model evaluation for insulin resistance). Type 2 diabetes develops when the pancreas' Islets of Langerhans fail to produce enough insulin. Insulin resistances arise when the body's cells do not react to the effects of insulin in the way that they should. Another factor that may contribute to the blood glucose lowering action is delayed stomach emptying, which prevents absorption and transport of glucose. Gastric emptying could also be linked to the galactomannan concentration in fenugreek, which forms a gel and is similarly responsible for weight loss. Furthermore, owing to more concentration of fibers, either total or mucilaginous fibers, fenugreek might be linked to another mechanism in lowering blood glucose (Najdi et al., 2019).

The seed extract of fenugreek enhanced glucose uptake by upregulating the mRNA expression levels of glucose transporter (GLUT-2) and sterol regulatory element-binding protein (Singh et al., 2017b; Keservani et al., 2015), according to new research. Fenugreek seed extract also enhanced the activity of glycogen kinase and glycogen synthase enzymes via altering insulin signaling pathways downstream. In L6C11 muscle cells, fenugreek seed extract increased intracellular creatinine levels, resulting in insulin mimicking characteristics. The peroxisome proliferator-activated receptor-γ (PPAR-γ), and CCAAT/enhancer-binding protein (C/EBPδ), its target genes glucose transporter-4, lipoprotein lipase, and adipocyte protein 2, all increased their mRNA expression levels in response to diosgenin which is one of the main contents of fenugreek seed (Nagulapalli et al., 2017).

8.3.5.4 GREEN TEA

It is a hot beverage prepared by a process called steeping or brewing or decoction. The brewing process involves boiling leaves and buds of *Camellia sinensis* and then served as a hot drink. The beverage is discovered in China and spread over Asia and then all over the globe. A number of types of green tea found that are based on the variety of *Camellia sinensis* and offer several health benefits like enhanced insulin activity, superior glucose management, avoidance of type 2 diabetes, and lesser danger of CVD (Keservani et al., 2016a; Khan & Mukhtar, 2013; Anna, 2018).

Green tea was known to contain poly-phenols having antioxidant potential. The chief antioxidant is called epigallo-catechin gallate (EGCG) that is believed to impart all the health benefits including prevention and control of diabetes. The details of the diabetes preventive role of green tea were reported in a study conducted in Japan. Participants who consumed 6 or even more cups of green tea every day had a 33% reduced risk of getting type 2 diabetes than those who consumed one cup each week, as per this investigation (Anna, 2018). Besides preventive role green tea also offer the role of management of diabetes in active cases of DM. As per the data of comprehensive review, consumption of green always show a direct lowering effect on major health indicator of diabetes like glucose level, A1C level and fasting glucose level (Kai et al., 2013).

8.4 CONCLUSION

Diabetes mellitus is a heterogeneous set of metabolic disorders of fat and protein characterized by elevated blood sugar/glucose levels. Different organizations like USDA, WHO, IDF, and the Canadian Diabetes Association (CDA) had also admitted that it is prevailing rapidly and affecting people globally. In addition to this, all organizations also recommend that people who want to avoid type 2 diabetes or manage diabetes or its complications should eat appropriate foods like whole grains, fruits (Keservani et al.,

2016b), vegetables, and low-fat milk and exercise regularly. Furthermore, despite the several difficulties the nutritional research that is going on in regard to diet and its effect on diabetes put out certain recommendations and concepts which are evidence-based and will benefit doctors, patients, and the general public. There are still certain areas of doubt and debate, and further study is needed to settle them. In concluding remark, it is possible to mention that person wish to prevent or manage diabetes should follow a balanced food and supplement diet. The balanced dietary recommendation includes the incorporation of minerals, antioxidants, dietary fibers, vitamins, and a few phyto foods (Keservani et al., 2017; Keservani et al., 2020).

In minerals Vanadium, Magnesium, Chromium, and Selenium are vital. Although all antioxidants are vital, omega fatty acids and alpha-lipoic acid are the most important. Both soluble and insoluble fibers are suggested in dietary fibers (Keservani et al., 2010a, b), but soluble fibers have a significant function in the prevention and managing diabetes, therefore cereals, whole grains, fruits, and vegetables should be considered vital in the diet. The role of vitamins is significant, though there are gaps in research regarding its very sound role both water-soluble and oil-soluble vitamins must be included as a supplement in managing or preventing diabetes. A few important Phyto foods include *Syzygium cumini, Momordica charantia, Trigonella foenum-graecum, Camellia sinensis* (green tea), and many more like this are significant in the management of diabetes.

KEYWORDS

- **antioxidants**
- **diabetes**
- **dietary fibers**
- **micronutrients**
- **phyto-foods**
- **supplements**
- **vitamins**

REFERENCES

A Harvard Health article, *Vitamins and Minerals, Are You Getting What You Need*? https://www.helpguide.org/harvard/vitamins-and-minerals.htm (accessed on 28 January 2023).

Alberto, M., (2008). Clinical and social impact of the diabetes mellitus epidemic. *Nefrologia, 28*(3), 241–359.

American Diabetes Association, (2008). Nutrition recommendations and interventions for diabetes, a position statement of the American diabetes association. *Diabetes Care, 31*(1), S61–S78.

Anna, S., (2018). *Green Tea and Diabetes Management*. Healthline newsletter [online]. https://www.healthline.com/health/diabetes/green-tea-and-diabetes (accessed on 28 January 2023).

Bai, L., Li, X., He, L., Zheng, Y., Lu, H., Li, J., Zhong, L., et al., (2019). Antidiabetic potential of flavonoids from traditional Chinese medicine: A review. *Am. J. Chin. Med., 47*(5), 933–957.

Barbagallo, M., & Dominguez, L. J., (2015). Magnesium and type 2 diabetes. *World J. Diabetes, 6*(10), 1152–1157.

Biodiversity India. *India Biodiversity Portal*, https://indiabiodiversity.org/species/show/264707 (accessed on 28 January 2023).

Bradley, R., & Walter, B., (2012). *Diabetes Action Research and Education Foundation*. https://diabetesaction.org/article-alpha-lipoic-acid acid (accessed on 28 January 2023).

Brun, P. J., Yang, K. J., Lee, S. A., Yuen, J. J., & Blaner, W. S., (2013). Retinoids: Potent regulators of metabolism. *Biofactors, 39*(2), 151–163.

Campbell, A. P., (2010). Diabetes and dietary supplements. *Clin. Diabetes, 28*(1), 35–39.

Caren, E. S., & Katherine, L. T., (2011). Health benefits of cereal fiber: A review of clinical trials. *Nutr. Res. Rev., 24*(1), 118–131.

Chandraguptala, S. G., Khalid, I., Muthuluri, T., Dantala, S., & Tavares, M., (2020). Diabetes and prediabetes prevalence among young and middle-aged adults, and geographic differences in India- national family health survey. *Epidemiology and Health, 42*, e2020065.

Chewcharat, A., Chewcharat, P., Rutirapong, A., & Papatheodorou, S., (2020). The effects of omega-3 fatty acids on diabetic nephropathy: A meta-analysis of randomized controlled trials. *PLoS One, 15*(2), e0228315.

China Faces 'Diabetes Epidemic' Research Suggest, (2010). BBC. http://news.bbc.co.uk/2/hi/asia-pacific/8587032.stm (accessed on 28 January 2023).

Chunye, C., Yuan, Z., Jing, X., Hongting, Z., Jun, L., Rong, F., Wenyi, Z., et al., (2016). Therapeutic effects of soluble dietary fiber consumption on type 2 diabetes mellitus. *Exp. Ther. Med., 12*(2), 1232–1242.

Crans, D. C., Henry, L. R., Cardiff, G., & Posner, B. I., (2019). Developing vanadium as an antidiabetic or anticancer drug: A clinical and historical perspective. *Met. Ions Life Sci., 19*, 203–230.

Diana, R., & Kristeen, C. (2021). *10 Fiber-Rich Foods for Your Diabetes Diet*. Everyday Health Newsletter. https://www.everydayhealth.com/hs/type-2-diabetes-live-better-guide/fiber-rich-foods-pictures/ (accessed on 28 January 2023).

Dong, J. Y., Xun, P., He, K., & Qin, L. Q., (2011). Magnesium intake and risk of type 2 diabetes: Meta-analysis of prospective cohort studies. *Diabetes Care, 34*(9), 2116–2122.

Elizabeth, W., (2021). *How Fiber Helps Manage Diabetes*. https://www.verywellhealth.com/soluble-and-insoluble-fiber-1087462 (accessed on 28 January 2023).

Emily, C., (2019). *Why Is Vitamin B Complex Important, and Where Do I Get It?* https://www.healthline.com/health/food-nutrition/vitamin-b-complex (accessed on 28 January 2023).

Gammone, M. A., Riccioni, G., Parrinello, G., & D'Orazio, N., (2019). Omega-3 polyunsaturated fatty acids: Benefits and endpoints in sport. *Nutrients, 11*(1), 46.

Gavrilov, V., Harman-Boehm, I., Amichay, D., Tessler, G., Shuster, T., Friger, M., & Gorodischer, R., (2012). Kidney function and retinol status in type 2 diabetes mellitus patients. *Acta Diabetol., 49*(2), 137–143.

Gillespie, K. M., (2006). Type 1 diabetes: Pathogenesis and prevention. *Can. Med. Assoc. J. [Online], 175*(2), 165–170. https://pubmed.ncbi.nlm.nih.gov/16847277/ (accessed on 28 January 2023).

Gloria, Y. Y., David, M. E., Roger, B. D., & Russel, L. P., (2002). Use of complementary and alternative medicine among persons with diabetes mellitus: Results of a national survey. *Am. J. Public Health, 92*, 1648–1652.

Griffin, R. M., (2020). *Alpha-Lipoic Acid.* WebMD, Diabetes. https://www.webmd.com/diabetes/supplement-guide-alpha-lipoic-acid (accessed on 28 January 2023).

Hannah, E. B., & Frank, E., (2008). Nutritional supplementation for type 2 diabetes: A systematic review. *Ophthalmic Physiol. Opt., 28*, 503–523.

Hannon, B. A., Fairfield, W. D., Adams, B., Kyle, T., Crow, M., & Thomas, D. M., (2020). Use and abuse of dietary supplements in persons with diabetes. *Nutr. Diabetes, 10*(14), 1–12.

Hartweg, J., Farmer, A. J., Holman, R. R., & Neil, A., (2009). Potential impact of omega-3 treatment on cardiovascular disease in type 2 diabetes. *Curr. Opin. Lipidol., 20*, 30–38.

Helmstadter, A., (2008). *Syzygium cumini* (L.) SKEELS (*Myrtaceae*) against diabetes-125 years of research. *Pharmazie, 63*, 91–101.

Hsin-Jung, H., Michio, K., & Hitoshi, S., (2020). Beneficial effects of vitamin K status on glycemic regulation and diabetes mellitus: A mini-review. *Nutrients, 12*(8), 2485.

Hye, J. Y., Dae, Y. K., Min, J. K., Suna, K., Da-Sol, K., & Sunmin, P., (2012). Jerusalem artichoke and chungkookjang additively improve insulin secretion and sensitivity in diabetic rats. *Nutrition and Metabolism [Online]., 9*, 112. https://nutritionandmetabolism.biomedcentral.com/articles/10.1186/1743-7075-9-112#citeas (accessed on 28 January 2023).

International Diabetes Federation, (2019). *IDF Diabetes Atlas* (9th edn.). Brussels: Belgium. https://www.diabetesatlas.org (accessed on 28 January 2023).

Itsiopoulos, C., Marx, W., Mayr, H. L., Tatucu-Babet, O. A., Dash, S. R., George, E. S., Trakman, G. L., et al., (2018). The role of omega-3 polyunsaturated fatty acid supplementation in the management of type 2 diabetes mellitus: A narrative review. *J. Nutr. Intermed. Metab., 14*, 42–51.

Jahangir, M., (2019). Pathophysiology of diabetes. *Epidemiology of Diabetes* (pp. 57–73). Elsevier Inc.

Jain, A. B., & Jain, V. A., (2012). Vitamin E, its beneficial role in diabetes mellitus (DM) and its complications. *J. Clin. Diagn. Res., 6*(10), 1624–1628.

Jeffrey, S., Samraj, P. I., & Raj, B. S., (2021). The role of alpha-lipoic acid supplementation in the prevention of diabetes complications: A comprehensive review of clinical trials. *Curr. Diabetes Rev.* [Online early access] doi: 10.2174/1573399817666210118145550. Published Online: https://pubmed.ncbi.nlm.nih.gov/33461470/ (accessed on 28 January 2023).

Jenny, E. K., & Karin, E. B., (2016). Impact of diabetes mellitus. *Arterioscler. Thromb. Vasc. Biol., 36*(6), 1049–1053.

Juan, A. P., Angel, G. S., Esther, S., Inmaculada, R., Antonio, V., Francisco, J. B., Antonio, E., et al., (2007). A MUFA-rich diet improves posprandial glucose, lipid, and GLP-1 responses in insulin-resistant subjects. *J. Am. Coll. Nutr., 26*(5), 434–444.

Kaczor, T., (2020). Highlighting alpha lipoic acid in diabetes. *Nat. Med. J., 12*(5).

Kai, L., Rui, Z., Bin, W., Ka, C., Lin-Ying, S., Jun-Dong, Z., & Man-Tian, M., (2013). Effect of green tea on glucose control and insulin sensitivity: A meta-analysis of 17 randomized controlled trials. *Am. J. Clin. Nutr., 98*(2), 340–348.

Kamrul-Hasan, A. B. M., Islam, A., Islam, M., & Selim, S., (2017). Vitamins and type 2 diabetes mellitus. *Journal of Clinical Diabetology, 4*, 3–9.

Karalis, D. T., (2019). The beneficiary role of selenium in type II diabetes: A longitudinal study. *Cureus, 11*(12), e6443.

Kathleen, M. Z. (2022). *The Benefits of Vitamin C: What Can Vitamin C Do for Your Health?* Diet & Weight Management. https://www.webmd.com/diet/features/the-benefits-of-vitamin-c#1 (accessed on 28 January 2023).

Keservani, R. K., & Sharma, A. K., (2014). Flavonoids: Emerging trends and potential health benefits. *Journal of Chinese Pharmaceutical Sciences, 23*(12), 815.

Keservani, R. K., Kesharwani, R. K., Sharma, A. K., Vyas, N., & Chadoker, A., (2010b). Nutritional supplements: An overview. *International Journal of Current Pharmaceutical Review and Research, 1*(1), 59–75.

Keservani, R. K., Kesharwani, R. K., Vyas, N., Jain, S., Raghuvanshi, R., & Sharma, A. K., (2010a). Nutraceutical and functional food as future food: A review. *Der Pharmacia Lettre, 2*(1), 106–116.

Keservani, R. K., Sharma, A. K., & Jarouliya, U., (2015). Protein and peptide in drug targeting and its therapeutic approach. *Ars Pharmaceutica (Internet), 56*(3), 165–177.

Keservani, R. K., Sharma, A. K., & Kesharwani, R. K., (2016a). Nutraceutical and functional foods for cardiovascular health. In: *Food Process Engineering* (pp. 257–278, 291–312). Apple Academic Press, CRC Press. ISBN: 9781771884020.

Keservani, R. K., Sharma, A. K., & Kesharwani, R. K., (2016b). Medicinal effect of nutraceutical fruits for the cognition and brain health. *Scientifica,* 10. Article ID 3109254. doi: 10.1155/2016/3109254.

Keservani, R. K., Sharma, A. K., & Kesharwani, R. K., (2017). An overview and therapeutic applications of nutraceutical and functional foods. *Recent Advances in Drug Delivery Technology,* 160–201. ISBN:9781522507543.

Keservani, R. K., Sharma, A. K., & Kesharwani, R. K., (2020). *Nutraceuticals and Dietary Supplements: Applications in Health Improvement and Disease Management*. CRC Press. ISBN: 9781771888738.

Khan, N., & Mukhtar, H., (2013). Tea and health: Studies in humans. *Curr. Pharm. Des., 19*(34), 6141–6147.

Kim, S. K., Jung, J., Jung, H. J., Yoon, N., Kang, S. S., Roh, G. S., & Hahm, J. R., (2020). Hypoglycemic efficacy and safety of *Momordica charantia* (bitter melon) in patients with type 2 diabetes mellitus. *Complement. Ther. Med., 52*, 102524.

Kotnik, P., Fischer-Posovszky, P., & Wabitsch, M., (2011). RBP4: A controversial adipokine. *Eur. J. Endocrinol., 165*(5), 703–711.

Learn the Genetics of Diabetes. https://diabetes.org/diabetes/genetics-diabetes (accessed on 28 January 2023).

Li, X., Bi, X., Wang, S., Zhang, Z., Li, F., & Zhao, A. Z., (2019). Therapeutic potential of ω-3 polyunsaturated fatty acids in human autoimmune diseases. *Front. Immunol., 10*, 2241.

Liu, Z., Gong, J., Huang, W., & Dong, H., (2021). The effect of *Momordica charantia* in the treatment of diabetes mellitus: A review. *Evid. Based Complement. Altern. Med., 1*(560), 1–14.

Lopez, G., Ros, G., Periago, M. J., Martinez, M. C., & Ortuno, J., (1996). Relationship between physical and hydration properties of soluble and insoluble fiber of artichoke. *J. Agric. Food Chem., 44*(9), 2773–2778.

Magda, I. M., Enas, E., & Meram, M. B., (2016). The effect of vitamin D supplementation on glycemic control and lipid profile in patients with type 2 diabetes mellitus. *J. Am. Coll. Nutr., 35*(5), 399–404.

Manna, P., & Kalita, J., (2016). Beneficial role of vitamin K supplementation on insulin sensitivity, glucose metabolism, and the reduced risk of type 2 diabetes: A review. *Nutrition, 32*(7, 8), 732–739.

Mark, L. D., & Adrienne, J. D., (2013). Hass avocado composition and potential health effects. *Crit. Rev. Food Sci. Nutr., 53*(7), 738–750.

Mathieu, C., Gysemans, C., Giulietti, A., & Bouillon, R., (2005). Vitamin D and diabetes. *Diabetologia, 48*(7), 1247–1257.

Mayo Clinic Staff. *Dietary Fiber: Essential for a Healthy Diet*. Healthy Lifestyle Nutrition and healthy eating. https://www.mayoclinic.org/healthy-lifestyle/nutrition-and-healthy-eating/in-depth/fiber/art-20043983 (accessed on 28 January 2023).

Mayo Clinic. Patient care and health information. *Diseases and Conditions*. Diabetes. https://www.mayoclinic.org/diseases-conditions/diabetes/symptoms-causes/syc-20371444 (accessed on 28 January 2023).

McCulloch, M., (2018). *10 Supplements to Help Lower Blood Sugar*. Nutrition [online] https://www.healthline.com/nutrition/blood-sugar-supplements (accessed on 28 January 2023).

McKenzie, H., (2012). Fiber facts about cereal. *Today's Dietitian [online], 14*(12), 30. https://www.todaysdietitian.com/newarchives/121112p30.shtml (accessed on 28 January 2023).

Mikulic, M., (2018). *Total Global Dietary Supplements Market Size 2016–2022*. https://www.statista.com/statistics/828514/total-dietary-supplements-market-sizeglobally/ (accessed on 28 January 2023).

Miranda, H., (2007). *Selenium Supplements: Diabetes Risk?* WebMD. Diabetes. News. https://www.webmd.com/diabetes/news/20070709/selenium-supplements-diabetes-risk (accessed on 28 January 2023).

Moradi, B., Abbaszadeh, S., Shahsavari, S., Alizadeh, M., & Beyranvand, F., (2018). The most useful medicinal herbs to treat diabetes. *Biom. Res. Ther., 5*(8), 2538–2551.

Nagulapalli, V. K. C., Swaroop, A., Bagchi, D., & Bishayee, A., (2017). A small plant with big benefits: Fenugreek (*Trigonella foenum-graecum* Linn.) for disease prevention and health promotion. *Mol. Nutr. Food Res., 61*(6), 1–26.

Najdi, R. A., Hagras, M. M., Kamel, F. O., & Magadmi, R. M., (2019). A randomized controlled clinical trial evaluating the effect of *Trigonella foenum-graecum* (fenugreek) versus glibenclamide in patients with diabetes. *Afri. Health Sci., 19*(1), 1594–1601.

National Center for Complementary and Integrative Health. National Institute of Health. *Diabetes and Dietary Supplements*. https://www.nccih.nih.gov/health/diabetes-and-dietary-supplements (accessed on 28 January 2023).

National Center for Complementary and Integrative Health. National Institute of Health, Health Information, *Omega-3 Supplements: In Depth*. https://www.nccih.nih.gov/health/omega3-supplements-in-depth (accessed on 28 January 2023).

National Institutes of Health Office of Dietary Supplements. U.S. Department of Health and Human Services. https://ods.od.nih.gov/factsheets/Magnesium-Consumer/#h3 (accessed on 28 January 2023).

National Institutes of Health Office of Dietary Supplements. U.S. Department of Health and Human Services. https://ods.od.nih.gov/factsheets/Chromium-HealthProfessional/ (accessed on 28 January 2023).

National Institutes of Health Office of Dietary Supplements. U.S. Department of Health and Human Services. https://ods.od.nih.gov/factsheets/Selenium-HealthProfessional/ (accessed on 28 January 2023).

National Institutes of Health Office of Dietary Supplements. U.S. Department of Health and Human Services. https://ods.od.nih.gov/factsheets/Omega3FattyAcids-HealthProfessional/ (accessed on 28 January 2023).

Natto, Z. S., Yaghmoor, W., Alshaeri, H. K., & Van, D. T. E., (2019). Omega-3 fatty acids effects on inflammatory biomarkers and lipid profiles among diabetic and cardiovascular disease patients: A systematic review and meta-analysis. *Sci. Rep., 9*, 1–10.

Navarro-Alarcon, M., & Cabrera-Vique, C., (2008). Selenium in food and the human body: A review. *Sci Total Environ., 400*(1–3), 115–141.

Nimesh, S., & Ashwlayan, V. D., (2018). Nutraceuticals in the management of diabetes mellitus. *Pharm. Pharmacol. Int. J., 6*(2), 114–120.

Nirmala, P. V. P., & Iris, J. J., (2020). Dietary fiber from whole grains and their benefits on metabolic health. *Nutrients, 12*(10), 3045.

Panchal, S. K., Wanyonyi, S., & Brown, L., (2017). Selenium, vanadium, and chromium as micronutrients to improve metabolic syndrome. *Curr. Hypertens. Rep., 19*, 10.

Patil, J. K., & Patel, M. R., (2012). Pharmacognostic and phytochemical investigation of *Benincasa hispida* (Thunb.) Cogn. fruit. *Pharma Science Monitor an International Journal of Pharmaceutical Sciences, 3*(1), 146–156.

Patrick, J. M., Wayne, H. F., Robert, J. W., Sheila, M. W., Sylvia, A., Anne, R. R., & Elizabeth, A. B., (2004). Effect of high-dose vitamin E on insulin resistance and associated parameters in overweight subjects. *Diabetes Care, 27*(9), 2166–2171.

Pullakhandam, R., Palika, R., Ghosh, S., & Reddy, G. B., (2012). Contrasting effects of type 2 and type 1 diabetes on plasma RBP4 levels: The significance of transthyretin. *IUBMB Life, 64*(12), 975–982.

Rao, A. S., Hegde, S., Pacioretty, L. M., DeBenedetto, J., & Babish, J. G., (2020). *Nigella sativa* and *Trigonella foenum-graecum* supplemented chapatis safely improve HbA1c, body weight, waist circumference, blood lipids, and fatty liver in overweight and diabetic subjects: A twelve-week safety and efficacy study. *J. Med. Food., 23*(9), 905–919.

Raquel, V., Yu-Tang, G., Qi, D., Gong, Y., Hui, C., Honglan, L., Wei, Z., & Xiao, O. S., (2009). Dietary calcium and magnesium intakes and the risk of type 2 diabetes: The shanghai women's health study. *Am. J. Clin. Nutr., 89*, 1059–1067.

Rebecca, B. T., (2019). *Types of Diabetes Mellitus*. https://www.webmd.com/diabetes/guide/types-of-diabetes-mellitus (accessed on 28 January 2023).

Rodriguez, M. M., Simental, M. L. E., Zambrano, G. G., & Guerrero, R. F., (2011). The role of magnesium in type 2 diabetes: A brief based-clinical review. *Magnes. Res., 24*(4), 156–162.

Roxana, V., Guadarrama-Lopez, A. L., Martinez-Carrillo, B. E., & Benitez-Arciniega, A. D., (2015). Vitamins and type 2 diabetes mellitus. *Endocr. Metab. Immune. Disord. Drug Targets, 15*(1), 54–63.

Sandoiu, A., (2017). *Omega-3s May Help to Treat Type 1 Diabetes.* Medical News Today. https://www.medicalnewstoday.com/articles/316756 (accessed on 28 January 2023).

Saurabh, N., & Vrish, D. A., (2018). Nutraceuticals in the management of diabetes mellitus, *Pharm. Pharmacol. Int. J., 6*(2), 114–120.

Scibior, A., Pietrzyk, L., Plewa, Z., & Skiba, A., (2020). Vanadium: Risks and possible benefits in the light of a comprehensive overview of its pharmacotoxicological mechanisms and multi-applications with a summary of further research trends. *J. Trace Elem. Med. Biol. 61*, 1–25.

Shahbandeh, M., (2019). *U.S. Sales of Vitamins and Nutritional Supplements Manufacturing 2018–2019*. https://www.statista.com/statistics/235801/retail-sales-of-vitamins-andnutritional-supplements-in-the-us/ (accessed on 28 January 2023).

Sharon, Y., Jane, S., & Nissa, M., (2018). Nutritional supplements for the prevention of diabetes mellitus and its complications. *J. Nutr. Intermed. Metab., 14*, 16–21.

Shaun, A. M., Michelle, A. K., & Glenn, D. W., (2021). Effects of vitamin C supplementation on glycemic control and cardiovascular risk factors in people with type 2 diabetes: A GRADE-assessed systematic review and meta-analysis of randomized controlled trials. *Diabetes Care, 44*(2), 618–630.

Singh, P., Kesharwani, R. K., & Keservani, R. K., (2017a). Antioxidants and vitamins: Roles in cellular function and metabolism. In: *Sustained Energy for Enhanced Human Functions and Activity* (pp. 385–407). Academic Press. ISBN:9780128054130.

Singh, P., Kesharwani, R. K., & Keservani, R. K., (2017b). Protein, carbohydrates, and fats: Energy metabolism. In: *Sustained Energy for Enhanced Human Functions and Activity* (pp. 103–115). Academic Press. ISBN:9780128054130.

Starr, R. R., (2015). Too little, too late: Ineffective regulation of dietary supplements in the United States. *Am. J. Public Health, 105*(3), 478–485.

Statistics About Diabetes, (2017). American Diabetes Association. www.diabetes.org/diabetes-basics/statistics/ (accessed on 28 January 2023).

Terri D., (2021). *Early Signs and Symptoms of Diabetes*. https://www.webmd.com/diabetes/guide/understanding-diabetes-symptoms (accessed on 28 January 2023).

The Nutrition Source. Harvard TH. Chan public health school. https://www.hsph.harvard.edu/nutritionsource/vitamin-e/ (accessed on 28 January 2023).

Trevino, S., Diaz, A., Sanchez-Lara, E., Sanchez-Gaytan, B. L., Perez-Aguilar, J. M., & Gonzalez-Vergara, E., (2019). Vanadium in biological action: Chemical, pharmacological aspects, and metabolic implications in diabetes mellitus. *Biol. Trace Elem. Res., 188*, 68–98.

Vladimir, S., Magomed, S., Tatiana, S., & Andrey, N., (2017). Nutritional supplements for control of diabetes. *J. Excip. Food Chem., 8*(2), 31–38.

Walsh, J. (2022). *Vanadium and Diabetes, Benefit or Harm?* Diabetesnet.com https://www.diabetesnet.com/vanadium-diabetes-benefit-or-harm/ (accessed on 28 January 2023).

WebMD, Vitamins and Supplements. *Alpha-Lipoic Acid*. https://www.webmd.com/vitamins/ai/ingredientmono-767/alpha-lipoic-acid (accessed on 28 January 2023).

Weinstock, R. S., Nathan, D. M., & Mulder, J. E., (2020). *Patient Education: Diabetes Mellitus Type 1: Overview (Beyond the Basics)*. Uptodate [online] https://www.uptodate.com/contents/diabetes-mellitus-type-1-overview-beyond-the-basics (accessed on 28 January 2023).

William, T., & Cefalu, F. B. H., (2004). Role of chromium in human health and in diabetes. *Diabetes Care, 27*(11), 2741–2751.

Winkler, C., Wirleitner, B., Schroecksnadel, K., Schennach, H., & Fuchs, D., (2006). Beer down-regulates activated peripheral blood mononuclear cells *in vitro*. *Int. Immunopharmacol., 6*(3), 390–395.

World Health Organization. https://www.who.int/news-room/fact-sheets/detail/diabetes (accessed on 28 January 2023).

Yeung, S., Soliternik, J., & Mazzola, N., (2018). Nutritional supplements for the prevention of diabetes mellitus and its complications. *J. Nutr. Intermed. Metab., 14*, 16–21.

Yingting, C., Shiqi, Z., Evan, A., & Zumin, S., (2018). Dietary magnesium-to-iron intake ratios and risk of impaired fasting glucose in Chinese adults: The prospective Jiangsu nutrition study (JIN). *J. Nutr. Intermed. Metab., 14*, 22–28.

Zulcafli, A. S., Lim, C., Ling, A. P., Chye, S., & Koh, R., (2020). Antidiabetic potential of *Syzygium* sp.: An overview. *Yale J. Biol. Med., 93*(2), 307–325.

CHAPTER 9

ROLE OF FOOD SUPPLEMENTS IN OBESITY

RINA H. SURYAWANSHI,[1] HEMANT P. SURYAWANSHI,[2] and BHUSHAN R. RANE[3]

[1]*NTV'S Sharada Junior College, Joganipada, Maharashtra, India*

[2]*PG College of Pharmaceutical Science and Research, Chaupale, Maharashtra, India*

[3]*Shri D.D. Vispute College of Pharmacy and Research Center, Devad-Vichumbe, Panvel, Navi Mumbai, Maharashtra, India*

ABSTRACT

The goal of using food supplements and many nutraceuticals is to regulate body weight. A recent analysis looked at the most common weight-loss supplements, categorizing them by the major effects for which they were studied. The effects of these drugs on the intestinal flora, whether direct or indirect, may also contribute to their effectiveness. New eating habits, as well as current production and consumption patterns, have an impact on one's health, the environment, and society. Obesity, osteoporosis, cancer, diabetes, allergies, and dental disorders affect the majority of the world's population. In addition, developed countries face issues such as aging populations, high-energy foods, and imbalanced diets. The use of food supplements in the prevention and treatment of health disorders, particularly in the gastrointestinal tract. Due to its involvement in nutritional, immunologic, and physiological processes, certain components of the gut microflora play a role in the host's health. The studies on food intake and weight control are summarized in this chapter, with a focus on diet recommendations that can help prevent obesity and its further complications.

Food Supplements and Dietary Fiber in Health and Disease. Bhushan R. Rane, Raj K. Keservani, Durgesh Singh, Nayan A. Gujarathi, and Ashish S. Jain, (Eds.)
© 2024 Apple Academic Press, Inc. Co-published with CRC Press (Taylor & Francis)

9.1 INTRODUCTION

Having psychological, social, cultural, genetic, physiological, metabolic, and behavioral factors, obesity is a complex chronic condition. The prevalence of overweight and obesity is increasing worldwide, in both emerging and industrialized nations (Obesity, 2015; Yazdi, 2015).

Excess body fat has accumulated to such a level in obesity that it can have a negative influence on health (Obesity, 2015). When a person's body mass index (BMI), which is calculated by dividing a person's weight by the square of their height, exceeds 30 kg/m^2, they are considered obese. Overweight is defined as a body mass index of 25 to 30 kg/m^2 (Obesity, 2015). Lower values are used in some Eastern Asian countries (Kanazawa, 2005). Obesity is linked to a number of diseases and ailments, including cardiovascular disease, type 2 diabetes, obstructive sleep apnea, some types of cancer, osteoarthritis, and asthma (Haslam, 2005). As a result, obesity has been linked to a reduction in life expectancy.

While a high BMI is a risk factor, it has not been proven to be a direct cause of diseases caused by nutrition, exercise, or environmental variables (Chiolero, 2018). Obesity raises the risk of depression, and depression is one of the leading causes of obesity (Luppino, 2010). Diet, exercise, mechanization, urbanization, genetic sensitivity, medicines, mental health difficulties, economic policies, endocrine disruption, and exposure to endocrine disrupters are all factors that contribute to obesity (Obesity, 2015; Yazdi, 2015; Kassotis, 2020; Bleich, 2008).

Obesity prevention necessitates a multifaceted approach that includes community, family, and individual treatments (Obesity, 2015; Chiolero, 2018). Diet and exercise are the most common treatments suggested by doctors (Haslam, 2005). Reduced energy-dense foods, such as those heavy in fat or sugar, and increased dietary fiber consumption can improve diet quality (Obesity, 2015). Medications can be used in conjunction with a healthy diet to control appetite or fat absorption (Yanovski, 2014). If diet, exercise, and medicine don't work, a gastric balloon or surgery may be used to reduce the size of the stomach or the length of the intestines, making you feel full faster and decreasing your ability to absorb nutrients from food (Colquitt, 2014; Imaz I, 2008).

Obesity is a primary cause of death in both adults and children around the world, and its prevalence is increasing (Obesity, 2015; Encyclopedia, 2015). In 2015, 600 million adults (12%) and 100 million children were obese in 195 countries (Afshin, 2017). Obesity is more common in women than in males (Obesity, 2015). Obesity is one of the 21st century's most important public health challenges (Dibaise, 2013). Numerous medical organizations, including the American Medical Association and the American Heart Association, recognized obesity as a disease in 2013 (Jensen, 2014; Pollack, 2013; Weinstock, 2013).

Obesity is a condition in which a person's excess body fat has accumulated to the point where it is potentially hazardous to their health (WHO 2009). The waist-hip ratio and total cardiovascular (Keservani et al., 2016a) risk factors are utilized to measure fat distribution, while the BMI is used to characterize it. BMI has a direct relationship with both percentage and total body fat (Gray, 1991). BMI is computed by dividing the subject's weight by the square of their height, as follows:

$$BMI = W/h^2$$

where, W is the weight and h is the height.

The BMI scale is usually expressed in kilograms per square meter of height.

i. **Severe Obesity:** BMI $\geq$ 35 or 40 kg/m^2.
ii. **Morbid Obesity:** BMI of $\geq$ 35 kg/m^2 and or $\geq$ 40–44.9 kg/m^2.
iii. **Super Obesity:** BMI of $\geq$ 45 or 50 kg/m^2.

Because Asian populations have lower BMIs than Caucasians, obesity has been redefined in numerous nations. For example, obesity in Japan is defined as a BMI of more than 25 kg/m^2 (Kanazawa, 2005), whereas obesity in China is defined as a BMI of more than 28 kg/m^2 (Bei-Fan, 2002).

9.2 MORTALITY

Obesity is one of the leading causes of death worldwide (Barness, 2007; Mokdad, 2004; Allison, 1999). According to various research, mortality risk is lowest in nonsmokers with a BMI of 20–25 kg/m^2 and highest in current smokers with a BMI of 24–27 kg/m^2 (Aune, 2016; Whitlock, 2009; Di Angelantonio, 2016; Calle, 1999; Pischon, 2008). According to a 2013 review, grade 1 obesity, defined as a BMI of 30–34.9, was not connected to a higher risk of death than normal weight, but overweight, defined as a BMI of 25–29.9, was linked to "reduced" mortality than normal weight, defined as a BMI of 18.5–24.9 (Flegal, 2013). The link between waist-to-hip and waist-to-height ratios and mortality is stronger than previously thought

(Carmienke, 2013). In Asians, the chance of negative health effects increases between 22 and 25 kg/m^2 (WHO, 2004). A BMI of higher than 32 kg/m^2 was connected to a twofold death rate among women over a 16-year period (Manson, 1995). Obesity is expected to cause 1,11,909 to 3,65,000 fatalities each year in the United States and 1 million (7.7%) deaths in Europe (Haslam, 2005; Allison, 1999; Tsigos, 2008; Fried, 2007). Obesity reduces life expectancy by six to seven years on average (Haslam, 2005), by two to four years with a BMI of 30–35 kg/m^2, and by 10 years with extreme obesity (BMI 40 kg/m^2) (Haslam, 2005; Whitlock, 2009).

9.3 MORBIDITY

Obesity puts you at risk for a number of physical and mental ailments. The metabolic syndrome (Haslam, 2005) is a set of medical diseases that includes type 2 diabetes, high blood pressure, high cholesterol, and high triglyceride levels (Grundy, 2004).

There are two sorts of health effects: those produced by an increase in fat mass, such as osteoarthritis, obstructive sleep apnea, and social stigmatization, and those caused by an increase in fat cell number, such as diabetes, cancer, cardiovascular disease, and non-alcoholic fatty liver disease (Haslam, 2005; Bray, 2004). Insulin resistance can be exacerbated by increased body fat, which changes the body's insulin response. Inflammation is also triggered by excess fat (Shoelson, 2007; Shoelson, 2006).

9.4 COMPLICATIONS OF OBESITY

Angina pectoris, myocardial infarction (Lu, 2014), congestive heart failure (Haslam, 2005; Aune, 2016), hypertension (Haslam, 2005), hypercholesterolemia (Haslam, 2005), deep vein thrombosis (Darvall, 2007), stretch marks, and cellulitis (Yosipovitch, 2007), diabetes mellitus (*Haslam, 2005*). Related to reproductive system polycystic ovarian syndrome, birth defects, menstrual disorders, infertility (*Haslam, 2005*), complications during pregnancy (*Haslam, 2005; Arendas, 2008*), erectile dysfunction (*Corona, 2014*). Stroke, depression in women (*Haslam, 2005*), migraines (*Bigal, 2008*), idiopathic intracranial hypertension (*Wall, 2008*), gastroesophageal reflux, fatty liver, cholelithiasis (*Dibaise, 2013*). Colorectal, pancreatic, gallbladder, esophageal, kidney, leukemia, malignant melanoma (*Basen, 2011*), and hepatocellular carcinoma (*Dibaise, 2013*). Related to Obstructive sleep apnea, obesity hypoventilation syndrome, asthma (*Haslam, 2005; Poulain, 2006*), augmented complications during general anesthesia (*Haslam, 2005*). Urinary incontinence (*Hunskaar, 2008*), renal failure (Ejerblad, 2006). Gouty arthritis (Aune, 2014), osteoarthritis (Haslam, 2005), and lower back pain (Molenaar, 2008).

9.5 CAUSES

The carbohydrate-insulin hypothesis proposes that eating processed, high-glycemic-load carbohydrates produces hormonal changes in the body that enhance calorie deposition in adipose tissue, stimulate appetite, and decrease energy expenditure (Ludwig, 2018). According to the calorie is calorie hypothesis, the majority of instances of obesity are caused by a combination of excessive food energy intake and a lack of physical activity (Lau, 2007). Genetics, medical factors, and psychological disorders account for a small number of cases (Bleich, 2008). In a 2016 study, excess food was found as the primary culprit (Bojanowska, 2016; Levitsky, 2019).

9.5.1 LIFESTYLE

Worldwide, there has been a major shift toward employment that are less physically demanding (Ness-Abramof, 2006), and at least 30% of the global population does not get enough exercise. This is because of an increase in the usage of mechanized transportation and labor-saving technology in the home (Ness-Abramof, 2006). As a result of decreasing walking and physical education, children's levels of physical activity appear to be declining (Salmon, 2007). In both children and adults, there is a relationship between television and mobile phone viewing time and the risk of obesity (Gortmaker, 1996; Vioque, 2000; Tucker, 1991).

9.5.2 GENETICS

Obesity, like many other medical conditions, is caused by a complex interplay of genetic and environmental factors (Albuquerque, 2017). Obesity is caused by polymorphisms in numerous genes that influence hunger and metabolism when there is enough dietary energy. As of 2006, more than 41 of these sites in the human genome have been linked to the development of obesity when a favorable environment is available (Poirier, 2006).

9.5.3 OTHER ILLNESSES

Some physical and mental disorders, as well as the drugs used to treat them, can worsen obesity. Several rare genetic syndromes, hypothyroidism, Cushing's syndrome, and growth hormone deficiency are among the medical factors that elevate the risk of obesity (Rosén, 1993). Patients with psychiatric diseases are more likely to be overweight or obese than people without mental illnesses (Chiles, 2010).

9.5.4 SOCIAL FACTORS

Many explanations have been put out to explain the connection between BMI and socioeconomic status. In industrialized nations, it is believed that the wealthy can afford more nutrient-dense food, are under greater social pressure to maintain a healthy weight, and have access to more opportunities that require a higher level of physical fitness.

The ability to purchase food, high energy expenditure from physical labor, and cultural values that promote a larger body size are all assumed to play a role in the observed trends in emerging countries (McLaren, 2007). Obesity appears to be connected to stress and a feeling of social inferiority (Wilkinson, 2009; Bjorntorp, 2001; Goodman, 2003). Smoking has a significant impact on one's weight. Those who quit smoking gain an average of 4.4 kilograms for males and 5.0 kilograms for women over the course of 10 years (Flegal, 1995). Obesity rates are rising in developing countries as a result of urbanization. Early-life malnutrition is thought to play a role in the rising obesity rates in developing nations (Caballero, 2001).

9.5.5 GUT BACTERIA

The study of infectious agents' effects on metabolism is still in its infancy. It has been shown that fat and lean persons have different gut flora. There is proof that gut flora affects metabolic potential. This observable shift is believed to confer an increased capacity for energy harvesting, which fuels obesity. Obesity has not yet been proven to be these alterations; direct cause or result in a conclusive manner (DiBaise, 2008).

9.5.6 OTHER FACTORS

Other factors include the use of antibiotics in youngsters has also been linked to an increased risk of obesity later in life (Cox, 2015). In humans and a variety of animal species, a link between viruses and obesity has been discovered (Falagas, 2006).

9.6 ROLE OF FOOD SUPPLEMENTS

Not only do diet quality and quantity matter in the prevention of obesity, but also willpower plays an important role.

It is no secret that the quantity of calories people consume has a direct impact on their weight: eat the same number of calories that the body burns over time, and your weight will remain stable. When you consume more calories than your body burns, you gain weight. When you eat less, you lose weight. But what about the source of calories: does it make a difference if they come from fat, protein, or carbohydrate? What foods, whole grains or potato chips, do you prefer? Dietary restrictions, such as the Mediterranean diet or the "Twinkie" diet? What about the timing and location of calorie consumption: Is it true that having breakfast makes it simpler to maintain a healthy weight? Is it more difficult if you eat at fast food restaurants? Foods and eating patterns that protect against heart disease, stroke, diabetes, and other chronic illnesses have been studied extensively. The good news is that many of the foods that help prevent diseases, such as whole grains, vegetables, fruits (Keservani et al., 2016b), and nuts, also appear to aid with weight loss. Many of the foods that increase illness risk, refined grains, and sugary drinks, for example, also contribute to weight gain. According to conventional opinion, because a calorie is a calorie regardless of where it comes from, the greatest advice for weight loss is to eat less and exercise more. However, new research reveals that certain meals and eating habits make it simpler to control calories, while others make people more inclined to overeat.

9.6.1 MACRONUTRIENTS

The percentage of calories from fat, protein, and carbohydrates does not appear to matter for weight loss when patients eat regulated meals in laboratory research. There may be some benefits to a higher protein, lower carbohydrate approach in studies where participants may pick what they eat. However, the quality and food sources of these nutrients matter more than their relative quantity in the diet when it comes to chronic disease prevention. And, according to new studies, the same lesson about diet quality also applies to weight loss.

9.6.1.1 FAT

Low fat diets have long been promoted as a means of maintaining a healthy weight and overall health. But the data isn't there: in the United States, the percentage of calories from fat in people's diets has decreased over the last 30 years, while obesity rates have risen dramatically (Willett, 2002; Melanson, 2009). Clinical investigations have shown that following a low-fat diet does not make losing weight any simpler than following a moderate- or high-fat diet. In reality, study participants who eat moderate or high fat diets lose the same amount of weight as those who eat low fat diets, if not more in certain cases (Sacks, 2009; Shai, 2008). Low-fat diets don't appear to offer any additional health benefits when it comes to disease prevention (Howard, 2006).

Low-fat diets are generally high in carbohydrate, especially from quickly absorbed foods like white bread and white rice. Weight gain, diabetes, and heart disease are all linked to diets high in these items.

The type of fat people eat is considerably more essential than the amount for their health, and there's some evidence that the same is true for weight loss (Field, 2007; Koh-Banerjee, 2003; Thompson, 2001; Mozaffarian, 2011). Increased consumption of unhealthy fats, trans fats in particular, but also saturated fats was linked to weight gain in the Nurses' Health Study, which followed 42,000 middle-aged and older women for eight years but not increased consumption of healthy fats monounsaturated and polyunsaturated fats was not (Field, 2007).

9.6.1.2 PROTEIN

Higher protein diets appear to have some weight loss benefits, however, only in short-term tests; in longer-term research, high-protein diets appear to perform equally well as other diets (Sacks, 2009; Shai, 2008). Because high-protein diets are typically low in carbohydrates and high in fat, it's difficult to distinguish the advantages of eating more protein from the advantages of eating more fat or less carbohydrate. However, there are a few reasons why consuming more protein-based calories may help you lose weight:

i. **More Satiety:** When people consume protein, they feel fuller on fewer calories than when they eat carbohydrates or fat (Halton, 2004).
ii. **Greater Thermic Effect:** Protein requires more energy to process and store than other macronutrients, which may help people burn more calories each day (Halton, 2004, Westerterp, 2009).
iii. **Improved Body Composition:** Protein appears to aid in the preservation of lean muscle mass during weight reduction, which can help boost the energy-burned side of the energy balance equation (Westerterp, 2009).

Diets that are higher in protein and lower in carbohydrates enhance blood lipid profiles and other metabolic markers, which may help to prevent heart disease and diabetes (Shai, 2008; Furtado, 2008; Appel, 2005). However, some high-protein foods are better for you than others: Red meat and processed meat consumption has been linked to an increased risk of heart disease, diabetes, and colon cancer (Bernstein, 2010; Aune, 2009; Pan, 2011).

The risk of heart disease and diabetes appears to be reduced when red, and processed meat is replaced with almonds, legumes, fish, or chicken (Bernstein, 2010; Pan, 2011). According to a recent study from the Harvard School of Public Health, this food regimen may also aid with weight loss. For up to 20 years, researchers studied the eating and lifestyle habits of 1,20,000 men and women to see how tiny changes contributed to weight increase over time (Mozaffarian, 2011). Over the course of the trial, people who ate more red and processed meat acquired more weight, about a pound every four years. Over the duration of the trial, people who ate more nuts gained about a half pound less every four years.

9.6.1.3 CARBOHYDRATES

In the short term, lower carbohydrate, higher protein diets may help you lose weight (Sacks, 2009; Shai, 2008). However, carbohydrate quality is far more essential than carbohydrate quantity when it comes to preventing weight gain and chronic disease.

White rice, white bread, white pasta, processed morning cereals, and other foods manufactured with milled, refined grains are high in rapidly absorbed carbohydrates. Potatoes and fizzy drinks are also bad for you. They have a high glycemic index and glycemic load, as the scientific word goes. Such foods generate rapid spikes in blood sugar and insulin, which can cause hunger to surge and lead to overeating in the short term, and raise the risk of weight gain, diabetes, and heart disease in the long term (Abete, 2010; Barclay, 2008; Mente, 2009).

People who increased their use of French fries, potatoes, potato chips, sugary drinks, and refined grains gained an extra 3.4, 1.3, 1.0, and 0.6 pounds per four years, respectively, in the diet and lifestyle modification research (Mozaffarin, 2011). People who consumed fewer of these foods gained less weight.

9.6.2 *SPECIFIC FOODS*

There is mounting evidence that certain food choices can aid weight loss. The good news is that many of the foods that aid weight loss also aid in the prevention of heart disease, diabetes, and other chronic illnesses. Conversely, foods and beverages that promote weight gains, such as refined carbohydrates and sugary drinks, also promote chronic disease.

9.6.3 *WHOLE GRAINS, FRUITS, AND VEGETABLES*

Whole grains, whole wheat, brown rice, barley, and other similar grains are absorbed more slowly than refined grains, especially in their less processed versions. As a result, they have a kinder influence on blood sugar and insulin, which may aid in the prevention of hunger. The same may be said for the majority of fruits and vegetables. These "low carbohydrate" foods offer a plethora of health benefits, as well as evidence that they can help prevent weight gain.

The evidence for weight loss is stronger in whole grains than in fruits and vegetables (Koh-Banerjee, 2004; Liu, 2003; Ledoux, 2011). The Harvard School of Public Health's nutrition and lifestyle change study found that people who ate more whole grains, whole fruits, and vegetables gained less weight throughout the course of the 20-year study—0.4, 0.5, and 0.2 pounds less every four years, respectively (Mozaffarin, 2011).

Naturally, the calories in whole grains, fruits, and vegetables do not vanish. When people increase their intake of certain items, they are likely to reduce their intake of calories from other foods. Fiber, which slows digestion and helps to decrease hunger, may be to blame for the weight-loss advantages of these foods. Water is abundant in fruits and vegetables, which may help people, feel full on fewer calories.

9.6.4 NUTS

Nuts are heavy in fat and contain a lot of calories, so they were formerly considered a no-no for dieters. Nuts, it turns out, do not induce weight gain and may even aid with weight control, possibly because they are high in protein and fiber, both of which might make individuals feel fuller and less hungry (Mozaffarin, 2011; Mattes, 2008; Bes-Rastrollo, 2007; Bes-Rastrollo, 2009). Another incentive to include nuts in a healthy diet is that people who eat them on a regular basis are less likely to suffer heart attacks or die from heart disease than those who do not (Mente, 2009).

9.6.5 DAIRY PRODUCTS

The dairy industry in the United States has actively pushed the weight-loss benefits of milk and other dairy products, mostly based on findings from short-term research it has funded (Zemel, 2000; Zemel, 2004). However, a recent assessment of nearly 50 randomized trials found no evidence that eating a lot of dairy or calcium helps you lose weight (Lanou, 2008). Similarly, most long-term follow-up studies have revealed no evidence that dairy or calcium protects against weight gain (Phillips, 2003; Rajpathak, 2006; Snijder, 2008; Boon, 2005), and one teenage study found that excessive milk intake was linked to a higher BMI (Berkey, 2005).

The Harvard School of Public Health recently published a dietary and lifestyle modification study that found that persons who increased their yogurt intake gained less weight; increases in milk and cheese intake, on the other hand, did not appear to promote weight loss or gain. It's likely that the good bacteria in yogurt can help you lose weight, but further research is needed.

9.6.6 SUGAR-CONTAINING BEVERAGES

Sugary drinks have been shown to raise the risk of weight gain, obesity, and diabetes: (Vartanian, 2007; Malik, 2009; Hu FB, 2010). "Clear connections of soft drink use with higher calorie intake and body weight," according to a systematic review and meta-analysis of 88 research (Vartanian, 2007). According to a more recent meta-analysis, the body mass index of children and adolescents increases by 0.08 units for every additional 12-ounce serving of sugary beverage ingested each day (Malik, 2009). Another meta-analysis discovered that persons who use sugared beverages on a regular basis have a 26% higher chance of getting type 2 diabetes than those who consume sugared beverages infrequently (Hu FB, 2010) New study reveals that drinking a lot of sugary drinks raises your risk of heart disease (Malik, 2010).

Sugary beverages, like refined grains and potatoes, are abundant in quickly digestible carbohydrates. According to research, when carbohydrates are provided in liquid form rather than solid form, they are less satiating, and people do not eat less to compensate for the increased calories (Pan, 2011).

These studies on sugary drinks are concerning, especially given that children and adults are consuming increasing amounts of them: In the 1970s, sugared beverages accounted for around 4% of daily calorie intake in the United States, but by 2001, they accounted for about 9% (Hu FB, 2010) According to the most recent data, half of Americans consume some form of sugared beverage on any given day, 25% consume at least 200 calories from sugared beverages, and 5% consume at least 567 calories from sugared drinks, which is the equal of four cans of sugary soda (Ogden, 2008).

The good news is that research on both children and adults has shown that reducing sugary drinks can help people lose weight (Chen, 2009; Ebbeling, 2006). Sugary drinks have emerged as a key focus for obesity control, spurring debate over policy approaches such as soda taxes (Brownell, 2009).

9.6.7 FRUIT JUICE

It's worth noting that fruit juices aren't a superior weight-loss alternative to sugar-sweetened beverages. Fruit juices, even those that are 100% fruit juice with no added sugar, have the same amount of sugar and calories as sugary beverages ounce for ounce. It's no wonder, however, that a recent Harvard School of Public Health study that followed the food and lifestyle habits of 1,20,000 men and women for up to 20 years discovered that those who increased their fruit juice intake acquired more weight over time than those who didn't (Mozaffarian, 2011). Pediatricians and public health experts advise children and adults to drink only a modest glass of fruit juice each day, if at all.

9.6.8 ALCOHOL

Despite the fact that most alcoholic beverages have more calories per ounce than sugar-sweetened drinks, there is no conclusive evidence that moderate drinking causes weight gain. While a recent diet and lifestyle modification study indicated that participants who drank more alcohol gained more weight over time, the results varied depending on the type of alcohol consumed (Mozaffarian, 2011). Previously, most prospective studies found no difference in weight increase over time between light-to-moderate drinkers and nondrinkers or that light-to-moderate drinkers acquired less weight than nondrinkers (Wang, 2010; Liu, 1994; Wannamethee, 2004; Lewis, 1997; Bes-Rastrollo, 2006).

9.7 DIET PATTERN

People do not consume nutrients or foods on their own. They consume meals that fit into a larger eating pattern, and experts are looking at whether certain diets or meal patterns aid in weight loss or promote weight gain. Over the last three decades, both the size of portions and the consumption of fast food have expanded considerably. Fast food, for example, provides a higher percentage of calories to children in the United States than school food (Poti, 2011), and these developments are assumed to be contributing to the obesity pandemic.

9.7.1 DIETARY PATTERNS

"Prudent" eating patterns, which include whole grains, vegetables, and fruits, have been associated to obesity, but "Western-style" dietary patterns, which include more red or processed meat, sugared drinks, sweets, refined carbohydrates, or potatoes, have been linked to obesity (Schulze, 2006; Newby, 2004; Schulz, 2005; Newby, 2003). A Western-style diet has also been linked to an increased risk of heart disease, diabetes, and other chronic illnesses.

Following a Mediterranean-style diet, which has been shown to reduce the risk of chronic disease (Sofi, 2010) looks to be beneficial for weight loss as well. The traditional Mediterranean diet contains more fat (approximately 40% of calories) than the usual American diet (34% of calories (Wright, 2010) but the majority of the fat comes from olive oil and other plant sources. Fruits, vegetables, nuts, legumes, and fish are also abundant in the diet. In most (but not all) studies, those who followed a Mediterranean-style diet had reduced obesity rates or lost more weight, according to a 2008 systematic review (Buckland, 2008). However, there is no single "Mediterranean" diet, and studies typically utilize multiple definitions, necessitating more research.

9.7.2 *BREAKFAST AND MEAL FREQUENCY*

There is some evidence that skipping breakfast increases the risk of weight gain and obesity in children, particularly teenagers, but the evidence is stronger in children, especially teenagers, than in adults (Dietary, 2010). In the United States, meal frequency and snacking have increased over the last 30 years. On average, youngsters consume 27% of their daily calories from snacks, largely from sweets and sugary drinks, but also from salty snacks and candies. However, the findings on the association between meal frequency, snacking, and weight control have been contradictory, and additional research is needed (Dietary, 2010).

9.8 PORTION SIZE

Portion sizes have increased among adults and children since the 1970s, both for food eaten at home and food eaten away from home (Nielsen, 2003). People eat more when they are provided greater servings, according to short-term research. In one experiment, moviegoers were given large or medium-sized buckets of stale popcorn; despite the fact that they did not appreciate the flavor of the popcorn, those who received large containers ate around 30% more popcorn than those who received medium-sized containers (Wansink, 2005). Another study found that those who were offered larger beverages drank much more, but their subsequent food consumption did not reduce (Rolls, 2007). Another study found that when consumers were given greater portion sizes, they ate more, with no decrease in subsequent food intake (Ello, 2005). The argument that larger portion sizes lead to obesity has an intuitive appeal, but long-term prospective research would help to reinforce this hypothesis.

9.9 FAST FOOD

Fast food is notorious for its enormous quantities, low pricing, high palatability, and high sugar content, and research shows that frequent fast food consumption leads to overeating and weight gain in teens and adults (Duffey, 2007; Duffey, 2009; Tayeras, 2005; French, 2000; Pereira, 2005; Rosenheck, 2008). For example, the CARDIA trial monitored 3,000 young adults for 13 years. People who consumed more fast food at the outset of the trial weighed around 13 pounds heavier on average than those who consumed the least fast food. They also had larger waist circumferences and higher triglyceride levels, as well as a two-fold increased risk of developing metabolic syndrome (Duffey, 2009). More research is needed to distinguish the effect of fast food consumption from the effect of the neighborhood in which people live or other individual characteristics that may make people more prone to consume fast food.

9.10 HEALTHY DIET CAN PREVENT OBESITY AND CHRONIC DISEASES

Weight gain in adulthood is usually modest, around a pound each year (Mozaffarian, 2011), too slow for most people to notice, but it can build up to a significant personal and national health issue over time. There's mounting evidence that the same healthy food choices and eating behaviors that help avoid heart disease, diabetes, and other chronic diseases may also help prevent weight gain:

- Choose entire foods that have been little processed, such as whole grains, vegetables, fruits, nuts, healthy protein sources (fish, poultry, legumes), and plant oils.
- Sugary drinks, refined cereals, potatoes, red and processed meats, and other highly processed foods, such as fast food, should be avoided.

Though each diet adjustment may have a minor impact on weight control, when taken together, the changes could have a significant impact over time and across society (*Mozaffarian, 2011*). Because people's food choices are influenced by their surroundings, governments must encourage policy and environmental reforms that increase the availability and marketing of healthy foods while decreasing the availability and marketing of unhealthy meals.

9.11 CONCLUSION

This chapter demonstrates that various natural ingredients often used as food supplements and nutraceuticals can have a prebiotic impact in humans, contributing to weight loss as well as other physiological consequences not related to weight loss (Keservani et al., 2010a, b, 2017, 2020).

Overall, this chapter discusses nutraceuticals or food supplements, particularly the importance of eating appropriate diets, health issues associated with failure to follow known healthy eating models, development of new nutraceuticals and food supplements with novel health benefits, and elucidation of these products' mechanisms of action. An appropriate diet leads to a healthy, properly functioning GI tract, which leads to proper human physiology, and thus healthy living or obesity control; otherwise, the opposite is true. For the ultimate objective of 'health for everyone,' it is necessary to model new eating patterns using existing information to control obesity and further complications.

KEYWORDS

- **body mass index**
- **carbohydrates**
- **food supplement**
- **gastrointestinal tract**
- **macronutrients**
- **morbidity**
- **nutraceuticals**
- **obesity**

REFERENCES

(2015). *Encyclopedia of Mental Health* (2nd edn., p. 158). Academic Press. ISBN 9780123977533.

(2015). *Obesity and Overweight Fact Sheet N°311*. WHO.

Abete, I., Astrup, A., Martinez, J. A., Thorsdottir, I., & Zulet, M. A., (2010). Obesity and the metabolic syndrome: Role of different dietary macronutrient distribution patterns and specific nutritional components on weight loss and maintenance. *Nutr. Rev., 68*, 214–231.

Afshin, A., Forouzanfar, M. H., Reitsma, M. B., Sur, P., Estep, K., & Lee, A., (2017). Health effects of overweight and obesity in 195 countries over 25 years. *The New England Journal of Medicine, 377*(1), 13–27. doi: 10.1056/NEJMoa1614362. PMC 5477817. PMID 28604169.

Albuquerque, D., Nóbrega, C., Manco, L., & Padez, C., (2017). The contribution of genetics and environment to obesity. *Br. Med. Bull., 123*(1), 159–173.

Allison, D. B., Fontaine, K. R., Manson, J. E., Stevens, J., & VanItallie, T. B., (1999). Annual deaths attributable to obesity in the United States. *JAMA, 282*(16), 1530–1538.

Appel, L. J., Sacks, F. M., Carey, V. J., et al., (2005). Effects of protein, monounsaturated fat, and carbohydrate intake on blood pressure and serum lipids: Results of the omni heart randomized trial. *JAMA, 294*, 2455–2464.

Arendas, K., Qiu, Q., & Gruslin, A., (2008). Obesity in pregnancy: Pre-conceptional to postpartum consequences. *J. Obstet. Gynaecol., 30*(6), 477–488.

Aune, D., Sen, A., Norat, T., Janszky, I., Romundstad, P., Tonstad, S., & Vatten, L. J., (2016). Body mass index, abdominal fatness, and heart failure incidence and mortality: A systematic review and dose-response meta-analysis of prospective studies. *Circulation, 133*(7), 639–649.

Aune, D., Ursin, G., & Veierod, M. B., (2009). Meat consumption and the risk of type 2 diabetes: A systematic review and meta-analysis of cohort studies. *Diabetologia, 52*, 2277–2287.

Barclay, A. W., Petocz, P., McMillan-Price, J., et al., (2008). Glycemic index, glycemic load, and chronic disease risk—A meta-analysis of observational studies. *Am. J. Clin. Nutr., 87*, 627–637.

Barness, L. A., Opitz, J. M., & Gilbert-Barness, E., (2007). Obesity: Genetic, molecular, and environmental aspects. *American Journal of Medical Genetics: Part A., 143A* (24), 3016–3034.

Basen-Engquist, K., & Chang, M., (2011). Obesity and cancer risk: Recent review and evidence. *Curr. Oncol. Rep., 13*(1), 71–76.

Bei-Fan, Z., (2002). Predictive values of body mass index and waist circumference for risk factors of certain related diseases in Chinese adults: Study on optimal cut-off points of body mass index and waist circumference in Chinese adults. *Asia Pac. J. Clin. Nutr., 11*(Suppl 8), S685–693.

Berkey, C. S., Rockett, H. R., Willett, W. C., & Colditz, G. A., (2005). Milk, dairy fat, dietary calcium, and weight gain: A longitudinal study of adolescents. *Arch Pediatr Adolesc Med., 159*, 543–550.

Bernstein, A. M., Sun, Q., Hu, F. B., Stampfer, M. J., Manson, J. E., & Willett, W. C., (2010). Major dietary protein sources and risk of coronary heart disease in women. *Circulation, 122*, 876–883.

Bes-Rastrollo, M., Sabate, J., Gomez-Gracia, E., Alonso, A., Martinez, J. A., & Martinez-Gonzalez, M. A., (2007). Nut consumption and weight gain in a Mediterranean cohort: The SUN study. *Obesity (Silver Spring), 15*, 107–116.

Bes-Rastrollo, M., Sanchez-Villegas, A., Gomez-Gracia, E., Martinez, J. A., Pajares, R. M., & Martinez-Gonzalez, M. A., (2006). Predictors of weight gain in a Mediterranean cohort:

The Seguimiento Universidad de Navarra study 1. *Am. J. Clin. Nutr., 83*, 362–370; quiz 94–5.

Bes-Rastrollo, M., Wedick, N. M., Martinez-Gonzalez, M. A., Li, T. Y., Sampson, L., & Hu, F. B., (2009). Prospective study of nut consumption, long-term weight change, and obesity risk in women. *Am. J. Clin. Nutr., 89*, 1913–1919.

Bigal, M. E., & Lipton, R. B., (2008). Obesity and chronic daily headache. *Curr Pain Headache Rep., 12*(1), 56–61.

Björntorp, P., (2001). Do stress reactions cause abdominal obesity and comorbidities? *Obes. Rev., 2*(2), 73–86.

Bleich, S., Cutler, D., Murray, C., & Adams, A., (2008). Why is the developed world obese? *Annual Review of Public Health (Research Support), 29*, 273–295. doi: 10.1146/annurev.publhealth.29.020907.090954. PMID 18173389.

Bojanowska, E., & Ciosek, J., (2016). Can we selectively reduce appetite for energy-dense foods? An overview of pharmacological strategies for modification of food preference behavior. *Curr. Neuropharmacol., 14*(2), 118–142.

Boon, N., Koppes, L. L., Saris, W. H., & Van, M. W., (2005). The relation between calcium intake and body composition in a Dutch population: The Amsterdam growth and health longitudinal study. *Am. J. Epidemiol., 162*, 27–32.

Bray, G. A., (2004). Medical consequences of obesity. *J. Clin. Endocrinol. Metab., 89*(6), 2583–2589.

Brownell, K. D., Farley, T., Willett, W. C., et al., (2009). The public health and economic benefits of taxing sugar-sweetened beverages. *N. Engl. J. Med., 361*, 1599–1605.

Buckland, G., Bach, A., & Serra-Majem, L., (2008). Obesity and the Mediterranean diet: A systematic review of observational and intervention studies. *Obes Rev., 9*, 582–593.

Caballero, B., (2001). Introduction. Symposium: Obesity in developing countries: Biological and ecological factors. *J. Nutr., 131*(3), 866S–870S.

Calle, E. E., Thun, M. J., Petrelli, J. M., Rodriguez, C., & Heath, C. W., (1999). Body-mass index and mortality in a prospective cohort of U.S. adults. *N. Engl. J. Med., 341*(15), 1097–1105.

Carmienke, S., Freitag, M. H., Pischon, T., Schlattmann, P., Fankhaenel, T., Goebel, H., & Gensichen, J., (2013). General and abdominal obesity parameters and their combination in relation to mortality: A systematic review and meta-regression analysis. *Eur. J. Clin. Nutr., 67*(6), 573–585.

Chen, L., Appel, L. J., Loria, C., et al., (2009). Reduction in consumption of sugar-sweetened beverages is associated with weight loss: The PREMIER trial. *Am. J. Clin. Nutr., 89*, 1299–1306.

Chiles, C., & Van-Wattum, P. J., (2010). Psychiatric aspects of the obesity crisis. *Psychiatr Times, 27*(4), 47–51.

Chiolero, A., (2018). Why causality, and not prediction, should guide obesity prevention policy. *The Lancet Public Health, 3*(10), e461–e462. doi: 10.1016/S2468-2667(18)30158-0. ISSN 2468-2667. PMID 30177480.

Colquitt, J. L., Pickett, K., Loveman, E., & Frampton, G. K., (2014). Surgery for weight loss in adults. *The Cochrane Database of Systematic Reviews (Meta-analysis, Review), 8*(8), CD003641. doi: 10.1002/14651858.CD003641.pub4. PMID 25105982.

Corona, G., Rastrelli, G., Filippi, S., Vignozzi, L., Mannucci, E., & Maggi, M., (2014). Erectile dysfunction and central obesity: An Italian perspective. *Asian J. Androl., 16*(4), 581–591.

Cox, L. M., & Blaser, M. J., (2015). Antibiotics in early life and obesity. *Nat. Rev. Endocrinol., 11*(3), 182–190.

Darvall, K. A., Sam, R. C., Silverman, S. H., Bradbury, A. W., & Adam, D. J., (2007). Obesity and thrombosis. *Eur. J. Vasc. Endovasc. Surg., 33*(2), 223–233.

Di Angelantonio, E., Bhupathiraju, S., Wormser, D., Gao, P., Kaptoge, S., & Berrington De, G. A., (2016). Body-mass index and all-cause mortality: Individual-participant-data meta-analysis of 239 prospective studies in four continents. *Lancet, 388*(10046), 776–786.

Dibaise, J. K., & Foxx-Orenstein, A. E., (2013). Role of the gastroenterologist in managing obesity. *Expert Review of Gastroenterology & Hepatology (Review), 7*(5), 439–451. doi: 10.1586/17474124.2013.811061. PMID 23899283. S2CID 26275773.

Dietary Guidelines for Americans Advisory Committee, (2010). Report of the DGAC on the Dietary Guidelines for Americans 2010.

Duffey, K. J., Gordon-Larsen, P., Jacobs, D. R. Jr., Williams, O. D., & Popkin, B. M., (2007). Differential associations of fast food and restaurant food consumption with 3-y change in body mass index: The coronary artery risk development in young adults study. *Am. J. Clin. Nutr., 85*, 201–208.

Duffey, K. J., Gordon-Larsen, P., Steffen, L. M., Jacobs. D. R., Jr., & Popkin, B. M., (2009). regular consumption from fast food establishments relative to other restaurants is differentially associated with metabolic outcomes in young adults. *J. Nutr., 139*, 2113–2118.

Ebbeling, C. B., Feldman, H. A., Osganian, S. K., Chomitz, V. R., Ellenbogen, S. J., & Ludwig, D. S., (2006). Effects of decreasing sugar-sweetened beverage consumption on body weight in adolescents: A randomized, controlled pilot study. *Pediatrics, 117*, 673–680.

Ejerblad, E., Fored, C. M., Lindblad, P., Fryzek, J., McLaughlin, J. K., & Nyrén, O., (2006). Obesity and risk for chronic renal failure. *Journal of the American Society of Nephrology, 17*(6), 1695–1702.

Ello-Martin, J. A., Ledikwe, J. H., et al., (2005). The influence of food portion size and energy density on energy intake: Implications for weight management. *Am. J. Clin. Nutr., 82*(1 Suppl), 236S–241S.

Falagas, M. E., & Kompoti, M., (2006). Obesity and infection. *Lancet, 6*(7), 438–446.

Field, A. E., Willett, W. C., Lissner, L., & Colditz, G. A., (2007). Dietary fat and weight gain among women in the nurses' health study. *Obesity (Silver Spring), 15*, 967–976.

Flegal, K. M., Kit, B. K., Orpana, H., & Graubard, B. I., (2013). Association of all-cause mortality with overweight and obesity using standard body mass index categories: A systematic review and meta-analysis. *JAMA, 309*(1), 71–82.

Flegal, K. M., Troiano, R. P., Pamuk, E. R., Kuczmarski, R. J., & Campbell, S. M., (1995). The influence of smoking cessation on the prevalence of overweight in the United States. *N. Engl. J. Med., 333*(18), 1165–1170.

French, S. A., Harnack, L., & Jeffery, R. W., (2000). Fast food restaurant use among women in the pound of prevention study: Dietary, behavioral and demographic correlates. *Int. J. Obes. Relat. Metab. Disord., 24*, 1353–1359.

Fried, M., Hainer, V., Basdevant, A., Buchwald, H., Deitel, M., Finer, N., Greve, J. W., et al., (2007). *Interdisciplinary European Guidelines for Surgery for Severe (Morbid) Obesity, 17*(2), 260–270. doi: 10.1007/s11695–007–9025–2.

Furtado, J. D., Campos, H., Appel, L. J., et al., (2008). Effect of protein, unsaturated fat, and carbohydrate intakes on plasma apolipoprotein B and VLDL and LDL containing apolipoprotein C-III: Results from the omni heart trial. *Am. J. Clin. Nutr., 87*, 1623–1630.

Geneeskunde (English abstract) (in Dutch), 152(45), 2457–2463.

Goodman, E., Adler, N. E., Daniels, S. R., Morrison, J. A., Slap, G. B., & Dolan, L. M., (2003). Impact of objective and subjective social status on obesity in a biracial cohort of adolescents. *Obes. Res., 11*(8), 1018–1026.

Gortmaker, S. L., Must, A., Sobol, A. M., Peterson, K., Colditz, G. A., & Dietz, W. H., (1996). Television viewing as a cause of increasing obesity among children in the United States, 1986–1990. *Arch Pediatr Adolesc Med., 150*(4), 356–362.

Gray, D. S., & Fujioka, K., (1991). Use of relative weight and body mass index for the determination of adiposity. *J. Clin. Epidemiol., 44*(6), 545–550.

Grundy, S. M., (2004). Obesity, metabolic syndrome, and cardiovascular disease. *J. Clin. Endocrinol. Metab., 89*(6), 2595–2600.

Halton, T. L., & Hu, F. B., (2004). The effects of high protein diets on thermogenesis, satiety and weight loss: A critical review. *J. Am. Coll. Nutr., 23*, 373–385.

Haslam, D. W., & James, W. P., (2005). Obesity. *Lancet (Review), 366*(9492), 1197–1209. doi: 10.1016/S0140-6736(05)67483-1. PMID 16198769. S2CID 208791491.

Howard, B. V., Manson, J. E., Stefanick, M. L., et al., (2006). Low-fat dietary pattern and weight change over 7 years: The women's health initiative dietary modification trial. *JAMA, 295*, 39–49.

Hu, F. B., & Malik, V. S., (2010). Sugar-sweetened beverages and risk of obesity and type 2 diabetes: Epidemiologic evidence. *Physiol. Behav., 100*, 47–54.

Hunskaar, S., (2008). A systematic review of overweight and obesity as risk factors and targets for clinical intervention for urinary incontinence in women. *Neurourol. Urodyn., 27*(8), 749–757.

Imaz, I., Martínez-Cervell, C., García-Alvarez, E. E., Sendra-Gutiérrez, J. M., & González-Enríquez, J., (2008). Safety and effectiveness of the intragastric balloon for obesity. A meta-analysis. *Obesity Surgery, 18*(7), 841–846. doi: 10.1007/s11695-007-9331-8. PMID 18459025. S2CID 10220216.

Jensen, M. D., Ryan, D. H., Apovian, C. M., Ard, J. D., & Comuzzie, A. G., (2013). American college of cardiology/American heart association task force on practice, guidelines., obesity, Society. 2013 AHA/ACC/TOS guideline for the management of overweight and obesity in adults: A report of the American college of cardiology/American heart association task force on practice guidelines and the obesity society. *Circulation, 129*(25 suppl. 2), S102–138. doi: 10.1161/01.cir.0000437739.71477.ee.

Kanazawa, M., Yoshiike, N., Osaka, T., Numba, Y., Zimmet, P., & Inoue, S., (2005). Criteria and classification of obesity in Japan and Asia-Oceania. Nutrition and fitness: Obesity, the metabolic syndrome, cardiovascular disease, and cancer. *World Review of Nutrition and Dietetics, 94*, 1–12. doi: 10.1159/000088200. ISBN 978-3-8055-7944-5. PMID 16145245. S2CID 19963495.

Kassotis, C. D., Vandenberg, L. N., Demeneix, B. A., Porta, M., Slama, R., & Trasande, L., (2020). Endocrine-disrupting chemicals: Economic, regulatory, and policy implications. *The Lancet Diabetes & Endocrinology, 8*(8), 719–730. doi: 10.1016/S2213-8587(20)30128-5. ISSN 2213-8587. PMC 7437819. PMID 32707119.

Keservani, R. K., Kesharwani, R. K., Sharma, A. K., Vyas, N., & Chadoker, A., (2010b). Nutritional supplements: An overview. *International Journal of Current Pharmaceutical Review and Research, 1*(1), 59–75.

Keservani, R. K., Kesharwani, R. K., Vyas, N., Jain, S., Raghuvanshi, R., & Sharma, A. K., (2010a). Nutraceutical and functional food as future food: A review. *Der Pharmacia Lettre, 2*(1), 106–116.

Keservani, R. K., Sharma, A. K., & Kesharwani, R. K., (2016a). Nutraceutical and functional foods for cardiovascular health. In: *Food Process Engineering* (pp. 257–278, 291–312). Apple Academic Press, CRC Press. ISBN: 9781771884020.

Keservani, R. K., Sharma, A. K., & Kesharwani, R. K., (2016b). Medicinal effect of nutraceutical fruits for the cognition and brain health. *Scientifica,* 10. Article ID 3109254, doi: 10.1155/2016/3109254.

Keservani, R. K., Sharma, A. K., & Kesharwani, R. K., (2017). An overview and therapeutic applications of nutraceutical and functional foods. *Recent Advances in Drug Delivery Technology,* 160–201. ISBN:9781522507543.

Keservani, R. K., Sharma, A. K., & Kesharwani, R. K., (2020). *Nutraceuticals and Dietary Supplements: Applications in Health Improvement and Disease Management*. CRC Press. ISBN: 9781771888738.

Koh-Banerjee, P., Chu, N. F., Spiegelman, D., et al., (2003). Prospective study of the association of changes in dietary intake, physical activity, alcohol consumption, and smoking with 9-y gain in waist circumference among 16 587 US men. *Am. J. Clin. Nutr., 78*, 719–727.

Koh-Banerjee, P., Franz, M., Sampson, L., et al., (2004). Changes in whole-grain, bran, and cereal fiber consumption in relation to 8-y weight gain among men. *Am. J. Clin. Nutr., 80*, 1237–1245.

Lanou, A. J., & Barnard, N. D., (2008). Dairy and weight loss hypothesis: An evaluation of the clinical trials. *Nutr. Rev., 66*, 272–279.

Lau, D. C., Douketis, J. D., Morrison, K. M., Hramiak, I. M., Sharma, A. M., & Ur, E., (2007). 2006 Canadian clinical practice guidelines on the management and prevention of obesity in adults and children [summary]. *CMAJ., 176*(8), S1–13.

Ledoux, T. A., Hingle, M. D., & Baranowski, T., (2011). Relationship of fruit and vegetable intake with adiposity: A systematic review. *Obes Rev., 12*, e143–150.

Levitsky, D. A., Sewall, A., Zhong, Y., Barre, L., Shoen, S., Agaronnik, N., LeClair, J. L., et al., (2019). Quantifying the imprecision of energy intake of humans to compensate for imposed energetic errors: A challenge to the physiological control of human food intake. *Appetite, 133*, 337–343.

Lewis, C. E., Smith, D. E., Wallace, D. D., Williams, O. D., Bild, D. E., & Jacobs, D. R. Jr., (1997). Seven-year trends in body weight and associations with lifestyle and behavioral characteristics in black and white young adults: The CARDIA study. *Am. J. Public Health, 87*, 635–642.

Liu, S., Serdula, M. K., Williamson, D. F., Mokdad, A. H., & Byers, T. A., (1994). Prospective study of alcohol intake and change in body weight among US adults. *Am. J. Epidemiol., 140*, 912–920.

Liu, S., Willett, W. C., Manson, J. E., Hu, F. B., Rosner, B., & Colditz, G., (2003). Relation between changes in intakes of dietary fiber and grain products and changes in weight and development of obesity among middle-aged women. *Am. J. Clin. Nutr., 78*, 920–927.

Ludwig, D. S., & Ebbeling, C. B., (2018). The carbohydrate-insulin model of obesity: Beyond calories in, calories out. *JAMA, 178*(8), 1098.

Luppino, F. S., De Wit, L. M., Bouvy, P. F., Stijnen, T., Cuijpers, P., Penninx, B. W., & Zitman, F. G., (2010). Overweight, obesity, and depression: A systematic review and meta-analysis of longitudinal studies. *Archives of General Psychiatry, 67*(3), 220–229. doi: 10.1001/archgenpsychiatry.2010.2. PMID 20194822.

Malik, V. S., Popkin, B. M., Bray, G. A., Despres, J. P., Willett, W. C., & Hu, F. B., (2010). Sugar-sweetened beverages and risk of metabolic syndrome and type 2 diabetes: A meta-analysis. *Diabetes Care, 33*, 2477–2483.

Malik, V. S., Willett, W. C., & Hu, F. B., (2009). Sugar-sweetened beverages and BMI in children and adolescents: Reanalyzes of a meta-analysis. *Am. J. Clin. Nutr., 89*, 438–439.

Mattes, R. D., Kris-Etherton, P. M., & Foster, G. D., (2008). Impact of peanuts and tree nuts on body weight and healthy weight loss in adults. *J. Nutr., 138*, 1741S–1745S.

McLaren, L., (2007). Socioeconomic status and obesity. *Epidemiol. Rev., 29*, 29–48.

Melanson, E. L., Astrup, A., & Donahoo, W. T., (2009). The relationship between dietary fat and fatty acid intake and body weight, diabetes, and the metabolic syndrome. *Ann. Nutr. Metab., 55*, 229–243.

Mente, A., Koning, L., Shannon, H. S., & Anand, S. S., (2009). A systematic review of the evidence supporting a causal link between dietary factors and coronary heart disease. *Arch. Intern. Med., 169*, 659–669.

Mokdad, A. H., Marks, J. S., Stroup, D. F., & Gerberding, J. L., (2004). Actual causes of death in the United States, 2000. *JAMA, 291*(10), 1238–1245.

Molenaar, E. A., Numans, M. E., Van, A. E. J., & Grobbee, D. E., (2008). Considerable comorbidity in overweight adults: Results from the Utrecht health project. *Nederlands Tijdschrift Voor.*

Mozaffarian, D., Hao, T., Rimm, E. B., Willett, W. C., & Hu, F. B., (2011). Changes in diet and lifestyle and long-term weight gain in women and men. *N. Engl. J. Med., 364*, 2392–2404.

Ness-Abramof, R., & Apovian, C. M., (2006). Diet modification for treatment and prevention of obesity. *Endocrine, 29*(1), 5–9.

Newby, P. K., Muller, D., Hallfrisch, J., Andres, R., & Tucker, K. L., (2004). Food patterns measured by factor analysis and anthropometric changes in adults. *Am. J. Clin. Nutr., 80*, 504–513.

Newby, P. K., Muller, D., Hallfrisch, J., Qiao, N., Andres, R., & Tucker, K. L., (2003). Dietary patterns and changes in body mass index and waist circumference in adults. *Am. J. Clin. Nutr., 77*, 1417–1425.

Nielsen, S. J., & Popkin, B. M., (2003). Patterns and trends in food portion sizes, 1977–1998. *JAMA, 289*, 450–453.

Ogden, C. L., Kit, B. K., Carroll, M. D., & Park, S., (2011). *Consumption of Sugar Drinks in the United States, 2005–2008.* Hyattsville, MD: National Center for Health Statistics.

Pan, A., & Hu, F. B., (2011). Effects of carbohydrates on satiety: Differences between liquid and solid food. *Curr. Opin. Clin. Nutr. Metab. Care, 14*, 385–390.

Pan, A., Sun, Q., Bernstein, A. M., et al., (2011). Red meat consumption and risk of type 2 diabetes: 3 cohorts of US adults and an updated meta-analysis. *Am. J. Clin. Nutr., 94*(4), 1088–1096.

Pereira, M. A., Kartashov, A. I., Ebbeling, C. B., et al., (2005). Fast-food habits, weight gain, and insulin resistance (the CARDIA study): 15-year prospective analysis. *Lancet, 365*, 36–42.

Phillips, S. M., Bandini, L. G., Cyr, H., Colclough-Douglas, S., Naumova, E., & Must A., (2003). Dairy food consumption and body weight and fatness were studied longitudinally over the adolescent period. *Int. J. Obes. Relat. Metab. Disord., 27*, 1106–1113.

Piernas, C., & Popkin, B. M., (2011). Food portion patterns and trends among U.S. children and the relationship to total eating occasion size, 1977–2006. *J. Nutr., 141*, 1159–1164.

Pischon, T., Boeing, H., Hoffmann, K., Bergmann, M., & Schulze, M., (2008). General and abdominal adiposity and risk of death in Europe. *N. Engl. J. Med., 359*(20), 2105–2120.

Poirier, P., Giles, T. D., Bray, G. A., Hong, Y., Stern, J. S., Pi-Sunyer, F. X., & Eckel, R. H., (2006). Obesity and cardiovascular disease: Pathophysiology, evaluation, and effect of weight loss. *Arterioscler Thromb. Vasc. Biol., 26*(5), 968–976.

Pollack, A., (2013). *A.M.A. Recognizes Obesity as a Disease*. The New York Times.

Popkin, B. M., & Duffey, K. J., (2010). Does hunger and satiety drive eating anymore? Increasing eating occasions and decreasing time between eating occasions in the United States. *Am. J. Clin. Nutr., 91*, 1342–1347.

Poti, J. M., & Popkin, B. M., (2011). Trends in energy intake among US children by eating location and food source, 1977–2006. *J. Am. Diet Assoc., 111*, 1156–1164.

Poulain, M., Doucet, M., Major, G. C., Drapeau, V., Sériès, F., Boulet, L. P., Tremblay, A., & Maltais, F., (2006). The effect of obesity on chronic respiratory diseases: Pathophysiology and therapeutic strategies. *CMAJ., 174*(9), 1293–1299.

Rajpathak, S. N., Rimm, E. B., Rosner, B., Willett, W. C., & Hu, F. B., (2006). Calcium and dairy intakes in relation to long-term weight gain in US men. *Am. J. Clin. Nutr., 83*, 559–566.

Rolls, B. J., Roe, L. S., et al., (2007). The effect of large portion sizes on energy intake is sustained for 11 days. *Obesity (Silver Spring), 15*(6), 1535–1543.

Rosén, T., Bosaeus, I., Tölli, J., Lindstedt, G., & Bengtsson, B. A., (1993). Increased body fat mass and decreased extracellular fluid volume in adults with growth hormone deficiency. *Clin. Endocrinol., 38*(1), 63–71.

Rosenheck, R., (2008). Fast food consumption and increased caloric intake: A systematic review of a trajectory towards weight gain and obesity risk. *Obes. Rev., 9*, 535–547.

Sacks, F. M., Bray, G. A., Carey, V. J., et al., (2009). Comparison of weight-loss diets with different compositions of fat, protein, and carbohydrates. *N. Engl. J. Med., 360*, 859–873.

Salmon, J., & Timperio, A., (2007). Prevalence, trends and environmental influences on child and youth physical activity. Pediatric fitness. *J. Sports Sci. Med., 50*, 183–199.

Schulz, M., Nothlings, U., Hoffmann, K., Bergmann, M. M., & Boeing, H., (2005). Identification of a food pattern characterized by high-fiber and low-fat food choices associated with low prospective weight change in the EPIC-Potsdam cohort. *J. Nutr., 135*, 1183–1189.

Schulze, M. B., Fung, T. T., Manson, J. E., Willett, W. C., & Hu, F. B., (2006). Dietary patterns and changes in body weight in women. *Obesity (Silver Spring), 14*, 1444–1453.

Shai, I., Schwarzfuchs, D., Henkin, Y., et al., (2008). Weight loss with a low-carbohydrate, Mediterranean, or low-fat diet. *N. Engl. J. Med., 359*, 229–241.

Shoelson, S. E., Herrero, L., & Naaz, A., (2007). Obesity, inflammation, and insulin resistance. *Gastroenterology, 132*(6), 2169–2168.

Shoelson, S. E., Lee, J., & Goldfine, A. B., (2006). Inflammation and insulin resistance. *J. Clin. Invest., 116*(7), 1793–1801.

Snijder, M. B., Van, D. R. M., Stehouwer, C. D., Hiddink, G. J., Heine, R. J., & Dekker, J. M., (2008). A prospective study of dairy consumption in relation to changes in metabolic risk factors: The Hoorn study. Obesity *(Silver Spring), 16*, 706–709.

Sofi, F., Abbate, R., Gensini, G. F., & Casini, A., (2010). Accruing evidence on benefits of adherence to the Mediterranean diet on health: An updated systematic review and meta-analysis. *Am. J. Clin. Nutr., 92*, 1189–1196.

Taveras, E. M., Berkey, C. S., Rifas-Shiman, S. L., et al., (2005). Association of consumption of fried food away from home with body mass index and diet quality in older children and adolescents. *Pediatrics, 116*, e518–524.

Thompson, A. K., Minihane, A. M., & Williams, C. M., (2011). Trans fatty acids and weight gain. *Int. J. Obes. (Lond), 35*, 315–324.

Tsigos, C., Hainer, V., Basdevant, A., Finer, N., Fried, M., Mathus-Vliegen, E., Micic, D., et al., (2008). Management of obesity in adults: European clinical practice guidelines. *Obes. Facts, 1*(2), 106–16.

Tucker, L. A., & Bagwell, M., (1991). Television viewing and obesity in adult females. *Am. J. Public Health, 81*(7), 908–911.

Vartanian, L. R., Schwartz, M. B., & Brownell, K. D., (2007). Effects of soft drink consumption on nutrition and health: A systematic review and meta-analysis. *Am. J. Public Health, 97*, 667–675.

Vioque, J., Torres, A., & Quiles, J., (2000). Time spent watching television, sleep duration and obesity in adults living in Valencia, Spain. *Int. J. Obes. Relat. Metab. Disord., 24*(12), 1683–1688.

Wall, M., (2008). Idiopathic intracranial hypertension (pseudotumor cerebri). *Curr. Neurol. Neurosci. Rep., 8*(2), 87–93.

Wang, L., Lee, I. M., Manson, J. E., Buring, J. E., & Sesso, H. D., (2010). Alcohol consumption, weight gain, and risk of becoming overweight in middle-aged and older women. *Arch. Intern. Med., 170*, 453–461.

Wannamethee, S. G., Field, A. E., Colditz, G. A., & Rimm, E. B., (2004). Alcohol intake and 8-year weight gain in women: A prospective study. *Obes. Res., 12*, 1386–1396.

Wansink, B., & Kim, J., (2005). Bad popcorn in big buckets: Portion size can influence intake as much as taste. *J. Nutr. Educ. Behav., 37*, 242–245.

Weinstock, M., (2013). *The Facts About Obesity*. H & HN. American Hospital Association.

Westerterp-Plantenga, M. S., Nieuwenhuizen, A., Tome, D., Soenen, S., & Westerterp, K. R., (2009). Dietary protein, weight loss, and weight maintenance. *Annu. Rev. Nutr., 29*, 21–41.

Whitlock, G., Lewington, S., Sherliker, P., Clarke, R., Emberson, J., Halsey, J., Qizilbash, N., et al., (2009). Body-mass index and cause-specific mortality in 900 000 adults: Collaborative analyses of 57 prospective studies. *Lancet, 373*(9669), 1083–1096.

WHO. (2022). *Physical Inactivity: A Global Public Health Problem.* World Health Organization.

Wilkinson, R., & Pickett, K., (2009). The spirit level: Why more equal societies almost always do better. *London: Allen Lane.*, 91–101.

Willett, W. C., & Leibel, R. L., (2002). Dietary fat is not a major determinant of body fat. *Am. J. Med., 113*(Suppl 9B), 47S–59S.

Wright, J. D., & Wang C. Y., (2010). *Trends in Intake of Energy and Macronutrients in Adults from 1999–2000 Through 2007–2008.* Hyattsville, MD: National Center for Health Statistics.

Yanovski, S. Z., & Yanovski, J. A., (2014). Long-term drug treatment for obesity: A systematic and clinical review. *JAMA (Review), 311*(1), 74–86. doi: 10.1001/jama.2013.281361. PMC 3928674. PMID 24231879.

Yazdi, F. T., Clee, S. M., & Meyre, D., (2015). Obesity genetics in mouse and human: Back and forth, and back again. *PeerJ, 3*, e856. doi: 10.7717/peerj.856. PMC 4375971. PMID 25825681.

Yosipovitch, G., DeVore, A., & Dawn, A., (2007). Obesity and the skin: Skin physiology and skin manifestations of obesity. *J. Am. Acad. Dermatol., 56*(6), 901–16, quiz 917–920.

Zemel, M. B., Shi, H., Greer, B., Dirienzo, D., & Zemel, P. C., (2000). Regulation of adiposity by dietary calcium. *FASEB J., 14*, 1132–1138.

Zemel, M. B., Thompson, W., Milstead, A., Morris, K., & Campbell, P., (2004). Calcium and dairy acceleration of weight and fat loss during energy restriction in obese adults. *Obes. Res., 12*, 582–590.

CHAPTER 10

ROLE OF FOOD SUPPLEMENTS IN CANCER

SHASHIKANT B. BAGADE,[1] PUNAM D. BAGAD,[2] PRATIKSHA R. AHER,[2] RUPALI A. PATIL,[2] and PRASHANT L. PINGALE[2]

[1]*Department of Pharmaceutical Chemistry, SVKM's NMIMS School of Pharmacy and Technology Management, Shirpur, Maharashtra, India*

[2]*Gokhale Education Society's Sir Dr. M. S. Gosavi College of Pharmaceutical Education and Research, Nashik, Maharashtra, India*

ABSTRACT

A "food supplement" is a component intended to replenish food that includes or contains one or more of the nutritional components listed below. Except for therapeutic supplements, dietary supplements are considered food under the Dietary Supplement Health and Education Act of 1994. Cancer patients should make sure they are eating healthily and maintaining a healthy weight. Good nutrition is especially important because the disease and its therapies might alter an eating habit. Most dietary guidelines emphasize eating a variety of vegetables, fruits, and whole-grain products. Oxidative damage generated by chemotherapy in cancer patients may be protected by the use of antioxidants. Antioxidants interact with free radicals and neutralize them, preventing them from causing harm to others. There is controversy over whether antioxidants should be used in combination with chemotherapy. The relationship between antioxidants and chemotherapy mostly depends on whether the patient is undergoing antioxidant therapy, such as antioxidant therapy or immuno-on-antibody therapy. In people with some forms of cancer, more antioxidants can protect normal tissue without compromising tumor control. Protein is an essential nutrient that aids in growth, tissue repair, and immune system health. Cancer

Food Supplements and Dietary Fiber in Health and Disease. Bhushan R. Rane, Raj K. Keservani, Durgesh Singh, Nayan A. Gujarathi, and Ashish S. Jain, (Eds.)
© 2024 Apple Academic Press, Inc. Co-published with CRC Press (Taylor & Francis)

patients require more protein than usual to mend tissues and fight infections. Some dietary supplements can help reduce the risk of some diseases. As long as they don't take too much, the majority of people can consume supplements without harm. However, they are not risk-free and can have adverse effects, particularly for those receiving cancer treatment. Supplements and drugs used before and after surgery may interact.

10.1 INTRODUCTION

A "food supplement" is a component (besides tobacco) intended to replenish food that includes or contains one or more of the nutritional components listed below: a vitamin, a mineral, an herb or other botanical, an amino acid, a concentrate, metabolite, constituent, extract, or a combination of these (Halsted, 2003).

Food supplements must be clearly labeled as such and intended for consumption, not as a replacement for regular food or as a single component of a meal. A nutritional supplement cannot be approved or permitted for evaluation as a novel medication, antibiotic, or biologic unless it has already been marketed as a food or nutritional supplement. Dietary supplements are considered food under the Dietary Supplement Health and Education Act of 1994, except for therapeutic supplements (Binda et al., 2020).

Cancer patients who believe nutritional supplements have anticancer and antitoxic characteristics use them frequently. The results of the vast majority of large-scale, randomized cancer prevention experiments have been negative. Beta-carotene has been linked to an increased risk of lung and stomach cancer in studies. Vitamin E and beta-carotene have been proven to reduce radiation damage but increase recurrence in people with head and neck cancer. The use of nutritional supplements during cancer treatment is still up for debate. Vitamin and mineral supplements should not be used in place of prescription medication (Harvie, 2014; Grobar et al., 2016).

10.2 FOOD SUPPLEMENTS AND THE NEED IN CANCER THERAPY

Consumption of a sufficient diet to receive the nutrients and calories is usually not an issue in good health. Cancer patients should make sure they are eating healthily and maintaining a healthy weight. Good nutrition is especially important because the disease and its therapies might alter an eating habit. Most dietary guidelines emphasize eating a variety of vegetables, fruits, and whole-grain products. They can also influence the body which tolerates and utilizes nutrition. They may require high-fat, high-calorie diets or thick, chilly foods such as ice cream or milkshakes to maintain their weight (Tuso et al., 2013).

People with cancer typically experience nausea, vomiting, diarrhea, and a loss of appetite after chemotherapy or radiation treatments, resulting in a reduced intake of dietary elements and weight loss (Norman et al., 2003). Individualized nutrition counseling is critical during therapy, according to experts, to avoid unwanted weight loss or increase. Supplementing with important vitamins and minerals may appear to be beneficial, but this is not always the case. Patients should consult their doctors before taking any supplements, as food interactions with the medication may impair the therapy's success. Essential macronutrients, vitamins, and minerals, as well as non-essential nutrients including phytochemicals, hormones, and herbs, are all included in dietary supplements (Evert et al., 2019).

The process through which food is taken and utilized by the body for development, health, and tissue replacement is known as nutrition. The patient can feel better and stay stronger by eating the right meals. Eating and drinking enough meals and liquids to provide the body with critical nutrients constitutes a healthy diet (Cencic et al., 2010).

Vitamins, minerals, amino acids, fatty acids, and other compounds can be provided as pills, tablets, capsules, liquids, and other forms of food supplements. Supplements can only be legally sold with an adequate daily dose recommendation and a warning statement to protect customers' health (Hassan et al., 2020) (Figure 10.1).

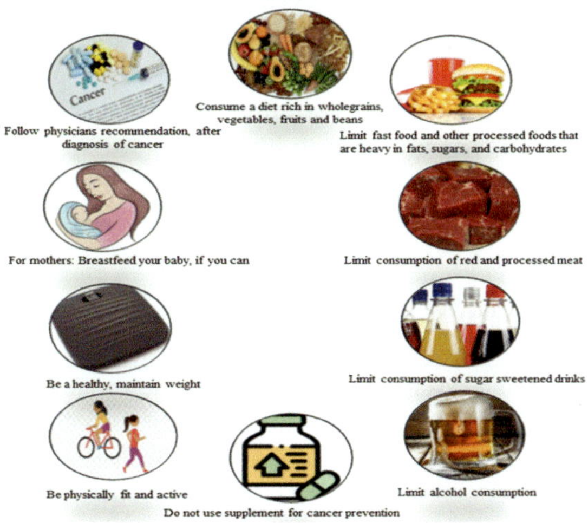
Cancer
Consume a diet rich in wholegrains, vegetables, fruits and beans
Follow physicians recommendation, after diagnosis of cancer
Limit fast food and other processed foods that are heavy in fats, sugars, and carbohydrates
For mothers: Breastfeed your baby, if you can
Limit consumption of red and processed meat
Be a healthy, maintain weight
Limit consumption of sugar sweetened drinks
Be physically fit and active
Limit alcohol consumption
Do not use supplement for cancer prevention

FIGURE 10.1 Cancer prevention recommendation by World Cancer Research Foundation. *Source: World Cancer Research Fund, American Institute for Cancer Research.*

10.3 DIETARY ANTIOXIDANTS IN CANCER TREATMENT

Antioxidants interact with free radicals and neutralize them, preventing them from causing harm to others. Antioxidants that arise naturally in the body are known as endogenous antioxidants. Exogenous sources, such as the diet, provide the body with the antioxidant balance it requires. Antioxidants protect against oxidative free radicals by interacting with them and destroying them, which makes them useful in adjuvant chemotherapy (Pham-Huy et al., 2008). Beta-carotene, lycopene, and vitamins A, C, and E are examples of dietary antioxidants (alpha-tocopherol). Oxidative damage generated by chemotherapy in cancer patients may be protected by the use of antioxidants. Anti-tumor drugs stimulate the production of free radicals, which results in cellular harm and tumor cell demise. As a result, antioxidants are avoided throughout treatment for fear of jeopardizing the medication's effectiveness (Kurutas et al., 2015).

Many integrative practitioners, on the other hand, advise the use of free radical scavenger supplements to help patients tolerate potentially more effective chemotherapy doses, resulting in better tumor response and survival rates. As a result, there is controversy over whether or not antioxidants should be used in combination with chemotherapy (Block & Gyllenhaal, 2005).

Chemotherapy medications generate an increase in oxidative stress by activating the stress response mechanism. Oxidative stress inhibits cell reproduction, which is when chemotherapy kills cancer cells. To minimize oxidative stress and improve chemotherapeutic efficacy, a minimal number of free radical scavengers are used at optimal doses (Singh et al., 2018).

Antioxidants, or their precursors, can have a variety of effects on human health, and antioxidants have several effects as well. Various antioxidant effects vary in chemotherapy, and variation in impact is dependent on quantity. Individualized nutritional therapy based on antioxidants may be useful in reducing pharmaceutical toxicity and thus increasing therapeutic efficacy (Ferdous & Yusof, 2021) (Table 10.1).

TABLE 10.1 The American Institute for Cancer Research: Recommendations on Dietary Supplements in Cancer Therapy (Norman et al., 2003)

Individual or combined antioxidant supplementation of cancer patients receiving current treatments over their RDA or AI cannot be advised as safe or effective.
A high dose of antioxidants is not recommended as the main therapy as they may be hazardous to normal cells owing to prooxidant action or may benefit cancer cells.
The evidence isn't strong enough to recommend vitamin E administration for people undergoing chemotherapy or radiation therapy.

During traditional therapy, over-supplementation is not advised. Patients with cancer should eat a balanced diet that includes at least the RDA of vitamin C and no more than twice that amount.

Large doses of β-carotene should be avoided by patients.

At this time, there is insufficient evidence to provide generalized or specific recommendations about the use of selenium.

Because of the limited research on antioxidant interactions, it is difficult to provide broad recommendations for antioxidant combinations.

Supplements containing soy isoflavones are not suggested because the levels in these supplements are typically far larger than what may be gained from diet.

Cancer patients and healthy persons can both benefit from the advised AI for polyunsaturated fatty acids.

Making vitamin D3 recommendations for people with cancer is impossible.

A daily multivitamin with DRI-level supplements can be taken safely as part of a well-balanced diet, WHO says.

10.3.1 VITAMIN E

As per the research carried out, vitamin E is being used in the treatment of disorders such as Alzheimer's and cancer. Its main function is to neutralize free radicals and so protect cells. Vitamin E is abundant in plant oils, eggs, almonds, green leafy vegetables, and whole grains.

Vitamin E helps the immune system and endothelial cells function by preventing the generation of reactive oxygen species caused by fat oxidation. Vitamin E refers to a set of eight fat-soluble antioxidants that includes alpha-, beta-, gamma-, and delta-tocopherol (Liu et al., 2018).

Vitamin E supplements may increase the risk of certain types of strokes, according to clinical trials. Evidence on whether it can cut cancer risk is equally divided. Antioxidant, anti-inflammatory, and anti-proliferative effects of vitamin E have all been linked to its anti-cancer properties (Sharifi-Rad et al., 2020).

Vitamin E has been linked to a reduced risk of prostate cancer; it does not affect the risk of other malignancies. To study the role of vitamin E in cancer prevention, Alkhenizan & Hafez (2007) conducted a meta-analysis of randomized controlled trials.

Vitamin E appears to lower the incidence of prostate and colorectal cancer among male smokers. The first results of the SELECT (Selenium and Vitamin E Cancer Prevention Research) trial suggest that eating vitamin E alone or in combination with selenium for five years did not affect prostate cancer incidence. Vitamin E has the potential to interact with a variety of conditions. Vitamin E and selenium supplements do not protect against prostate cancer, according to a study. If patients with a history of heart disease take vitamin E supplements, they may be more likely to die (Klein et al., 2012; Hatfield & Gladyshev, 2009).

10.3.2 VITAMIN C

Ascorbic acid is a water-soluble vitamin C found in many fruits (Keservani et al., 2016b) and vegetables. It's necessary for a lot of physiologic activities like collagen and catecholamine creation, as well as carnitine and peptide synthesis. Scurvy can be caused by a lack of it (Padayatty & Levine 2016).

Supplemental consumption of vitamin C may shorten the length and severity of the common cold, but the effect is minor unless the person is under extreme physical stress. In ambulatory patients infected with SARS-CoV-2, high-dose vitamin C alone or in combination with zinc did not reduce symptom duration (Thomas et al., 2021).

Supplemental vitamin C did not diminish the risk of coronary heart disease in large-scale randomized trials. Data on the effects of prophylactic vitamin C for lowering blood pressure are mixed. Other data suggest shorter hospital stays, shorter mechanical ventilation, and lower atrial fibrillation rates (Hemilä & Chalker, 2019).

Supplemental vitamin C supplementation reduced the incidence of cervical cancer but did not prevent gastrointestinal, prostate, or lung cancers or influence death. Vitamin C levels in the blood were linked to a decreased risk of gastrointestinal cancer, most likely due to its protective actions against carcinogenic nitroso compounds (Gaziano et al., 2009).

Vitamin C is a powerful antioxidant with anti-inflammatory and immune-boosting properties. There is still a lack of experimental and epidemiologic evidence linking vitamin C to cancer risk. More clinical trials are needed to assess whether high dose vitamin C has an additive effect in cancer patients (Chambial et al., 2013).

Vitamin C taken orally differs from vitamin C administered intravenously (via a vein). This has reignited interest in vitamin C's potential as a cancer treatment. In well-designed, randomized, controlled trials of vitamin C in pill form, there were no such advantages for cancer patients (Padayatty et al., 2004).

Free radicals cause oxidative damage, which ascorbic acid protects against. It improves endothelium-dependent vasodilation by inactivating nitric oxide. Oral ingestion of dietary or supplementary forms results in plasma concentrations less than 0.1 mM. In cancer cells, this causes DNA damage and ATP depletion (Ladurner et el., 2012).

Vitamin C restored normal function in leukemic cells by compensating for Tet2 mutations. High-dose vitamin C has been shown to prevent breast cancer cells from spreading. The presence of intracellular iron, copper, and an increase in p53 activity may all contribute to cancer cells' preferential oxidative cytotoxic effects (Linowiecka et al., 2020).

Vitamin C may have chemopreventive benefits at doses greater than the current suggested dietary limit of 60 mg/d without producing toxicity. It is also used to prevent chronic diseases caused by oxidative stress, such as a tumor, heart disease, hypertension, stroke, and neurological disorders (Traber & Stevens, 2011).

1. **Vitamin C in Cancer:** Vitamin C has been shown to enhance immunological function, inhibit nitrosamine production, and block carcinogen metabolic activation. Carcinogenesis is promoted by epigenetic processes like inflammation and the suppression of gap junction intercellular communication (GJIC), which could be mediated by ROIs (Carr & Maggini, 2017).
2. **Anti-Inflammatory Action:** Vitamin C has been found to diminish the inflammation generated by ROIs, reducing the risk of stomach cancer. The scavenging of mucosal oxygen radicals and the suppression of the production of carcinogenic nitrosamines may be part of vitamin C's anti-carcinogenic actions (Bhattacharyya et al., 2014).
3. **Restoration of Cell-to-Cell Communication:** Cell-to-cell communication inhibition is significantly linked to carcinogenic progression, especially tumor promotion. GJIC is also inhibited by hydrogen peroxide, a renowned tumor promoter. As a result, we believe that vitamin C's chemopreventive benefits in carcinogenesis are linked to its antioxidant properties and protection against inflammation (Sovadinová et al., 2021).

10.3.3 β-CAROTENE

Beta-carotene is a pigment that gives fruits and vegetables their color. It is present in plants. It is converted to vitamin A in the human body (retinol).

Vitamin A is necessary for healthy vision and eye health, as well as a strong immune system, skin, and mucous membranes. Too much beta carotene can be detrimental to smokers (Gilbert, 2013).

β-Carotene is a kind of vitamin A and an antioxidant. It defends the body from free radicals, which are harmful chemicals. This damage can lead to a variety of chronic ailments over time. Consuming more antioxidant-rich foods has been shown to enhance the immune system.

Carotenoids, such as β-carotene, have been demonstrated to lower cancer risk in the diet (Lobo et al., 2010).

- It protects cells from oxidative or free radical damage by acting as an antioxidant.
- Boosting cellular defense systems, which could include tumor-specific antigens; and/or Stimulating cell-to-cell communication, which may protect cells against malignant transformation and proliferation.
- Formulating retinoic acid, which regulates gene expression (especially in people with low preformed retinol consumption).

Cigarette smoke is very oxidative, and it has been demonstrated that it depletes carotenoids in the blood. As a result, β-carotene in smokers' airways may be more susceptible to oxidative damage, perhaps resulting in a pro-oxidant state that promotes cancer (Shin et al., 2020).

The association between dietary β-carotene and tumor protection may be due to something other than β-carotene, such as another carotenoid or chemical combination in the meal.

It's also likely that nutritional supplementation and higher amounts of β-carotene can give reduce or change the positive role of β-carotene in the diet. Though high quantities of cellular oxidants can harm cells, they are required for a range of defense functions, including apoptosis, phagocytosis, and the cytochrome P-450 complex's detoxification responses. Antioxidants taken in excess can inhibit more cellular oxidants than are needed, interfering with their beneficial effects (Black et al., 2020).

Benefits of β-carotene in cancer prevention:

1. **Dietary β-Carotene:** Food high in carotenoids is likely to protect against lung, mouth, throat, and laryngeal malignancy. Nutritional carotene was linked to a lower danger of esophageal cancer but not of prostate or non-melanoma skin malignancies (Fiedor & Burda, 2014).
2. **Breast Malignancy:** Blood levels of beta-carotene, lutein, and total carotenoids have the strongest links to a reduced risk of breast

cancer. Breast tumors that are estrogen receptor-negative (ER-) have a stronger link than ER+ tumors (Bakker et al., 2016).

3. **Lung Malignancy:** High-dose beta-carotene supplements are thought to raise the risk of lung malignancy in the present and previous smokers. Previous studies have shown that intake and serum levels of beta-carotene and total carotenoids are linked to decreased danger of lung cancer (Black et al., 2020).
4. **Prostate Malignancy:** Lycopene has been related to less danger of cancer, although the evidence isn't conclusive. The AICR/WCRF study found no link between lycopene and prostate cancer risk. An additional study found a reduced danger of advanced stage and aggressive prostate malignancy (Wei & Giovannucc, 2012).

10.3.4 SELENIUM

Selenium is a trace mineral found in Brazil nuts, seafood, meats, cereals, and grains. It's a part of the antioxidant enzyme glutathione peroxidase, which protects cells and DNA from harm. As a result, it's being studied for the prevention of diseases including cancer, heart disease, and rheumatoid arthritis, all of which are caused or worsened by cellular damage. Although selenium is required for appropriate immune system function, it is unknown if higher-than-normal selenium levels might boost the immune system. Long-term selenium consumption has been linked to an increased risk of some cancers (Hariharan & Dharmaraj, 2020).

Selenium is a naturally occurring element that most people acquire from their diet, but it's also found in the air, water, and nutritional supplements. Selenium can be found in many different forms. Selenium comes in several chemical forms, each with its unique biological effect. According to a few observational studies dating back to the late 1960s, people with high levels of selenium in their food or body tissues had a lower cancer risk, and laboratory trials revealed that selenium might restrict cancer cell proliferation (Kieliszek, 2019).

Role of selenium in the prevention of cancer:

1. **Selenium in Beginning and Progression of Carcinogenesis:** The main effects of selenium substances in the subsequent stages of carcinogenesis are thought to be due to their pro-oxidative properties. Redox cycling and ROS generation are the key sources of action.

Thiol oxidation is also caused by redox-active selenium metabolites like selenide (Kuršvietienė et al., 2020).

2. **Effect of Selenium in Progression and Metastasis:** Selenium may influence tumor progression and metastasis, according to some evidence. Selenite reduces the expression of matrix metalloproteinase-2 and -9, which inhibits the invasion of human fibrosarcoma cells. The GPX1 genotype affects the stage of bladder cancer tumors and is connected to urinary tumor growth (Chen et al., 2013).
3. **Selenium in Breast Cancer:** Tight junctions are critical for maintaining cell integrity and controlling paracellular diffusion and permeability. In epithelial cells, tight junctions serve as adhesive complex, holding cells together. Selenium appears to maintain cell structure, reduce cell motility, and limit cell migration and invasion (Zihni et al., 2016).
4. **Colorectal Malignancy:** SBP1 is a marker for colon tumor differentiation. A decrease in SBP1 expression is linked to a bad prognosis. GPX2 was found to boost HT29 human colon adenocarcinoma cell growth while inhibiting cell migration and invasion (Clerici et al., 2021).
5. **Melanoma:** Selenium may be used to control the spread of melanoma. In mice, nutritional selenite and Selenomethionine supplementation lowers the frequency of metastatic disease. A blend of high-Se separated soy proteins showed a similar effect to adding Se compounds in reducing metastasis (Kieliszek and Błażejak, 2016).

Selenite therapy reduced HIF-1, VEGF, and IL-18, all of which are known to influence cell motility. Cell viability was lowered by 20% with 20 M selenite. Selenite decreased cell migration in a dose-dependent manner without impacting cell survival (Chen et al., 2013).

10.3.5 MULTIVITAMIN AND MINERAL SUPPLEMENTS

Despite their clinical manifestations, cancers share many risks and etiologic variables, including age, alcohol use, smoking status, poor diet, sedentary behavior, and obesity. Inflammation and oxidative stress, both of which are ideal targets for vitamin and mineral supplements, appear to account for at least part of the overlap in risk factors between illnesses (Rock et al., 2020). Another possible mechanism for cancer genesis is a lack of control over methionine metabolism and methylation of a variety of biological substrates.

Antioxidant and anti-inflammatory capabilities, as well as the ability to influence methionine metabolism, are found in several dietary supplements. This has been used to justify the use of dietary supplements as a cancer-prevention strategy (Wanders et al., 2020).

Vitamin E protects against oxidized LDL, which is particularly atherogenic. Water-soluble antioxidants like vitamin C are essential to keep vitamin E in its antioxidant or reduced state. Low amounts of vitamin B12 and folate, both of which are involved in DNA synthesis, can lead to methionine insufficiency, which leads to abnormal DNA synthesis and carcinogenesis (Goszcz et al., 2015). Vitamin E (alpha-tocopherol), zinc, and vitamin A are thought to reduce inflammation. Increased levels of homocysteine, an amino acid generated by the demethylation of methionine, have been linked to an increased risk of coronary heart disease events. While vitamin A has an upper limit because high dosages can cause toxicity, beta-carotene has not been proved to induce toxicity and hence has no upper limit. Such interactions, as well as their causes and impacts, are frequently unknown or understudied. Multivitamins cannot replace a well-balanced diet that contains a variety of unprocessed foods. The molecular structure of single vitamin supplements may differ significantly from that of complete foods, thus altering biological effects (Zaric et al., 2020; Fernández-Sanz et al., 2019).

10.3.6 COMBINATION OF ANTIOXIDANTS DURING CANCER TREATMENT

Two types of antioxidant doses may be used to categorize data on the effect of antioxidants in cancer therapy. Both normal and malignant cells are protected by the prophylactic dose. The therapeutic dose inhibits the growth of cancer cells but not normal cells (Yasueda et al., 2016).

Antioxidants may help minimize some types of chemotherapy-related toxicity, but they may do so by interfering with the efficacy of standard treatment. Some researchers believe typical antioxidant concentrations are insufficient to counteract the increased synthesis of reactive oxygen metabolites, promoting cell proliferation and malignant development (Forman & Zhang, 2021).

The relationship between antioxidants and chemotherapy mostly depends on whether the patient is receiving conventional chemotherapy with or without radiation, as well as whether they are undergoing an antioxidant therapy such as antioxidant therapy or a form of immuno-on-antibody therapy (Pucci et al., 2019).

Extra antioxidants can protect normal tissue without impairing tumor control in individuals with certain types of cancer, but studies are inconclusive on whether they should be added to regular chemotherapy. Antioxidants do not interfere with chemotherapy and augment chemotherapy's cytotoxic effect, according to a recent review (Singh et al., 2018).

According to the American Institute for Cancer Research, cancer patients should eat more fruits and vegetables (AICR). According to the AICR, patients should only take a daily multivitamin-multimineral pill with antioxidants below the tolerable upper intake level (Norman et al., 2003).

10.3.7 DIETARY SUPPLEMENTS WITHOUT ANTIOXIDANTS CHARACTERISTICS

Although the effects of nonantioxidant supplements on the efficiency of chemotherapy regimens are controversial, many cancer patients take them. Among them are soy meals and goods (n–3 fatty acids and vitamin D) (Sahin et al., 2019).

10.3.7.1 SOY PROTEINS AND ISOFLAVONES

Soy isoflavones, also known as phytoestrogens, have been shown to inhibit estrogen's detrimental effects on breast and endometrial cancer. This is because they have a slight estrogenic effect and are popular in Asian nations where soy products are widely consumed.

Clinical studies have revealed that soy phytoestrogens cause epithelial cell proliferation in premenopausal women's breasts, which could be a precursor to cancer. In epidemiological research, relationships between soy diets and isoflavones with breast cancer incidence varied. Some found protective correlations, while others found none (Gómez-Zorita et al., 2020).

The USFDA has approved the health claim that eating 25 grams of soy protein per day lowers the risk of heart disease. Soy protein is the highest quality protein derived from the plant kingdom, and it is consumed as an essential by two-thirds of the world's population (Rizzo & Baroni, 2018).

According to the American Institute of Cancer Research (AICR), there is inadequate data to support claims that consuming soy can help prevent breast cancer. Isoflavone supplements are not suggested because the levels of isoflavones in them are usually significantly higher than what may be gained through diet (Messina, 2016).

Phytoestrogens inhibit enzymes that inactivate natural estrogens, potentially resulting in higher levels of active estrogen. Soy isoflavones may be protective throughout adulthood only if consumed during infancy or puberty. In case-control studies, high soy consumption in childhood was connected to a decreased incidence of breast cancer in adulthood (Desmawati & Sulastri, 2019).

It is unclear whether soy isoflavones are useful in preventing or treating human prostate cancer. Soy phytoestrogens have antiestrogenic properties in the uterus, although pilot research demonstrated no reduction in estrogen-mediated endometrial activation. Prostate cancer is uncommon in Asian countries where soy products are widely consumed (Kim, 2021).

10.3.7.2 POLYUNSATURATED FATTY ACIDS

Human cancer growth control is still a hotly debated topic. The mechanisms underpinning fatty acid effects on tumor growth and carcinogenesis are unknown. Prostaglandin E2, which is produced from (n–6) fatty acids, has been proven to promote tumor growth. Omega-3 fatty acids, particularly docosahexaenoic acid, may make breast cancers more sensitive to cytotoxic medicines like doxorubicin. Several clinical studies have looked into the effects of (n–3) fatty acid supplementation on cancer patients, with positive results (Freitas & Campos 2019).

Polyunsaturated fatty acids (PUFAs) like omega-3 and omega-6 play significant roles in cell membrane structure, fluidity, and signaling. EPA and DHA, two omega-3 polyunsaturated fatty acids, are best acquired from fatty cold-water fish such as salmon (Balic et al., 2020).

DHA and EPA are two types of omega-3 fatty acids. Pro-inflammatory eicosanoids are reduced, while inflammation-resolving derivatives are increased. Disrupt oncogenic protein signaling by disrupting lipid rafts in the plasma membrane. Increased breast cancer gene expression (BRCA 1/2, phosphatase, and tensin homolog) (Fabian et al., 2015).

High dietary intakes of EPA and DHA were linked to a 25% reduction in breast cancer recurrence and a 25% reduction in overall mortality. One cause could be the augmentation of some forms of chemotherapeutic cytotoxicity, which has been found when DHA and anthracyclines are given together (D'Eliseo & Velotti, 2016).

Normal growth and development, as well as the treatment of cancer and other disorders, require dietary fat. According to AICR recommendations, dietary fat should account for 30% of total energy consumption. Cancer patients and healthy persons are advised to ingest the recommended adequate intake (AI) of polyunsaturated fatty acids (Bojková et al., 2020).

10.3.7.3 VITAMIN D-3

In recent years, researchers have been looking for biological regulators of cancer cells that limit proliferation, promote differentiation into a latent, dedifferentiated state, and stimulate cell death. Several research projects have combined vitamin D-3 (cholecalciferol) analogs with radiation (Huang et al., 2019).

Vitamin D-3 has been shown to prevent tumor growth in a range of cell types, including breast cancer cells. Increased dietary calcium and vitamin D, according to research, may play a role in the chemoprevention of colon and breast cancer. These analogs are still in the experimental stage and cannot be recommended for cancer patients at this time (Jeon & Shin, 2018).

There is no scientific proof that fruits and vegetables are harmful to cancer patients who are undergoing treatment. According to the World Health Organization, taking a multivitamin-multimineral supplement containing important minerals can be used safely as part of a balanced dietary regimen (Neuhouser et al., 2009).

10.4 PROTEINS AS NUTRITION IN CANCER TREATMENT

Protein is necessary for growth, tissue repair, and the maintenance of our immune systems. Fish, poultry, lean red meat, eggs, low-fat dairy products, nuts, and nut butter are all good sources of protein for people who are battling cancer (Hoffman & Falvo, 2004).

Protein is an essential nutrient that aids in growth, tissue repair, and immune system health. When the body lacks protein, it breaks down muscles to give the energy it requires. This increases the amount of time it takes to recover from an illness and reduces the body's resistance to infection. Cancer patients require more protein than usual to mend tissues and fight infections (Carbone & Pasiakos, 2019).

This protein is coupled with nanobubbles of phospholipid dioleoyl phosphatidylserine, a fat molecule. The new agent can locate cancer cells and kill them without harming healthy tissue.

This drug may be particularly beneficial in treating glioblastoma and other malignant brain tumors because fat nanoparticles can cross the blood-brain barrier (Davis et al., 2019).

1. **Peptides as Anticancer Drug Candidates:** Peptides are fragments of larger protein molecules. There are signs that peptide therapy could be useful in cancer treatment. Clinical trials with Cilengitide, Trebananib, NGR-hTNF, Tyroserleutide, and other peptides are under clinical trial (Marqus et al., 2017).
2. **Cell-Penetrating Peptides:** These are peptides that permeate the cell membrane and affect crucial intracellular proteins involved in the regulation of cancer growth. Well-known CP peptides have been synthesized using heparin-, RNA-, or DNA-binding proteins, antibiotic or viral proteins, and a wide range of natural proteins (Xie et al., 2020).
3. **An Anti-Cancer Drug:** It is being studied as an intravenous bolus in patients with stage IV cancer who have refractory metastatic solid tumors. The medicine reduces angiogenesis and, as a result, tumor cell proliferation by lowering the phosphorylation of VEGFR-2, FAK, and AKT22 in tumor cells (Volz et al., 2020).
4. **Anticancer Potential of Bacterial Proteins:** The protein azurin from *P. aeruginosa* could be exploited as an anticancer medication. Antibacterial agents include immunotoxins, the mAbs described in Table 10.2, and bacterial proteins such as MPT63 from *Mycobacterium bovis* (Nguyen & Nguyen, 2016).

TABLE 10.2 Marketed Monoclonal Antibodies (MAb)

MAb Name	Market Name	Target Site	Type of Cancer Treated	FDA Approval
Pertuzumab	Perjeta®	HER2	Metastatic breast cancer	2012
Ipilimumab	Yervoy®	CTLA-4	Melanoma	2011
Ofatumumab	Arzerra®	CD20	Chronic lymphocytic leukemia	2009
Panitumumab	Vectibix®	EGFR	Colorectal carcinoma	2006
Cetuximab	Erbitux®	EGFR	Colorectal cancer	2004
Bevacizumab	Avastin®	VEGF	Metastatic colorectal cancer	2004
Ibritumomab	Zevalin®	CD20	B-cell non-Hodgkin lymphoma	2002
Alemtuzumab	Campath®	CD52	Chronic lymphocytic leukemia	2001
Trastuzumab	Herceptin®	HER2	Metastatic breast cancer	1998
Rituximab	Rituxan®	CD20	Chronic lymphocytic leukemia	1997

10.5 CARBOHYDRATES AS NUTRITION IN CANCER TREATMENT

Carbohydrates are an important source of energy for physical activity and organ function. To have a balanced diet, it is critical to ingest the proper amount of carbs. Fruits, vegetables, and whole grains, as well as bread, potatoes, rice, cereals, maize, peas, and beans, are the finest sources of carbs. For energy, cancer cells require a lot of glucose-much more than normal cells. This is because cancer cells metabolize carbohydrates differently and less effectively than normal, healthy cells. Normally, cells burn glucose for energy using oxygen (Liberti & Locasale, 2016).

Cancer cells, on the other hand, often live in a low-oxygen environment due to their excessive growth and tight packing and have adapted to break down sugars in the absence of oxygen, a process known as anaerobic metabolism. Unfortunately, anaerobic metabolism is substantially less efficient than aerobic or oxygen-based sugar metabolism. As a result, cancer cells may require up to 40 times the quantity of glucose than normal cells with proper oxygen levels due to generating the same amount of energy (Vander Heiden et al., 2009).

The liver breaks down proteins and fats to produce additional glucose to meet high sugar demand in cancer. As a result, the tumor's high energy needs may explain why cancer patients frequently experience weight loss and weariness (Yee et al., 2020).

One goal of cancer nutritional therapy is to decrease the amount of excess glucose available to cancer while ensuring that the brain and other important systems are not harmed. Maintaining even blood sugar levels and preventing glucose spikes, which supply more sugars for the tumor to use, is one strategy that can help with this (Duan et al., 2014).

Blood sugar management can be done with a variety of tools. Although the glycemic index and a low-carbohydrate diet are well-known methods, a whole-food diet may be more convenient and successful (Evert et al., 2019).

10.6 HERBS AND PHYTONUTRIENTS AS NUTRITION IN CANCER TREATMENT

Secondary metabolites of plants and their semisynthetic derivatives are now widely used in anticancer medication therapy. Consume meals high in antioxidants and phytonutrients, which help clean and protect the body's cells. Colored plant meals, such as fruits and vegetables, easily incorporate these nutrients. Consider the various hues as a guide to which foods are best (Seca & Pinto, 2018) (Figure 10.2).

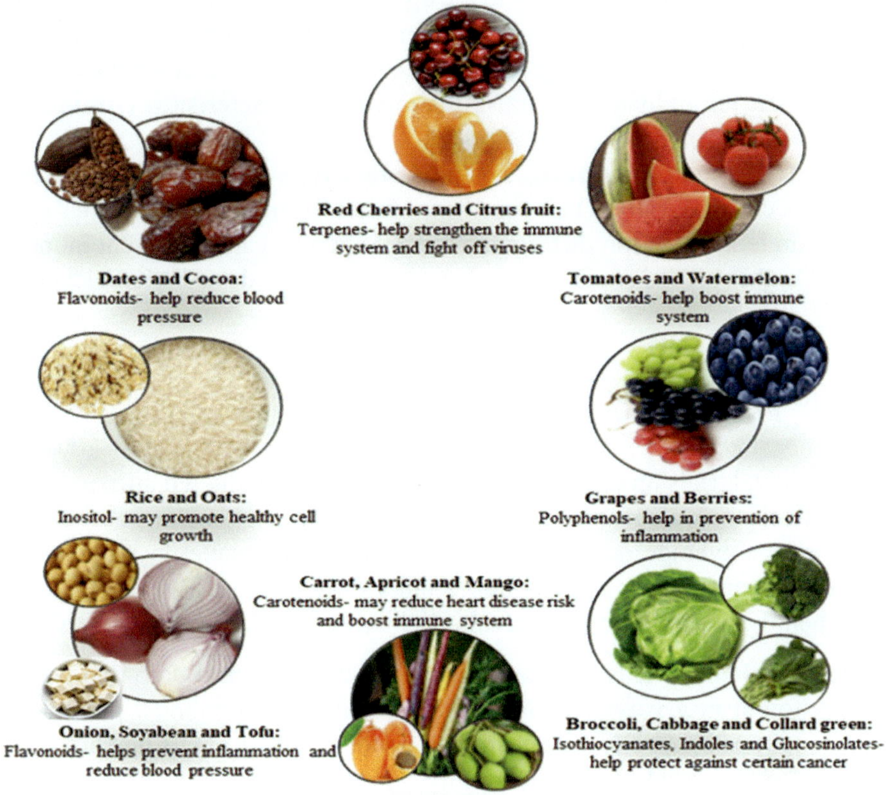
Red Cherries and Citrus fruit:
Terpenes- help strengthen the immune system and fight off viruses
Dates and Cocoa:
Flavonoids- help reduce blood pressure
Tomatoes and Watermelon:
Carotenoids- help boost immune system
Rice and Oats:
Inositol- may promote healthy cell growth
Grapes and Berries:
Polyphenols- help in prevention of inflammation
Carrot, Apricot and Mango:
Carotenoids- may reduce heart disease risk and boost immune system
Onion, Soyabean and Tofu:
Flavonoids- helps prevent inflammation and reduce blood pressure
Broccoli, Cabbage and Collard green:
Isothiocyanates, Indoles and Glucosinolates- help protect against certain cancer

FIGURE 10.2 Phytonutrient sources: Colorful fruits and vegetables.

10.6.1 TERPENES

Terpenes are a broad group of chemical compounds with distinctive odors. Many plants, primarily conifers, produce them. Terpenoids are hydrocarbons with functional groups attached to them. Many terpenes could have functioned as a type of defense (Cox-Georgian et al., 2019):

1. **Diterpenes:** Taxanes are diterpenes produced by the Taxus plant that is commonly employed as chemotherapeutic drugs. Because they are poorly soluble in water, they pose challenges in the manufacture of pharmaceuticals. Taxol is a powerful anti-cancer medicine that

has been licensed by the US FDA to treat a range of malignancies (Škubník et al., 2021).

2. **Triterpenes and Triterpenoids:** Triterpenes have the chemical formula C30H48 and are made up of six isoprene units. Triterpenoids are found in therapeutic plants in large quantities. Several triterpenoids have been suggested as potential anticancer treatments due to their antioxidant and anti-inflammatory characteristics (Aminfar et al., 2019).
3. **Triterpene Saponins:** Saponins are a type of plant glycoside that occurs naturally. Their significant foam-forming characteristics in an aqueous solution distinguish them. Saponins can be present in many higher plants' roots, tubers, leaves, flowers, and seeds (Kregiel et al., 2017).

10.6.2 PHENOLS AND POLYPHENOLS

Many clinical trials on cancer prevention have been conducted utilizing plant polyphenols such as curcumin and resveratrol. Flavonoids alone account for 1–2 g of the average daily consumption. Flavonoids make up the majority of fruits, vegetables, oils, and humectants 60% and 30% of total dietary polyphenols, respectively (Keservani & Sharma, 2014; Janabi et al., 2020):

1. **Chalcones:** It is an aromatic ketone with a central core that can be found in a variety of important biological compounds. They are a group of polyphenolic chemicals generated from plants that belong to the flavonoid class. Their antibacterial, antiviral, anti-inflammatory, antioxidant, and anticancer properties have been attributed to chalcones (Jasim et al., 2021).
2. **Anthocyanins:** Also known as anthocyans – are pH-dependent water-soluble vacuolar pigments that range in hue from red to purple to blue. They can be found in higher plants in various parts like leaves, stems, roots, flowers, and fruits (Khoo et al., 2017).
3. **Flavanones:** Citrus fruits and juice have been investigated for their potential role in the prevention of cardiovascular disease (Keservani et al., 2016a, 2017, 2020) and cancer. Flavanones, the polyphenols found in citrus fruits, are principally responsible for these beneficial effects. Hesperetin, naringenin, eriodictyol, and isosakuranetin are all found in cucumbers (Testai & Calderone, 2017).

4. **Flavanols:** Flavan-3-ols are composed of two benzene rings (A- and B-rings) as well as a dihydropyran heterocycle (the C-ring). Catechins operate as antioxidants by scavenging free radicals, chelating redox-active transition metal ions, inhibiting pro-oxidant enzymes, and activating antioxidant enzymes. Epigallocatechin gallate (EGCG), an antioxidant, inhibits the occurrence and spread of cancer in a range of organs, including the liver, stomach, skin, lungs, mammary gland, and colon. EGCG has a lot of potential in cancer prevention due to its safety, low cost, and bioavailability (Truong & Jeong, 2021).
5. **Flavones:** Apigenin is a flavonoid that can be found in a variety of foods, including fruits, vegetables, and spices. It has many chemo-preventive qualities, including the ability to induce apoptosis, limit cancer cell proliferation, and participate in angiogenesis. Lutein has been proven to inhibit tumor cell growth in human skin, liver, and ovarian cancer cells (Patra et al., 2021).
6. **Flavonols:** The flavonoid quercetin is found in the highest concentration in foods. It is most abundantly available in apples, berries, and grapes, as well as onions and broccoli, tea, and red wine. This flavonol has been shown to have antiproliferative properties in a variety of circumstances, including breast cancer (Salehi et al., 2020).
7. **Myricetin:** These found in fruits, vegetables, and red wine, is the next flavonol with anticancer properties. This compound has been shown to inhibit the invasion and migration of human lung adenocarcinoma cells. A study found that myricetins caused apoptosis in human leukemia cell lines (Kopustinskiene et al., 2020).
8. **Kaempferol:** It is a flavonol found in a variety of plants, including tea, broccoli, grapefruit, brussels sprouts, apples, and others. On numerous types of cancer, this chemical has antioxidant, anti-inflammatory, and anticancer properties. It has been shown to stop the human invasive breast cancer cell line from invading (Jideani et al., 2021).
9. **Curcuminoids:** The major curcuminoid found in turmeric, which belongs to the ginger family, is curcumin. For ages, it has been used to cure a wide range of illnesses. Curcumin decreased HepG2 cell proliferation in head and neck cancer patients by causing apoptosis (Singh et al., 2020).
10. **Stilbenoids:** These are C6-C2-C6 stilbene derivatives that have been hydroxylated. They are secondary metabolites that can be found in a

wide variety of plant groups. The levels of trans-resveratrol in grapes and grape skins used in winemaking are high (Valletta et al., 2020; Rienth et al., 2021).

11. **Galic Acid:** It is a hydroxybenzoic acid that can be found in a range of foods such as red fruits, black radish, onions, and fresh tea leaves. In many types of cancer cells, gallic acid has anti-invasive and anti-metastatic effects. It could be utilized to treat stomach cancer metastases as a prophylactic and therapeutic agent (Abotaleb et al., 2020).
12. **Tannis:** It is a bitter, astringent polyphenolic substance found in plants. Pentagalloylglucose and geraniin were the most active tannins. Geraniin has been isolated from Geranium thunbergii dry leaves (Yoshida et al., 2018).

10.6.3 POLYSACCHARIDES

Polysaccharides are biopolymers composed of monosaccharides with straight or branched side chains connected by glycosidic linkages. The majority of polysaccharides generated from higher plants are harmless and have few adverse effects. They are great prospects for immunomodulatory and anticancer treatments with little toxicity. In immunomodulatory and anticancer actions, the kind of connection between saccharide units appears to be crucial. β-1,3-glucans, β-1,6-glucans, and β-1,3-glucans, as well as various additional glycosidic linkages, are found in the majority of anticancer polysaccharides (Sindhu et al., 2021; Górska et al., 2021).

The Actinidia (Actinidiaceae) family contains approximately 58 species that are widely spread across Asia. Some Actinidia species, such as *A. macrosperma*, are used in traditional medicine as health foods and medical commodities. The anticancer and immunomodulatory activities of four polysaccharides extracted and purified from *A. eriantha* roots could be affected (Zhang et al., 2019).

Rhizomaarisaematis is a bitter, fiery, pungent, and toxic plant that develops from the rhizome of *Pinelliapedatisecta*. This polysaccharide has been shown in animal experiments to significantly inhibit tumor growth (Fan et al., 2020; Huang et al., 2011).

Rhodiola rosea L. is a Crassulaceae plant that grows in Europe, Asia, the Arctic, and mountainous areas of North America. The rhizome and roots have long been used in Russian and Chinese folk medicine (Li et al., 2017).

A ginseng polysaccharide injection has been developed in China as a beneficial adjuvant for cancer patients receiving irradiation and chemotherapy. By increasing immune processes and inducing apoptosis, polysaccharides from the plant have anti-tumor and anti-proliferative properties (Hoffman et al., 2020; Riaz et al., 2019).

In tropical and subtropical climes, the tea plant (*Camellia sinensis*) is mostly grown. Green tea protects the body from a variety of malignancies when consumed regularly. Tea polysaccharides contain anti-inflammatory, antioxidant, anticancer, and hypoglycemic properties (Kochman et al., 2021; Musial et al., 2020; Sánchez et al., 2020).

10.7 WATER IN CANCER TREATMENT

Drinking enough water throughout therapy can aid the recovery process go more smoothly. Anti-cancer treatment and some drugs may also induce extreme dehydration as a side effect.

Water is one of the most vital nutrients for bodily detoxification and cancer prevention. This liquid is a vital component of the body's cells, supplying sustenance to all of the body cells. The majority of internal activities, such as maintaining a healthy body temperature, removing pollutants, and preserving joint health, are supported by water (Maggini et al., 2018).

Water also keeps things flowing in the intestines. It aids in the passage of food and promotes proper digestion. Water eliminates toxins from the body, avoids accumulation, and so protects the colon and rectum from diseases like colorectal cancer (Vancamelbeke & Vermeire, 2017).

Drinking more water and eating more water-rich meals can help body cells grow, live, and reproduce healthily. This can aid in the prevention of cancer in the colon, bladder, and breast tissue (Donaldson, 2004).

10.8 DIETARY SUPPLEMENT SAFETY CONSIDERATIONS

Dietary supplement manufacturers are accountable for safeguarding that their products are safe and that their labeling is accurate. Dietary supplement manufacturers must ensure that their products are of high quality, that they are free of toxins and impurities, and that they are labeled correctly. Some dietary supplements (Keservani et al., 2010a, b) can help reduce the risk of some diseases. Most people can use supplements safely as long as they don't take too much. But they are not safe and can have risks, especially for people who are getting cancer treatment (Glisson et al., 2011).

Supplements can cause complications for patients who are undergoing cancer therapy in a variety of ways. Consider the following scenario.

When consumed during radiation treatment, some dietary supplements might induce skin irritation and severe responses. Before taking any supplement, one should consult a doctor while undergoing radiation treatment.

Some supplements may interact with medications used before and after surgery or raise the risk of certain adverse effects, such as bleeding and infection in those who need surgery. Other medications can harm the heart and brain, causing difficulties during and after surgery (Toshkova et al., 2017).

Chemotherapy patients who take nutritional supplements may be at an increased risk of side effects. Some supplements can interfere with how chemotherapy is broken down in the body, making it less effective or increasing unwanted effects (Singh et al., 2018).

Many cancer doctors advise consumers to avoid dietary supplements while undergoing cancer therapy because of these concerns. However, if a patient decides to take supplements, should talk to the doctor or cancer care team beforehand. They can assist in determining whether or not a product is suitable (Rock et al., 2012).

10.9 FUTURE PERSPECTIVES

Nutritional advice may aid cancer patients in obtaining critical nutrients such as protein (Keservani et al., 2015; Singh et al., 2017b), vitamins (Singh et al., 2017), and minerals. It can also assist them in maintaining a healthy weight. A registered dietitian (RD) or nutritionist (RDN) is the best source of nutritional advice for cancer patients.

Dietitians and other nutrition professionals can assist patients in developing a diet that matches unique nutritional requirements (Evert et al., 2019). Among their suggestions could be:

- Vitamins and minerals that are missing out on;
- To assist in achieving the objective, liquid nutritional supplements and snacks are available;
- Feeding tubes or nutritional supplementation according to the body's needs.

Advances in molecularly targeted medicines and immunotherapy have transformed cancer treatment. More advances in cancer treatment are on the way. In the future, not only will it be feasible to molecularly describe a patient's cancer cells, but it will also be possible to use the cellular components of their tumor to offer treatment options (Malone et al., 2020).

The search for new cancer therapeutic targets, such as those involved in cancer cell survival, development, and dissemination, as well as drug resistance mechanisms, which is a major cause of treatment failure in patients, is now underway (Zhang et al., 2020).

Saposin C, a synthetically generated human lysosomal protein, is used in Bexion Pharmaceuticals' investigational cancer treatment (Sandin et al., 2021).

The objective of the National Cancer Institute (NCI) is to increase the effectiveness and utilization of cancer medicines by figuring out how to combine therapies and avoid severe side effects (Choudhari et al., 2020). The National Cancer Institute funds research into precision radiotherapy and techniques to reduce the impact of radiation harm on normal tissues (Bauman et al., 2020).

KEYWORDS

- **adequate intake**
- **estrogen receptor-negative**
- **gap junction intercellular communication**
- **nutritional supplementation**
- **polyunsaturated fatty acids**
- **saposin C**

REFERENCES

Abotaleb, M., Liskova, A., Kubatka, P., & Büsselberg, D., (2020). Therapeutic potential of plant phenolic acids in the treatment of cancer. *Biomolecules, 10*(2), 221.

Alkhenizan, A., & Hafez, K., (2007). The role of vitamin E in the prevention of cancer: A meta-analysis of randomized controlled trials. *Annals of Saudi Medicine, 27*(6), 409–414.

Aminfar, Z., Rabiei, B., Tohidfar, M., & Mirjalili, M. H., (2019). Identification of key genes involved in the biosynthesis of triterpenic acids in the mint family. *Scientific Reports, 9*(1), 1–15.

Bakker, M. F., Peeters, P. H., Klaasen, V. M., Bueno-De-Mesquita, H. B., Jansen, E. H., Ros, M. M., Travier, N., et al., (2016). Plasma carotenoids, vitamin C, tocopherols, and retinol and the risk of breast cancer in the European prospective investigation into cancer and nutrition cohort, 2. *The American Journal of Clinical Nutrition, 103*(2), 454–464.

Balić, A., Vlašić, D., Žužul, K., Marinović, B., & BukvićMokos, Z., (2020). Omega-3 versus omega-6 polyunsaturated fatty acids in the prevention and treatment of inflammatory skin diseases. *International Journal of Molecular Sciences, 21*(3), 741.

Baumann, B. C., Mitra, N., Harton, J. G., Xiao, Y., Wojcieszynski, A. P., Gabriel, P. E., Zhong, H., et al., (2020). Comparative effectiveness of proton vs photon therapy as part of concurrent chemoradiotherapy for locally advanced cancer. *JAMA Oncology, 6*(2), 237–246.

Bhattacharyya, A., Chattopadhyay, R., Mitra, S., & Crowe, S. E., (2014). Oxidative stress: An essential factor in the pathogenesis of gastrointestinal mucosal diseases. *Physiological Reviews, 94*(2), 329–354.

Binda, S., Hill, C., Johansen, E., Obis, D., Pot, B., Sanders, M. E., Tremblay, A., & Ouwehand, A. C., (2020). Criteria to qualify microorganisms as "probiotic" in foods and dietary supplements. *Frontiers in Microbiology, 11*, 1662.

Black, H. S., Boehm, F., Edge, R., & Truscott, T. G., (2020). The benefits and risks of certain dietary carotenoids that exhibit both anti-and pro-oxidative mechanisms—A comprehensive review. *Antioxidants, 9*(3), 264.

Block, K. I., & Gyllenhaal, C., (2005). Commentary: The pharmacological antioxidant amifostine—Implications of recent research for integrative cancer care. *Integrative Cancer Therapies, 4*(4), 329–351.

Bojková, B., Winklewski, P. J., & Wszedybyl-Winklewska, M., (2020). Dietary fat and cancer—Which is good, which is bad, and the body of evidence. *International Journal of Molecular Sciences, 21*(11), 4114.

Cancer Prevention Recommendation. By World Cancer Research Foundation. Accessed from: https://www.wcrf.org/diet-and-cancer/cancer-prevention-recommendations/ (accessed on 28 January 2023).

Carbone, J. W., & Pasiakos, S. M., (2019). Dietary protein and muscle mass: Translating science to application and health benefit. *Nutrients, 11*(5), 1136.

Carr, A. C., & Maggini, S., (2017). Vitamin C and immune function. *Nutrients, 9*(11), 1211.

Cencic, A., & Chingwaru, W., (2010). The role of functional foods, nutraceuticals, and food supplements in intestinal health. *Nutrients, 2*(6), 611–625.

Chambial, S., Dwivedi, S., Shukla, K. K., John, P. J., & Sharma, P., (2013). Vitamin C in disease prevention and cure: An overview. *Indian Journal of Clinical Biochemistry, 28*(4), 314–328.

Chen, Y. C., Prabhu, K. S., & Mastro, A. M., (2013). Is selenium a potential treatment for cancer metastasis? *Nutrients, 5*(4), 1149–1168.

Choudhari, A. S., Mandave, P. C., Deshpande, M., Ranjekar, P., & Prakash, O., (2020). Phytochemicals in cancer treatment: From preclinical studies to clinical practice. *Frontiers in Pharmacology, 10*, 1614.

Clerici, S. P., Peppelenbosch, M., Fuhler, G., Consonni, S. R., & Ferreira-Halder, C. V., (2021). Colorectal cancer cell-derived small extracellular vesicles educate human fibroblasts to stimulate migratory capacity. *Frontiers in Cell and Developmental Biology, 9.*

Cox-Georgian, D., Ramadoss, N., Dona, C., & Basu, C., (2019). Therapeutic and medicinal uses of terpenes. In: *Medicinal Plants* (pp. 333–359). Springer, Cham.

D'Eliseo, D., & Velotti, F., (2016). Omega-3 fatty acids and cancer cell cytotoxicity: Implications for multi-targeted cancer therapy. *Journal of Clinical Medicine, 5*(2), 15.

Davis, H. W., Vallabhapurapu, S. D., Chu, Z., Vallabhapurapu, S. L., Franco, R. S., Mierzwa, M., Kassing, W., et al., (2019). Enhanced phosphatidylserine-selective cancer therapy with irradiation and SapC-DOPS nanovesicles. *Oncotarget, 10*(8), 856.

Desmawati, D., & Sulastri, D., (2019). Phytoestrogens and their health effect. *Open Access Macedonian Journal of Medical Sciences, 7*(3), 495.

Donaldson, M. S., (2004). Nutrition and cancer: A review of the evidence for an anti-cancer diet. *Nutrition Journal, 3*(1), 1–21.

Duan, W., Shen, X., Lei, J., Xu, Q., Yu, Y., Li, R., Wu, E., & Ma, Q., (2014). Hyperglycemia, a neglected factor during cancer progression. *BioMed Research International, 2014.*

Evert, A. B., Dennison, M., Gardner, C. D., Garvey, W. T., Lau, K. H. K., MacLeod, J., Mitri, J., et al., (2019). Nutrition therapy for adults with diabetes or prediabetes: A consensus report. *Diabetes Care, 42*(5), 731–754.

Fabian, C. J., Kimler, B. F., & Hursting, S. D., (2015). Omega-3 fatty acids for breast cancer prevention and survivorship. *Breast Cancer Research, 17*(1), 1–11.

Fan, Y., Ma, Z., Zhao, L., Wang, W., Gao, M., Jia, X., Ouyang, H., & He, J., (2020). Anti-tumor activities and mechanisms of traditional Chinese medicines formulas: A review. *Biomedicine & Pharmacotherapy, 132*, 110820.

Ferdous, U. T., & Yusof, Z. N. B., (2021). Medicinal prospects of antioxidants from algal sources in cancer therapy. *Frontiers in Pharmacology, 12*, 157.

Fernández-Sanz, P., Ruiz-Gabarre, D., & García-Escudero, V., (2019). Modulating effect of diet on Alzheimer's disease. *Diseases, 7*(1), 12.

Fiedor, J., & Burda, K., (2014). Potential role of carotenoids as antioxidants in human health and disease. *Nutrients, 6*(2), 466–488.

Forman, H. J., & Zhang, H., (2021). Targeting oxidative stress in disease: Promise and limitations of antioxidant therapy. *Nature Reviews Drug Discovery*, 1–21.

Freitas, R. D., & Campos, M. M., (2019). Protective effects of omega-3 fatty acids in cancer-related complications. *Nutrients, 11*(5), 945.

Gaziano, J. M., Glynn, R. J., Christen, W. G., Kurth, T., Belanger, C., MacFadyen, J., Bubes, V., et al., (2009). Vitamins E and C in the prevention of prostate and total cancer in men: The physicians' health study II randomized controlled trial. *JAMA, 301*(1), 52–62.

Gilbert, C., (2013). What is vitamin A and why do we need it? *Community Eye Health, 26*(84), 65.

Glisson, J. K., Minor, D. S., Walker, L. A., & Gurley, B. J., (2011). Dietary supplements: Safety issues and quality control. *Archives of Internal Medicine, 171*(5), 476, 477.

Gómez-Zorita, S., González-Arceo, M., Fernández-Quintela, A., Eseberri, I., Trepiana, J., & Portillo, M. P., (2020). Scientific evidence supporting the beneficial effects of isoflavones on human health. *Nutrients, 12*(12), 3853.

Górska, S., Maksymiuk, A., & Turło, J., (2021). Selenium-containing polysaccharides—Structural diversity, biosynthesis, chemical modifications and biological activity. *Applied Sciences, 11*(8), 3717.

Goszcz, K., Deakin, S. J., Duthie, G. G., Stewart, D., Leslie, S. J., & Megson, I. L., (2015). Antioxidants in cardiovascular therapy: Panacea or false hope? *Frontiers in Cardiovascular Medicine, 2*, 29.

Grober, U., Holzhauer, P., Kisters, K., Holick, M. F., & Adamietz, I. A., (2016). Micronutrients in oncological intervention. *Nutrients, 8*(3), 163.

Halsted, C. H., (2003). Dietary supplements and functional foods: 2 sides of a coin? *The American Journal of Clinical Nutrition, 77*(4), 1001S–1007S.

Hariharan, S., & Dharmaraj, S., (2020). Selenium and selenoproteins: It's role in regulation of inflammation. *Inflammopharmacology, 28*(3), 667–695.

Harvie, M., (2014). Nutritional supplements and cancer: Potential benefits and proven harms. *American Society of Clinical Oncology Educational Book, 34*(1), e478–e486.

Hassan, S., Egbuna, C., Tijjani, H., Ifemeje, J. C., Olisah, M. C., Patrick-Iwuanyanwu, K. C., Onyeike, P. C., & Ephraim-Emmanuel, B. C., (2020). Dietary supplements: Types, health benefits, industry and regulation. In: *Functional Foods and Nutraceuticals* (pp. 23–38). Springer, Cham.

Hatfield, D. L., & Gladyshev, V. N., (2009). The outcome of selenium and vitamin E cancer prevention trial (SELECT) reveals the need for better understanding of selenium biology. *Molecular Interventions, 9*(1), 18.

Hemilä, H., & Chalker, E., (2019). Vitamin C can shorten the length of stay in the ICU: A meta-analysis. *Nutrients, 11*(4), 708.

Hoffman, J. R., & Falvo, M. J., (2004). Protein–which is best? *Journal of Sports Science & Medicine, 3*(3), 118.

Hoffman, R. D., Li, C. Y., He, K., Wu, X., He, B. C., He, T. C., & Gao, J. L., (2020). Chinese herbal medicine and its regulatory effects on tumor related T cells. *Frontiers in Pharmacology, 11*, 492.

Huang, C. F., Yang, R. S., Liu, S. H., Hsieh, P. C., & Lin-Shiau, S. Y., (2011). Evidence for improved neuropharmacological efficacy and decreased neurotoxicity in mice with traditional processing of Rhizoma Arisaematis. *The American Journal of Chinese Medicine, 39*(05), 981–998.

Huang, R., Xiang, J., & Zhou, P., (2019). Vitamin D, gut microbiota, and radiation-related resistance: A love-hate triangle. *Journal of Experimental & Clinical Cancer Research, 38*(1), 1–10.

Janabi, A. H. W., Kamboh, A. A., Saeed, M., Xiaoyu, L., BiBi, J., Majeed, F., Naveed, M., et al., (2020). Flavonoid-rich foods (FRF): A promising nutraceutical approach against lifespan-shortening diseases. *Iranian Journal of Basic Medical Sciences, 23*(2), 140.

Jasim, H. A., Nahar, L., Jasim, M. A., Moore, S. A., Ritchie, K. J., & Sarker, S. D., (2021). Chalcones: Synthetic chemistry follows where nature leads. *Biomolecules, 11*(8), 1203.

Jeon, S. M., & Shin, E. A., (2018). Exploring vitamin D metabolism and function in cancer. *Experimental & Molecular Medicine, 50*(4), 1–14.

Jideani, A. I., Silungwe, H., Takalani, T., Omolola, A. O., Udeh, H. O., & Anyasi, T. A., (2021). Antioxidant-rich natural fruit and vegetable products and human health. *International Journal of Food Properties, 24*(1), 41–67.

Keservani, R. K., & Sharma, A. K., (2014). Flavonoids: Emerging trends and potential health benefits. *Journal of Chinese Pharmaceutical Sciences, 23*(12), 815.

Keservani, R. K., Kesharwani, R. K., Sharma, A. K., Vyas, N., & Chadoker, A., (2010b). Nutritional supplements: An overview. *International Journal of Current Pharmaceutical Review and Research, 1*(1), 59–75.

Keservani, R. K., Kesharwani, R. K., Vyas, N., Jain, S., Raghuvanshi, R., & Sharma, A. K., (2010a). Nutraceutical and functional food as future food: A review. *Der Pharmacia Lettre, 2*(1), 106–116.

Keservani, R. K., Sharma, A. K., & Jarouliya, U., (2015). Protein and peptide in drug targeting and its therapeutic approach. *Ars Pharmaceutica (Internet), 56*(3), 165–177.

Keservani, R. K., Sharma, A. K., & Kesharwani, R. K., (2016a). Nutraceutical and functional foods for cardiovascular health. In: *Food Process Engineering* (pp. 257–278, 291–312). Apple Academic Press, CRC Press. ISBN: 9781771884020.

Keservani, R. K., Sharma, A. K., & Kesharwani, R. K., (2016b). Medicinal effect of nutraceutical fruits for the cognition and brain health. *Scientifica,* 10. Article ID 3109254. doi: 10.1155/2016/3109254.

Keservani, R. K., Sharma, A. K., & Kesharwani, R. K., (2020). *Nutraceuticals and Dietary Supplements: Applications in Health Improvement and Disease Management*. CRC Press. ISBN: 9781771888738.

Khoo, H. E., Azlan, A., Tang, S. T., & Lim, S. M., (2017). Anthocyanidins and anthocyanins: Colored pigments as food, pharmaceutical ingredients, and the potential health benefits. *Food & Nutrition Research, 61*(1), 1361779.

Kieliszek, M., & Błażejak, S., (2016). Current knowledge on the importance of selenium in food for living organisms: A review. *Molecules, 21*(5), 609.

Kieliszek, M., (2019). Selenium–fascinating microelement, properties and sources in food. *Molecules, 24*(7), 1298.

Kim, I. S., (2021). Current perspectives on the beneficial effects of soybean isoflavones and their metabolites for humans. *Antioxidants, 10*(7), 1064.

Klein, E. A., Thompson, I., Tangen, C. M., Lucia, M. S., Goodman, P., Minasian, L. M., Ford, L. G., et al., (2012). Vitamin E and the risk of prostate cancer: Updated results of the Selenium and Vitamin E Cancer Prevention Trial (SELECT). *Journal of Clinical Oncology 30*(5_suppl), 7.

Kochman, J., Jakubczyk, K., Antoniewicz, J., Mruk, H., & Janda, K., (2021). Health benefits and chemical composition of matcha green tea: A review. *Molecules, 26*(1), 85.

Kopustinskiene, D. M., Jakstas, V., Savickas, A., & Bernatoniene, J., (2020). Flavonoids as anticancer agents. *Nutrients, 12*(2), 457.

Kregiel, D., Berlowska, J., Witonska, I., Antolak, H., Proestos, C., Babic, M., Babic, L., & Zhang, B., (2017). Saponin-based, biological-active surfactants from plants. *Application and Characterization of Surfactants, 183*.

Kuršvietienė, L., Mongirdienė, A., Bernatonienė, J., Šulinskienė, J., & Stanevičienė, I., (2020). Selenium anticancer properties and impact on cellular redox status. *Antioxidants, 9*(1), 80.

Kurutas, E. B., (2015). The importance of antioxidants which play the role in cellular response against oxidative/nitrosative stress: Current state. *Nutrition Journal, 15*(1), 1–22.

Ladurner, A., Schmitt, C. A., Schachner, D., Atanasov, A. G., Werner, E. R., Dirsch, V. M., & Heiss, E. H., (2012). Ascorbate stimulates endothelial nitric oxide synthase enzyme activity by rapid modulation of its phosphorylation status. *Free Radical Biology and Medicine, 52*(10), 2082–2090.

Li, Y., Pham, V., Bui, M., Song, L., Wu, C., Walia, A., Uchio, E., Smith-Liu, F., & Zi, X., (2017). *Rhodiola rosea* L.: An herb with anti-stress, anti-aging, and immunostimulating properties for cancer chemoprevention. *Current Pharmacology Reports, 3*(6), 384–395.

Liberti, M. V., & Locasale, J. W., (2016). The Warburg effect: How does it benefit cancer cells? *Trends in Biochemical Sciences, 41*(3), 211–218.

Linowiecka, K., Foksinski, M., & Brożyna, A. A., (2020). Vitamin C transporters and their implications in carcinogenesis. *Nutrients, 12*(12), 3869.

Liu, Z., Ren, Z., Zhang, J., Chuang, C. C., Kandaswamy, E., Zhou, T., & Zuo, L., (2018). Role of ROS and nutritional antioxidants in human diseases. *Frontiers in Physiology, 9*, 477.

Lobo, V., Patil, A., Phatak, A., & Chandra, N., (2010). Free radicals, antioxidants and functional foods: Impact on human health. *Pharmacognosy Reviews, 4*(8), 118.

Maggini, S., Pierre, A., & Calder, P. C., (2018). Immune function and micronutrient requirements change over the life course. *Nutrients, 10*(10), 1531.

Malone, E. R., Oliva, M., Sabatini, P. J., Stockley, T. L., & Siu, L. L., (2020). Molecular profiling for precision cancer therapies. *Genome Medicine, 12*(1), 1–19.

Marqus, S., Pirogova, E., & Piva, T. J., (2017). Evaluation of the use of therapeutic peptides for cancer treatment. *Journal of Biomedical Science, 24*(1), 1–15.

Messina, M., (2016). Soy and health update: Evaluation of the clinical and epidemiologic literature. *Nutrients, 8*(12), 754.

Musial, C., Kuban-Jankowska, A., & Gorska-Ponikowska, M., (2020). Beneficial properties of green tea catechins. *International Journal of Molecular Sciences, 21*(5), 1744.

Neuhouser, M. L., Wassertheil-Smoller, S., Thomson, C., Aragaki, A., Anderson, G. L., Manson, J. E., Patterson, R. E., et al., (2009). Multivitamin use and risk of cancer and cardiovascular disease in the women's health initiative cohorts. *Archives of Internal Medicine, 169*(3), 294–304.

Nguyen, C., & Nguyen, V. D., (2016). Discovery of azurin-like anticancer bacteriocins from human gut microbiome through homology modeling and molecular docking against the tumor suppressor p53. *BioMed Research International, 2016.*

Norman, H. A., Butrum, R. R., Feldman, E., Heber, D., Nixon, D., Picciano, M. F., Rivlin, R., et al., (2003). The role of dietary supplements during cancer therapy. *The Journal of Nutrition, 133*(11), 3794S–3799S.

Padayatty, S. J., & Levine, M., (2016). Vitamin C: The known and the unknown and Goldilocks. *Oral Diseases, 22*(6), 463–493.

Padayatty, S. J., Sun, H., Wang, Y., Riordan, H. D., Hewitt, S. M., Katz, A., Wesley, R. A., & Levine, M., (2004). Vitamin C pharmacokinetics: Implications for oral and intravenous use. *Annals of Internal Medicine, 140*(7), 533–537.

Patra, S., Nayak, R., Patro, S., Pradhan, B., Sahu, B., Behera, C., Bhutia, S. K., & Jena, M., (2021). Chemical diversity of dietary phytochemicals and their mode of chemoprevention. *Biotechnology Reports*, e00633.

Pham-Huy, L. A., He, H., & Pham-Huy, C., (2008). Free radicals, antioxidants in disease and health. *International Journal of Biomedical Science: IJBS, 4*(2), 89.

Pucci, C., Martinelli, C., & Ciofani, G., (2019). Innovative approaches for cancer treatment: Current perspectives and new challenges. *Ecancermedicalscience, 13.*

Riaz, M., Rahman, N. U., Zia-Ul-Haq, M., Jaffar, H. Z., & Manea, R., (2019). Ginseng: A dietary supplement as an immune-modulator in various diseases. *Trends in Food Science & Technology, 83*, 12–30.

Rienth, M., Vigneron, N., Darriet, P., Sweetman, C., Burbidge, C., Bonghi, C., Walker, R. P., et al., (2021). Grape berry secondary metabolites and their modulation by abiotic factors in a climate change scenario: A review. *Frontiers in Plant Science, 12*, 262.

Rizzo, G., & Baroni, L., (2018). Soy, soy foods and their role in vegetarian diets. *Nutrients, 10*(1), 43.

Rock, C. L., Doyle, C., Demark-Wahnefried, W., Meyerhardt, J., Courneya, K. S., Schwartz, A. L., Bandera, E. V., et al., (2012). Nutrition and physical activity guidelines for cancer survivors. *CA: A Cancer Journal for Clinicians, 62*(4), 242–274.

Rock, C. L., Thomson, C., Gansler, T., Gapstur, S. M., McCullough, M. L., Patel, A. V., Andrews, K. S., et al., (2020). American cancer society guidelines for diet and physical activity for cancer prevention. *CA: A Cancer Journal for Clinicians, 70*(4), 245–271.

Sahin, I., Bilir, B., Ali, S., Sahin, K., & Kucuk, O., (2019). Soy isoflavones in integrative oncology: Increased efficacy and decreased toxicity of cancer therapy. *Integrative Cancer Therapies, 18*, 1534735419835310.

Salehi, B., Machin, L., Monzote, L., Sharifi-Rad, J., Ezzat, S. M., Salem, M. A., Merghany, R. M., et al., (2020). Therapeutic potential of quercetin: New insights and perspectives for human health. *ACS Omega, 5*(20), 11849–11872.

Sánchez, M., González-Burgos, E., Iglesias, I., Lozano, R., & Gómez-Serranillos, M. P., (2020). The pharmacological activity of *Camellia sinensis* (L.) Kuntze on metabolic and endocrine disorders: A systematic review. *Biomolecules, 10*(4), 603.

Sandin, S. I., Gravano, D. M., Randolph, C. J., Sharma, M., & De Alba, E., (2021). Engineering of saposin C protein chimeras for enhanced cytotoxicity and optimized liposome binding capability. *Pharmaceutics, 13*(4), 583.

Seca, A. M., & Pinto, D. C., (2018). Plant secondary metabolites as anticancer agents: Successes in clinical trials and therapeutic application. *International Journal of Molecular Sciences, 19*(1), 263.

Sharifi-Rad, M., Anil, K. N. V., Zucca, P., Varoni, E. M., Dini, L., Panzarini, E., Rajkovic, J., et al., (2020). Lifestyle, oxidative stress, and antioxidants: Back and forth in the pathophysiology of chronic diseases. *Frontiers in Physiology, 11*, 694.

Shin, J., Song, M. H., Oh, J. W., Keum, Y. S., & Saini, R. K., (2020). Pro-oxidant actions of carotenoids in triggering apoptosis of cancer cells: A review of emerging evidence. *Antioxidants, 9*(6), 532.

Sindhu, R. K., Goyal, A., Das, J., Choden, S., & Kumar, P., (2021). Immunomodulatory potential of polysaccharides derived from plants and microbes: A narrative review. *Carbohydrate Polymer Technologies and Applications, 2*, 100044.

Singh, A., Shafi, Z., Mahto, S. K., Yadav, S., & Sankhwar, R., (2020). Role and application of curcumin as an alternative therapeutic agent. *Adv. Microb. Res.*

Singh, K., Bhori, M., Kasu, Y. A., Bhat, G., & Marar, T., (2018). Antioxidants as precision weapons in war against cancer chemotherapy induced toxicity–exploring the armory of obscurity. *Saudi Pharmaceutical Journal, 26*(2), 177–190.

Singh, P., Kesharwani, R. K., & Keservani, R. K., (2017b). Protein, carbohydrates, and fats: Energy metabolism. In: *Sustained Energy for Enhanced Human Functions and Activity* (pp. 103–115). Academic Press. ISBN:9780128054130.

Škubník, J., Pavlíčková, V., Ruml, T., & Rimpelová, S., (2021). Current perspectives on taxanes: Focus on their bioactivity, delivery and combination therapy. *Plants, 10*(3), 569.

Sovadinová, I., Upham, B. L., Trosko, J. E., & Babica, P., (2021). Applicability of scrape loading-dye transfer assay for non-genotoxic carcinogen testing. *International Journal of Molecular Sciences, 22*(16), 8977.

Testai, L., & Calderone, V., (2017). Nutraceutical value of citrus flavanones and their implications in cardiovascular disease. *Nutrients, 9*(5), 502.

Thomas, S., Patel, D., Bittel, B., Wolski, K., Wang, Q., Kumar, A., Il'Giovine, Z. J., et al., (2021). Effect of high-dose zinc and ascorbic acid supplementation vs usual care on symptom length and reduction among ambulatory patients with SARS-CoV-2 infection: The COVID A to Z randomized clinical trial. *JAMA Network Open, 4*(2), e210369-e210369.

Toshkova, Y., Tarpomanova, T., Filkova, S., & Yeremiev, K., (2017). Safety of dietary supplements- A review article. *Asian Journal of Science and Technology, 8*(3), 4530–4535.

Traber, M. G., & Stevens, J. F., (2011). Vitamins C and E: Beneficial effects from a mechanistic perspective. *Free Radical Biology and Medicine, 51*(5), 1000–1013.

Truong, V. L., & Jeong, W. S., (2021). Cellular defensive mechanisms of tea polyphenols: Structure-activity relationship. *International Journal of Molecular Sciences, 22*(17), 9109.

Tuso, P. J., Ismail, M. H., Ha, B. P., & Bartolotto, C., (2013). Nutritional update for physicians: Plant-based diets. *The Permanente Journal, 17*(2), 61.

Valletta, A., Iozia, L. M., & Leonelli, F., (2021). Impact of environmental factors on stilbene biosynthesis. *Plants, 10*(1), 90.

Vancamelbeke, M., & Vermeire, S., (2017). The intestinal barrier: A fundamental role in health and disease. *Expert Review of Gastroenterology & Hepatology, 11*(9), 821–834.

Vander, H. M. G., Cantley, L. C., & Thompson, C. B., (2009). Understanding the Warburg effect: The metabolic requirements of cell proliferation. *Science, 324*(5930), 1029–1033.

Volz, C., Breid, S., Selenz, C., Zaplatina, A., Golfmann, K., Meder, L., Dietlein, F., et al., (2020). Inhibition of tumor VEGFR2 induces serine 897 EphA2-dependent tumor cell invasion and metastasis in NSCLC. *Cell Reports, 31*(4), 107568.

Wanders, D., Hobson, K., & Ji, X., (2020). Methionine restriction and cancer biology. *Nutrients, 12*(3), 684.

Wei, M. Y., & Giovannucci, E. L., (2012). Lycopene, tomato products, and prostate cancer incidence: A review and reassessment in the PSA screening era. *Journal of Oncology, 2012.*

Xie, J., Bi, Y., Zhang, H., Dong, S., Teng, L., Lee, R. J., & Yang, Z., (2020). Cell-penetrating peptides in diagnosis and treatment of human diseases: From preclinical research to clinical application. *Frontiers in Pharmacology, 11*, 697.

Yasueda, A., Urushima, H., & Ito, T., (2016). Efficacy and interaction of antioxidant supplements as adjuvant therapy in cancer treatment: A systematic review. *Integrative Cancer Therapies, 15*(1), 17–39.

Yee, L. D., Mortimer, J. E., Natarajan, R., Dietze, E. C., & Seewaldt, V. L., (2020). Metabolic health, insulin, and breast cancer: Why oncologists should care about insulin. *Frontiers in Endocrinology, 11*, 58.

Yoshida, T., Yoshimura, M., & Amakura, Y., (2018). Chemical and biological significance of oenothein B and related ellagitannin oligomers with macrocyclic structure. *Molecules, 23*(3), 552.

Zaric, B. L., Radovanovic, J. N., Gluvic, Z., Stewart, A. J., Essack, M., Motwalli, O., Gojobori, T., & Isenovic, E. R., (2020). Atherosclerosis linked to aberrant amino acid metabolism and immunosuppressive amino acid catabolizing enzymes. *Frontiers in Immunology, 11.*

Zhang, F., Yan, Z., Xu, Y., & Lin, H., (2019). The complete chloroplast genome of *Actinidia* fulvicoma. *Mitochondrial DNA Part B, 4*(2), 4089–4090.

Zhang, Z., Zhou, L., Xie, N., Nice, E. C., Zhang, T., Cui, Y., & Huang, C., (2020). Overcoming cancer therapeutic bottleneck by drug repurposing. *Signal Transduction and Targeted Therapy, 5*(1), 1–25.

Zihni, C., Mills, C., Matter, K., & Balda, M. S., (2016). Tight junctions: From simple barriers to multifunctional molecular gates. *Nature Reviews Molecular Cell Biology, 17*(9), 564–580.

CHAPTER 11

ROLE OF FOOD SUPPLEMENTS IN CHD

AMITKUMAR R. DHANKANI,[1] BHUSHAN R. RANE,[2] MANSI A. DHANKANI,[1] AKASH S. JAIN,[1] DIVAKAR R. PATIL,[1] SANDIP A. TADVI,[1] and SUNILA A. PATIL[1]

[1]*P.S.G.V.P. Mandal's College of Pharmacy, Shahada, Nandurbar, Maharashtra, India*

[2]*Shri D.D. Vispute College of Pharmacy and Research Center, Devad-Vichumbe, Panvel, Navi Mumbai, Maharashtra, India*

ABSTRACT

Cardiovascular disease (CVD) has overcome as the top cause of mortality worldwide, and it is an increasing public health concern. Dietary variables are crucial in the etiology of CVD and may influence CVD risk to a great extent, although they have received much less attention. The preventive benefits of dietary supplements in the prevention of Coronary Heart Disease have sparked a surge of interest. There has been a paradigm shift in nutritional epidemiology in the last decade, with researchers looking at connections between dietary habits and health. Specific dietary methods to address cardiovascular risk factors, such as the Dietary Approaches to Stop Hypertension diet and Therapeutic Lifestyle Changes, are based on food-based principles and have been demonstrated to be beneficial in treating hypertension and hypercholesterolemia, respectively. As a result, these diets considerably lower the risk of coronary heart disease. On the impact of foods and dietary supplements on the risk of coronary heart disease, a number of

Food Supplements and Dietary Fiber in Health and Disease. Bhushan R. Rane, Raj K. Keservani, Durgesh Singh, Nayan A. Gujarathi, and Ashish S. Jain, (Eds.)
© 2024 Apple Academic Press, Inc. Co-published with CRC Press (Taylor & Francis)

reviews and research papers have been published. The function of numerous diets and food supplements in the prevention of coronary heart disease has been discussed here.

11.1 INTRODUCTION

Obesity, diabetes, and cardiovascular ailment are all key causes of death rate. Cardiac disorders are the primary reason of death in the US, affecting 80 million people (Kashiwagi& L., 2012). Coronary artery disease is another name for coronary heart disease. The coronary arteries (heart arteries) are responsible for the flow of blood to cardiac muscles. Plaque (deposited fatty substance) obliterates the arteries of the heart in coronary heart disease, and blood platelets can bind to these affected zones, obstructing the flow of blood. This can cause ischemia (oxygen deprivation to cells of cardiac muscles) or ischemic stroke (Torpy, 2009).

The expense of not spending in coronary heart diseases prophylaxis and management is predicted to surpass $47 trillion globally over the next few 25 years (QuiaraLovatti et al., 2019). In the United States, 16.8 million individuals are believed to have severe coronary heart disease (CHD); 9.8 millions of those individuals have unstable angina, and around 8 million have suffered a heart attack. In the United States, CHD's projected direct and indirect financial impact in the year 2009 was $165.4 billion. In 2002, over 16.7 million fatalities globally (as compared to around 5 million deaths due to TB, HIV, and malaria combined) were attributable to cardiovascular disease, with 80% of these fatalities occurring in the developing world (Cassar et al., 2009).

In 2030, coronary heart disease is likely to assassinate 23.4 million individuals. Furthermore, cardiovascular disease affects people at an earlier phase in the developing domain, which might have a severe impact on the workforce and economic output (World Health Organization, 2004).

Nutrition, in general, is undeniably important in the prevention of CHD. In the last century, we've come a long way in understanding the impact of nutrition in CHD. Data on food ingestion trends and biological studies that indicated relationships between frequency of coronary heart disease and lipid ingestion around and inside the nations provided the first evidence (Bhupathiraju & Tucker, 2011).

The American Heart Association suggests that nutrition abundant in fruits, vegetables, whole grains, and meals with high amounts of fiber, as well as lean meats and fowl, moderate seafood intake, milk goods which are free from fat or having low fat content, and restricting saturated fat, trans fat, and cholesterol (Kashiwagi, 2012).

More research is being done on nutrition and the function of dietary supplements (Keservani et al., 2015; Keservani et al., 2016;) in averting CHD across the globe. Hence, the American Heart association's policy contains both, lifestyle and diet as a key aspect in reducing CHD among common populance (Lichtenstein et al., 2006).

Because culinary habits are one of the risk factors for CVD's that can be altered or controlled, a worldwide approach established on understanding of the relevance of elements that can cause CHD, in diverse geographical regions and cultural groups is required to successfully avert diseases (Basnet et al., 2020). As a result, the significance of nutritional supplements and diet in avoiding Coronary Heart Disease is critical.

11.2 POTENTIAL RISK FACTORS

The Framingham Heart Study's first findings in the early 1960s were the first to explicitly define factors that can cause risk of CHD. The Framingham Heart Study (FHS) was the pioneer to define the terminology "risk factors" in CHD, publishing its findings in 1957. There are a number of threat elements for CHD. Few, out of them, could be treated or controlled but not all of them can be managed. The discoveries were absolutely remarkable (Hajar, 2017) (Figure 11.1).

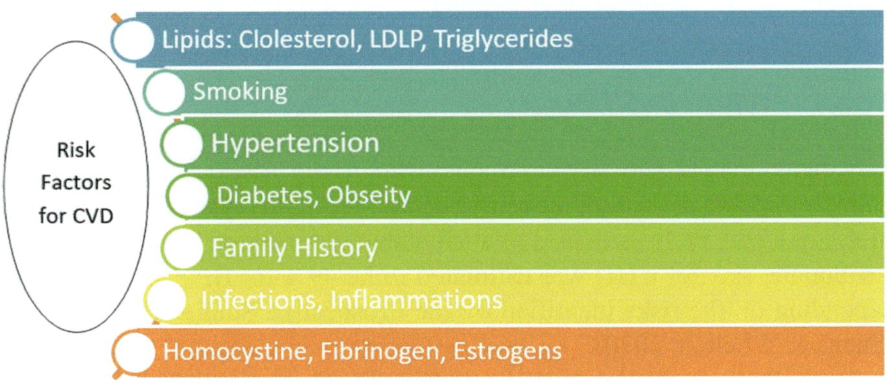

FIGURE 11.1 Potential risk factors of CHD.

11.2.1 LIPIDS

Several meta-analyzes and evaluations have emphasized the link amid Triglyceride concentration and the threat of CHD in common populace, with ansurge in TG level being concomitant with a greater threat of CHD events (Ye et al., 2019). Now that high density lipoprotein cholesterol (HDL-C) being recognized as having a vital role in atherosclerosis by the medical profession, increasing HDL-C has become a common treatment method for lowering CHD rates (Gordon et al., 1989).

11.2.2 SMOKING

Tobacco use is the biggest avoidable reason for mortality in the US and a key contributor to CHD. Smoking has a significant number of effects on the CVS and hazard causing elements related to coronary system. Acute increase in BP and vascular resistance in coronary arteries, decreased oxygen supply, aggregation of platelets, increase in fibrinogen, and lowering of HDL are all negative consequences (Rigotti & Pasternak, 1996). Several researchers have looked at the impact of smoking on serum lipids throughout the last 40 years. As per WHO, smoking seems to be accountable for 10% of all CVD cases (Messner & Bernhard, 2014). In the year 2000, smoking was responsible for more than one out of every 10 fatalities globally due to cardiovascular disease. The advancement of alterations caused by atherosclerosis with narrowing of the lumen of arteries and creation of a prothrombotic state, which leads to the risk of thrombosis (acute), are general processes by which smoking causes cardiovascular events (Prevention (US) et al., 2010).

11.2.3 HYPERTENSION

Elevated blood pressure (BP) or hypertension is the hazard element for CHD with the greatest indication for causation and the highest prevalence of exposure. For CHD, early estimates of attributable risk were as high as 25%. The attributable risk for CHD was estimated to be 49% for BP$\geq$ 115/75 mmHg depending on the risks identified by the Prospective Studies Collaboration (Fuchs & Whelton, 2020).

Both illnesses are linked by a number of pathophysiological pathways. Hypertension causes endothelial malfunction, worsens atherosclerosis and also makes atherosclerotic plaques more unstable. Hypertrophy of the Left ventricles, a common consequence of hypertension, reduces 'coronary flow reserve' and elevates myocardial oxygen demand, each of which leads to myocardial ischemia. Clinical signs of CHD (angina, myocardial infarction) are common in hypertensive individuals, whether related to coronary atherosclerosis or a diminished coronary reserve (Escobar, 2002). Injury to the endothelium impairs the creation and release of nitric oxide, a strong vasodilator, along with the buildup of ROS and other inflammation causing agents, all of which gives contribution to the growth of atherosclerosis, formation of thrombus, &arterial occlusion (Olafiranye et al., 2011).

11.2.4 DIABETES

Around 8.8% of the globe's demographic is impacted by diabetes. According to the forecasting done by International Diabetes Federation, by 2040, the number of diabetics would have risen to 642 million. In diabetics, coronary heart disease (CHD) is the main reason of fatality and disability (Einarson et al., 2018). Kannel and McGee first showed that people of all age groups having diabetes are at a greater risk of CHD as compared to those who are not diabetic (defined at the time by random blood sugar of 150 mg/dL [8.3 mmol/L]). It was in Framingham Heart Study, which was a seminal piece of research, published in 1979. Diabetes mellitus affects women more than males when it comes to cardiovascular morbidity and mortality (Low Wang et al., 2016).

Endothelial dysfunction, hypercoagulability, and platelet dysfunction appear to be implicated, with hyperglycemia being the most prevalent cause (Chiha et al., 2012). Furthermore, diabetes is linked to an inflammatory and pro-thrombotic milieu, which exacerbates atherosclerotic plaque disruption and thrombosis. Increased blood sugar level and Insulin resistance both facilitates endothelial cell dysfunction and increased free radicals. This can hasten the development of atherosclerosis. Insulin resistance and increased blood sugar level have a direct influence on thrombosis, which also includes a larger amount of clotting factors and anti-fibrinolytic proteins, as well as a more lysis-resistant fibrin network and increased platelet activation. It is generally understood that strengthening glycemic control reduces microvascular consequences in both type 1 and type 2 diabetes (King & Grant, 2016).

11.2.5 OBESITY

Overweight and corpulence are recognized by WHO as aberrant or extreme fat deposition that offers a health hazard. Severe corpulence and becoming overweight are major concern markers for a wide range of chronic diseases. These diseases may include cardiovascular disorders like coronary heart disease (Obesity, n.d.). The body mass index (BMI) is now used to assess overweight and corpulent persons (Poirier et al., 2006). It is determined by BMI, which is calculated by dividing a person's weight (in kilos) by the square of his or her height (in meters) (Akil & Ahmad, 2011). Adults with a BMI of 25.0 to 29.9 kg/m^2 are supposed to be overweight; on the other hand, those with a BMI of $\geq$ 30.0 kg/m^2 are considered corpulent (Poirier et al., 2006). There is a lot of epidemiologic data that there is a link between being overweight or obese and having a Coronary Heart Disease (Katta et al., 2021).

Hormones and peptides are also involved in the cardiovascular problems linked with obesity and endothelial dysfunction, coagulation activation, insulin resistance, coronary calcification, inflammation, renin angiotensin, and sympathetic nervous system activation are only a few examples. Adiponectin is a peptide generated in adipose tissue that is highly found in lean, healthy persons but gets dysregulated in obese people (Cercato & Fonseca, 2019) (Figure 11.2).

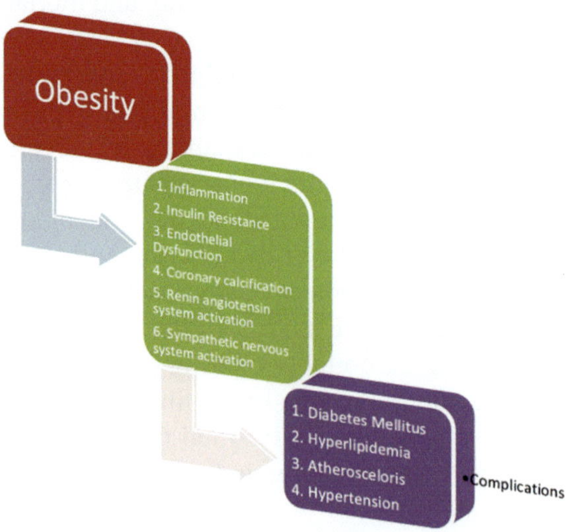

FIGURE 11.2 Mechanisms and complications of obesity in CHD.

11.2.6 FAMILY HISTORY

Premature coronary heart disease (CHD) in the family is considered as an established threat in CHD occurrences (Nasir et al., 2007). Regardless of the usual threat considerations, a familial past of cardiovascular disorders is attributed with 1.5 to 2.0 times increased threat of CHD, underscoring the role of genetic factors in disease susceptibility (Safarova et al., 2016). Bachman et al., in a study, found that coronary heart disease diagnosed before the age of 50 years was allied to a clinically meaningful rise in the lifetime threat of CHD death. These findings may be beneficial to clinicians, since they provide a larger context in which to examine the implications of early CHD identification on CHD mortality risk over time (Bachmann et al., 2012).

11.2.7 HOMOCYSTEINE

Since its discovery in 1932, homocysteine has been the subject of considerable debate. Because of its molecular resemblance to cysteine, it was given the name homocysteine. Hyperhomocysteinemia is a disorder in which an unusually high amount of homocysteine is present in the blood (more than 15 μmol/L) (Ganguly & Alam, 2015) (Figure 11.3).

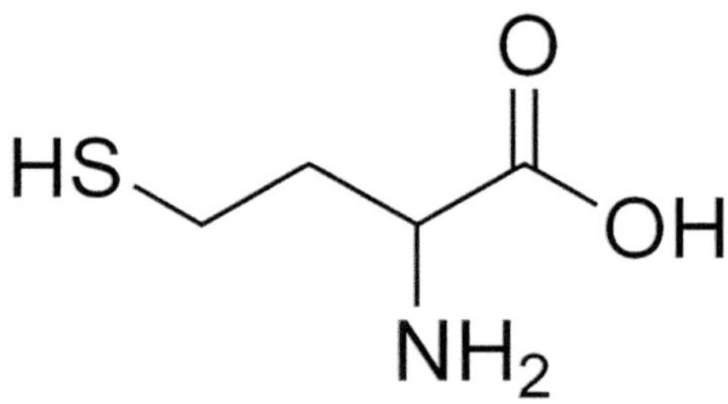

FIGURE 11.3 Structure of homocysteine.

Hyperhomocysteinemia is linked as a threat to a numerous of ailments, along with cardiovascular and neurological problems (Tinelli et al., 2019). Based on clinical results in two individuals with homocystinuria caused by separate inborn metabolic abnormalities, McCully postulated in 1969 that homocysteine increases atherosclerosis (Hortin, 2006).

Hyperhomocysteinemia is hazardous to the endothelial layer because it promotes vascular smooth muscle cell growth, enhances platelet agglomeration, and affects the fibrinolysis and coagulation pathway, either individually or in combination with other risk elements to create a prothrombotic milieu. It stimulates clotting factors V, X, and XII, as well as inhibiting protein C and cell-surface thrombomodulin activation, as well as modulating tissue plasminogen activator binding to its endothelial receptor, annexin II. Oxidation, nitrosylation, homocysteinylation, and hypomethylation are among the proposed toxicity pathways (Perna et al., 2003). As per meta-analysis study, homocysteine increases the hazard of coronary heart ailment by 60% in fully-grown males and 80% in fully-grown females for every 5 μM upsurge in plasma. Another meta-analysis research found a seven-time-upsurge in a fatality in individuals with hyperhomocysteinemia when compared to healthy controls (Lai & Kan, 2015).

11.2.8 FIBRINOGEN

The function of fibrinogen amount in the prognosis of atherosclerotic progression and CHD occurrences has been investigated in several research (Song et al., 2015). Fibrinogen has a significant impact in development of atherosclerosis through platelet aggregation, fibrin cross linking and helps to increase blood viscosity, as a thromboplastic and inflammatory marker. Fibrinogen was found to be not only an indicator of cardiovascular disorders that aren't yet clinical like calcification of arteries of the heart and *Arteria carotis* intima-media thickness, but it was also linked to the progression of CHD, increase in blood pressure, stroke, and cardiovascular events that are hazardous or unfavorable, in previous studies (Liu et al., 2020). Fibrinogen has a considerable influence on the conglomeration of blood, rheological properties of blood, and platelet aggregation, as well as having direct effects on the protective membrane of vessels. Finally, fibrinogen is a key protein in the acute phase. All of these occurrences may shed light on the pathophysiological processes at work (Ernst, 1993). Observational studies demonstrate that a 1 g/L rise in plasma fibrinogen is linked to a two-fold increase in coronary heart disease, and fibrinogen levels may predict the onset, course, and adverse outcome of coronary artery disease (CAD). However, the association between circulating levels of plasma fibrinogen and CHD threat is unknown (Song et al., 2015).

11.2.9 INFECTIONS

A lot of research has looked into the probable link between persistent infections and CHD (Roeters van Lennep, 2002). Chronic infections have a pathophysiological environment in similar with persistent inflammatory condition. Several bacterial and viral infections demonstrated that they are responsible for having significant influence on vascular endothelial cells as well as having indirect effect through the generation of cytokines. Both these hasten significantly the plaque formation (Pothineni et al., 2017). The majority of these researches concern *Helicobacter pylori, Chlamydia pneumonia,* Human Immunodeficiency Virus (HIV), hepatitis C virus, influenza A virus, cytomegalovirus (CMV), and *Porphyromonas gingivalis* (Pothineni et al., 2017; Roeters van Lennep, 2002). A large number of research have discovered evidence of a link between *C. pneumoniae* antibodies and CHD (Roeters van Lennep, 2002). The SARS CoV-2 is the causative agent for COVID-19 infection. It infects the cells via angiotensin-converting enzyme 2 receptors. As a result of infection, more than 7% of patients suffering from COVID-19 infection also suffers from cardiovascular disorders (Clerkin et al., 2020).

11.2.10 INFLAMMATION

The pathway which regulates inflammation is particularly crucial in the process of atheroscloris development. Inflammation is commonly regarded as a major contributory element in the pathogenesis of CHD (Shrivastava et al., 2015). The underlying pathophysiology of coronary heart disease (CHD) is atherosclerosis, which is a disease that causes inflammation. Inflammation is having a significant role in the instability as well as rupture of atherosclerotic plaques, resulting in acute cardiac problems, at both the local and systemic levels (Madjid & Willerson, 2011). Tumour necrosis factor (TNF-α) and interleukin-6 are the cytokines which mediate inflammation and also are the principal cause for release of C-reactive protein in the liver. C-reactive protein is a substandard inflammatory indicator, and current research proposes that it may be a factor in the etiology of atherosclerotic plaques in humans (Pai et al., 2004). CRP is having a part in the generation of lesions caused due to atheroscloris. It is due to the inhibition of formation of enzymes like prostacyclin synthase and nitric oxide synthase. Also, it binds to the low-density lipoprotein-cholesterol and enhances the absorption by phagocytes, a vital step in generation of atherosclerosis (Shrivastava et al., 2015).

11.2.11 PSYCHOSOCIAL FACTORS

Psychosocial variables including stress, adversity, socioeconomic position, depression, and anxiety are linked to general health and, in particular, cardiovascular health (Peterson, 2020). Although most of Coronary Heart Disease investigations has focused on selection of livelihood and biological risk factors, few evidence suggests that psychosocial and psychatriac issues have a significant influence on the disease's onset, advancement, duration, and prognosis (Khayyam-Nekouei et al., 2013).

Extreme stressful circumstances like worry, anger, sadness, etc., may cause plaque rupturing, which can lead to an immediate myocardial infarction, due to the acute reaction of stress hormones, the immunity, and the coagulation system (Albus et al., 2019). People who suffer from insomnia objectively are three times more likely to develop the arterial hypertension (Bathgate et al., 2016). From a psychophysiological standpoint, stimulation of the renin–angiotensin pathway, particularly the angiotensin II which acts as a neuromodulator, causes oxidative stress in the CNS, which is interceded by the nicotinamide adenine dinucleotide phosphate (NADPH) oxidase, which not only causes hypertension but also causes worsening of mood and anxiety (Albus et al., 2019) (Figure 11.4).

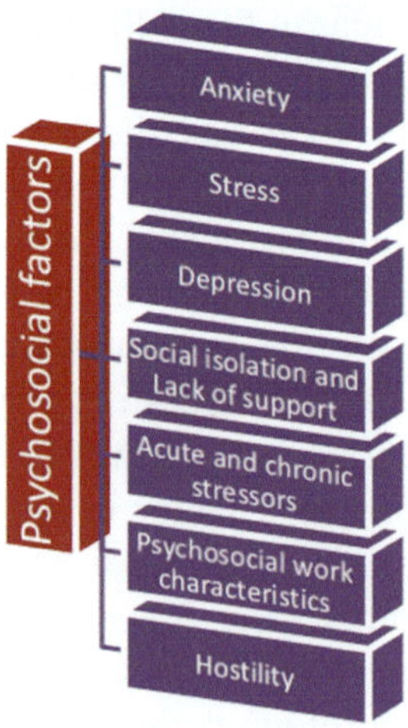

FIGURE 11.4 Various psychosocial factors in CHD.

11.2.12 ESTROGENS

Estrogen affects the cardiovascular system in a pleiotropic manner (Murphy, 2011). When compared to men, epidemiological studies show that women before menopause are slightly shielded in opposition to the progression of CVD. In comparison to males of similar age, females had a lower incidence of CHD. As the frequency and acerbity of CHD increases in females after menopause, sex hormone levels are linked to female protection against CHD, and the frequency of coronary heart disease (CHD) is higher in early-aged females who underwent surgical removal of ovaries as compared to those with healthy ovaries. Taken together, these findings have prompted a lot of concentration in the role of female sex hormones in cardioprotection. Study of several years into female sex hormones has revealed that estrogen (E2), the major sex hormone found in females, is cardioprotective by a number of different ways (Iorga et al., 2017; Ueda et al., 2021). Estrogen influences metabolism, vascular function, insulin sensitivity, the inflammatory response, cardiac myocyte and stem cell survival, and the development of hypertrophy, among other things. Estrogen activates estrogen receptors (ER), which can affect genetic expression in the nucleus or abruptly stimulate kinase signaling in cytosol, mediating these consequences on the cardiovascular system (Murphy, 2011).

11.3 FOODS HAVING ROLE IN CHD

11.3.1 FISH

Fish is a main part of a food regime since it is helpful for coronary heart diseases (de Goede et al., 2010). According to modern survey, it has been recommended that a large amount of fish ingestion is related with a lower possibility of Heart attack, hypertension, atherosclerosis, and stroke (Ahmad Jayedi et al., 2010; Yang et al., 2016; Zhao et al., 2019). In particular, fish content is enriched unsaturated fatty acids with a long chain, i.e., omega-3 fatty acid (n–3 LCPUFAs) (Zuchi et al., 2010). Recent three perspectives of epidemiological studies are having evidence; that fish consumption helps to reduce mortality from CHD (Kromann & Green, 1980; Newman et al., 1993). Omega-3 fatty acid helps to reduce the triglyceride level and also has an anti-inflammatory effect (Ajith& Jayakumar, 2018).

There is further evidence that omega-3 fats and fish oil help significantly to reduce the size of infarct as assessed by the Q-wave frequency (Landmark et al., 1998). LDL cholesterol level was not significantly higher in those who ate a lot of fish than in those who consumed less amounts of fish, according to the findings, whether in a crude or age-gender adjusted analysis and showed a considerable rise in HDL-C, proving the benefits of fish consumption in preventing CHD. HDL-C has a well-documented anti-atherosclerotic action (Abbott et al., 1988).

The therapeutic properties of polyunsaturated fatty acid (omega-3 fatty acids) on CHD in both people having well before cardio-vascular events and healthy people have recently been reported, providing data through randomized controlled trials (RCTs). Supplements of Omega-3 fats are seen by RCTs to diminish cardiac events and slow the course of plaque formation among people with coronary artery disease. More study is required to prove and explain the medicinal benefits of n–3 essential fats supplementation in the prevention and treatment of diseases. Current findings have shed light on the effect of omega-3 fats impact on cardiac function (including prevent and treat abnormal heartbeats), cerebral perfusion (cardiac mechanics), and vascular function. According to Stone, three population-based prospective epidemiological studies found that men who eat part of fish regularly used to have a decreased threat of cardiovascular disease death risk than those who did not (Kris-Etherton et al., 2002). Fish ingestion stayed connected to lower danger of among all, myocardial infarction, and stroke death across various countries in an ecological analysis conducted by Zhang and their coworkers (Zhang et al., 1999).

11.3.2 VEGETABLE AND FRUIT

Several perspectives of scientific studies evaluated that consumption of sufficient amount of fruits and vegetables are very crucial components recommended for balanced nutrition than their protecting action in coronary vascular disease (CVD) (Dauchet et al., 2009). Fruits and vegetables have a variety of nutrients in them, like Potassium, folate, vitamins, fibers, and other phenolic compounds which are some of the protective components (Van Duyn & Pivonka, 2000). Those elements works by reducing oxidative stress, enhancing the profile of lipid, reduction of blood pressure in hypertensives, boosting sensitivity to insulin, or improving clot formation, among other things. A detailed working comprehension of the fruit-vegetable connection between diet and heart disease hazard might be immensely helpful to health practitioners based on patient safety and quality of care (Dauchet et al.,

2006). Isolated dietary components may lose their bioactivity, behave differently than entire foods, or require extra ingredients, from the whole diet to function properly (Hennekens et al., 1996). Age, caloric consumption, BMI, physical activity score, smoking, alcohol usage, and supplement use were all taken into account when determining the relationship between dietary variables and mortality (Tucker et al., 2005).

11.3.3 NUTS AND LEGUMES

Nuts are full of nutrients that contains good source of unsaturated fat, vitamins, minerals proteins, vitamins, as well as fibers, which play a vital role in a balance food there in U.S., day by day increased to intake of these foods 0.5 to 0.75 portions/day (de Souza et al., 2007; Rehm et al., 2017). Nuts include a substantial quantity of bioavailable antioxidants, such as tocopherol, as well as bioactive components, such as phytochemicals, phytoestrogens, and phytosterols, which can protect the heart through a variety of pathways. The ingestion of the Dietary Approaches to Stop Hypertension (DASH) dietary pattern revealed that nuts are cardioprotective, as well as good for hypertension (Sabate & Wien, 2013). The phytosterols in nuts may help to restrict dietary cholesterol absorption and recirculation of intrinsic bile lipoprotein in the gut mucosa that might be connected to lower plasma cholesterol and CVD prevention (Ostlund Jr., 2002).

Plant proteins, such as those found in peas, lupins, cowpeas, jack beans, chickpeas, lentils, or soybeans, have grown progressively famous in recent years even as function of their therapeutic characteristics (Bouchenak & Lamri-Senhadji, 2013; Bazzano et al., 2008; Jayathilake et al., 2018). Legumes were shown to help in the management and cure of a numerous disorders, including cardiovascular and gastrointestinal problems (Elmaliklis et al., 2019). The ingestion of legumes regularly has been proven to lower cholesterol level, bad cholesterol, as well as TG levels while increasing good cholesterol (Bazzano et al., 2008). The mortality rate is diminished by 8% for every 20 grams of beans taken (Kabagambe et al., 2005). If the comparison done among the persons who only eat beans once a week and those who eat them more than four times in a week, those who eat them more than four times in a week will have 22% decline in the hazards of myocardial infarction as well as an 11% reduction in the hazards of cardiovascular disease (Flight & Clifton, 2006).

11.3.4 SOY PROTEIN

A soy product has long been the focus of Eastern diets, and their application in soy-based goods and functional meals enhanced with soy extracts has recently increased their importance in western diets. Protein makes up approximately 35–40% of the soybean. The United States Food and Drug Administration, a federal agency of the Department of Health, and Human Services, recognized consumption of soy protein has been allied to improved health in coronary disease risk, depending on soy protein's cholesterol-lowering impact, which could contribute toward a decreased cardiovascular risk (FDA, 1999).

Soy has been shown in several studies to improve plasma lipid levels. In patients without coronary heart disease, 47 grams ingestion of soy protein everyday led to 9% reduction in entire cholesterol, 13% decrease in bad lipid, and 10.5% drop in triglycerides, according to 38 clinical trials that were reviewed in a meta-analysis (Hodges et al., 1967; Anderson et al., 1995). An excellent study of research published in the journal "Nutrients" attempted to address these soy's have "pleiotropic" properties. Soy is helpful on hypertension, hyperglycemia, inflammatory indicators, as well as fattiness, according to Dam Ramdath et al. (2017). It subsequently found that soy contents non-protein also affects by reducing blood lipid levels. The review also suggested soy components like protein, phytic acid, fiber, lecithin, and saponins do not show a hypotensive effect.

All soya flours contains isoflavones which is having hypocholesterolemic effects. In humans, isoflavones have a weak estrogenic impact. Lower LDL cholesterol and higher HDL cholesterol are two positive effects of estrogen's (Crouse JR III et al., 1999). Saponins, which are contained in soy protein, are heat-stable molecules which might help lower cholesterol by stimulating bile excretion (Oakenfull, 1986).

11.3.5 WHOLE GRAIN

Current American dietary guidelines promote an increase in grain consumption to avoid coronary vascular disease. However, the actual volume of whole grains that should have been consumed is not indicated (US Department of Health and Human Services & US Department of Agriculture, 1995). These instructions were based on the premise that substituting carbohydrates for fats would elevate plasma lipids, decreasing the hazard of cardiovascular disease (American Heart Association, 1996). Grains are one of the world's most popular fundamental foods, providing 56% energies and 50% of protein. The majority of nutritional advisers suggest consuming whole grains every day. Endosperm, germ, bran, fiber, B vitamins, and trace minerals are all important components of whole grain nutrition (iron, magnesium, and zinc, etc.) have already been related to lower incidence of diabetes, cardiovascular diseases, then fatness (Aune et al., 2016). Furthermore, whole grains, provide protein with healthy fats in addition to carbohydrates or might contain specific and helpful compositions of minerals, oxidative protective agents, phytonutrients, or fiber (Slavin, 1994).

Consumption of whole grains varies greatly by population. In the Nordics region, bread of grains is the key source in the United States, whole grains are popular, whole grain bread then the breakfast cereals are primary sources of whole grains; in Africa, brown rice, unrefined maize, and sorghum are the primary sources of whole grains; and also in Asia, brown rice is the primary source of whole grains, despite the fact that white rice is consumed in the majority of Asian countries. We performed a literature evaluation with meta-study of whole-grain ingesting in relation to cardiovascular disorder, cerebrovascular disorder, heart disease, cancer, and death due to all factors, along with the less common causes of mortality like lung problems, communicable disease, hyperglycemia, nerve problem, then all non-coronary heart disorder, non-neurovascular diseases. The researchers wanted to know how strong and how prolong the drug action association amongst whole-grain consumption then the outcomes were (Aune et al., 2016).

"All adults should eat at least half of their grains as whole grains," according to the United States and Canadian guidelines, which corresponds to at least two or three servings of whole grains per day (Oldways Whole Grains Council). Whereas in Northern countries, it is encouraged to consume foods 75 g of whole grain (dry basis), which approximately converts to around 250 gm of whole-grain products (fresh and dry weight) each day (eight servings) (Kyrø et al., 2012).

11.3.6 DARK CHOCOLATE

Numerous research surveys stated that higher consumption of dietary flavonoids is connected with decreased incidence of cardiovascular event, In comparison to champagne, black coffee, grapefruit juice, pears, and dark chocolate which includes a high level of flavonoids (Lee et al., 2017). Flavonoids, in particular flavonol, can be found in dark chocolate (catechin, epicatechin, and procyanidins), which can assist in the protection from heart ailment (Ried et al., 2012). Various studies have also shown that chocolate possesses bioactive substances like polyphenols, as well as unsaturated fats, proteins, amines, vitamins, minerals, and others in lower levels, have all been demonstrated to have cardioprotective effects. Chocolate is a popular meal for enjoyment because of its special texture and flavor. However, these have been re-evaluated as a supply for useful bioactive chemicals for several years. The caloric content of dark chocolate is estimated to be 515–593 kcal/100 g (Sperkowska et al., 2021). The meta-analysis and three additional single-blinded RCTs found that daily chocolate-eating can help lowers hypertension in a small duration. For 15 days, a small group of hypertensive adults with hyperglycemia but still no diabetes was given whichever 0.1 kg of high flavonol content dark chocolate as well as 0.1 kg of non-flavonol containing white chocolate. In comparison to white chocolate and dark chocolate dramatically decrease systolic as well as diastolic blood pressure (Taubert et al., 2007). Flavonoids (Keservani & Sharma, 2014; Keservani et al., 2017, 2020), a type of antioxidant found in many of these foods, have generated a significant level of concern for their probabilities to reduce risk of Cardiac disease. Chocolate's potential benefits on CVD (Keservani et al., 2016) should be investigated because cocoa products have more antioxidant capacity and polyphenols each serve overall tea or red wines. Chocolate was used as a therapeutic cure for a long time and is now being recommended by drug therapy as a strategy to prevent a variety of chronic ailments (Ding et al., 2006). Numerous research findings have shown that Cocca product has considerable effects on cardiovascular disease, high blood pressure, heart failure, hypercholesterolemia, inflammation, oxidative stress, and platelet activities, all of which are mediated by diverse pathways (Senturk, 2015) (Figures 11.5 and 11.6).

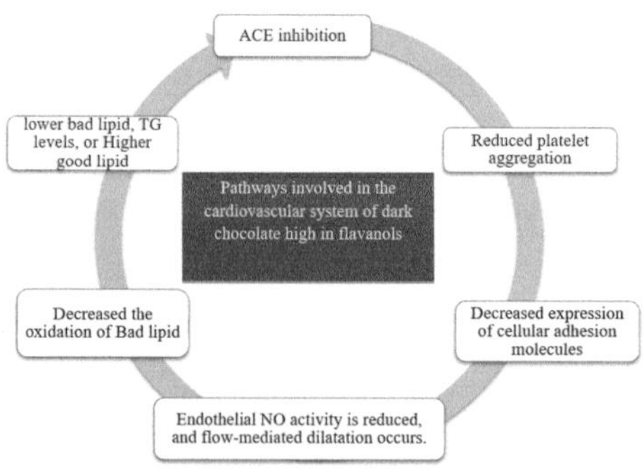

FIGURE 11.5 Pathways involved in the cardiovascular system of dark chocolate high in flavanols.

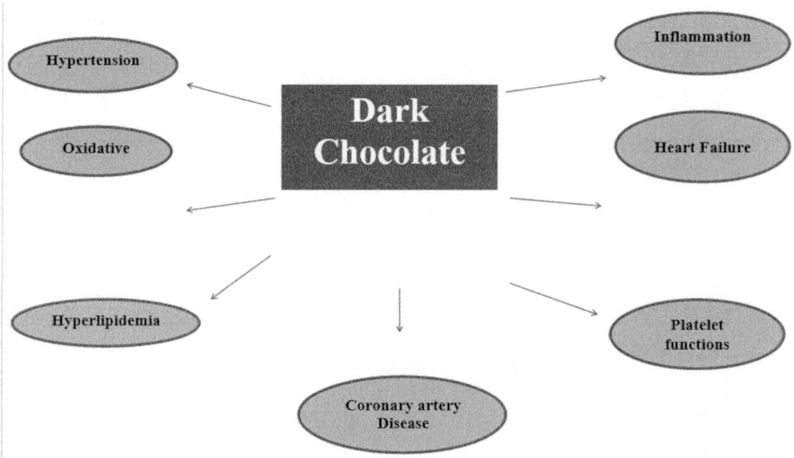

FIGURE 11.6 The effect of dark chocolate on cardiovascular system.

11.3.7 COFFEE AND TEA

There has been a lot of research done on the connection between coffee and tea drinking on cardiovascular disease. While most prior cohort researches indicate no relation between coffee and cardiovascular disease (CVD), more recent findings have already been conflicting. Although case-control research showed the link between coffee intake and the hazard of heart disorders, future group research found that people who drink more coffee have reduced threat of heart disease. Moreover, various studies found that in both more and less coffee consumption was allied to a greater threat of CHD when compared to moderate coffee consumption (Lopez-Garcia et al., 2006).

Coffee is made by roasted Coffee seeds (beans), an evergreen plant native to Africa. It is one of the regularly taken drinks on the planet. Coffee contains a lot of caffeine in it (Grioni et al., 2015). According to several epidemiological research, diabetes, dementia, mental disease, disorders of the metabolism and fatty liver illness can be prevented by adequate amount of caffeine, coffee, and tea use (Gaeini et al., 2019).

Health Canada's, the United States Food and Drug Administration's (FDA, 2012), the European Food Safety Authority's (EFSA, 2015), and, most recently, the United States Nutritional Guidelines for America' views (USDHHS & USDA, 2015) concluded that the consumption of moderate amount caffeine, i.e., 0.4 gm/day is never linked by harmfulness, cardiac impacts, calcium concentrations and bone health are also affected. Figure

11.7 assesses the scientific writings on caffeine and its potential cardiovascular effects (Turnbull et al., 2017).

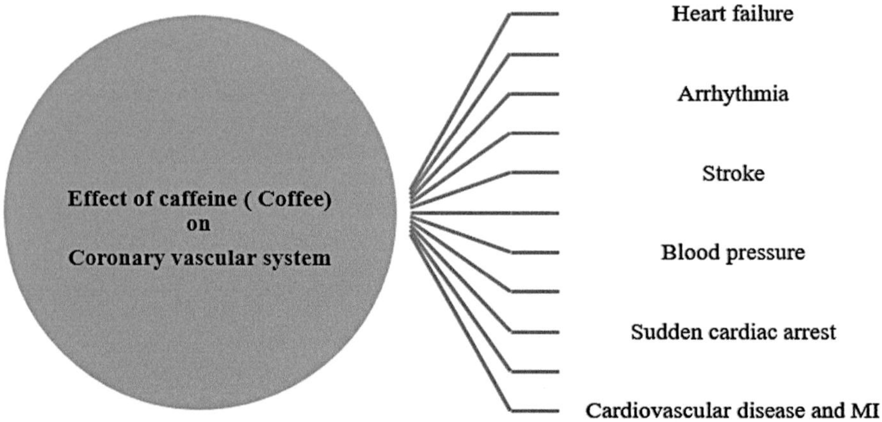

FIGURE 11.7 Effect of caffeine (coffee) on coronary vascular system.

Tea is the second most popular drink globally. Due to the large intake, even minor impacts in individuals can have a significant impact on the health of the general public. Tea's polyphenolic flavonoids were connected to a decrease in the threat of developing cardiovascular disease. Atherosclerotic plaques in the circulatory system include oxidized low-density lipoproteins (Shaikh et al., 1988). Those who consumed at least three mugs of black tea every day had a lesser threat of cardiovascular disease and stroke, according to human population research (Larsson et al., 2013; & Arab et al., 2009). Especially compared to non-consumers, young people who consume few cups of tea per day may reduce the threat overall mortality from cardiovascular disease through 8–12% and their threat of all-cause fatality by 4–6%, as shown in a 2020 evaluation. Over 65-year-olds who drank an 8-ounce cup of tea use to have a 10% decline in chance of dying with cardiovascular disease (Chung et al., 2020). Drinking tea was shown to have substantial advantages of heart health, which includes lowering of cardiovascular containing decreasing the rate of cardiac problem occurrences, lowering the development of the disease, reducing LDL-C, and reducing blood pressure – with benefits can be shown with as low as one as one cup per day upto six cups per day (Miller et al., 2016). According to Harvard research, the threat of MI was reduced by 44% in people that drink more black tea on a daily basis (Sesso et al., 1999). Adults who consumed more than twice mugs of green tea per day lowered the threat by mortality from CVD by 22–23%, according to a big population based research conducted and listed in the Journal of the American Medical Association (Kuriyama et al., 2006).

11.3.8 POLYPHENOL COMPOUND (RED WINE)

Varieties of food, for example, olive oil, cocoa, tea, coffee, and red wine contains polyphenols and has been examined to decide whether their consumption might change cardio-vascular disease (CVD) hazard. Recent proof have shown that the use of polyphenols may also cut down the threat of CVD (Christy C. Tangney & Rasmussen, 2013). Red wine is high in polyphenols such as proanthocyanidins (PAs), catechins, anthocyanosides (ACs), stilbenes, and other phenolics. A variety of fruits and vegetables contains anthocyanosides (ACs) which is a flavonoid. They add texture to red wines along with red and black grape skins (Bosisio et al., 2004; Taylor et al., 2009). Classification of polyphenols is given in Figure 11.8.

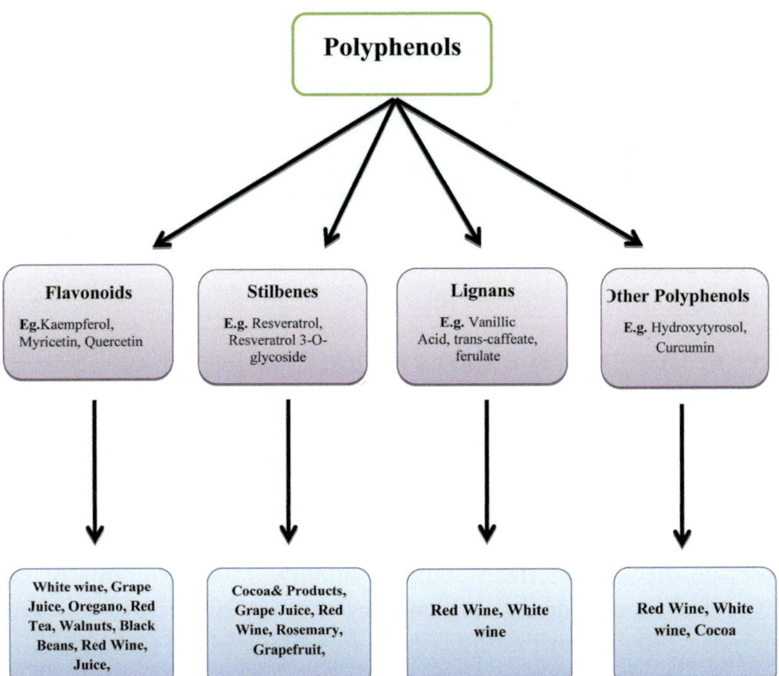

FIGURE 11.8 Classification of polyphenols.

Red wine polyphenols (RWPs) have now been found to have numerous biological activities, including the suppression of platelet aggregation, Vaso-relaxing action, lipid metabolism regulation, and prevention of low-density lipoprotein oxidation (Borriello et al., 2010; Maxwell et al., 1994; Frankel et al., 1993). The health advantages of normal red wine intake are based on a wide range of activities. The biological mechanisms of red wine stilbenes (trans-resveratrol) have attracted a lot of attention (Bhat et al., 2001; Chun-Fu et al., 2013; Id et al., n.d.). Polyphenols also contribute to endothelial cell antioxidant defense by directly lowering nicotinamide adenine dinucleotide phosphate oxidase production as well as effect. Finally, polyphenols increase the free-radical scavengers' effects of an additional enzymes like catalase (Steffen et al., 2008). The production of ROS in the arterial lumen, peroxynitrite, a potent low-density lipoprotein scavenger derived via superoxide and nitric oxide, is one example, is the main trigger for endothelial damage, which results in a significant inflammatory reaction (Borriello et al., 2010). The findings for these antioxidant effects come mostly from *in vitro* studies. Red wine and other phenols contain a stilbene called resveratrol; it protects LDL against oxidation caused by peroxynitrite (Borriello et al., 2010). The expression of thioredoxin was found to be boosted by resveratrol, a cellular protein reductase that is crucial for preserving the redox condition in muscle cells. Resveratrol is an antioxidant that protects against oxidative damage not only through direct antioxidant activity, but also through upregulation of additional endogenous antioxidant mechanisms (Ahsan et al., 2009). In smooth muscle cells in the heart and aorta, resveratrol boosts superoxide dismutase, catalase, and glutathione peroxidase development (Spanier, 2009; Ungvari et al., 2010).

11.3.9 PLANT STEROLS AND STANOLS

Cholesterol-lowering activity is the identity of plant sterols and stanols and this was found way back in the 1950s. Preliminary studies assessed the efficacy of high doses of plant sterols such as campesterol, stigmasterol, and b-sitosterol, which are found abundantly in pine trees and veggie fats and oils. The average diet of American contains roughly 250 milligrams of sterols, while vegetarians take double of that (Hasler et al., 2000). A typical Western diet includes 200–500 milligrams of saturated fat with up to 500 milligrams of phyto-sterols, out of that plant sterols contributed for 200–400 milligrams, but plant stanols contributed for barely 50 milligrams (Bo et al., 2009; Köhler et al., n.d.). They are non-nutritive substances naturally present in plants that vary from cholesterol in the structure just slightly by presence of methyl or an ethyl group at C-24. Saturated plant sterols having a double bond in the sterol ring are known as plant stanols. Plant stanols are produced when plant sterols are saturated. Estimates for plant sterol absorption in the intestine vary from 0.4 to 5% and from 0.02 to 0.3% for their saturated equivalents. As a result, concentrations of plant stanol in serum are approximately tenfold less than serum levels of plant sterol (Fransen et al., 2007; Köhler et al., n.d.; Pinsdorf et al., 2010; Weingärtner et al., 2016). Elevated lipid levels have long been considered a danger for cardiovascular ailment (Baigent et al., 2005). Phyto-stanols are saturated sterol derivatives such as sitostanol, have been shown in research to decrease lipid more effectively than plant sterols due to their higher capacity to diminish intestinal absorption of cholesterol while remaining essentially unabsorbed. As a result, dietary fat seemed to be a more excellent tool for carrying phyto-stanols to the small intestine, a technique was devised to esterify and solubilize plant stanols in meals high in fat without disrupting the characteristics of the foodstuff (Esters, 2018; Hasler et al., 2000). Consumption of phytosterols in gram amounts has been reported to prevent absorption of cholesterol and is among the ancient treatment approaches for hypercholesterolemia (Patel, 2008). In Finland, stanol esters including margarine have been on the market since 1995. A significant clinical experiment done in Finland in 1995 showed that a margarine in phyto-stanol ester may reduce total and low-density lipoprotein lipid levels by 10% and 14%, slightly in hypercholesterolemic individuals (Artiainen, 1995). Since then, several other experiments have scientifically proved the effectiveness of phyto-stanol esters and sterols in the treatment of high cholesterol (Hendriks et al., 1999; Iii, 2000). In 2000 on September 8, the FDA declared about permitting the use of potential health benefits for the relationship among phyto-sterol/stanol esters and a lower chance of coronary heart disease (Iii, 2000).

11.3.10 VITAMIN C

Vitamin C is also known as ascorbic acid fairly effective antioxidant loses electrons and a water-soluble vitamin (Bhupathiraju & Tucker, 2011). Harman proposed anti-aging theory in which he stated that the vitamin C is a potent antioxidant (Singh et al., 2017a, b) for free radicals present in the body (Bhupathiraju & Tucker, 2011; Harman, 1956). Ascorbic acid helps in further development of nitric oxide of the endothelium, which, thus, expands the wall of the vessels by relaxing them, decreasing circulatory strain (d'Uscio et al., 2003; Moser & Chun, 2016). Besides, ascorbic acid might ward off apoptosis of myocytes and helps to maintain plaques more robust if there are chances that atherosclerosis has grown (Siow et al., 1999).

11.3.11 VITAMIN E

Vitamin E is generally soluble in fat and occurs in eight distinct forms. Tocopherols and tocotrienols are the two primary classes of vitamin E, which are further subdivided into alpha, beta, delta, and gamma forms with somewhat different chemical structures (Christine C. Tangney, 1997). The most ubiquitous and physiologically bioactive form of vitamin E is alpha-tocopherol, and it is also believed that if there is any form which meets all the human dietary needs then it is Alpha-tocopherol (Dutta & Dutta, 2003; Christine C. Tangney, 1997). Vitamin supplements often include Acetate and succinates which are synthetic isomers of α-tocopherol. In contrast, one of the most usual types of vitamin E found in the human food supplement is γ-tocopherol (Brigelius-Flohé et al., 2002). Several dietary sources have been identified as providing a considerable quantity of vitamin E. Vitamin E-rich foods include salad dressing, margarine, mayonnaise, and Snack foods with added vitamin E. On the other hand, The majority of fruits and vegetables have less amount of vitamin E. Certain dry drupes and seeds, notably, almonds, groundnut, and sunflower seeds, seem to be good source of vitamin E (Dutta & Dutta, 2003). The maximum daily amount of vitamin E for just an fully grown human is 15 mg (Dutta & Dutta, 2003). Many experiments have shown the Vitamin E's influence on atherosclerosis. In 2001, Ferre et al. have investigated the impact of various antiatherogenic increased-fat, relatively low-cholesterol foods on lipid peroxidation in the liver and antioxidants systems in apo E-deficient mice. Where they made 5 groups of 80 apolipoprotein E-deficient mice. They were regularly fed chayote gourd, chayote gourd plus coconut, chayote gourd plus palm, chayote gourd plus olive oil, as well as chayote gourd along with sunflower oil. A few weeks later, mouse livers were extracted and alpha-tocopherol in the liver, lipid peroxidation, and oxidative enzyme activities were determined. Furthermore, the Atheromatous size of fat deposits in the mouse aortas was determined. The researchers discovered that foods high in vitamin E (olive and sunflower oil) supplement diet protect against hepatic lipid peroxidation.

Additionally, they found that foods enriched with olive, palm, or sunflower oil was linked with a reduction in the extent of atherosclerotic plaques in the aorta (Ferré et al., 2001). Another experiment carried out by Thomas et al. studied vita E and Co q10 antiatherogenic effects in apo E-deficient Mice were given high-lipid meals to eat Containing 0.2% vita-E, 0.5% Coenzyme Q10, or 0.2% vita-E + 0.5% Co Q10 for 24 weeks. They discovered that serum obtained from animals given Coenzyme Q10 or vita-E + Coenzyme Q10 was more immune to *in vitro* lipid peroxidation than plasma from control animals. Mice given vita-E and Coenzyme Q10 had considerably lower levels of tissue lipid hydroperoxides. As compared to the control group mice, all treatment groups showed effectively decreased aortic cholesterol. Animals that were given vitamin E and CoQ10 had relatively low levels of atherosclerosis in the root of the aorta, the arch, and thoracic aorta. Animals treated solely with vitamin E have far less atherosclerosis at the aortic root (Thomas et al., 2001). This concludes that vitamin E has some effect on the body by lowering the risk of disease.

11.3.12 CAROTENOIDS

Carotenoids are among the most common natural colors, with over 700 unique components identified thus far (Kaulmann & Bohn, 2014). Nevertheless, only around 50 molecules from the diet can be consumed and used by humans (Mueller & Boehm, 2011). They are classified into two types: xanthophylls (which include O_2) and carotenes (which are pure hydrocarbons that don't contain O_2). Luteins, zeaxanthins, and beta-cryptoxanthins are examples of xanthophyll, whereas carotene includes alpha-carotenes, lycopenes, and beta-carotenes. These chemicals are the source of the red, oranges, and yellow pigments observed in plants and certain animals (Stahl & Sies, 2003). Their long pi-electron system that is conjugated of units of isoprene defines them (Kaulmann & Bohn, 2014). Carotenoids can serve as antioxidants by directly reducing singlet oxygen or by interacting with free radicals (Bohn, 2008). In 1999, Kritchevsky did perform diet epidemiologic research, and its findings indicate ineffective in establishing the donation of certain carotenoids to ailment hazard. Since nutritional principles of different carotenoids were formerly unknown, most research focused on nutritional total pro-vitamin A carotenoid ingestion (predominantly b-carotene). He performed six studies on dietary carotenoids and coronary heart disease; four out of six examined provitamin A carotenoid ingestion, one measured ingestion of carotenoids-rich fruitlets and vegetable, and single measured consumption among all five carotenoids (alpha and beta-carotene, luteins, lycopenes, and cryptoxanthins). Five researchers suggested that people who consumed more carotenoids had decreased relative risk of coronary events (Gaziano et al., 1995; Pandey et al., 1995; Teitelbaum et al., 1993). However, only two of them could eliminate the possibility (Gaziano et al., 1995; Teitelbaum et al., 1993). In research of 1,299 senior Massachusetts residents, researchers examined the total servings of six carotenoid-rich food categories and discovered that individuals in top 25% of intake possessed considerably decreased risk of fatal MI (RR 50.27). In addition, the chapter compares individuals who consumed one serving of each of the six food groups every 24 hrs against the others who ate fewer than just one serving every 24 hrs. Carrots and/or squash (RR 50.40) and salads and/or green leafy vegetables (RR 50.40) had opposite connections with risk of CVD mortality (RR 50.49). This study shows the relation between the consumption of carotenoids and CHD that is chances can be reduced by dietary food consumption.

KEYWORDS

- **body mass index**
- **cardiovascular disease**
- **coronary heart disease**
- **diet**
- **food supplements**
- **Framingham heart study**
- **high density lipoprotein cholesterol**

REFERENCES

Abbott, R. D., Wilson, P. W., Kannel, W. B., & Castelli, W. P., (1988). High density lipoprotein cholesterol, total cholesterol screening, and myocardial infarction. The Framingham study. *Arteriosclerosis, 8*(3), 207–211.

Ahsan, M. K., Lekli, I., Ray, D., Yodoi, J., & Das, D. K., (*2009*). Redox regulation of cell survival by the thioredoxin superfamily: An implication of redox gene therapy in the heart. *Antioxidants and Redox Signaling, 11*(11), 2741–2758.

Ajith, T. A., & Jayakumar, T. G., (2018). Omega-3 fatty acids in coronary heart disease: Recent updates and future perspectives. *Clin. Exp. Pharmacol. Physiol., 46*(1), 11–18.

Akil, L., & Ahmad, H. A., (2011). Relationships between obesity and cardiovascular diseases in four Southern States and Colorado. *Journal of Health Care for the Poor and Underserved, 22*(4 Suppl), 61–72.

Albus, C., Waller, C., Fritzsche, K., Gunold, H., Haass, M., Hamann, B., Kindermann, I., et al., (2019). Significance of psychosocial factors in cardiology: Update 2018: Position paper of the German cardiac society. *Clinical Research in Cardiology, 108*(11), 1175–1196.

Anderson, J. W., Johnstone, B. M., & Cook-Newell, M. E., (1995). Meta-analysis of the effects of soy protein intake on serum lipids. *N. Engl. J. Med., 333*(5), 276–282.

Arab, L., Liu, W., & Elashoff, D., (2009). Green and black tea consumption and risk of stroke: A meta-analysis. *Stroke, 40*(5), 1786–1792.

Artiainen, E. R. V., (1995). Reduction of serum cholesterol with sitostanol-ester margarine in a mildly hypercholesterolemic population. *The New England Journal of Medicine, 333*(20), 1308–1312.

Aune, D., Keum, N., Giovannucci, E., Fedness, L. T., Boffetta, P., Greenwood, D. C., Tonstad, S., et al., (2016). Whole grain consumption and risk of cardiovascular disease, cancer, and all cause and cause specific mortality: Systematic review and dose-response meta-analysis of prospective studies. *BMJ, 353*, i2716.

Bachmann, J. M., Willis, B. L., Ayers, C. R., Khera, A., & Berry, J. D., (2012). Association between family history and coronary heart disease death across long-term follow-up in men: The cooper center longitudinal study. *Circulation, 125*(25), 3092–3098.

Baigent, C., Keech, A., Kearney, P. M., Blackwell, L., Buck, G., Pollicino, C., Kirby, A., et al., (2005). Cholesterol treatment trialists' (CTT) Collaborators. Efficacy and safety of cholesterol-lowering treatment: Prospective meta-analysis of data from 90,056 participants in 14 randomized trials of statins. *Lancet, 366*(9493), 1267–1278.

Basnet, T. B., Sriijana, G. C., Basnet, R., & Neupane, B., (2020). Dietary nutrients of relative importance associated with coronary artery disease: Public health implication from random forest analysis. *PLOS One, 15*(12).

Bathgate, C. J., Edinger, J. D., Wyatt, J. K., & Krystal, A. D., (2016). Objective but not subjective short sleep duration associated with increased risk for hypertension in individuals with insomnia. *Sleep, 39*(5), 1037–1045.

Bazzano, L., Tees, M. T., & Nguyen, C. H., (2008). Effect of non-soy legume consumption on cholesterol levels: A meta-analysis of randomized controlled trial. *Circulation, 118*(18), S1122.

Bhat, K. P. L., Kosmeder, II. J. W., & Pezzuto, J. M., (2001). Biological effects of resveratrol. *Forum Review, 3*(6), 1041–1064.

Bhupathiraju, S. N., & Tucker, K. L., (2011). Coronary heart disease prevention: Nutrients, foods, and dietary patterns. *Clinica Chimica Acta; International Journal of Clinical Chemistry, 412*(17, 18), 1493–1514.

Bohn, T., (2008). Bioavailability of non-provitamin a carotenoids. *Current Nutrition & Food Science, 4*(4), 240–258.

Borriello, A., Cucciolla, V., Ragione, F. D., & Galletti, P., (2010). Dietary polyphenols: Focus on resveratrol, a promising agent in the prevention of cardiovascular diseases and control of glucose homeostasis. *Nutrition, Metabolism and Cardiovascular Diseases, 20*(8), 618–625.

Bosisio, E., Agli, M. D., & Busciala, A., (2004). Vascular effects of wine polyphenols. *Cardiovasc Res., 63*(4), 593–602.

Bouchenak, M., & Lamri-Senhadji, M., (2013). nutritional quality of legumes, and their role in cardiometabolic risk prevention: A review. *J. Med. Food., 16*(3), 185–198.

Brigelius-Flohé, R., Kelly, F. J., Salonen, J. T., Neuzil, J., Zingg, J. M., & Azzi, A., (2002). The European perspective on vitamin E: Current knowledge and future research. *American Journal of Clinical Nutrition, 76*(4), 703–716.

Cassar, A., Holmes, D. R., Rihal, C. S., & Gersh, B. J., (2009). Chronic coronary artery disease: Diagnosis and management. *Mayo Clinic Proceedings, 84*(12), 1130–1146.

Center for Disease Control and Prevention (US); National Center for Chronic Disease Prevention and Health Promotion (US); Office on Smoking and Health (US), (2010). Atlanta (GA). In: *How Tobacco Smoke Causes Disease: The Biology and Behavioral Basis for Smoking-Attributable Disease: A Report of the Surgeon General*. Centers for Disease Control and Prevention (US).

Cercato, C., & Fonseca, F. A., (2019). Cardiovascular risk and obesity. *Diabetology & Metabolic Syndrome, 11*(1), 74.

Chiha, M., Njeim, M., & Chedrawy, E. G., (2012). Diabetes and coronary heart disease: A risk factor for the global epidemic. *International Journal of Hypertension, 2012*, 1–7.

Chun-fu, W. U., Jing-yu, Y., Fang, W., & Xiao-xiao, W., (2013). Resveratrol: Botanical origin, pharmacological activity and applications. *Chinese Journal of Natural Medicines, 11*(1), 1–15.

Chung, M., Zhao, N., Wang, D., Shams-White, M., Karlsen, M., Cassidy, A., Ferruzzi, M., et al., (2020). Dose-response relation between tea consumption and risk of cardiovascular disease and all-cause mortality: A systematic review and meta-analysis of population-based studies. *Adv. Nutr., 11*(4), 790–814.

Clerkin, K. J., Fried, J. A., Raikhelkar, J., Sayer, G., Griffin, J. M., Masoumi, A., Jain, S. S., et al., (2020). COVID-19 and cardiovascular disease. *Circulation, 141*(20), 1648–1655.

Crouse, J. R. III., Morgan, T., Terry, J. G., Ellis, J., Vitolins, M., & Burke, G. L., (1999). A randomized trial comparing the effect of casein with that of soy protein containing varying amounts of isoflavones on plasma concentrations of lipids and lipoproteins. *Arch. Intern. Med., 159*(117), 2070–2076.

d'Uscio, L. V., Milstien, S., Richardson, D., Smith, L., & Katusic, Z. S., (2003). Long-term vitamin C treatment increases vascular tetrahydrobiopterin levels and nitric oxide synthase activity. *Circulation Research, 92*(1), 88–95.

Dan, R. D., Padhi, E. M. T., Sarfaraz, S., Renwick, S., & Duncan, A. M., (2017). Beyond the cholesterol-lowering effect of soy protein: A review of the effects of dietary soy and its constituents on risk factors for cardiovascular disease. *Nutrients, 9*(4), 324.

Dauchet, L., Amouyel, P., & Dallongeville, J., (2009). Fruits, vegetables and coronary heart disease. *Nat. Rev. Cardiol., 6*, 599–608.

Dauchet, L., Amouyel, P., Hercberg, S., & Dallongeville, J., (2006). Fruit and vegetable consumption and risk of coronary heart disease: A meta-analysis of cohort studies. *J. Nutr., 136*(10), 2588–2593.

De Goede, J., Geleijnse, J. M., Boer, J. M. A., Kromhout, D., & Verschuren, W. M. M., (2010). Marine (n-3) fatty acids, fish consumption, and the 10-year risk of fatal and nonfatal coronary heart disease in a large population of Dutch adults with low fish intake. *J. Nutr., 140*(5), 1023–1028.

De Souza, R. G. M., Schincaglia, R. M., Pimentel, G. D., & Mota, J. F., (2017). Nuts and human health outcomes: A systematic review. *Nutrients, 9*(12), 1311.

Ding, E. L., Hutfless, S. M., Ding, X., & Girotra, S., (2006). Chocolate and prevention of cardiovascular disease: A systematic review. *Nutr. Metab., 3*(2), 1–12.

Dutta, A., & Dutta, S. K., (2003). Vitamin e and its role in the prevention of atherosclerosis and carcinogenesis: A review. *Journal of the American College of Nutrition, 22*(4), 258–268.

Einarson, T. R., Acs, A., Ludwig, C., & Panton, U. H., (2018). Prevalence of cardiovascular disease in type 2 diabetes: A systematic literature review of scientific evidence from across the world in 2007–2017. *Cardiovascular Diabetology, 17*(1), 83.

Elmaliklis, I. N., Liveri, A., Ntelis, B., Paraskeva, K., Goulis, I., & Koutelidakis, A., (2019). Increased functional food's consumption and Mediterranean diet adherence may have a protective effect in the appearance of gastrointestinal diseases: A case–control study. *Medicines, 6*(2), 50.

Ernst, E., (1993). The role of fibrinogen as a cardiovascular risk factor. *Atherosclerosis, 100*(1), 1–12.

Escobar, E., (2002). Hypertension and coronary heart disease. *Journal of Human Hypertension, 16*(S1), S61–S63.

Esters, P. S., (2018). *Recent Advances in Nutritional Sciences the Cholesterol-Lowering Action of Plant Stanol Esters* (pp. 2109–2112). American Society for Nutritional Sciences.

FDA, (1999). Food labeling health claims: Soybean protein and coronary heart disease final rule. *Federal Reg., 57*, 699–635.

Ferré, N., Camps, J., Paul, A., Cabré, M., Calleja, L., Osada, J., & Joven, J., (2001). Effects of high-fat, low-cholesterol diets on hepatic peroxidation and antioxidants in apolipoprotein E-deficient mice. *Molecular and Cellular Biochemistry, 218*(1, 2), 165–169.

Flight, I., & Clifton, P., (2006). Cereal grains and legumes in the prevention of coronary heart disease and stroke: A review of the literature. *Eur. J. Clin. Nutr., 60*(10), 1145–1159.

Frankel, E. N., Kanner, J., German, J. B., Parks, E., & Kinsella, J. E., (1993). Inhibition of oxidation of human low-density lipoprotein by phenolic substances in red wine. *Lancet, 341*(8843), 454–457.

Fransen, H. P., Jong, N. De., Wolfs, M., Verhagen, H., Verschuren, W. M., Bergmann, K. V., Plat, J., & Mensink, R. P., (2007). Customary use of plant sterol and plant stanol enriched margarine is associated with changes in serum plant sterol and stanol concentrations in humans 1, 2. *J. Nutr., 137*(5), 1301–1306.

Fuchs, F. D., & Whelton, P. K., (2020). High blood pressure and cardiovascular disease. *Hypertension, 75*(2), 285–292.

Gaeini, Z., Bahadoran, Z., Mirmiran, P., & Azizi, F., (2019). Tea, coffee, caffeine intake and the risk of cardio-metabolic outcomes: Findings from a population with low coffee and high tea consumption. *Nutr. Metab., 16*(1), 28.

Ganguly, P., & Alam, S. F., (2015). Role of homocysteine in the development of cardiovascular disease. *Nutrition Journal, 14*, 6.

Gaziano, J. M., Manson, J. E., Branch, L. G., Colditz, G. A., Willett, W. C., & Buring, J. E., (1995). A prospective study of consumption of carotenoids in fruits and vegetables and decreased cardiovascular mortality in the elderly. *Annals of Epidemiology, 5*(4), 255–260.

Gil-Izquierdo, A., Penalvo, J. L., Gil, J. I., Medina, S., Horcajada, M. N., Lafay, S., Silberberg, M., et al., (2012). Soy isoflavones and cardiovascular disease epidemiological, clinical and – omics perspectives. *Curr. Pharm. Biotechnol., 13*(5), 624–631.

Gordon, D. J., Probstfield, J. L., Garrison, R. J., Neaton, J. D., Castelli, W. P., Knoke, J. D., Jacobs, D. R., et al., (1989). High-density lipoprotein cholesterol and cardiovascular disease. four prospective American studies. *Circulation, 79*(1), 8–15.

Grioni, S., Agnoli, C., Sieri, S., Pala, V., Ricceri, F., Giovanna, M., Saieva, C., et al., (2015). Espresso coffee consumption and risk of coronary heart disease in a large Italian cohort. In: Vinciguerra, M., (ed.), *PLOS One, 10*(5), e0126550.

Hajar, R., (2017). Risk factors for coronary artery disease: Historical perspectives. *Heart Views, 18*(3), 109.

Harman, D., (1956). Aging: A theory on free radical radiation chemistry. *J. Gerontol., 11*, 298–300.

Hasler, C. M., Kundrat, S., & Wool, D., (2000). Functional foods and cardiovascular disease. *Curr. Atheroscler. Rep., 2*(6), 467–475.

Hendriks, H. F. J., Weststrate, J. A., Van, V. T., & Meijer, G. W., (1999). Spreads enriched with three different levels of vegetable oil sterols and the degree of cholesterol lowering in normocholesterolaemic and mildly hypercholesterolaemic subjects. *Eur. J. Clin. Nutr., 53*(4), 319–327.

Hennekens, C. H., Buring, J. E., Manson, J. E., Tampfer, M., Rosner, B., Cook, N. R., Belanger, C., et al., (1996). Lack of effect of long-term supplementation with β-carotene on the incidence of malignant neoplasms and cardiovascular disease. *N. Engl. J. Med., 334*(18), 1145–1149.

Hodges, R. E., Krehl, W. A., Stone, D. B., & Lopez, A., (1967). Dietary carbohydrates and low cholesterol diets: Effects on serum lipids of man. *Am. J. Clin. Nutr., 20*(2), 198–208.

Hortin, G. L., (2006). Homocysteine: Clinical significance and laboratory measurement. *Laboratory Medicine. 37*(9), 551–553.

Iii, P., (2000). Standards for privacy of individually identifiable health information. *Department of Health and Human, 65*, 82462–82829.

Iorga, A., Cunningham, C. M., Moazeni, S., Ruffenach, G., Umar, S., & Eghbali, M., (2017). The protective role of estrogen and estrogen receptors in cardiovascular disease and the controversial use of estrogen therapy. *Biology of Sex Differences, 8*(1), 33.

Jayathilake, C., Visvanathan, R., Deen, A., Bangamuwage, R., Jayawardana, B. C., Nammi, S., & Liyanage, R., (2018). Cowpea: An overview on its nutritional facts and health benefits. *J. Sci. Food Agric., 98*(13), 4793–4806.

Jayedi, A., Zargar, M. S., & Shab-Bidar, S., (2018). Fish consumption and risk of myocardial infarction: A systematic review and dose-response meta-analysis suggests a regional difference. *Nutr. Res., 62*, 1–12.

Kabagambe, E. K., Baylin, A., Ruiz-Narvarez, E., Siles, X., & Campos, H., (2005). Decreased consumption of dried mature beans is positively associated with urbanization and nonfatal acute myocardial infarction. *J. Nutr., 135*(7), 1770–1775.

Kashiwagi, S., & Paul, L., (2012). Dietary supplements and cardiovascular disease: What is the evidence and what should we recommend? In: Gasparyan, A. Y., (ed.). *Cardiovascular Risk Factors*. In-Tech.

Katta, N., Loethen, T., Lavie, C. J., & Alpert, M. A., (2021). Obesity and coronary heart disease: Epidemiology, pathology, and coronary artery imaging. *Current Problems in Cardiology, 46*(3), 100655.

Kaulmann, A., & Bohn, T., (2014). Carotenoids, inflammation, and oxidative stress-implications of cellular signaling pathways and relation to chronic disease prevention. *Nutrition Research, 34*(11), 907–929.

Keservani, R. K., & Sharma, A. K., (2014). Flavonoids: Emerging trends and potential health benefits. *Journal of Chinese Pharmaceutical Sciences, 23*(12), 815.

Keservani, R. K., Kesharwani, R. K., & Sharma, A. K., (2015). Pulmonary and respiratory health: Antioxidants and nutraceuticals. In: Debasis, B., Harry, G. P., & Anand, S., (eds.), *Nutraceutical and Functional Foods in Human Life and Disease Prevention* (pp. 279–295). Boca Raton, Fl. CRC Press, Taylor and Francis, Chapter 17. ISBN: 9781482237214.

Keservani, R. K., Sharma, A. K., & Kesharwani, R. K., (2016a). Nutraceutical and functional foods for cardiovascular health. In: *Food Process Engineering* (pp. 257–278, 291–312). Apple Academic Press, CRC Press. ISBN: 9781771884020.

Keservani, R. K., Sharma, A. K., & Kesharwani, R. K., (2017). An overview and therapeutic applications of nutraceutical and functional foods. *Recent Advances in Drug Delivery Technology,* 160–201. ISBN:9781522507543.

Keservani, R. K., Sharma, A. K., & Kesharwani, R. K., (2020). *Nutraceuticals and Dietary Supplements: Applications in Health Improvement and Disease Management*. CRC Press. ISBN: 9781771888738.

Khayyam-Nekouei, Z., Neshatdoost, H., Yousefy, A., Sadeghi, M., & Manshaee, G., (2013). Psychological factors and coronary heart disease. *ARYA Atherosclerosis, 9*(1), 102–111.

King, R. J., & Grant, P. J., (2016). Diabetes and cardiovascular disease: Pathophysiology of a life-threatening epidemic. *Herz., 41*(3), 184–192.

Köhler, J., Teupser, D., Elsässer, A., & Weingärtner, O., (2017). sterol enriched functional food and atherosclerosis. *Br. J. Pharmacol., 174*(11), 1281–1289.

Krauss, R. M., Deckelbaum, R. J., Ernst, N., Fisher, E., Howard, B. V., Knopp, R. H., Kotchen, T., et al., (1996). American heart association. Dietary guidelines for healthy American adults a statement for health professionals from the nutrition committee. *Circulation, 94*(7), 1795–1800.

Kris-Etherton, P. M., Harris, W. S., & Appel, L. J., (2002). Fish consumption, fish oil, omega-3 fatty acids, and cardiovascular disease. *Circulation, 106*(21), 2747–2757.

Kromann, N., & Green, A., (1980). Epidemiological studies in the Upernavik district, Greenland. Incidence of some chronic diseases 1950–1974. *Acta. Medica Scand., 208*(5), 401–406.

Kuriyama, S., Shimazu, T., Ohmori, K., Kikuchi, N., Nakaya, N., Nishino, Y., Tsubono, Y., & Tsuji, I., (2006). Green tea consumption and mortality due to cardiovascular disease, cancer, and all causes in Japan: The Ohsaki study. *JAMA, 296*(10), 1255–1265.

Kyrø, C., Skeie, G., Dragsted, L. O., Christensen, J., Overvad, K., Hallmans, G., Johansson, I., et al., (2012). Intake of whole grain in Scandinavia: Intake, sources and compliance with new national recommendations. *Scand. J. Public Health, 40*(1), 76–84.

Lai, W. K. C., & Kan, M. Y., (2015). Homocysteine-induced endothelial dysfunction. *Annals of Nutrition and Metabolism, 67*(1), 1–12.

Landmark, K., Abdelnoor, M., Kilhovd, B., & Dorum, H. P., (1998). Eating fish may reduce infarct size and the occurrence of Q wave infarcts. *Eur. J. Clin. Nutr., 52*(1), 40–44.

Landmark, K., Abdelnoor, M., Urdal, P., Dorum, H. P., Borge, N., & Refvem, H., (1998). Use of fish oils appears to reduce infarct size as estimated from peak creatine kinase and lactate dehydrogenase activities. *Cardiology, 89*, 94–102.

Larsson, S. C., Virtamo, J., & Wolk, A., (2013). Black tea consumption and risk of stroke in women and men. *Ann. Epidemiol., 23*(3), 157–160.

Lee, Y., Berryman, C. E., West, S. G., Chen, C. O., Blumberg, J. B., Lapsley, K. G., Pretsen, A. G., et al., (2017). Effects of dark chocolate and almonds on cardiovascular risk factors in overweight and obese individuals: A randomized controlled-feeding trial. *J. Am. Heart*

Assoc., 6(12), e005162. doi: 10.1161/JAHA.116.005162. PMID: 29187388; PMCID: PMC5778992.

Lichtenstein, A. H., Appel, L. J., Brands, M., Carnethon, M., Daniels, S., Franch, H. A., Franklin, B., et al., (2006). Diet and lifestyle recommendations revision 2006: A scientific statement from the American heart association nutrition committee. *Circulation, 114*(1), 82–96.

Liu, S. L., Wu, N. Q., Shi, H. W., Dong, Q., Dong, Q., Gao, Y., Guo, Y. L., & Li, J. J., (2020). Fibrinogen is associated with glucose metabolism and cardiovascular outcomes in patients with coronary artery disease. *Cardiovascular Diabetology, 19*(1), 36.

Lopez-Garcia, E., Van, D. R. M., Willett, W. C., Rimm, E. B., Mannson, J. E., Stampfer, M. J., Rexrode, K. M., & Hu, F. B., (2006). Coffee consumption and coronary heart disease in men and women: A prospective cohort study. *Circulation, 113*(17), 2045–2053.

Low, W. C. C., Hess, C. N., Hiatt, W. R., & Goldfine, A. B., (2016). Clinical update: Cardiovascular disease in diabetes mellitus: Atherosclerotic cardiovascular disease and heart failure in type 2 diabetes mellitus – mechanisms, management, and clinical considerations. *Circulation, 133*(24), 2459–2502.

Madjid, M., & Willerson, J. T., (2011). Inflammatory markers in coronary heart disease. *British Medical Bulletin, 100*(1), 23–38.

Maxwell, S., Cruickshank, A., & Thorpe, G., (1994). Red wine and antioxidant activity in serum. In: *The Lancet, 344*(8916), 193–194.

Messner, B., & Bernhard, D., (2014). Smoking and cardiovascular disease: Mechanisms of endothelial dysfunction and early atherogenesis. *Arteriosclerosis, Thrombosis, and Vascular Biology, 34*(3), 509–515.

Miller, P. E., Zhao, D., Frazier-Wood, A. C., Michos, E. D., Averill, M., Sandfort, V., Burke, G. L., et al., (2017). Associations of coffee, tea, and caffeine intake with coronary artery calcification and cardiovascular events. *The American Journal of Medicine, 130*(2), 188–197.

Moser, M. A., & Chun, O. K., (2016). Vitamin C and heart health: A review based on findings from epidemiologic studies. In: *International Journal of Molecular Sciences, 17*(8), 1328.

Mueller, L., & Boehm, V., (2011). Antioxidant activity of β-carotene compounds in different *in vitro* assays. *Molecules, 16*(2), 1055–1069.

Murphy, E., (2011). Estrogen signaling and cardiovascular disease. *Circulation Research, 109*(6), 687–696.

Nasir, K., Budoff, M. J., Wong, N. D., Scheuner, M., Herrington, D., Arnett, D. K., Szklo, M., et al., (2007). Family history of premature coronary heart disease and coronary artery calcification: Multi-ethnic study of atherosclerosis (MESA). *Circulation, 116*(6), 619–626.

Newman, W., Middaugh, J., Propst, M., Rogers, D., & Newman, P., (1993). Atherosclerosis in Alaska natives and non-natives. *Lancet, 341*(8852), 1056–1057.

Obesity. Retrieved from: https://www.who.int/westernpacific/health-topics/obesity (accessed on 28 January 2023).

Olafiranye, O., Zizi, F., Brimah, P., Jean-louis, G., Makaryus, A. N., McFarlane, S., & Ogedegbe, G., (2011). Management of hypertension among patients with coronary heart disease. *International Journal of Hypertension, 2011*, 1–6.

Oldways Whole Grains Council, http://wholegrainscouncil.org/whole-grains-101/whole-grain-guidelines-worldwide (accessed on 28 January 2023).

Ostlund, Jr. R. E., (2002). Phytosterols in human nutrition. *Annu. Rev. Nutr., 22*, 533–549.

Pai, J. K., Pischon, T., Ma, J., Manson, J. E., Hankinson, S. E., Joshipura, K., Curhan, G. C., et al., (2004). Inflammatory markers and the risk of coronary heart disease in men and women. *New England Journal of Medicine, 351*(25), 2599–2610.

Pandey, D. K., Shekelle, R., Selwyn, B. J., Tangney, C., & Stamler, J., (1995). Dietary vitamin c and β-carotene and risk of death in middle-aged men: The western electric study. *American Journal of Epidemiology, 142*(12), 1269–1278.

Patel, S. B., (2008). Plant sterols and stanols: Their role in health and disease dietary sterols normal physiology. *Journal of Clinical Lipidology, 2*(2), 11–19.

Perna, A. F., Ingrosso, D., Lombardi, C., Acanfora, F., Satta, E., Cesare, C. M., Violetti, E., et al., (2003). Possible mechanisms of homocysteine toxicity. *Kidney International, 63*, S137–S140.

Peterson, P. N., (2020). JAHA spotlight on psychosocial factors and cardiovascular disease. *Journal of the American Heart Association, 9*(9), e017112.

Pinsdorf, T., Rogacev, K. S., Blo, L., Grenner, Y., Weinga, O., Fliser, D., Laufs, U., et al., (2010). The relationships of markers of cholesterol homeostasis with carotid intima-media thickness. *PLoS One, 5*(10), e13467.

Poirier, P., Giles, T. D., Bray, G. A., Hong, Y., Stern, J. S., Pi-Sunyer, F. X., & Eckel, R. H., (2006). Obesity and cardiovascular disease: Pathophysiology, evaluation, and effect of weight loss. *Arteriosclerosis, Thrombosis, and Vascular Biology, 26*(5), 968–976.

Pothineni, N. V. K., Subramany, S., Kuriakose, K., Shirazi, L. F., Romeo, F., Shah, P. K., & Mehta, J. L., (2017). Infections, atherosclerosis, and coronary heart disease. *European Heart Journal, 38*(43), 3195–3201.

QuiaraLovatti, A., Samuel, B. C., & DarÍzy, F. S., (2019). Role of nutraceuticals in the prevention and treatment of hypertension and cardiovascular diseases. *Journal of Hypertension and Management, 5*(1), 037.

Rehm, C. D., Penalvo, J. L., Afshin, A., & Mozaffarian, D., (2016). Dietary intake among US adults 1999–2012. *JAMA, 315*(23), 2542–2553.

Ried, K., Sullivan, T. R., Fakler, P., Frank, O. R., & Stocks, N. P., (2012). Effect of cocoa on blood pressure. *Cochrane Database Syst. Rev., 4*(4), Cd008893.

Rigotti, N. A., & Pasternak, R. C., (1996). Cigarette smoking and coronary heart disease: Risks and management. *Cardiology Clinics, 14*(1), 51–68.

Roeters, V. L. J., (2002). Risk factors for coronary heart disease: Implications of gender. *Cardiovascular Research, 53*(3), 538–549.

Sabaté, J., & Wien, M., (2013). Consumption of nuts in the prevention of cardiovascular disease. *Curr. Nutr. Rep., 2*(4), 258–266.

Safarova, M. S., Bailey, K. R., & Kullo, I. J., (2016). Association of a family history of coronary heart disease with initiation of statin therapy in individuals at intermediate risk: Post hoc analysis of a randomized clinical trial. *JAMA Cardiology, 1*(3), 364–366.

Senturk, T., (2015). The mysterious light of dark chocolate. *Turk Kardiyol Dernegi Arsivi-Arch Turk Soc. Cardiol., 43*(2), 199–207.

Sesso, H. D., Gaziano, J. M., Buring, J. E., & Hennekens, C. H., (1999). Coffee and tea intake and the risk of myocardial infarction. *Am. J. Epidemiol, 149*(2), 162–167.

Shaikh, M., Martini, S., Quiney, J. R., Baskerville, P., La, Ville, A. E., Browse, N. L., Duffield, R., et al., (1988). Modified plasma-derived lipoproteins in human atherosclerotic plaques. *Atherosclerosis, 69*(2, 3), 165–172.

Shrivastava, A. K., Singh, H. V., Raizada, A., & Singh, S. K., (2015). C-reactive protein, inflammation, and coronary heart disease. *The Egyptian Heart Journal, 67*(2), 89–97.

Sidhu, G. S., & Oakenfull, D. G., (1986). A mechanism for the hypocholesterolemic activity of saponins. *Br. J. Nutr., 55*(3), 643–649.

Singh, P., Kesharwani, R. K., & Keservani, R. K., (2017a). Antioxidants and vitamins: Roles in cellular function and metabolism. In: *Sustained Energy for Enhanced Human Functions and Activity* (pp. 385–407). Academic Press. ISBN:9780128054130.

Singh, P., Kesharwani, R. K., & Keservani, R. K., (2017b). Protein, carbohydrates, and fats: Energy metabolism. In: *Sustained Energy for Enhanced Human Functions and Activity* (pp. 103–115). Academic Press. ISBN:9780128054130.

Siow, R. C. M., Richards, J. P., Pedley, K. C., Leake, D. S., & Mann, G. E., (1999). Vitamin C protects human vascular smooth muscle cells against apoptosis induced by moderately oxidized LDL containing high levels of lipid hydroperoxides. *Arteriosclerosis, Thrombosis, and Vascular Biology, 19*(10), 2387–2394.

Slavin, J. L., (1994). Whole grains and health: Separating the wheat from the chaff. *Nutrition Today, 29*(4), 6–10.

Snopek, L., Mlcek, J., Sochorova, L., Baron, M., Hlavacova, I., Jurikova, T., Kizek, R., et al., (2018). Contribution of red wine consumption to human health protection. *Molecules, 23*(7), 1684.

Song, B., Shu, Y., Xu, Y. N., & Fu, P., (2015). Plasma fibrinogen lever and risk of coronary heart disease among Chinese population: A systematic review and meta-analysis. *International Journal of Clinical and Experimental Medicine, 8*(8), 13195–13202.

Spanier, G., (2009). Resveratrol reduces endothelial oxidative stress by modulating the gene expression of superoxide dismutase 1 (SOD1), glutathione peroxidase 1 (GPx1) and NADPH oxidase subunit (NOX4) the gene expression of superoxide dismutase 1 (SOD1), glutathio. *J. Physiol. Pharmaco, 60*(4), 111–116.

Sperkowska, B., Murawska, J., Przybylska, A., Gackowsi, M., Kruszewaski, S., Durmowicz, M., & Rutkowaska, D., (2021). Cardiovascular effects of chocolate and wine—Narrative review. *Nutrients, 13*(12), 4269.

Stahl, W., & Sies, H., (2003). Antioxidant activity of carotenoids. *Molecular Aspects of Medicine, 24*(6), 345–351.

Steffen, Y., Gruber, C., Schewe, T., & Sies, H., (2008). Mono-O-methylated flavanols and other flavonoids as inhibitors of endothelial NADPH oxidase. *Archives of Biochemistry and Biophysics, 469*(2), 209–219.

Tangney, C. C., & Rasmussen, H. E., (2013). Polyphenols, inflammation, and cardiovascular disease. *Curr. Atheroscler. Rep., 15*(5), 324.

Tangney, Christine, C., (1997). Vitamin E and cardiovascular disease. *Nutrition Today, 32*(1), 13–22.

Taubert, D., Roesen, R., & Schömig, E., (2007). Effect of cocoa and tea intake on blood pressure: A meta-analysis. *Arch, Intern, Med., 167*(7), 626–634.

Taylor, P., Francis, F. J., & Markakis, P. C., (2009). Food colorants: Anthocyanins. *Critical Reviews in Food Science and Nutrition, 28*(4), 273–314.

Teitelbaum, J. S., Zatorre, R. J., Carpenter, S., Gendron, D., Evans, A. C., Gjedde, A., & Cashman, N. R., (1990). Neurologic sequelae of domoic acid intoxication due to the ingestion of contaminated mussels. *N. Engl. J. Med., 322*(25), 1781–1787.

Thomas, S. R., Leichtweis, S. B., Pettersson, K., Croft, K. D., Mori, T. A., Brown, A. J., & Stocker, R., (2001). Dietary co-supplementation with vitamin E and coenzyme Q10 inhibits atherosclerosis in apolipoprotein E gene knockout mice. *Arteriosclerosis, Thrombosis, and Vascular Biology, 21*(4), 585–593.

Tinelli, C., Di Pino, A., Ficulle, E., Marcelli, S., & Feligioni, M., (2019). Hyperhomocysteinemia as a risk factor and potential nutraceutical target for certain pathologies. *Frontiers in Nutrition, 6*, 49.

Torpy, J. M., (2009). Coronary heart disease risk factors. *JAMA, 302*(21), 2388.

Tucker, K. L., Hallfrisch, J., Qiao, N., Muller, D., Andres, R., & Fleg, J. L., (2005). The combination of high fruit and vegetable and low saturated fat intakes is more protective against mortality in aging men than is either alone: The Baltimore longitudinal study of aging. *J. Nutr., 135*(3), 556–561.

Turnbull, D., Rodricks, J. V., Mariano, G. F., & Chowdhury, F., (2017). Caffeine and cardiovascular health. *Regul. Toxicol. Pharmacol., 89*, 165–185.

Ueda, K., Fukuma, N., Adachi, Y., Numata, G., Tokiwa, H., Toyoda, M., Otani, A., et al., (2021). Sex differences and regulatory actions of estrogen in cardiovascular system. *Frontiers in Physiology, 12*, 738218.

Ungvari, Z., Bagi, Z., Feher, A., Recchia, F. A., Sonntag, W. E., Pearson, K., Cabo, R. De., & Csiszar, A., (2010). Resveratrol confers endothelial protection via activation of the antioxidant transcription factor Nrf2. *American Journal of Physiology: Heart and Circulatory Physiology, 299*(1), 18–24.

US Department of Health and Human Services, US Department of Agriculture, (1995). *Dietary Guidelines for Americans* (4th edn.). Washington, DC: US Government Printing Office.

Van, D. M. A., & Pivonka, E., (2000). Overview of the health benefits of fruit and vegetable consumption for the dietetics professional: Selected literature. *J. Am. Diet. Assoc., 100*(12), 1511–1521.

Weingärtner, O., Bogeski, I., Kummerow, C., Schirmer, S. H., Husche, C., Vanmierlo, T., Wagenpfeil, G., et al., (2016). Plant sterol ester diet supplementation increases serum plant sterols and markers of cholesterol synthesis, but has no effect on total cholesterol levels. *Journal of Steroid Biochemistry and Molecular Biology, 169*, 219–225.

Weingärtner, O., Böhm, M., & Laufs, U., (2009). Controversial role of plant sterol esters in the management of hypercholesterolaemia. *Eur. Heart J., 30*(4), 404–409.

World Health Organization, (2004). *A Race Against Time: The Challenge of Cardiovascular Disease in Developing Economies* (pp. 1–87). Trustees of Columbia University in the City of New York.

Yang, B., Shi, M. Q., Li, Z. H., Yang, J. J., & Li, D., (2016). Fish, long-chain n-3 PUFA and incidence of elevated blood pressure: A meta-analysis of prospective cohort studies. *Nutrients, 8*(1), 58.

Ye, X., Kong, W., Zafar, M. I., & Chen, L. L., (2019). Serum triglycerides as a risk factor for cardiovascular diseases in type 2 diabetes mellitus: A systematic review and meta-analysis of prospective studies. *Cardiovascular Diabetology, 18*(1), 48.

Zhang, J., Sasaki, S., Amano, K., & Kesteloot, H., (1999). Fish consumption and mortality from all causes, ischemic heart disease, and stroke: An ecological study. *Prev. Med., 28*(5), 520–529.

Zhao, W., Tang, H., Yang, X., Luo, X., Wang, X., Shao, C., & He, J., (2019). Fish consumption and stroke risk: A meta-analysis of prospective cohort studies. *J. Stroke Cerebrovasc. Dis., 28*(3), 604–611.

Zuchi, C., Ambrosio, G., Lüscher, T. F., & Landmesser, U., (2010). Nutraceuticals in cardiovascular prevention: Lessons from studies on endothelial function: Nutraceuticals in cardiovascular prevention. *Cardiovasc. Ther., 28*(4), 187–201.

CHAPTER 12

ROLE OF FOOD SUPPLEMENTS IN GUT HEALTH

NITIN RAJENDRA SHIRSATH and LAXMIKANT R. ZAWAR

H.R. Patel Institute of Pharmaceutical Education and Research, Karwand Naka, Shirpur, Maharashtra, India

ABSTRACT

Food is a basic need in our life that provides nutritional benefits and contributes to the maintenance of normal health. In addition to providing essential nutrients, functional foods protect humans from various disorders. The human gastrointestinal system is containing a population of 500–1000 distinct bacteria species in appropriate amount. These foods also help to maintain a healthy gut microbiota and promote health in a variety of ways. A healthy gut microbiota protects against gastrointestinal disorders such as infection and inflammatory bowel syndromes. Food supplements like probiotics, prebiotics, polyunsaturated fatty acids, phytochemicals, and micronutrients play an important role in maintaining normal gastrointestinal microflora. Probiotics prevent and treat a wide range of gastrointestinal problems, including antibiotic-associated diarrhea. Prebiotics are indigestible dietary substances that improve the health and well-being of the hosts by stimulating the growth, composition, and activity of microflora in the gastrointestinal system. In this chapter, we have described the role of various dietary food supplement that helps in maintaining of normal gut health.

Food Supplements and Dietary Fiber in Health and Disease. Bhushan R. Rane, Raj K. Keservani, Durgesh Singh, Nayan A. Gujarathi, and Ashish S. Jain, (Eds.)
© 2024 Apple Academic Press, Inc. Co-published with CRC Press (Taylor & Francis)

12.1 NORMAL FLORA

The normal flora of a human being contains a small number of eukaryotic fungi and protists, but bacteria are the most abundant and visible microbial components. Approximately 1014 bacteria are found in the human body on a regular basis. Normal flora helps to maintain a healthy gut microbiota and improve health in a variety of ways. A healthy gut microbiota protects against gastrointestinal disorders such as infection and inflammatory bowel syndromes, etc. (Baron, 1996).

12.2 GASTROINTESTINAL FLORA

The gastrointestinal tract's microflora is important for the host's morphological, physiological, and immunological development. It boosts the immune system to respond quickly to pathogen infection. Microflora prevents harmful or pathogenic bacteria from colonizing the gut through bacterial antagonis (HAENEL, 1970). Bacteroides, Butyrivibrio, Fusobacterium, Bifidobacterium, Lactobacillus, and Eubacterium, are among the families represented. Enterococcus and Escherichia coli make up less than 1% of all microbes in the colon. Anaerobes outnumber facultative anaerobes and microaerophiles in a 1000:1 ratio (Mestecky & Russell, 1998). The dominant flora, which makes up 90% of the population and is primarily made up of bifidobacteria and lactobacilli, is more diverse and contains potentially pathogenic species.

12.3 GUT MICROBIOTA

The gastrointestinal system of human is containing a population of 500–1000 distinct bacteria species that coexist in an appropriate amount. Bacteria are thought to contribute for 35–50% of the volume of the human colon. They may be Lactobacillus, Eubacterium, Clostridium, and Veillonella, etc. Bifidobacterium and Lactobacillus species are the most common bacterial strains with favorable characteristics. The intestine's main microbial composition has been found to be consistent throughout time during adulthood, and each individual's microbial patterns are distinct (Ley, Peterson et al., 2006). However, several external factors such as genetics, age, birth delivery method, nutrition, antibiotic treatments, and other microorganisms such as probiotics has impact on gut microbiota. The digestive tract of a baby appears sterile, yet a microbial population forms soon after birth (Foster-Nyarko &

Pallen, 2022). Microbes from the mother's gastrointestinal tract, as well as those from the environment, colonize the infant's gastrointestinal tract shortly after delivery. A newborn's microbiota develops quickly and is initially influenced by the mother's microbiota, the manner of birth, the environment at birth, and cleanliness, before being influenced by feeding habits and the infant's environment. In the human body, the intestine is sites that contact with exogenous agents (viruses, bacteria, and allergies). The gut microbiota has an impact on human health by influencing the gut defense barrier, immunological function, and nutrient utilization (Neophytou & Pitsouli, 2022). Maintaining a healthy balance among the bacteria species found in the human gut is critical. When this balance is upset, the host-microbe connection can deteriorate and lead to disease. Furthermore, microbiome variations have been linked to an increased risk of certain disorders such as inflammatory bowel disease, irritable bowel disease, and antibiotic-associated diarrhea, as well as allergies, obesity, and diabetes. As a result, maintaining microbiota balance is critical for maintaining and promoting health (Kogut, 2022).

12.4 INTESTINAL MICROBIOTA'S FUNCTION

It can be thought of as an active "organ" that participates in a variety of functions, including improving nutrient bioavailability and degrading non-digestible dietary components, supplying nutrients, and removing damaging, poisonous, and non-nutritive substances. Although microbiota participated in some metabolic processes (Prasanth, Malar, et al., 2022).

12.5 FOOD

Food is a basic need in our lives that satisfies nutritional requirements and aids in the maintenance of health. Many experts are investigating the link between diet and health. Nutritional science is the study of the effects of food and its components on human and animal growth, metabolism, health, and disease resistance, as well as psychological effects associated to eating. Nutritional science has progressed from the prevention of nutritional deficiencies to the incorporation of required nutrition in foods and high-quality products known as functional foods (Shenoy, Buttar, et al., 2022). Carotenoids, dietary fiber, fatty acids, flavonoids, phenolic acids, plant stanols and sterols, polyols, prebiotics, probiotics, phytoestrogens, soy protein, vitamins, and minerals are among the potentially beneficial components found in these functional foods, which are either naturally present in food or added as supplements. Fruits, vegetables, soya, grains, pulses, animal protein, and milk are used to make these dietary products, which are high in nutritional content and give health benefits. Functional foods are foods that improve health in addition to providing basic nutrients. These foods have the potential to improve health in different ways (Ahmed, Vasas, et al., 2022). The increased desire to use foods to help prevent chronic illnesses or maximize health is the primary motivation for purchasing functional foods. The global sales of functional products containing probiotic bacteria have increased dramatically over the last two decades, making it one of the fastest growing food categories, with a compound annual growth rate of 8.6% in the 10 years leading up to 2012 (Palanivelu, Thanigaivel, et al., 2022). The introduction of probiotics has marked a significant advancement in the food business. In the last two decades, researchers have looked at the health benefits of several diets. This trend has resulted in a rise in the manufacture of functional foods containing active ingredients such as prebiotics, probiotics, and synbiotics. Due to scientific data supporting the premise that maintaining a healthy gut microbiota protects against gastrointestinal disorders such as infection and inflammatory bowel syndromes, probiotics are commonly utilized as food supplements. Fruits and vegetables are high in antioxidants, vitamins, dietary fibers, and minerals, making them healthful foods. Fruit juices have a well-established market as a functional drink, and they must be drunk on a regular basis to reap the full benefits of probiotics (Nobre, Simões, et al., 2022).

Claesson et al. (2012) explained that the intestinal microbiota composition correlated to occurrence of some diseases, including obesity and inflammatory diseases. The microbiota of elderly people differs from that of younger adults in terms of inter-individual variance. His findings support a link between food, microbiota, and health status, and suggest that diet-driven microbiome changes may play a role in varied rates of health deterioration as people age (Claesson, Jeffery, et al., 2012).

12.5.1 FUNCTIONAL FOODS

Functional foods are described by the National Academy of Sciences Food and Nutrition Board as "any modified food or food ingredient that may provide a health advantage in addition to the traditional nutrients it contains." They are defined by the International Life Sciences Institute as "foods that give a health advantage beyond basic nutrition due to the presence of physiologically active components." Functional foods are defined by the American Dietetic Association as foods that are "whole, fortified, enriched, or improved," and they must be consumed as "part of a varied diet on a regular basis, at effective levels for consumers to enjoy their potential health benefits." Functional foods, according to the Academy of Nutrition and Dietetics (AND), are "whole foods, fortified, enriched, or improved foods that have a potentially favorable influence on health when consumed as part of a diverse diet on a regular basis, at effective levels." Functional foods, according to the FDA, are foods or nutrients that cause significant physiological changes in the body that are distinct from those connected with their role as nutrition (Villaño, Gironés-Vilapana, et al., 2022). The primary function of food is to provide adequate nutrients to meet metabolic requirements in the human body while also creating a sense of satisfaction and well-being to the consumer (Shenoy, Buttar, et al., 2022). Food may have multiple physiological functions in addition to providing nutritional demands, and may play a negative or positive impact in specific disorders. Functional foods were created to promote a sense of well-being, improve health, and lower the risk of disease (Manassi, de Souza et al., 2022). A wide range of functional foods, such as probiotic, prebiotic, and synbiotic foods, as well as foods enriched with antioxidants, isoflavones, phytosterols, anthocyanins, and fat-reduced, sugar-reduced, or salt-reduced foods, have recently been developed and are now being produced all over the world. Probiotic functional foods are the first choice among these foods for their favorable impact on human health. Dairy probiotic foods and non-dairy probiotic foods are the two types of probiotic functional foods (Misra, Mohanty, et al., 2022). Probiotics are live microorganisms that provide a health benefit to the host when given in appropriate proportion. Probiotic microorganisms have been progressively integrated into dairy dishes as nutritional supplements in recent years (Zawistowski & Kopeć 2022).

Functional food items are foods that have been fortified with compounds that help to improve or maintain one's health. Food products fortified with unique substances that have physiological health benefits were originally referred to as "functional food" in Japan in the 1980s. Previously, vitamin and mineral supplements such as vitamin C, vitamin E, folic acid, zinc, iron, and calcium were used in the development of functional food items (Hadi, Amani, et al., 2022). Following that, the attention switched to foods enriched with various micronutrients, such as omega-3 fatty acids, phytosterol, and soluble fiber, to promote excellent health and illness prevention. Several products are now available on the market, including fortified margarines, psyllium, spinach, kale, collard greens, and whole oat products. Diet providing nutritional demands, may affect numerous physiological activities and play a negative or positive effect in some disorders. As a result, in Japan, the development of novel food products containing biologically active chemicals, dubbed functional food, was explored in order to lower the risk of such illness. Functional foods are foods that include one or more substances that have important or limited roles in the body, such as increasing welfare and health or lowering the risk of diseases like hypertension, diabetes, cancer, osteoporosis, and heart disease (Adetuyi et al., 2022). Rinninella et al. (2019) described that the gut microbiota content is affected by food components, which influence its abundance and diversity. On the one hand, a high-protein, saturated-fat, sugar, and salt diet may favor pathogenic bacteria over beneficial bacteria, thereby disrupting the intestinal barrier. Intake of omega-3 fatty acids, polyphenols, and vitamins appear to influence gut flora and so promote health. They study the effects of specific food and various dietary patterns on gut microbiota composition in order to determine the best diet for gut microbiota regulation (Rinninella, Cintoni, et al., 2019).

12.5.2 INDIAN TRADITIONAL FUNCTIONAL FOOD

Our forefathers devised various diets in order to survive, then eventually enriched them through extended empirical tests including locally accessible food items that therapeutically complement and support one another. The traditional eating habits of each Indian area are essentially a reflection of its culture. Diet has an important part in both preventive and therapeutic medicine in Indian culture. Food's therapeutic power has been a long-held belief in India for many generations. These Indian traditional cuisines are based on several indigenous medical systems that were the natural approach to achieve bodily and mental wellness, but their origin is unknown (Bagchi, 2014).

Numerous health effects associated with functional food consumption have been demonstrated in epidemiological randomized clinical trials conducted in various countries, including cancer risk reduction, improved heart health, immune system stimulation, reduction of menopausal symptoms, anti-inflammatory effects, blood pressure reduction, vision maintenance, and antibacterial effect (Watson, Singh, et al., 2018). Cardiovascular illnesses, metabolic diseases, neurodegenerative diseases, and cancer were shown to be 4.4 times less common in Indian adults than in the same age group in the United States.

Traditional Indian cuisine is "functional" because it provides high levels of dietary fiber, antioxidants, and probiotics (curds and fermented batter products). These traditional Indian cuisines have a synergistic impact due to the chemical variety of the ingredients. Traditional Indian diets, which are primarily plant-based, are high in natural dietary fiber and low in fat, both of which help to minimize the risk of coronary heart disease. The health benefits may include ensuring normal physiological functions in the body, such as improving gastrointestinal health, enhancing the immune system, improving skeletal health, lowering oxidative stress, lowering the risk of cardiovascular diseases, and possibly preventing diabetes (Keservani et al., 2010).

12.5.3 TRADITIONAL FUNCTIONAL FOOD

These are the foods that have been given by adding new components or modifying original ingredients. Foods containing functional ingredients (Keservani et al., 2010) or bacterial strains may be defined as functional foods; however, they are not traditional functional foods. These foods are not medicines, but rather a type of diet that may have disease-prevention properties when ingested as part of a regular diet. A functional ingredient is a food ingredient that affects its host in a specific manner to have a positive influence on health. Traditional functional food naturally contains one or more functional components (Choudhary & Tandon, 2009). The active ingredients are discussed in subsections.

12.5.3.1 PROBIOTICS

These are a single or mixed culture of living microorganisms that, when administered in sufficient amounts, improve the host's intestinal microbial balance, increase colonization resistance to infections, and improve immune responses (Sakamoto, Igarashi, et al., 2001). The bacteria that are currently used in probiotic solutions are diverse, i.e., *Lactobacillus bulgaricus*, *Lactobacillus salivarius*, *Lactobacillus acidophilus*, *Lactobacillus casei*, *Lactobacillus helveticus*, *Streptococcus thermophilus*, *Enterococcus faecium*, and *Bifidobacterium* spp., are the most common type of bacteria used as probiotics (Lesbros-Pantoflickova, Corthesy-Theulaz, et al., 2007).

Beneficial microorganisms with specialized roles in the human gut, which may be employed in foods or supplements to improve health and prevent and treat diseases, are gaining popularity. Specific bacteria's protective effect against gastrointestinal infections and illnesses, as well as the underlying mechanisms, have been widely researched (Reuben, Elghandour, et al., 2022). Because of their health-promoting benefits, specific Lactobacillus, Bifidobacterium, and Propionibacterium strains have been introduced as probiotics in food products (Misra, Mohanty, et al., 2022). A probiotic is a "live microbe that gives a health benefit to the host when administered in suitable levels" (Reque & Brandelli, 2022). Originally, probiotics were employed to impact animal and human health by modulating the gut flora. Currently, the effects of certain live microbial dietary ingredients on human health are being researched in food matrices as well as single or mixed culture preparations (Yadav, Kumari, et al., 2022).

Many physiological activities, ranging from energy control and cognitive processes to toxin neutralization and pathogen immunity, are regulated by the gut microbiota (Guslandi, 2022). As a result, changes in the gut microbiota's composition have been linked to the development of a variety of chronic disorders. Recent advances in the study of gut microbiota have revealed that intestinal bacteria play an important role in the development of a variety of diseases. Prebiotics and probiotics may have used in maintaining health and immune-related disorders (Shehata, Yalçın, et al., 2022).

According to a study by Roberfroid et al. (2010), Apart from protein fermentation, bacterial secondary metabolism might produce hazardous chemicals. A prebiotic impact should not boost the proteolytic microbiota, reducing overall bacterial metabolism creation (Roberfroid, Gibson, et al., 2010). Rolfe et al. (2000) suggested that probiotics will improve gut health. Escherichia coli, Streptococcus sp., Enterococcus sp., Bacteroides sp., Bacillus sp., Propionibacterium sp., and different fungi are among the organisms utilized as probiotics in humans. Several bacterial strains are mixed together in some probiotic formulations. Probiotics have been studied for their ability to prevent and treat a wide range of gastrointestinal problems, including antibiotic-associated diarrhea. They looked at a variety of methods that probiotics use to improve gut health, including immune activation, competition for restricted nutrients, suppression of epithelial and mucosal adhesion, inhibition of epithelial invasion, and the synthesis of antimicrobial compounds (Rolfe, 2000).

12.5.3.1.1 Mechanism Action of Probiotics as Food Supplement and Health Benefits

Probiotic microorganisms are thought to benefit the host's health, but the exact method by which they do so is uncertain. Much research on the mechanism by which probiotics protect the host from intestinal diseases have been reported. The following are the mechanisms of probiotics:

- Production of inhibitory compounds such as organic acids and bacteriocins that inhibit both G "+" and G "–" bacteria.
- Pathogens are inhibited by probiotics sticking to gut epithelial surfaces and inhibiting adhesion sites.
- Pathogens are inhibited by probiotics because they consume the nutrients that pathogens require.
- Immune stimulation, both particular and nonspecific. Specific cell wall components or cell layers are hypothesized to act as adjuvants, boosting the humoral immune response.
- Intestinal diseases are avoided when toxin receptors on the intestinal mucosa are degraded. Suppression of toxin generation, lowering of gut pH, and virulence attenuation are some of the other methods proposed.

12.5.3.2 Prebiotics

Prebiotics are indigestible dietary substances that improve the health and well-being of the hosts by stimulating the growth, composition, and activity of microflora in the gastrointestinal system (Singh, Zapata, et al., 2018). Prebiotics are resistant to stomach acidity, enzyme hydrolysis, and probiotic fermentation. Fructooligosaccharides, inulin, oligofructose, lactulose, and galactooligosaccharides are some of the prebiotics discovered. Prebiotics, in general, have promising health effects, such as enhancing gut microbiota by increasing probiotic growth and inhibiting harmful microbes. Nondigestible carbohydrates, such as inulin and oligofructose, change various indicators, including gastrointestinal transit speed, experimentally induced neoplasia, and colonic microflora, suggesting they may improve quality of life and disease resistance in both people and animals (Singh, Zapata, et al., 2018).

Prebiotics use intestinal microflora to create short-chain fatty acids, which lowers the risk of gastrointestinal disease, cancer, and cardiovascular disease while also improving lipid profiles. A food item must not be hydrolyzed or absorbed in the upper gastrointestinal system in order to be categorized as a prebiotic. Rather, it must be fermented selectively by one or a small number of potentially beneficial bacteria found in the colon, such as Bifidobacteria and Lactobacilli, which are encouraged to develop and become metabolically active. Prebiotics must be able to change the microflora of the colon to a healthy state, such as increasing the amount of helpful species while decreasing pathogenic germs (Scott, Gratz, et al., 2013).

Fructooligosaccharides (FOS) and inulin are two well-known prebiotic chemicals that boost the activity of beneficial living active cultures, improve mineral absorption, and suppress pathogenic bacteria in the digestive tract. Inulin aids in the digestion of high-protein diets, slows fat absorption, provides roughage to prevent constipation, remains in the digestive tract to provide satiety without carrying extra calories, lowers blood cholesterol and triglycerides, aids in diabetic blood glucose control, and lowers the risk of colon cancer (David, Maurice, et al., 2014).

Probiotics and prebiotics play distinct functions in human nutrition, mostly involving the modification of microbial populations or activities in the human GI tract. Increased immunological function, improved colonic integrity and duration of intestinal infections, down-regulated allergic reaction, and improved digestion and elimination are all benefits of regular probiotic or prebiotic use (de Paulo Farias, de Araújo et al., 2019).

Furthermore, dietary fiber, which includes non-starch polysaccharides such cellulose, dextrins, chitins, pectins, beta-glucans, and waxes, as well as lignin, can control the transit time through the gut, offering benefits similar to inulin-type fructans. Many foods, such as cereal and nuts, contain these chemicals. They're also susceptible to bacterial fermentation, which can alter bacterial populations, especially the quantity of bifidobacteria and lactobacilli. These dietary soluble fibers have been found to have additional health benefits, such as enhancing gut barrier function *in vitro* and *in vivo*, which may be due in part to their impact on microbiota composition.

He et al. (2017) suggested that gut microbiota plays a key role in the onset and progression of metabolic syndromes. Plasma glucose, hunger, serum lipids, and pro-inflammation have all been shown to be influenced by gut bacteria. Prebiotics and probiotics lower plasma glucose, weight loss, serum lipid levels, and improved insulin resistance (He & Shi, 2017).

Vieira et al. (2013) described that many elements, including dietary components and commensal microorganisms, have an impact on the gut immune system. Nutrients that alter gut immunity, as well as techniques that affect microbial composition to reestablish a healthy gut microbial population, are being developed as new therapeutic approaches to treat a variety of inflammatory illnesses. Although probiotics and prebiotics have shown promise in clinical and animal studies as treatments for a variety of diseases, a better understanding of the molecular mechanisms underlying the direct and indirect effects on the gut immune response will allow for better and possibly more efficient disease treatment. Prebiotics and probiotics are innovative treatment techniques that modulate the microbial makeup and gut immune responses of the host, according to his study (Vieira, Teixeira, et al., 2013).

Toward et al. (2012) explained that certain changes in the colonic microbiota occur as people get older, and these changes can have an impact on their health. Bifidobacteria populations, for example, are known to decline significantly at the age of 55–65 years. Bifidobacteria are known harmful microbe inhibitors, and a decrease in their activity may increase infection susceptibility. They showed that prebiotic galactooligosaccharides can have a significant impact on bifidobacteria in the gut flora of elderly people (Toward, Montandon et al., 2012).

12.5.3.3 Synbiotics

Both probiotics and prebiotics have been found to have beneficial effects on birds' guts. Synbiotics are formed when probiotics and prebiotics are mixed (Pusceddu, El Aidy, et al., 2015). Because the health-promoting organism's specialized substrate is accessible for fermentation, this combination may help it survive and remain in the guts of birds (Lee, You, et al., 2020).

According to the study by Rupa et al. (2012), the gastrointestinal (GI) tract is home to a staggering number of bacterial species, each of which has a significant impact on the biology, function, physiology, and immunological response of the host. The study described that the individuals have different GI microbiota compositions, which are regulated by a variety of external and internal factors including food, antibiotic use, and host genetics, all of which influence health and disease outcomes (Rupa & Mine, 2012).

12.5.3.4 Polyunsaturated Fatty Acids (PUFAs)

PUFAs are fatty acids that have more than one double bond between them and are separated by a single methylene group (Horigome, Okubo, et al., 2019). In animals and people, PUFA-rich diets have been proven to improve immunological function, blood pressure, cholesterol, and triglyceride levels, and cardiovascular function. The adult microbiome isn't particularly rich in genes involved in fatty acid metabolism (Bellenger, Bellenger, et al., 2021), although there have been reports of PUFA interactions with the indigenous microbiota and probiotics, which could impact their biological activities (El-Salhy, Hatlebakk, et al., 2019). Lactobacillus bacteria can use PUFAs supplied into the growing medium to produce a variety of products (Danneskiold-Samsøe, Barros, et al., 2019). The treatment of PUFAs also improved Lactobacillus adherence to the jejunal mucosa of gnotobiotic piglets, implying that these fatty acids may affect the intestinal levels of this bacterial group (Plamada & Vodnar, 2022). Lactic acid bacteria prevailed among Gram-positive bacteria within epithelial mucosa in fish-fed PUFA-rich diets, suggesting that dietary fatty acids influence the attachment sites for the gastrointestinal microbiota, presumably by changing the fatty acid content of the intestine wall (Catalkaya, Venema, et al., 2020). Lactic acid bacteria prevailed among Gram-positive bacteria within epithelial mucosa in fish-fed PUFA-rich diets, suggesting that dietary fatty acids influence the attachment sites for the gastrointestinal microbiota, presumably by changing the fatty acid content of the intestine wall. The administration of an infant formula fortified with Bifidobacterium Bb-12 or Lactobacillus GG to 15 infants with atopic eczema had some benefits on plasma lipids in a short clinical trial (Plamada & Vodnar, 2022). Probiotic treatment lowered alpha-linolenic acid (18:3 n–3) proportions in neutral lipids, while only Bifidobacterium Bb-12 supplementation increased alpha-linolenic acid proportions in phospholipids. As a result, the evidence suggests that some probiotic physiological effects may be linked to interactions between probiotics and dietary PUFA, albeit more research is needed to confirm this concept *in vivo*. Fu et al. (2021) say that omega-3 polyunsaturated fatty acids (omega-3 PUFAs) are necessary fatty acids that people should get from food and have health advantages. Omega-3 PUFAs (docosahexaenoic acid (DHA) have diverse impacts on intestinal immunological tolerance and gut microbiota maintenance, in addition to affecting the structure and function of cell membranes. The importance of omega-3 polyunsaturated fatty acids (PUFAs) in maintaining the equilibrium between gut immunity and gut microbiota was explored. They concluded that the gut immune system is modulated by the microbiota through omega-3 PUFAs. Omega-3 supplementation can be tailored to specific pathways in order to prevent and treat intestinal illnesses, which could aid researchers in developing new diagnostic procedures (Fu, Wang, et al., 2021).

Coelho et al. (2019) described that energy intake, diet composition can affect gut microbiota. The contents of the gut microbiota may be affected by dietary fatty acids, which alter human metabolic health. The processes by which different types of FFA influence gut microbiota are still poorly understood, and there are few studies on the subject. Fatty acids can cause growth suppression or even bacterial mortality by interfering with energy production, inhibiting enzyme activity, impairing food absorption, and generating toxic chemicals in cells. Consumption of n–3 PUFAs causes beneficial modifications in the microbiota of obese people, bringing it closer to that of healthy people (Coelho, Cândido, et al., 2019).

12.5.3.5 Phytochemicals

Phytochemicals are non-nutrient bioactive plant molecules found in fruits, vegetables, and other plant foods that have been related to lower health-related problems (Carrera-Quintanar, Lopez Roa, et al., 2018). Carotenoids, phenolics, alkaloids, nitrogen-containing, and organosulfur compounds are some of the substances in this group that can be classified based on structural similarities. Because of their potential actions as antioxidants (Luo, Lin, et al., 2021), anti-inflammatory and immunomodulatory (Geldert, Abdo, et al., 2021), cardioprotective and anticarcinogenic, phenolics, flavonoids, and phytoestrogens have piqued interest (Geldert, Abdo, et al., 2021). Polyphenol bioavailability and effects are heavily reliant on their modification by certain gut microbiota components by glucosidase, esterase, dehydroxylation, and decarboxylation activities (Pérez-Burillo, Molino, et al., 2021). Polyphenols are often found in plant meals as a bound form, most commonly conjugated as glycosides, and the majority of them are digested by gut microbes, resulting in aglycone production (Aravind, Wichienchot, et al., 2021). Phenolics and flavonoids may also inhibit *L. rhamnosus*' ability to adhere to intestinal epithelial cells. Tea catechins have also been demonstrated to alter ileum mucin concentration, which may influence bacterial adherence and colonization (Cladis, Simpson, et al., 2021). As a result, polyphenols appear to have the potential to improve health by altering gut microbiota.

The gut microbiota and dietary phytochemicals play important roles in human health, according to Yin et al. (2019). Dietary phytochemicals, such as phenolics, carotenoids, and dietary fiber, have been shown to change the human gut microbiota in recent studies. Furthermore, both pathogenic and nonpathogenic bacteria have regulatory effects with phytochemicals, implying possible synergistic benefits in improving human gut health and preventing chronic diseases (Yin, Kuo, et al., 2019).

Wang et al. (2021) described the impact of dietary phytochemicals in regulating gut microbiota. Recent data suggests that dietary phytochemicals can help prevent and treat symptoms of Alzheimer's disease, a neurodegenerative disease that has been connected to the condition of the gut microbiota in recent years. His review seeks to offer the most recent evidence on phytochemicals' regulating role in the gut microbiota and its relevance to Alzheimer's disease, as well as summarize the processes that underpin these modulative effects (Wang, Lim, et al., 2021).

Dingeo et al. (2020) overviewed the importance of a healthy gut microbiota (GM) for a healthy lifestyle. The diversity of the GM is frequently diminished or altered in pathological situations, often toward an increased Firmicutes/Bacteroidetes ratio. The colonic fermentation of dietary fiber has been shown to increase the production of short chain fatty acids, such as propionate and butyrate, and improve gut epithelium integrity, such as tight junction functionality, while also stimulating the fraction of bacteria purported to have beneficial health effects, acting as prebiotics. However, a number of phytochemicals, many of which are linked to dietary fiber, have been postulated as potential GM modulators. They described the phytochemicals with antioxidant and anti-inflammatory effects that may benefit the GM (Dingeo, Brito, et al., 2020).

12.5.3.6 Fats

The amount and quality of dietary fat has an impact on the composition of the gut microbiota (Daniel, Gholami, et al., 2014). Saturated fatty acids (SFAs) are mostly found in mammalian animal products. Several animal studies found that mice on a high-fat diet (HFD)—specifically SFAs—had fewer Bacteroidetes and more Firmicutes and Proteobacteria (Serino, Luche, et al., 2012). Surprisingly, these changes can be reversed over time with a control diet. Bacillus bifidus levels were also shown to be lower in mice fed an HFD in another investigation (Biesalski, 2016). As a result, a high consumption of dietary fats, especially SFA, may cause intestinal dysbiosis. In addition, HFD-induced dysbiosis may result in changes to the intestinal barrier. Consumption of a high-SFA diet has been shown to boost the formation of SRB, resulting in a faulty mucus layer and increased intestinal inflammation, colitis scores (Portincasa, Bonfrate, et al., 2022).

12.5.3.7 Micronutrients

Micronutrients play a crucial role in forming the gut microbiota, which is an important mediator of their health-promoting effects (Karlsson, Fåk, et al., 2012). Vitamins and minerals are important for energy metabolism, cell development and differentiation, and immunological function (Yang, Liang, et al., 2020). All bacteria in the phyla Bacteroidetes, Fusobacteria, and Proteobacteria had the essential riboflavin and biotin production pathways. Furthermore, all Fusobacteria were expected to be vitamin B12 makers, with Bacteroidetes appearing to have the greatest number of anticipated B vitamin producers. Several studies showed that vitamins like vitamin D can affect the composition of the gut microbiota. Vitamin D, for example, has been shown to improve IBD symptoms by modifying the gut microbiota and boosting the prevalence of potentially helpful bacterial strains (Barra, Anhê, et al., 2021). Furthermore, researchers found that vitamin D was associated with higher Lachnobacterium but decreased Lactococcus in some work of infant gut microbiome at age 3–6 months, and proposed that these correlations may have long-term consequences for immune system regulation and asthma/allergic disease incidence (Mach & Clark, 2017).

12.5.3.8 Vegan and Vegetarian Diets

Vegetarians, unlike omnivores, avoid eating all sorts of meat and seafood. Vegans are vegetarians who avoid eating animal products such as eggs, milk, and dairy products, as well as honey (Barrett, Gomez-Arango, et al., 2018). Some of them found that vegetarians and vegans had higher ratios of Bacteroides/Prevotella, Clostridium clostridio forme, Klebsiella pneumonia, and Faecalibacterium-prausnitziiand lower ratios of Clostridium cluster XIVa and Bilophila wads (Tomova, Bukovsky, et al., 2019). Some studies reported that both vegans and vegetarians had lower counts of Bifidobacterium and Bacteroides species in their gut microbiota. It also demonstrates that vegetarian diets can reduce gut microbiota diversity but not SCFAs or methane levels (Wong et al., 2018).

12.6 CONCLUSION AND FUTURE PERSPECTIVES

Food is a basic need in our life that provides nutritional benefits and contributes to the maintenance of normal health. In addition to providing essential nutrients, functional foods protect human from various disorders. The human gastrointestinal system is containing a population of 500–1000 distinct bacteria species in appropriate amount. These foods also help to maintain a healthy gut microbiota and promote health in a variety of ways. These dietary products obtained from fruits, vegetables, soya, legumes, and milk. A healthy gut microbiota protects against gastrointestinal disorders such as infection and inflammatory bowel syndromes. Food supplements like probiotics, prebiotics, polyunsaturated fatty acids, phytochemicals, and micronutrients play an important role in maintaining normal gastrointestinal microflora. Probiotics are a single or mixed culture of living microorganisms that, when administered in sufficient amounts, improve the host's intestinal microbial balance, increase colonization resistance to infections, and improve immune responses. Probiotics also prevent and treat a wide range of gastrointestinal problems, including antibiotic-associated diarrhea. Prebiotics are indigestible dietary substances that improve the health and well-being of the hosts by stimulating the growth, composition, and activity of microflora in the gastrointestinal system. Prebiotics use intestinal microflora to create short chain fatty acids, which lowers the risk of gastrointestinal disease, cancer, and cardiovascular disease while also improving lipid profiles. Both pathogenic and nonpathogenic bacteria have regulatory effects with phytochemicals, indicating possible synergistic benefits in improving human gut health and preventing chronic diseases. Micronutrients also act as an important mediator of their health-promoting effects. In this chapter, we have described the role of various dietary food supplements that helps in maintaining of normal gut health.

There is a hope that functional food will protect from diseases and disorders through maintaining gut microbiota. By providing health and nutrition-containing food, it will be a new opportunity in the biomedical field to protection of human beings from various disorders.

KEYWORDS

- **alpha-linolenic acid**
- **docosahexaenoic acid**
- **food supplements**
- **fructooligo saccharides**
- **functional food**
- **gut microbiota**
- **polyunsaturated fatty acids**
- **prebiotics**

REFERENCES

Adetuyi, B. O., Odine, G. O., Olajide, P. A., Adetuyi, O. A., Atanda, O. O., & Oloke, J. K., (2022). Nutraceuticals: Role in metabolic disease, prevention and treatment. *World News of Natural Sciences, 42,* 1–27.

Ahmed, M. H., Vasas, D., Hassan, A., & Molnár, J., (2022). The impact of functional food in prevention of malnutrition. *Pharma. Nutrition,* 100288.

Aravind, S. M., Wichienchot, S., Tsao, R., Ramakrishnan, S., & Chakkaravarthi, S., (2021). Role of dietary polyphenols on gut microbiota, their metabolites and health benefits. *Food Research International, 142*, 110189.

Barra, N. G., Anhê, F. F., Cavallari, J. F., Singh, A. M., Chan, D. Y., & Schertzer, J. D., (2021). Micronutrients impact the gut microbiota and blood glucose. *Journal of Endocrinology, 250*(2), R1–R21.

Barrett, H. L., Gomez-Arango, L. F., Wilkinson, S. A., McIntyre, H. D., Callaway, L. K., Morrison, M., & Dekker, N. M., (2018). A vegetarian diet is a major determinant of gut microbiota composition in early pregnancy. *Nutrients, 10*(7), 890.

Bellenger, J., Bellenger, S., Bourragat, A., Escoula, Q., Weill, P., & Narce, M., (2021). *Intestinal Microbiota Mediates the Beneficial Effects of n-3 Polyunsaturated Fatty Acids During Dietary Obesity, 28*, 21.

Biesalski, H. K., (2016). Nutrition meets the microbiome: Micronutrients and the microbiota. *Annals of the New York Academy of Sciences, 1372*(1), 53–64.

Carrera-Quintanar, L., Lopez, R. R. I., Quintero-Fabián, S., Sánchez-Sánchez, M. A., Vizmanos, B., & Ortuño-Sahagún, D., (2018). Phytochemicals that influence gut microbiota as prophylactics and for the treatment of obesity and inflammatory diseases. *Mediators of Inflammation, 2018.*

Catalkaya, G., Venema, K., Lucini, L., Rocchetti, G., Delmas, D., Daglia, M., De Filippis, A., et al., (2020). Interaction of dietary polyphenols and gut microbiota: Microbial metabolism of polyphenols, influence on the gut microbiota, and implications on host health. *Food Frontiers, 1*(2), 109–133.

Chopra, A. S., Lordan, R., Horbańczuk, O. K., Atanasov, A. G., Chopra, I., Horbańczuk, J. O., Jóźwik, A., et al., (2022). The current use and evolving landscape of nutraceuticals. *Pharmacological Research, 175*, 106001.

Choudhary, R., & Tandon, R., (2009). Consumption of functional food and our health concerns. *Pakistan Journal of Physiology, 5*(1), 76–83.

Cladis, D. P., Simpson, A. M., Cooper, K. J., Nakatsu, C. H., Ferruzzi, M. G., & Weaver, C. M., (2021). Blueberry polyphenols alter gut microbiota & phenolic metabolism in rats. *Food & Function, 12*(6), 2442–2456.

Claesson, M. J., Jeffery, I. B., Conde, S., Power, S. E., O'connor, E. M., Cusack, S., Harris, H. M., et al., (2012). Gut microbiota composition correlates with diet and health in the elderly. *Nature, 488*(7410), 178–184.

Coelho, O. G. L., Cândido, F. G., & Alfenas, R. C. G., (2019). Dietary fat and gut microbiota: Mechanisms involved in obesity control. *Critical Reviews in Food Science and Nutrition, 59*(19), 3045–3053. doi: 10.1080/10408398.2018.1481821. Epub 2018, Jul 11. PMID: 29851507.

Danneskiold-Samsøe, N. B., Dias de Freitas Queiroz Barros H., Santos, R., Bicas, J. L., Cazarin, C. B. B., Madsen, L., Kristiansen, K., et al., (2019). Interplay between food and gut microbiota in health and disease. *Food Research International, 115*, 23–31. doi: 10.1016/j. foodres.2018.07.043. Epub 2018, Jul 30. PMID: 30599936.

De Cosmi, V., Mazzocchi, A., Agostoni, C., & Visioli, F., (2022). Fructooligosaccharides: From breast milk components to potential supplements. a systematic review. *Advances in Nutrition, 13*(1), 318–327.

De Paulo, F. D., De Araújo, F. F., Neri-Numa, I. A., & Pastore, G. M., (2019). Prebiotics: Trends in food, health and technological applications. *Trends in Food Science & Technology, 93*, 23–35.

Dingeo, G., Brito, A., Samouda, H., Iddir, M., La Frano, M. R., & Bohn, T., (2020). Phytochemicals as modifiers of gut microbial communities. *Food & Function, 11*(10), 8444–8471.

El-Salhy, M., Hatlebakk, J. G., & Hausken, T., (2019). Diet in irritable bowel syndrome (IBS): Interaction with gut microbiota and gut hormones. *Nutrients, 11*(8), 1824.

Foster-Nyarko, E., & Pallen, M. J., (2022). The microbial ecology of *Escherichia coli* in the vertebrate gut. *FEMS Microbiology Reviews,* 1–22.

Fu, Y., Wang, Y., Gao, H., Li, D., Jiang, R., Ge, L., Tong, C., & Xu, K., (2021). Associations among dietary omega-3 polyunsaturated fatty acids, the gut microbiota, and intestinal immunity. *Mediators of Inflammation, 2021.*

Geldert, C., Abdo, Z., Stewart, J., & HS, A., (2021). Dietary supplementation with phytochemicals improves diversity and abundance of honey bee gut microbiota. *Journal of Applied Microbiology, 130*(5), 1705–1720.

Guslandi, M., (2022). Probiotics and intestinal health. In. *Probiotics* (pp. 343–353). Elsevier.

Hadi, S., Amani, R., Tehrani, M. M., Hadi, V., Hejri, S., & Askari, G., (2022). Ready-to-use therapeutic food (RUTF) formulations with functional food and nutrient density for the treatment of malnutrition in crisis. *International Journal of Preventive Medicine, 13*(1), 16.

He, M., & Shi, B., (2017). Gut microbiota as a potential target of metabolic syndrome: The role of probiotics and prebiotics. *Cell & Bioscience, 7*(1), 1–14.

Horigome, A., Okubo, R., Hamazaki, K., Kinoshita, T., Katsumata, N., Uezono, Y., Xiao, J., & Matsuoka, Y., (2019). Association between blood omega-3 polyunsaturated fatty acids and the gut microbiota among breast cancer survivors. *Beneficial Microbes, 10*(7), 751–758.

Huang, R., He, K., Duan, X., Xiao, J., Wang, H., & Xiang, G., (2022). Changes of intestinal microflora in colorectal cancer patients after surgical resection and chemotherapy. *Computational and Mathematical Methods in Medicine,* vol. 2022, Article ID 1940846, 16 pages, 2022. https://doi.org/10.1155/2022/1940846.

Karlsson, F. H., Fak, F., Nookaew, I., Tremaroli, V., Fagerberg, B., Petranovic, D., Bäckhed, F., & Nielsen, J., (2012). Symptomatic atherosclerosis is associated with an altered gut metagenome. *Nature Communications, 3*(1), 1–8.

Keservani, R. K., Kesharwani, R. K., Vyas, N., Jain, S., Raghuvanshi, R., & Sharma, A. K., (2010). Nutraceutical and functional food as future food: A review. *Der Pharmacia Lettre., 2*(1), 106–116.

Kogut, M. H., (2022). Impact of the gut microbiota on the immune system. In. *Avian Immunology* (pp. 353–364). Elsevier.

Komanduri, M., Savage, K., Lea, A., McPhee, G., Nolidin, K., Deleuil, S., Stough, C., & Gondalia, S., (2022). The relationship between gut microbiome and cognition in older Australians. *Nutrients, 14*(1), 64.

Lee, S. H., You, H. S., Kang, H. G., Kang, S. S., & Hyun, S. H., (2020). Association between altered blood parameters and gut microbiota after synbiotic intake in healthy, elderly Korean women. *Nutrients, 12*(10), 3112.

Lesbros-Pantoflickova, D., Corthesy-Theulaz, I., & Blum, A. L., (2007). Helicobacter pylori and probiotics. *The Journal of Nutrition, 137*(3), 812S–818S.

Ley, R. E., Peterson, D. A., & Gordon, J. I., (2006). Ecological and evolutionary forces shaping microbial diversity in the human intestine. *Cell, 124*(4), 837–848.

Luo, J., Lin, X., Bordiga, M., Brennan, C., & Xu, B., (2021). Manipulating effects of fruits and vegetables on gut microbiota–a critical review. *International Journal of Food Science & Technology, 56*(5), 2055–2067.

Mach, N., & Clark, A., (2017). Micronutrient deficiencies and the human gut microbiota. *Trends in Microbiology, 25*(8), 607–610.

Manassi, C. F., De Souza, S. S., De Souza, H. G., Sartor, S., Lima, C. M. G., Miotto, M., Lindner, J. D. D., et al., (2022). Functional meat products: Trends in pro-, pre-, syn-, para-and post-biotic use. *Food Research International*, 111035.

Mestecky, J., & Russell, M., (1998). Passive and active protection against disorders of the gut. *Veterinary Quarterly, 20*(sup3), 83–87.

Misra, S., Mohanty, D., & Mohapatra, S., (2022). Food-based probiotics: Functional dietary ingredients. In: *Probiotics* (pp. 257–275). Elsevier.

Narayanan, A. P., Latika, A., Nair, A. S., Ajeesh, P., Kumar, N. S., & Babu, M., (2021). Role of gut microbiota in human health and diseases. *Current Nutrition & Food Science, 17*(4), 374–383.

Neophytou, C., & Pitsouli, C., (2022). How gut microbes nurture intestinal stem cells: A drosophila perspective. *Metabolites, 12*(2), 169.

Nobre, C., Simões, L. S., Gonçalves, D. A., Berni, P., & Teixeira, J. A., (2022). Fructooligosaccharides production and the health benefits of prebiotics. In: *Current Developments in Biotechnology and Bioengineering* (pp. 109–138). Elsevier.

Palanivelu, J., Thanigaivel, S., Vickram, S., Dey, N., Mihaylova, D., & Desseva, I., (2022). Probiotics in functional foods: Survival assessment and approaches for improved viability. *Applied Sciences, 12*(1), 455.

Perez-Burillo, S., Molino, S., Navajas-Porras, B., Valverde-Moya, Á. J., Hinojosa-Nogueira, D., López-Maldonado, A., Pastoriza, S., & Rufián-Henares, J. Á., (2021). An *in vitro* batch fermentation protocol for studying the contribution of food to gut microbiota composition and functionality. *Nature Protocols, 16*(7), 3186–3209.

Plamada, D., & Vodnar, D. C., (2022). Polyphenols—Gut microbiota interrelationship: A transition to a new generation of prebiotics. *Nutrients, 14*(1), 137.

Portincasa, P., Bonfrate, L., Vacca, M., De Angelis, M., Farella, I., Lanza, E., Khalil, M., et al., (2022). Gut microbiota and short chain fatty acids: Implications in glucose homeostasis. *International Journal of Molecular Sciences, 23*(3), 1105.

Prasanth, M. I., Malar, D. S., Kesika, P., Tencomnao, T., & Sivamaruthi, B. S., (2022). Impact of probiotic supplementation and the role of gut microbiome in obesity. In. *Probiotics* (pp. 297–319). Elsevier.

Pusceddu, M. M., El Aidy, S., Crispie, F., O'Sullivan, O., Cotter, P., Stanton, C., Kelly, P., et al., (2015). N-3 polyunsaturated fatty acids (PUFAs) reverse the impact of early-life stress on the gut microbiota. *PloS One, 10*(10), e0139721.

Reque, P. M., & Brandelli, A., (2022). An introduction to probiotics. In. *Probiotics* (pp. 1–17). Elsevier.

Reuben, R. C., Elghandour, M. M., Alqaisi, O., Cone, J. W., Márquez, O., & Salem, A. Z., (2022). Influence of microbial probiotics on ruminant health and nutrition: Sources, mode of action and implications. *Journal of the Science of Food and Agriculture, 102*(4), 1319–1340.

Rinninella, E., Cintoni, M., Raoul, P., Lopetuso, L. R., Scaldaferri, F., Pulcini, G., Miggiano, G. A. D., et al., (2019). Food components and dietary habits: Keys for a healthy gut microbiota composition. *Nutrients, 11*(10), 2393.

Roberfroid, M., Gibson, G. R., Hoyles, L., McCartney, A. L., Rastall, R., Rowland, I., Wolvers, D., et al., (2010). Prebiotic effects: Metabolic and health benefits. *British Journal of Nutrition, 104*(S2), S1–S63.

Rolfe, R. D., (2000). The role of probiotic cultures in the control of gastrointestinal health. *The Journal of Nutrition, 130*(2), 396S–402S.

Rupa, P., & Mine, Y., (2012). Recent advances in the role of probiotics in human inflammation and gut health. *Journal of Agricultural and Food Chemistry, 60*(34), 8249–8256.

Sakamoto, I., Igarashi, M., Kimura, K., Takagi, A., Miwa, T., & Koga, Y., (2001). Suppressive effect of *Lactobacillus gasseri* OLL 2716 (LG21) on *Helicobacter pylori* infection in humans. *Journal of Antimicrobial Chemotherapy, 47*(5), 709–710.

Scott, K. P., Gratz, S. W., Sheridan, P. O., Flint, H. J., & Duncan, S. H., (2013). The influence of diet on the gut microbiota. *Pharmacological Research, 69*(1), 52–60.

Serino, M., Luche, E., Gres, S., Baylac, A., Bergé, M., Cenac, C., Waget, A., et al., (2012). Metabolic adaptation to a high-fat diet is associated with a change in the gut microbiota. *Gut., 61*(4), 543–553.

Shehata, A. A., Yalçın, S., Latorre, J. D., Basiouni, S., Attia, Y. A., El-Wahab, A., Visscher, C., et al., (2022). Probiotics, prebiotics, and phytogenic substances for optimizing gut health in poultry. *Microorganisms, 10*(2), 395.

Shenoy, A., Buttar, H. S., Dicholkar, P., Kaur, G., & Chintamaneni, M., (2022). Role of nutraceuticals, functional foods, and spices in the management of metabolic syndrome and related disorders. In: *Functional Foods and Nutraceuticals in Metabolic and Non-Communicable Diseases* (pp. 583–601). Elsevier.

Singh, A., Zapata, R. C., Pezeshki, A., Reidelberger, R. D., & Chelikani, P. K., (2018). Inulin fiber dose-dependently modulates energy balance, glucose tolerance, gut microbiota, hormones and diet preference in high-fat-fed male rats. *The Journal of Nutritional Biochemistry, 59*, 142–152.

Tomova, A., Bukovsky, I., Rembert, E., Yonas, W., Alwarith, J., Barnard, N. D., & Kahleova, H., (2019). The effects of vegetarian and vegan diets on gut microbiota. *Frontiers in Nutrition, 6,* 47.

Toward, R., Montandon, S., Walton, G., & Gibson, G. R., (2012). Effect of prebiotics on the human gut microbiota of elderly persons. *Gut Microbes, 3*(1), 57–60.

Vieira, A. T., Teixeira, M. M., & Martins F. D. S., (2013). The role of probiotics and prebiotics in inducing gut immunity. *Frontiers in Immunology, 4*, 445.

Villano, D., Girones-Vilapana, A., Garcia-Viguera, C., & Moreno, D. A., (2022). Development of functional foods. In: *Innovation Strategies in the Food Industry* (pp. 193–207). Elsevier.

Wang, Y., Lim, Y. Y., He, Z., Wong, W. T., & Lai, W. F., (2021). Dietary phytochemicals that influence gut microbiota: Roles and actions as anti-Alzheimer agents. *Critical Reviews in Food Science and Nutrition,* 1–27.

Watson, R. R., Singh, R. B., & Takahashi, T., (2018). *The Role of Functional Food Security in Global Health*. Academic Press.

Wong, M. W., Yi, C. H., Liu, T. T., Lei, W. Y., Hung, J. S., Lin, C. L., Lin, S. Z., & Chen, C. L., (2018). Impact of vegan diets on gut microbiota: An update on the clinical implications. *Tzu-Chi Medical Journal, 30*(4), 200.

Yadav, M. K., Kumari, I., Singh, B., Sharma, K. K., & Tiwari, S. K., (2022). Probiotics, prebiotics and synbiotics: Safe options for next-generation therapeutics. *Applied Microbiology and Biotechnology,* 1–17.

Yang, Q., Liang, Q., Balakrishnan, B., Belobrajdic, D. P., Feng, Q. J., & Zhang, W., (2020). Role of dietary nutrients in the modulation of gut microbiota: A narrative review. *Nutrients, 12*(2), 381.

Yin, R., Kuo, H. C., Hudlikar, R., Sargsyan, D., Li, S., Wang, L., Wu, R., & Kong, A. N., (2019). Gut microbiota, dietary phytochemicals, and benefits to human health. *Current Pharmacology Reports, 5*(5), 332–344.

Zawistowski, J., & Kopec, A., (2022). Effect of functional food ingredients on nutrient absorption and digestion. In. *Nutrition and Functional Foods in Boosting Digestion, Metabolism, and Immune Health* (pp. 173–189).

CHAPTER 13

ROLE OF DIETARY FIBERS IN COLORECTAL CANCER

SURENDRA AGRAWAL,[1,2] PAYAL TIWARI,[1] and PRAVINA GURJAR[3]

[1]*Shobhaben Pratapbhai Patel School of Pharmacy and Technology Management, SVKM's NMIMS, Vile Parle, Mumbai, Maharashtra, India*

[2]*Datta Meghe College of Pharmacy, DMIHER, Sawangi Meghe, Wardha, India*

[3]*Sharadchandra Pawar College of Pharmacy, Otur, Pune, Maharashtra, India*

ABSTRACT

Colorectal cancer havoc is difficult to handle by the medical team and difficult to tolerate by the patients as it surpasses extremes of associated symptoms. It is always better to prevent the occurrence, but lifestyle changes have worsened the scenario. This chapter attempts to discuss the risk factors for the development of colon cancer, symptoms, and detection, as well as diagnosis methods for understanding the criticalities and role of dietary fiber in colon cancer. It also covers the different dietary fibers, and their role in preventive and therapeutic segments. Subsequently, HELGA cohort case study and research outcomes are outlined to conclude that the dietary fibers are effective in the treatment of colorectal cancer.

13.1 INTRODUCTION

Colon is the final part of the digestive tract also known as large bowel or large intestine that is part of digestive system or digestive tract, which helps

Food Supplements and Dietary Fiber in Health and Disease. Bhushan R. Rane, Raj K. Keservani, Durgesh Singh, Nayan A. Gujarathi, and Ashish S. Jain, (Eds.)
© 2024 Apple Academic Press, Inc. Co-published with CRC Press (Taylor & Francis)

in removing water and some nutrients and electrolytes out of the body from partially digested food. Most of the large intestine is made up of the colon, and they are further named according to which way the food is traveled through them, i.e., ascending colon, transverse colon, descending colon and sigmoid colon. The ascending and transverse colon section together are called the proximal colon and descending and sigmoid colon is called the distal colon (Ber et al., 2021; Sensoy, 2021).

The rectum is the final part of the large intestine that ends at the anus. The remaining food material, i.e., solid waste known as stool, that moves through colon, stored in rectum and gets eliminated out of the body through anus (Nidhi et al., 2016).

Colon cancer is caused when an healthy cell in lining of colon and rectum increases and goes out of control forming a thick mass, called tumor or polyps that is form on the inside of the colon. If polyps are not treated or removed on time, this might become a potentially life threatening cancer. This tumor can be either malignant or benign (Ahmed, 2020).

The chance of polyps turning into cancer depends on the type of polyps present:

1. **Adenomatous Polyps:** Adenomas are called pre-cancerous cells which are of three types:
   i. Tubular;
   ii. Villous; and
   iii. Tubulovillous.

   Finding and removing these adenomas or precancerous polyps on time may prevent colorectal cancer.
2. **Hyperplastic and Inflammatory Polyps:** These are the most common polyps but not precancerous. Colonic cancer with these types of polyps having large hyperplastic polyps can be detected by colorectal cancer screening with colonoscopy.
3. **Sessile Serrated Polyps (SSP) and Traditional Serrated Adenomas:** They are similar to adenomas and need special care for the treatment of this cancer (Islam et al., 2013; Kuipers et al., 2015; Pericleous et al., 2013).

13.1.1 TYPES OF COLORECTAL CANCER

Commonest colorectal cancer are adenocarcinomas which are present in the glandular tissues like colorectal and grow where in organs release substances in the body like digestive juice and other fluid present in the colon. Some subtypes of adenocarcinomas have also been detected like signet ring and mucinous which have worse prognosis than adenocarcinomas and other types of cancer (Harris & Ferguson, 1993; Nitsche et al., 2013). Different types of tumors found in colon and rectum are:

1. **Carcinoid Tumors:** There are neuroendocrine cells also present in the GI Tract which have similar action to that of nerve cells and endocrine cells which are called neuroendocrine tumors (NETs) (Detterbeck, 2010).
2. **Gastrointestinal Stromal Tumors (GISTs):** This starts from special cells in the wall of the colon known as interstitial cells of Cajol (ICCs). They are sometimes called the pacemaker of the gastro-intestinal tract as they signal the muscles present in the GI tract that contract to move food and liquid together. This type of cancer can be found anywhere in the digestive tract, but seen commonly in the colon (Corless et al., 2004).
   Cancer that starts in the squamous cells, which are flat cells that are liming parts of GI tracts in the upper part of the esophagus and end of the anus, this type of cancer is called squamous cell carcinomas (McDowell, 2006).
3. **Lymphomas:** This type of cancer is a cancer of immune system cells, they start with lymph nodes but in this case, it can also start in the colon, rectum or other organs. Non-Hodgkin lymphoma is cancer that starts in white blood cells known as lymphocytes which are part of the immune system (Lenz & Staudt, 2010).
   There are two types of non-Hodgkin's lymphoma that is (Armitage et al., 2009):
   i. B-cell lymphocytes (B cells); and
   ii. T-cell lymphocytes (T cells).
4. **Sarcomas:** This type of cancer starts in blood vessels, layers in the muscle and various connective tissues in the wall lining of the colon and the rectum. Sarcomas in the region of the colon and rectum are rarely seen (Banerjee et al., 2013).

13.1.2 RISK FACTORS OF COLORECTAL CANCER

A risk factor can be anything that increases the chance of getting the disease and affecting the body severely such as smoking, any medical or family history that leads to cancer and also the person's age (Lin, 2009).

A person with a history of inflammatory bowel disease which can be either ulcerative colitis or Crohn's disease which later risk in causing colorectal cancer. IBD if not treated and continued for longer period of time caused development in dysplasia which kills the cells in the lining of the colon and rectum and over the period of time turns inti cancer (Lukas, 2010).

According to the research, about 5% of people with colorectal cancer have an inherited gene that causes family cancer syndromes. An inherited syndrome that is linked to colorectal cancer is Lynch syndrome which is non-polyposis colorectal cancer familiar to adenomatous polyposis found in the history of colorectal cancer (Snyder & Hampel, 2019).

In adenomatous polyposis alteration in APC gene inherited in persons from their parents which accounts for about 1% of the total colorectal cancer cause (Hegde et al., 2014). This type of cancer may further lead to risk of stomach, liver, pancreas, and cancer of small intestines too. Figure 13.1 illustrates the genetic factors leading to colorectal cancer. There is also sub-type of adenomatous polyposis which are: Attenuated FAP, Gardner syndrome, and Turcot syndrome (Shussman & Wexner, 2014).

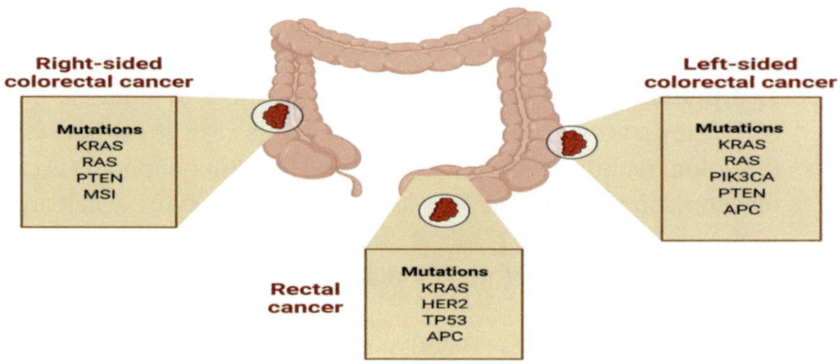

FIGURE 13.1 Genetic factors leading to colorectal cancer.

13.1.3 SPREAD OF COLORECTAL CANCER

Cancer in the form of polyps initially grows on the wall of the colon or rectum as it consists of various cell layers within them. Colorectal cancer starts within the mucosal layer that is the innermost layer of the cell and then grows outward and penetrates various cell lining layers (Bond, 2000; Tanaka, 2009).

If cancers are present in the walls of the colon and rectum, there are chances of to grow into the blood vessels and lymph vessels and thus later travel to lymph nodes or distant parts of the body (Leong et al., 2021). Figure 13.2 illustrates the spread of colorectal cancer.

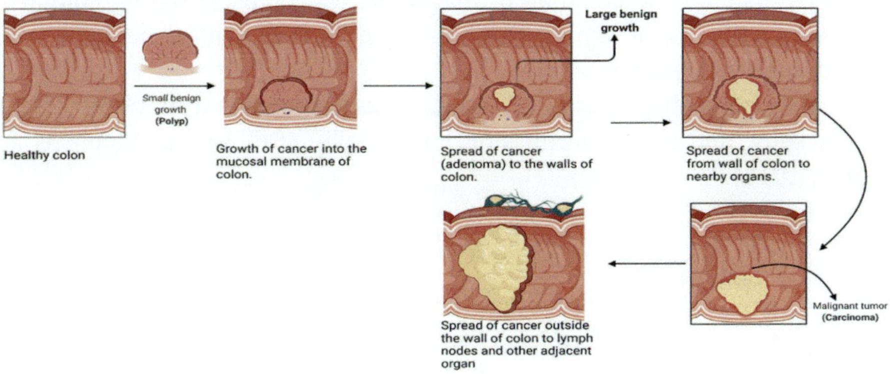

FIGURE 13.2 Spread of colorectal cancer.

Sign and symptoms of colorectal cancer (John et al., 2011):

- Changes is bowel habit causing diarrhea, stool narrowing, constipation;
- Rectal bleeding with deep red color;
- Abdominal pain and cramps;
- Unintended weight loss;
- Persistent abdominal discomfort;
- Weakness and fatigue;
- Rectal pressure or fullness;
- Anemia.

13.1.4 DETECTION AND DIAGNOSIS OF COLORECTAL CANCER

After showing the above sign and symptoms, doctors recommend stool test and check for occult blood, which is a major sign for colorectal cancer. Blood tests are recommended to check the complete blood count (CBC), check liver enzymes whether the cancer has spread to liver and test for tumor makers which is cell that is produced by colorectal cancer cells which is carcinoembryonic antigen (CEA) (Labianca & Merelli, 2010).

A diagnostic colonoscopy is the screening colonoscopy with a colonoscope to the entire length of the colon and rectum (Winawer, 2015).

Proctoscopy test is performed inside the rectum which has small video camera on the end, which is helps in measurement and the exact location of the colorectal cancer and its severeness (Birnbaum, 2019).

Biopsy is another screening or diagnostic test biopsied during colonoscopy, where the doctor removes a small piece of tissue with a special instrument through this scope.

Various other diagnosis is CT scan, ultrasound, MRI scan, chest X-ray, angiography, and positron emission tomography (PET) scan (Stephens & Aigner, 2016).

13.1.5 TREATMENTS

If cancer detected at the early stage, several surgical interventions are available and these are espoused based on the cancer size and patient's health (Pita-Fernandez et al., 2015; Thai et al., 2020):

1. **Polypectomy:** This a type of surgery where doctors remove polyps during the colonoscopy which is easier if cancer is small and completely contained in polyps and detected at the early stage.
2. **Endoscopic Mucosal Resection:** If the polyps are bigger than it is removed during colonoscopy using special tools to remove them along with small amount of inner lining of the colon, thus procedure called an endoscopic mucosal resection.
3. **Laparoscopic Surgery:** If colonoscopy procedure is not possible doctors go on to laparoscopic surgery in which small incisions are made in the abdominal wall and then perform surgery with the help of an instrument and attached camera to it which make it easier to detect and remove the polyps.
4. **Partial Colectomy:** In this the doctors remove a part of the colon along with the cancerous part on either side of the cancer.

Various methods such as chemotherapy, radiation therapy, immunotherapy, and certain targeted drug therapy are performed for advanced colon cancer (Mishra et al., 2013).

Palliative care is also called supportive care in which they aim to provide relief from the pain and other symptoms of colorectal cancer. There is a team focusing on improving quality of life for people and provide proper curative and other treatments that may help in relieving the health of the patients.

Proper dietary care is provided by a team focusing on the dietary fibers that may help in the treatment of colorectal cancer (Gulbake et al., 2016).

13.2 TYPES OF DIETARY FIBERS

There are two types of fiber found in the ample amount of all fruits and vegetables:

1. **Soluble Fiber:** These are found in plant cells that contain pectin, gums, and mucilage. Rich sources of soluble fibers are all the vegetables, fruits, barley, oats, soy, peas, lentils, etc. These play a major role in controlling bad cholesterol and help in the ease of constipation (Albuquerque et al., 2020). Soluble dietary fiber dissolves in water and also in the gastrointestinal fluids as it enters the stomach and the intestines. When entered it gets transformed into a gel-like mass which i later digested by the bacterias present in the large and small intestines (Blackwood et al., 2000; Mudgil & Barak, 2013). Soluble fibers include gums, pectins, psyllium, beta-glucans, and others. Insoluble fibers include lignin and cellulose (Chawla & Patil, 2010).
2. **Insoluble Fiber:** Cellulose, hemicellulose, and lignan are insoluble fiber that forms structural components of plant cells. They are majorly found in rice bran, corn bran, skins of fruits and vegetable, wheat bran, whole grains food, etc. It helps in bulking of feces and prevents constipation and various effects relating to hemorrhoids (Harris & Ferguson, 1993; JOHNSON & LUND, 2007). Insoluble dietary fiber does not dissolve in water as well as gastrointestinal fluid and remains almost unchanged as move through the GI tract. Benefits of insoluble fiber includes:
   i. **Preventing Constipation:** As an indigestible material, insoluble fiber sits in the gastrointestinal tract, absorbing fluid and sticking to other by-products of digestion that are ready to be formed into the stool. Its presence speeds up the movement and processing of waste, helping prevent gastrointestinal blockage and constipation or reduced bowel movements (Capuano, 2017).
   ii. **Lowering the Risk of Diverticular Disease:** By preventing constipation and intestinal blockages, insoluble fiber helps reduce the risk of developing small folds and hemorrhoids in the colon. It may also reduce the risk of colorectal cancer (Joye, 2020).

13.3 DIETARY FIBER PROVED EFFECTIVE IN PREVENTION AND TREATMENT OF COLORECTAL CANCER

13.3.1 BLACK BEANS

Black beans are classified under the legumes category, contains a high amount of protein and fiber content, and also contains various vitamins and minerals that provide health benefits to humans on consumption. The scientific name of black beans is Phaseolus vulgaris Linn belonging to the family Papilionaceae. Black beans are rich in carbohydrates and a good source of fiber, in the form of starch and fiber resistant which are slowly digested thus provide better health benefits (Singh, 2017).

13.3.2 PEAS

Scientific name of peas is Pisum sativum belonging to family Legume. Peas are used as flavoring agent and contains high amount of vitamins and various other nutrients such as high protein and good amount as fiber. Peas and legumes contains vitamin A, B1, B6 and vitamin C known and used in the maintaining bone health and in the treatment of osteoporosis (Venkidasamy et al., 2019).

13.3.3 SOYABEAN

Soyabean species are found in east Asia. Scientific name of soybean is Glycine max belonging to family Fabceae and subfamily Faboideae. Soyabean consist of dietary minerals and vitamins such as Vitamin B and Vitamin A (Azeem et al., 2015). These are processed further into soy milk, vegetable oils out of which tofu and tofu skins are beings prepared. They are highly rich in proteins and fibers that aid in the process of digestion (Zheng et al., 2020).

13.3.4 MUCILAGE

Mucilage is naturally occurring soluble fibers found majorly in oats, beans, flaxseed, soybeans, and various different fruits and vegetables. Rich source of mucilage type fiber is seed husk of Plantago ovate which is also known as psyllium seed gum or psyllium hydrocolloid (Kumar et al., 2017).

13.3.5 BETA GLUCAN

Beta glucans are naturally occurring polysaccharide derived from the cell wall of some bacteria, fungi, cereals, plants, and also from yeast. These consist of fermentable fiber, also called prebiotic fiber, found in the large intestine and helps increasing the fecal volume and affects the digestive function and in the maintenance of glucose and cholesterol. They are found in barley, soybeans, apples, bananas, oats, and a variety of oats (Ciecierska et al., 2019; de Graaff et al., 2018).

13.3.6 INULIN OLIGOFRUCTOSE

These are storage carbohydrates found in foods such as vegetables, fruits, and whole grains. They help in the growth of intestinal bifidobacterial and thus helps in maintenance of blood sugar and glucose levels. They are also used as flavoring agent in some as low-calorie foods and sweeteners (Kaur & Gupta, 2002).

13.3.7 PECTIN

Pectin are fibers that are found on fruits present in the primary and middle lamella of fruits and cell wall of some plants. Pectin when ingested increases the bulk of fecal as it expands and forms a gel like mass and thus felicitate digestion from the intestine (Zhang et al., 2015).

13.3.8 CELLULOSE

Cellulose fibers are made of esters and ethers of cellulose made from the bark of plants and some plant-based material. These are found in nuts, grains seeds and vegetables along with whole foods with or without skin or as whole seed intact. Intake of cellulose helps in the increase bowel movement in intestine and suggested, diet consisting of high cellulose results in decreasing the risk of colon cancer (Gill et al., 2018; Levi et al., 2001).

13.3.9 LIGNIN

Lignin are insoluble polysaccharide consisting of phenolic resin found majorly in fruits such as carrot, kiwi pear, apple, also some vegetables such as spinach, rhubarb, and kohlrabi (Potter, 1996; Yang et al., 2021).

13.3.10 RESISTANT STARCH

These are found naturally in foods, which can be either raw food, isolated or synthetically manufactured foods. These are found in grains, seeds, legumes, raw potatoes and rice both cooked and raw. They are known as friendly bacteria in the intestine increasing the health of individual by maintaining healthy gut bacteria and facilitate bowel movement (Dreher, 2018; Mehta et al., 2015).

13.4 DIETARY FIBER IN TREATMENT APPROACHES

13.4.1 HEALTHY GUT

The major benefit of including foods rich in fiber is the promotion of good and healthy digestive system. As peristalsis movement takes place smoothly eases the passage of food until excreted out of the body. Soluble fiber absorbs the water which bulks the feces and eases to move out of the gut, resulting in slow down of digestion process. Mechanism of dietary fibers to prevent disease risk in human gut microbiota, as consumption of fiber deprived diet causes degradation of host mucus membrane where it utilizes the host mucus glycoprotein as nutrients and destroys the mucus barrier to mucosal pathogens that leads to colorectal cancer, colitis diseases. It has also shown to decrease the incidence of inflammatory bowel disease (Chuwa et al., 2020; Lunn & Buttriss, 2007).

13.4.2 BLOOD CHOLESTEROL LOWERING

High cholesterol level in body gets deposited in the walls of arteries resulting in narrowing of blood vessels and resulting in cardiovascular diseases such as coronary heart disease, stroke, etc. Thus some studies provide data stating decrease the blood cholesterol level using food containing high fiber content (Appel & Group, 2009; Tosh & Yada, 2010).

13.4.3 WEIGHT MANAGEMENT

High diet fiber prevents in weight gain as soluble fiber forms gel that reduces the gastric emptying time and letting full for longer period of time and remain in transit time from intestine. High dense foods control hunger and keeps you satiated for longer period and also reduces absorption of sugar from intestine (Howarth et al., 2001).

13.4.4 REGULATION OF BLOOD GLUCOSE LEVELS

Fiber rich foods reduces the absorption of glucose in the from small intestine into the blood and controls urge of high insulin level in the blood and body (Weickert & Pfeiffer, 2008).

13.5.5 PREVENTION OF CANCER RISK

Use of dietary fiber such as cereal fiber of wholegrain foods are used in the prevention of cancer such causes decrease in the reduction of bowel cancer risk by increasing the bulk of the stool. The presence of fiber in the diet causes bacterial fermentation that produces short chain fatty acids that shows protective action against cancer. Studies also proves that high fiber intake at the age of adolescence and in early age of adulthood leads in prevention of breast cancer in women (Fernández et al., 2016).

13.5 RESEARCH ON THE ROLE OF DIETARY FIBERS IN COLORECTAL CANCER

There are studies that have demonstrated the reduction of colon cancer in the population with high diets which include high in total fiber and certain whole grain foods (Dahl & Stewart, 2015).

Studies on animal models showed an inhibitory effect of dietary fiber on the development of colonic cancer varying with the source and nature of the fiber used. These dietary fibers have also shown altering effects of dietary fibers on certain bacterial enzymes involved in the production and maturation of putative colon polyps causing cancer (Ferguson et al., 2004).

Intake of dietary fiber is a hypothesized mechanism to lower the risk and causes of colorectal cancer through various mechanisms such as diluting the fecal carcinogens, reducing the transit bowel time, alteration in the gut microbiota. Along with this mechanism there is production of short chain fatty acids that in result causes decrease in the pH of the colon or by adsorption of cytotoxic bile acids (Scharlau et al., 2009).

Cohort study performed to provide evidence associated with dietary fiber intake and association of colorectal cancer focussing on different sources of fibers and effects on specific tumor location. The study population consisted of three prospective cohorts in countries of Denmark, Norway, and Sweden. HELGA cohort study provided an opportune setting on giving data of a wide variety of intake of a range of cereals food and enables to show effects and differentiate between cereal foods with high or low fiber content (Nomura et al., 2007; Zhu et al., 2015).

This HELGA cohort consists of people of three different perspective:

i. The Norwegian Women and Cancer study (NOWAC);
ii. The Northern Sweden Health and Disease Study (NSHDS); and
iii. Danish Diet, Cancer, and Health study (DCH).

In this study, the Norwegian cohort population recruited only women, whereas the Northern and Danish diet included people both male and female but from specific areas in the country.

In all the cohort study the dietary fiber determination was Official method of analysis of the Association of Official Analytical Chemists (AOAC) method, the dietary variables of each group interest in the study where the total dietary fiber from majorly four sources: (i) vegetables; (ii) fruits; (iii) potatoes; and (iv) cereals and cereals foods.

Which was further divided into categories based on the amount of fiber content, whether it's low fiber content or high fiber content.

The HELGA cohort is usually followed for cancer incidence by information provided from National Cancer Registries, and cause of death registries. According to this data the overall colorectal cancer included the area of proximal and distal colon cancer which also include hepatic flexure, splenic flexure as well as overlapping lesion of colon whereas the rectum cancer included rectosigmoid junction (Kyrø et al., 2013).

According to the test analysis, the link between two variables viz-dietary fiber and incidence rate ratio of both colon and rectal cancer is provided by

Cox proportional hazards models. Test for interaction between the average intake of dietary fiber and sex or age or cohort study was performed, and related information provided. The quantitative variable was added linearly to Cox models for easier characterization, which increases the power of the test analysis.

Thus, two models were presented: i) An age-adjusted model and ii) multivariable model, which were adjusted such that information of subtype of fiber intake was assessed for colorectal risk factor leading to cancer from lifestyle questionnaires (Zhu et al., 2013).

There were incident of colon cancer diagnosed in HELGA cohort out of which major cases followed from Danish cohort having maximum reported colorectal cancer followed by Norwegian cohort, later followed by Swedish cohort. Among which, the number of colorectal cancer reported to women was significantly more than the number of men. This state the variable interaction between sex and intake of fiber provides significant data whereas variable of cohort country and fiber intake data was not more significant. The data of total cohort and colorectal cancer report were separately for men and women in Table 13.1. In comparison with the total male cohort and female cohort, colorectal cancer cases in males had higher total median intake of alcohol and processed meat the lifestyle of males included current smokers. The major cause for individual colon cancer was majorly due to smoking whereas colon cancer was current HRT users. The major sources of fiber intake in this cohort included a maximum number of cereals (56%) following fiber intake from vegetables (17%), intake from Fruits (16%) and from potatoes (11%).

For the multivariable model, for men and women, data corresponding to average intake of total and variable sources of fiber. The total fiber intake shows a lower risk of colorectal cancer among men in comparison to the highest to lowest intake as illustrated in Table 13.2. Intake of total cereal fiber and cereal related foods having high fiber intake is said to be associated to low risk fo cancer among men when compared to highest to lowest quartile intake and suggested, for women, increase in 2 g of total cereal fiber intake will significantly risk the chances of colorectal cancer. The potato fiber intake to risk of colorectal cancer in men was inversely related, whereas increased risk was observed for women when compared the highest to lowest potato fiber quartile intake. The analysis was also made in performed for the location of cancer including proximal and distal colon cancer showed an inverse correlation with distal colon cancer of increase in 10 g/day intake of fiber in men. It was observed, high risk of proximal colon cancer associated with dietary fiber found in potatoes, conversely the same intake of potato fiber was associated with lower risk of distal colon cancer. There was no significant data associated with rectal cancer in both men and women as mentioned in Table 13.3.

Data provided by Scandinavian cohort. Shows inverse relation between intake of dietary fiber and risk of colorectal cancer in men, it stated that intake of cereal specially ceral from food having higher content of dietary fiber was beneficially showing lowering the risk of overall cancer in men. This relation was also seen in women and having proximal colon cancer risk. HELGA and Scandinavian test all together provided number of advantages such as:

- HELGA cohorts including population and age-based data that directly links with National cancer registries to identify and fight incident cancer cases, as this data has clearly mentioned the incident cases, death, and immigration related to colorectal cancer.
- This study included a large number of populations having different cases and specifies the affected are of cancer that is proximal and distal colon cancer.
- This cohort study was successfully able to include various types of dietary fibers from different sources and enabling differentiation between cereal food containing high and low fiber content.
- The HELGA report is suggested for studying the relation of intake of cereal fiber and colorectal cancer as the results specify that 50% of the total fiber intake into test bos=dies provided high fiber content from cereals and cereals food.
- All three test of HELGA cohort was based on AOAC method providing a comparison of fiber content data.

Data was also obtained from FFQ who has also validated each three cohorts and its data stem are self-reported FFQs, which might be leading to some degree of misclassification.

There is also a linkage of healthy lifestyle apart from intake of dietary fiber along with other plant-based foods which impact the fiber intake and is in association with lifestyle factors (Barber et al., 2020).

Changes made in the consumption of folate in the cohort study along with the dietary fiber, knowing folate is said to be a weak link in total fiber intake. It was observed that higher risk of rectal cancer was associated in men on intake of fruit fiber, as fruits are a rich source of fiber and thus resultant higher risk of cancer were seen on adjustment of folate in the diet. No changes were as such made in the multivariable cohort studies model (Klurfeld, 2015).

All the data provided conclude that major changes were seen in men, which is further related to two different studies giving differentiation in men and women. There is as such no data provided for difference resulting in men and women data. It can be considered as hormonal factor that has significant role in the etiology of colon and rectum cancer as risk and preventive action taken may have different effect on men and women.

Results of total dietary risk and colorectal cancer is similar to those data provided by EPIC study, where in comparison of HELGA study only Danish and Swedish and Norwegian was excluded as low number of cases were observed from time of analysis.

The HELGA and Epic study both provide the data regarding dietary fiber intake effect on colorectal cancer differentiating in the number of prospective consider; the HELGA cohort has three prospective whereas the EPIC cohort included four prospective.

Another study performed by Park and their co-workers performed animal and human studies to prove the effect of dietary fibers supporting colorectal cancer showing inverse effect or prevent colorectal cancer (Park et al., 2005).

1. **Animal Studies:** These animal studies resulted in a conflicting effect on the occurrence of colorectal cancer as quantities of carcinogens used to induce tumors in animal models differed from each other. Various model resulted in no effect of dietary fiber due to the high amount of carcinogens that were unable to overcome the carcinogenic effects shown by the animals. Composition of food consumed by different experimental groups were kepts same with same amount of fats, vitamins, protein, and minerals. Carcinogens were administered after continuing the diet for several weeks and monitoring the effects.
   i. **Wheat Bran and Citrus Fiber with Azoxymethane (AOM) v/s Controlled Diet with Azoxymethane:** Experimental studies showed lower incidence of reported animals with tumor and showed decreased in the multiplicity of number of tumors and animals' rat with tumors. Whereas no effect of preventive action was seen in the controlled diet with AOM.
   ii. **Wheat Bran and Citrus Fiber with DMAB (3,2'-Dimethyl-4-Aminobiphenyl) v/s Controlled Diet with DMAB:** Animals when administered with DMAB also showed lower incidence of multiplicity of colon cancer whereas the control sample showed little or no effect with DMAB on prevention of colorectal cancer. A graphical representation of mutagenicity effect with

wheat bran and citrus fiber such as cellulose in comparison with control sample in Figure 13.3.

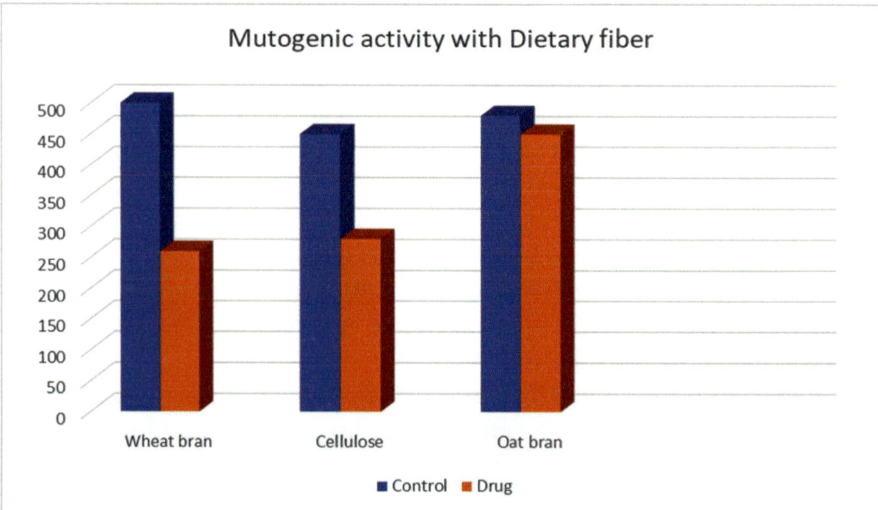

FIGURE 13.3 Mutagenicity effect with wheat bran and citrus fiber.

iii. **Use of Corn Bran with DMAB:** The experimental group when administered with corn bran and DMAB actually showed increased in the incidence of colorectal cancer and also showed increased multiplicity of colon tumor when compared to control diet with DMAB.

2. **Human Studies:** The studies performed to see the effect of fiber on animal fecal and certain bile acids on human, which significantly show a high risk of colorectal cancer.

Experimental design were similar to animal studies. Initially healthy volunteers were subjected to normal diet containing dietary fiber from wheat bran, oat fiber and cellulose fiber for the duration of 5 weeks and later subjected to 4-week with normal diet. After completion of individual diet, their stool samples checked for mutagens and bile acids.

This resulted in a decrease in the degree of mutagenic activity as well as bile acid concentration in experimental model consuming wheat bran and cellulose fiber supplements, whereas oat bran consumption did not significantly respond to the experimental change.

TABLE 13.1 Baseline Characteristics and Fiber Consumption Among the Total HELGA Cohort and Colorectal Cancer Cases, Separately for Men and Women

Observations	Men			Women		
	Total Cohort (n = 38852)	Cases of Colon Cancer (n = 312)	Cases of Rectal Cancer (n = 257)	Total Cohort (n = 69229)	Cases of Colon Cancer (n = 379)	Cases of Rectal Cancer (n = 220)
Age (yrs.)	54 (31–64)	59 (50–64)	59 (50–65	52 (40–63)	55 (45–64)	55 (45–64)
BMI (kg m^2)	26 (21–33)	26 (21–33)	26 (21–33)	24 (20–33)	25 (20–34)	25 (20–35)
Smoking Status (%)						
Never	36	28	20	42	40	39
Former	33	39	40	27	29	25
Current	31	33	40	31	31	36
Alcohol intake (g day^{-1})[1]	31	16	18	4	5	5
Red and processed meat (g day^{-1})[1]	107	118	118	64	71	69
Total fiber intake (g day^{-1})[1]	22	21	23	20	21	20
Vegetable fiber (g day^{-1})[1]	3	3	3	3	3	4
Fruit fiber (g day^{-1})[1]	2	2	3	3	3	3
Potato fiber (g day^{-1})[1]	3	2	3	2	2	2
Cereal fiber (g day^{-1})[1]	13	13	13	11	11	10
Low fiber cereal foods (g day^{-1})[1]	1	1	2	1	1	1
High fiber cereal foods (g day^{-1})[1]	11	10	11	9	10	9

TABLE 13.2 Incidence Rate Ratio of Colon Cancer in Men and Women in HELGA Cohort According to Daily Intake of 10 g day^{-1}

	Men				Women			
	Q2	**Q3**	**Q4**	**Linear**	**Q2**	**Q3**	**Q4**	**Linear**
Total Fiber								
Range/increment (g day^{-1})	>16.8–≤22.1	>22.1-≤28.1	>28.1	Per 10 g day	>15.4-≤19.6	>19.6-≤24.5	>24.5	Per 10 g day
Crude model	0.93	0.86	0.55	0.75	0.72	0.98	0.86	0.96
Multivariable model	0.93	0.86	0.55	0.74	0.73	0.99	0.87	0.99
Vegetable Fiber								
Range/increment (g day^{-1})	>1.4-≤2.8	>2.8-≤4.5	>4.5	Per 2 g day	>2.1-≤3.4	>3.4-≤5.0	>5.0	Per 2 g day
Crude model	1.12	0.98	0.80	0.91	1.07	0.89	1.05	1.00
Multivariable model	1.20	1.10	0.93	0.95	1.10	0.94	1.13	1.05
Fruit Fiber								
Range/increment (g day^{-1})	>1.0-≤2.2	>2.2-≤3.7	>3.7	Per 2 g day	>1.7-≤3.0	>3.0-≤4.9	>4.9	Per 2 g day
Crude model	0.71	0.65	0.69	0.91	1.15	0.91	0.97	1.04
Multivariable model	0.75	0.72	0.79	0.95	1.15	0.91	0.95	0.98
Potato Fiber								
Range/increment (g day^{-1})	>1.7-≤2.5	>2.5-≤3.7	>3.7	Per 2 g day	>1.1-≤2.0	>2.0-≤3.4	>3.4	Per 2 g day
Crude model	0.77	0.86	0.67	0.90	0.98	1.04	1.65	1.01
Multivariable model	0.76	0.85	0.65	0.89	0.97	1.03	1.59	1.15
Cereal Fiber								
Range/increment (g day^{-1})	>9.5-≤13.5	>13.5-≤17.8	>17.8	Per 2 g day	>7.5-≤10.7	>10.7-≤13.7	>13.7	Per 2 g day
Crude model	0.84	0.82	0.59	0.93	0.72	0.98	0.77	0.97
Multivariable model	0.87	0.87	0.66	0.94	0.71	0.96	0.75	0.97

TABLE 13.3 Incidence Rate Ratio of Rectal Cancer in Men and Women in HELGA Cohort According to Daily Intake of 10 g day^{-1}

Observations	Men				Women			
	Q2	**Q3**	**Q4**	**Linear**	**Q2**	**Q3**	**Q4**	**Linear**
Total Fiber								
Range/increment (g day^{-1})	>16.8-≤22.1	>22.1-≤28.1	>28.1	Per 10 g day	>15.4-≤19.6	>19.6-≤24.5	>24.5	Per 10 g day
Crude model	1.17	1.40	0.97	0.98	0.82	0.72	0.89	0.95
Multivariable model	1.24	1.54	1.11	1.02	0.85	0.77	0.97	0.99
Vegetable Fiber								
Range/increment (g day^{-1})	>1.4-≤2.8	>2.8-≤4.5	>4.5	Per 2 g day	>2.1-≤3.4	>3.4-≤5.0	>5.0	Per 2 g day
Crude model	1.09	1.03	1.08	1.03	1.51	1.53	1.30	1.01
Multivariable model	1.11	1.06	1.11	1.00	1.61	1.68	1.46	1.03
Fruit Fiber								
Range/increment (g day^{-1})	>1.0-≤2.2	>2.2-≤3.7	>3.7	Per 2 g day	>1.7-≤3.0	>3.0-≤4.9	>4.9	Per 2 g day
Crude model	0.99	1.11	1.19	0.99	1.08	0.74	1.12	0.99
Multivariable model	1.08	1.29	1.42	1.08	1.15	0.80	1.21	1.00
Potato Fiber								
Range/increment (g day^{-1})	>1.7-≤2.5	>2.5-≤3.7	>3.7	Per 2 g day	>1.1-≤2.0	>2.0-≤3.4	>3.4	Per 2 g day
Crude model	1.07	1.09	1.30	1.17	0.79	0.93	1.10	1.09
Multivariable model	1.09	1.12	1.33	1.01	0.82	0.96	1.12	0.98
Cereal Fiber								
Range/increment	>9.5-≤13.5	>13.5-≤17.8	>17.8	Per 2 g day	>7.5-≤10.7	>10.7-≤13.7	>13.7	Per 2 g day
Crude model	1.04	0.85	0.88	0.98	0.68	0.59	0.62	0.97
Multivariable model	1.06	0.89	0.94	0.98	0.69	0.60	0.64	0.98

13.6 CONCLUSION

The global rise in the incidences of colorectal cancer due to lifestyle changes and challenges in treatment strategy paved a path to look critically into the ways to prevent the occurrence. The ancient systems and modern science altogether declared the dietary fibers to be opted in the prevention and mitigation approaches. The success in the previous experiments demands alternatives fibers other than identified fibers to be explored for the same.

KEYWORDS

- **carcinoembryonic antigen**
- **colorectal cancer**
- **dietary fibers in cancer treatment**
- **gastrointestinal stromal tumors**
- **HELGA cohort case study**
- **neuroendocrine**
- **positron emission tomography**
- **soluble and insoluble dietary fibers**

REFERENCES

Ahmed, M., (2020). Colon cancer: A clinician's perspective in 2019. *Gastroenterology Research, 13*(1), 1.

Albuquerque, T. G., Nunes, M. A., Bessada, S. M., Costa, H. S., & Oliveira, M. B. P., (2020). Biologically active and health promoting food components of nuts, oilseeds, fruits, vegetables, cereals, and legumes. In: *Chemical Analysis of Food* (pp. 609–656). Elsevier.

Appel, L.J., & American Society of Hypertension Writing Group, (2009). ASH position paper: dietary approaches to lower blood pressure. *Journal of the American Society of Hypertension, 3*(5), 321–331.

Armitage, J. O., Coiffier, B., & Dalla-Favera, R., (2009). *Non-Hodgkin Lymphomas*. Lippincott Williams & Wilkins.

Azeem, S., Gillani, S. W., Siddiqui, A., Jandrajupalli, S. B., Poh, V., & Sulaiman, S. A. S., (2015). Diet and colorectal cancer risk in Asia–a systematic review. *Asian Pacific Journal of Cancer Prevention, 16*(13), 5389–5396.

Banerjee, R., Bandopadhyay, D., & Abilash, V., (2013). Epidemiology, pathology, types and diagnosis of soft tissue sarcoma: A research review. *Asian J. Pharm. Clin. Res., 6*(suppl 3), 18–25.

Barber, T. M., Kabisch, S., Pfeiffer, A. F., & Weickert, M. O., (2020). The health benefits of dietary fiber. *Nutrients, 12*(10), 3209.

Ber, Y., García-Lopez, S., Gargallo-Puyuelo, C. J., & Gomollón, F., (2021). Small and large intestine (II): Inflammatory bowel disease, short bowel syndrome, and malignant tumors of the digestive tract. *Nutrients, 13*(7), 2325.

Birnbaum, E., (2019). Ultrasonographic diagnosis of anorectal disease. In: *Shackelford's Surgery of the Alimentary Tract, 2 Volume Set* (Vol. 2, pp. 1713–1720). Elsevier.

Blackwood, A. D., Salter, J., Dettmar, P. W., & Chaplin, M. F., (2000). Dietary fiber, physicochemical properties and their relationship to health. *The Journal of the Royal Society for the Promotion of Health, 120*(4), 242–247.

Bond, J. H., (2000). Polyp guideline: Diagnosis, treatment, and surveillance for patients with colorectal polyps. *The American Journal of Gastroenterology, 95*(11), 3053.

Capuano, E., (2017). The behavior of dietary fiber in the gastrointestinal tract determines its physiological effect. *Critical Reviews in Food Science and Nutrition, 57*(16), 3543–3564.

Chawla, R., & Patil, G., (2010). Soluble dietary fiber. *Comprehensive Reviews in Food Science and Food Safety, 9*(2), 178–196.

Chuwa, C., Dhiman, A., Kathuria, D., Mwita, M., & Gautam, S., (2020). Food fibers a solution to combat noncommunicable diseases. *Nutr. Metab. Open Access. https://doi.org/10.29011/NMOA-105.100005.*

Ciecierska, A., Drywien, M., Hamulka, J., & Sadkowski, T., (2019). Nutraceutical functions of beta-glucans in human nutrition. *Roczniki Państwowego Zakładu Higieny, 70*(4).

Corless, C. L., Fletcher, J. A., & Heinrich, M. C., (2004). Biology of gastrointestinal stromal tumors. *Journal of Clinical Oncology, 22*(18), 3813–3825.

Dahl, W. J., & Stewart, M. L., (2015). Position of the academy of nutrition and dietetics: Health implications of dietary fiber. *Journal of the Academy of Nutrition and Dietetics, 115*(11), 1861–1870.

De Graaff, P., Govers, C., Wichers, H. J., & Debets, R., (2018). Consumption of β-glucans to spice up T cell treatment of tumors: A review. *Expert Opinion on Biological Therapy, 18*(10), 1023–1040.

Detterbeck, F. C., (2010). Management of carcinoid tumors. *The Annals of Thoracic Surgery, 89*(3), 998–1005.

Dreher, M. L., (2018). *Dietary Fiber in Health and Disease*. Springer.

Ferguson, L. R., Philpott, M., & Karunasinghe, N., (2004). Dietary cancer and prevention using antimutagens. *Toxicology, 198*(1–3), 147–159.

Fernández, J., Redondo-Blanco, S., Gutiérrez-del-Río, I., Miguélez, E. M., Villar, C. J., & Lombo, F., (2016). Colon microbiota fermentation of dietary prebiotics towards short-chain fatty acids and their roles as anti-inflammatory and anti-tumor agents: A review. *Journal of Functional Foods, 25*, 511–522.

Gill, S., Chater, P. I., Wilcox, M. D., Pearson, J. P., & Brownlee, I. A., (2018). The impact of dietary fibers on the physiological processes of the large intestine. *Bioactive Carbohydrates and Dietary Fiber, 16*, 62–74.

Gulbake, A., Jain, A., Jain, A., Jain, A., & Jain, S. K., (2016). Insight to drug delivery aspects for colorectal cancer. *World Journal of Gastroenterology, 22*(2), 582.

Harris, P. J., & Ferguson, L. R., (1993). Dietary fiber: Its composition and role in protection against colorectal cancer. *Mutation Research/Fundamental and Molecular Mechanisms of Mutagenesis, 290*(1), 97–110. https://doi.org/https://doi.org/10.1016/0027-5107(93)90037-G.

Hegde, M., Ferber, M., Mao, R., Samowitz, W., & Ganguly, A., (2014). ACMG technical standards and guidelines for genetic testing for inherited colorectal cancer (lynch syndrome, familial adenomatous polyposis, and MYH-associated polyposis). *Genetics in Medicine, 16*(1), 101–116.

Howarth, N. C., Saltzman, E., & Roberts, S. B., (2001). Dietary fiber and weight regulation. *Nutrition Reviews, 59*(5), 129–139.

Islam, R. S., Patel, N. C., Lam-Himlin, D., & Nguyen, C. C., (2013). Gastric polyps: A review of clinical, endoscopic, and histopathologic features and management decisions. *Gastroenterology & Hepatology, 9*(10), 640.

John, S., George, S., Primrose, J., & Fozard, J., (2011). Symptoms and signs in patients with colorectal cancer. *Colorectal Disease, 13*(1), 17–25.

JOHNSON, I. T., & LUND, E. K., (2007). Review article: Nutrition, obesity and colorectal cancer. *Alimentary Pharmacology & Therapeutics, 26*(2), 161–181. https://doi.org/https://doi.org/10.1111/j.1365-2036.2007.03371.x.

Joye, I. J., (2020). Dietary fiber from whole grains and their benefits on metabolic health. *Nutrients, 12*(10), 3045.

Kaur, N., & Gupta, A. K., (2002). Applications of inulin and oligofructose in health and nutrition. *Journal of Biosciences, 27*(7), 703–714.

Klurfeld, D. M., (2015). Research gaps in evaluating the relationship of meat and health. *Meat Science, 109*, 86–95.

Kuipers, E. J., Grady, W. M., Lieberman, D., Seufferlein, T., Sung, J. J., Boelens, P. G., Van De, V. C. J. H., & Watanabe, T., (2015). Colorectal cancer. *Nature Reviews: Disease Primers, 1*, 15065. doi: 10.1038/nrdp.2015.65. PMID: 27189416; PMCID: PMC4874655.

Kumar, D., Pandey, J., Kumar, P., & Raj, V., (2017). Psyllium mucilage and its use in pharmaceutical field: An overview. *Curr. Synthetic Sys. Biol., 5*(134), 1–7. doi:10.4172/2332–0737.1000134.

Kyrø, C., Skeie, G., Loft, S., Landberg, R., Christensen, J., Lund, E., Nilsson, L. M., et al., (2013). Intake of whole grains from different cereal and food sources and incidence of colorectal cancer in the Scandinavian HELGA cohort. *Cancer Causes & Control, 24*(7), 1363–1374.

Labianca, R., & Merelli, B., (2010). Screening and diagnosis for colorectal cancer: Present and future. *Tumori Journal, 96*(6), 889–901.

Lenz, G., & Staudt, L. M., (2010). Aggressive lymphomas. *New England Journal of Medicine, 362*(15), 1417–1429.

Leong, S. P., Pissas, A., Scarato, M., Gallon, F., Pissas, M. H., Amore, M., Wu, M., et al., (2021). The lymphatic system and sentinel lymph nodes: Conduit for cancer metastasis. *Clinical & Experimental Metastasis,* 1–19.

Levi, F., Pasche, C., Lucchini, F., & La Vecchia, C., (2001). Dietary fiber and the risk of colorectal cancer. *European Journal of Cancer, 37*(16), 2091–2096. https://www.sciencedirect.com/science/article/abs/pii/S0959804901002544?via%3Dihub (accessed on 28 January 2023).

Lin, O. S., (2009). Acquired risk factors for colorectal cancer. *Cancer Epidemiology,* 361–372.

Lukas, M., (2010). Inflammatory bowel disease as a risk factor for colorectal cancer. *Digestive Diseases, 28*(4, 5), 619–624.

Lunn, J., & Buttriss, J., (2007). Carbohydrates and dietary fiber. *Nutrition Bulletin, 32*(1), 21–64.

McDowell, J. D., (2006). An overview of epidemiology and common risk factors for oral squamous cell carcinoma. *Otolaryngologic Clinics of North America, 39*(2), 277–294.

Mehta, N., Ahlawat, S., Sharma, D., & Dabur, R., (2015). Novel trends in development of dietary fiber rich meat products—A critical review. *Journal of Food Science and Technology, 52*(2), 633–647.

Mishra, J., Drummond, J., Quazi, S. H., Karanki, S. S., Shaw, J., Chen, B., & Kumar, N., (2013). Prospective of colon cancer treatments and scope for combinatorial approach to enhanced cancer cell apoptosis. *Critical Reviews in Oncology/Hematology, 86*(3), 232–250.

Mudgil, D., & Barak, S., (2013). Composition, properties and health benefits of indigestible carbohydrate polymers as dietary fiber: A review. *International Journal of Biological Macromolecules, 61*, 1–6.

Nidhi, Rashid, M., Kaur, V., Hallan, S. S., Sharma, S., & Mishra, N., (2016). Microparticles as controlled drug delivery carrier for the treatment of ulcerative colitis: A brief review. *Saudi Pharm. J., 24*(4), 458–472. https://doi.org/10.1016/j.jsps.2014.10.001.

Nitsche, U., Zimmermann, A., Späth, C., Müller, T., Maak, M., Schuster, T., Slotta-Huspenina, J., et al., (2013). Mucinous and signet-ring cell colorectal cancers differ from classical adenocarcinomas in tumor biology and prognosis. *Annals of Surgery, 258*(5), 775.

Nomura, A. M., Hankin, J. H., Henderson, B. E., Wilkens, L. R., Murphy, S. P., Pike, M. C., Marchand, L. L., et al., (2007). Dietary fiber and colorectal cancer risk: The multiethnic cohort study. *Cancer Causes & Control, 18*(7), 753–764.

Park, Y., Hunter, D. J., Spiegelman, D., Bergkvist, L., Berrino, F., Van, D. B. P. A., Buring, J. E., et al., (2005). Dietary fiber intake and risk of colorectal cancer: A pooled analysis of prospective cohort studies. *JAMA, 294*(22), 2849–2857.

Pericleous, M., Mandair, D., & Caplin, M. E., (2013). Diet and supplements and their impact on colorectal cancer. *Journal of Gastrointestinal Oncology, 4*(4), 409–423. https://doi.org/10.3978/j.issn.2078-6891.2013.003.

Pita-Fernandez, S., Alhayek-Ai, M., Gonzalez-Martin, C., Lopez-Calvino, B., Seoane-Pillado, T., & Pertega-Diaz, S., (2015). Intensive follow-up strategies improve outcomes in nonmetastatic colorectal cancer patients after curative surgery: A systematic review and meta-analysis. *Annals of Oncology, 26*(4), 644–656.

Potter, J. D., (1996). Nutrition and colorectal cancer. *Cancer Causes Control, 7*(1), 127–146. https://doi.org/10.1007/bf00115644.

Scharlau, D., Borowicki, A., Habermann, N., Hofmann, T., Klenow, S., Miene, C., Munjal, U., Stein, K., & Glei, M., (2009). Mechanisms of primary cancer prevention by butyrate and other products formed during gut flora-mediated fermentation of dietary fiber. *Mutation Research/Reviews in Mutation Research, 682*(1), 39–53.

Sensoy, I., (2021). A review on the food digestion in the digestive tract and the used *in vitro* models. *Current Research in Food Science*.

Shussman, N., & Wexner, S. D., (2014). Colorectal polyps and polyposis syndromes. *Gastroenterology Report, 2*(1), 1–15.

Singh, N., (2017). *Pulses: An Overview* (Vol. 54, pp. 853–857). In Springer.

Snyder, C., & Hampel, H., (2019). Hereditary colorectal cancer syndromes. *Seminars in Oncology Nursing*.

Stephens, F. O., & Aigner, K. R., (2016). Investigations that may be useful in detecting cancer. In: *Basics of Oncology* (pp. 61–81). Springer.

Tanaka, T., (2009). Colorectal carcinogenesis: Review of human and experimental animal studies. *Journal of Carcinogenesis, 8*.

Thai, M. T., Phan, P. T., Hoang, T. T., Wong, S., Lovell, N. H., & Do, T. N., (2020). Advanced intelligent systems for surgical robotics. *Advanced Intelligent Systems, 2*(8), 1900138.

Tosh, S. M., & Yada, S., (2010). Dietary fibers in pulse seeds and fractions: Characterization, functional attributes, and applications. *Food Research International, 43*(2), 450–460.

Venkidasamy, B., Selvaraj, D., Nile, A. S., Ramalingam, S., Kai, G., & Nile, S. H., (2019). Indian pulses: A review on nutritional, functional and biochemical properties with future perspectives. *Trends in Food Science & Technology, 88*, 228–242.

Weickert, M. O., & Pfeiffer, A. F., (2008). Metabolic effects of dietary fiber consumption and prevention of diabetes. *The Journal of Nutrition, 138*(3), 439–442.

Winawer, S. J., (2015). The history of colorectal cancer screening: A personal perspective. *Digestive Diseases and Sciences, 60*(3), 596–608.

Yang, Y., Yang, L., Zhou, L., & Tang, S., (2021). A critical review of the effect of dietary fiber intake on the prevention of colorectal cancer in Eastern Asian Countries. *Journal of Healthcare Engineering, 2021,* Article ID 6680698, 8 pages, 2021. https://doi.org/10.1155/2021/6680698.

Zhang, W., Xu, P., & Zhang, H., (2015). Pectin in cancer therapy: A review. *Trends in Food Science & Technology, 44*(2), 258–271.

Zheng, L., Regenstein, J. M., Teng, F., & Li, Y., (2020). Tofu products: A review of their raw materials, processing conditions, and packaging. *Comprehensive Reviews in Food Science and Food Safety, 19*(6), 3683–3714.

Zhu, B., Sun, Y., Qi, L., Zhong, R., & Miao, X., (2015). Dietary legume consumption reduces risk of colorectal cancer: Evidence from a meta-analysis of cohort studies. *Scientific Reports, 5*(1), 1–7.

Zhu, Y., Wu, H., Wang, P. P., Savas, S., Woodrow, J., Wish, T., Jin, R., et al., (2013). Dietary patterns and colorectal cancer recurrence and survival: A cohort study. *BMJ Open, 3*(2), e002270.

PART III
Regulation and Miscellaneous

CHAPTER 14

BOTANICALS IN DIETARY SUPPLEMENTS AND FIBERS

RICHA GUPTA,[1] AJAY SINGH KUSHWAH,[1] and JAVESH KASHINATH PATIL[2]

[1]*Amar Shaheed Baba Ajit Singh Jujhar Singh Memorial College of Pharmacy (An Autonomous College), Bela, Ropar, Punjab, India*

[2]*PSGVP Mandal's College of Pharmacy, Shahada, Nandurbar, Maharashtra, India*

ABSTRACT

The word 'botanicals' is not a new term; everyone is very familiar with it. The difference is only that now it is not limited to just plant and their parts, but it includes plant constituents, plant preparations, secretions, and plant extractives too in the form of medicines, supplements, and formulations. So, with the advancements, the term *botanicals* is becoming wider and is used for various health, nutrition, and medicinal purposes. Botanicals are widely available in form of dietary supplements and have the benefit to supplement the diet with health benefits. These are easily available and are free from FDA regulations because these are included in the food category. Dietary supplements include various nutritional ingredients such as minerals, vitamins, proteins, amino acids, enzymes, herbs, herb extract, etc., and are available in all types of oral formulations. Many botanicals like Spirulina, Fenugreek, Soybean, Green tea, Flaxseed, Ginseng, Ginkgo, Garlic, and Echinacea role have been defined as dietary supplements. Likewise, dietary fibers are also very essential in our daily diet for improved digestion and a healthy body. The main applications of dietary fibers include maintenance

Food Supplements and Dietary Fiber in Health and Disease. Bhushan R. Rane, Raj K. Keservani, Durgesh Singh, Nayan A. Gujarathi, and Ashish S. Jain, (Eds.)
© 2024 Apple Academic Press, Inc. Co-published with CRC Press (Taylor & Francis)

of healthy weight, decreasing the risk of coronary heart disease, obesity, diabetes, and lowering the cholesterol level with a healthy digestive system. The botanicals which are rich in fiber are fruits, vegetables, whole grains, nuts, and dry fruits. These all are natural and generally have no side effects but care should be taken regarding the quality and quantity of any nature.

14.1 INTRODUCTION TO BOTANICALS

Herbs are playing a vital role for both nutrition and health purposes. According to data available around 2,50,000 flowering plant species are present on the earth, in which near about 85,000 species are using worldwide for their health benefits. According to a report given by World Health Organization (WHO), more than 80% of the world population believes in herbs and herbal products for various applications (Rane et al., 2020a, b, c; Sharma et al., 2020). Botanical is a wider term and generally includes a plant or plant part having some medicinal and aromatic value. But in a broad sense, it includes fresh or dried whole plant, any plant part, plant constituents, plant or plant part extracts, essential oils, resins, and other plant extractives or products that are useful as a nutritive or medicine or flavoring agent or for other purposes. So, herbs are a subpart of botanicals (Jiratchariyakul et al., 2013).

Being natural, Botanicals have become popular in recent years among consumers worldwide and maintaining top position of demand under food market. In most of the European countries, botanicals are considered under ingredients of food supplements and regulated by Food law, and in other countries; botanicals are taken as traditional medicine products, which are regulated under Drug law (Colombo et al., 2020). So the definition of Botanicals according to the European Safety Authority is "Botanicals means aromatic, medicinal, and cosmetic plants that can be used directly as such or processed in different forms to be included as food ingredients, food supplements, household products, cosmetics, animal feed, drugs, pesticides, medical devices, biological products and are regulated by different laws according to their use." Based on this definition by European legislation, products containing Botanicals are classified under three categories:

- Products regulated under pharmaceutical law such as conventional drugs, over the counter drugs, homeopathy, alternative medicine, and traditional medicine products.
- Products regulated under food law, such as fruits and vegetables, functional foods, traditional food, and food supplements.

- Other products, such as medical devices and formulations (Colombo et al., 2020).

So, botanicals cover a wide range of products concerned with maintenance & improvement in health and other purposes. According to a variety of functions, botanicals can use as well as prepare in different forms. These can be used either as such plant or its part in fresh or dried form, and the most common ways for preparation of botanicals include infusions, teas, tinctures, decoctions, and extract form. These are prepared by simple methods such as:

- Infusions and teas are made by addition of fresh or dry botanical in boiling water and let them steep for sufficient them. These can be consumed after filtering either hot or cold. An infusion is similar to tea but is a stronger preparation.
- A tincture can be prepared by soaking botanical in alcohol or water for a specified time. These are concentrated liquid preparation that can be preserved for further use. Tincture strength may vary according to drug and can be expressed as botanical to extract ratio (ratio of the weight of dried botanical used to the weight or volume of finished product).
- Some botanicals require more strong treatment to extract out the desired constituents. These botanicals are preferred to form in decoction form. For this, the raw material is added in water and brought to boil. Then it is allowed to heat for several minutes at lower heat. This long-time heating dissolves more constituents in water and gives a concentrated decoction that can be consumed either hot or cold.
- Botanicals can be prepared in the form of extract too. For this, the dry plant material is soaked in a particular solvent such as water or alcohol or other solvent suitable to the drug. The extract can be used after soaking either in concentrated liquid form or as dry extract for use in tablets and capsules.

These are some general methods to prepare botanicals. But botanicals can also be dispensed in form of modern medicine like tablets, capsules, ointment, soft gels, liquids, powders, gel caps, patches, etc., for different purposes (Kumadoh & Ofori-Kwakye, 2017).

14.1.1 DIETARY SUPPLEMENTS

Dietary supplements are the products that can supplement our diet and provide equal or more nutrients as compared. These are mostly obtained from natural sources so that they can be safe and have no side effects. Botanical dietary supplements, sometimes called herbals or herbal dietary supplements. These products are made from plants, plant parts, or plant extracts. They are meant to be consumed and contain one or more such ingredient that is meant to supplement the diet but not intended to replace a healthy diet. According to a nation wise survey by government, about 18% of adults are using natural dietary supplements.

Botanical dietary supplements are used in both traditional and complementary medicine. But to be considered under dietary supplement, a botanical must fulfill all the characteristics of the dietary supplement definition given by congress in "Dietary supplement Health and Education Act 1994." As per the act, a dietary supplement is a product (other than tobacco) that is intended to supplement the diet, and contains one or more ingredients that can be used in daily diet, such as vitamins, herbs, minerals, enzymes, amino acids, botanicals or their constituents and is intended to be taken by oral route as a pill, tablet, capsule, energy bars and drinks (Coppens et al., 2006).

So, botanical supplements are plants or plant parts used for medicinal purposes through the oral route of administration. These have medicinal benefits and may look like a drug, but these are regulated differently from pharmaceutical drugs. Generally, these are sold under the names like 'herbals,' 'herbal remedies,' and 'herbal medicines' or labeled as 'dietary supplement.' These all products do not require a lot of scientific research and testing to appear in the market for consumers. They even do not require approval from FDA as other drugs but FDA has the right to take legal action if any herbal supplement has received a sufficient number of side effects reports which describes the product as unsafe. The FDA can recommend withdrawal of that particular product from the market or to label it along with its side effects (Colombo et al., 2020). The following are some regulations according to Federal law regarding dietary supplements that should be considered before use:

- Every dietary supplement should be labeled as "dietary supplement," or as "calcium supplement," or "herbal supplement" that actually describes the dietary ingredient of that product.
- Dietary supplements do not require any safety approval from FDA before entering in market.
- According to law, a dietary supplement product label is not required to claim FDA's satisfaction that it is accurate from all points of view before this label is pasted on the product. Because the quantity of active ingredients is not similar in whole plant and a different method

of preparation (decoction, extraction, infusion, etc.) also results in quality variation. Sometimes herbs may contain some toxic elements, so it is difficult to claim the actual strength of herbal product.

- A dietary supplement product does not need prior approval from FDA, but its role starts after the product enters in the market. Because it is the FDA's duty to keep watch on any side effects or toxic/allergic symptoms appear after the product use. If any such case is reported, then FDA can take action against that product. Even FDA can prohibit misbranded or adulterated or spurious products.
- Federal Trade Commission has all the rights for promoting dietary supplements by advertising, exhibiting, and broadcasting on radio and television.
- FDA has certain rights to monitor safety issues regarding dietary supplements once they are in the market. It is mandatory for users, health care professionals and firms of dietary supplements to report any type of adverse reaction after use of product to the FDA. After this type of information, FDA has the right to review product information, composition mention on label, its packaging, prescribed doses and other indications related with product. FDA can stop product marketing till the case is resolved.
- It is required for any dietary supplement product before marketing to get certify from Consumer Laboratory (CL) for various evaluation parameters like product identity (authentic source), purity (free from adulterants), potency (amount of constituents/label composition) and consistency (similar product from one batch to another). The Consumer Lab certifies only the products that pass all standard tests.
- Legally, a dietary supplement product is not allowed to claim like "The product is useful in treatment of this particular disease or it is effective to reduce this disease symptom." A dietary supplement is only effective to maintain our general health and enhance immunity. These are not for treatment of any disease.
- FDA can validate the dietary supplement label claims as permitted by the resource mention. If a dietary supplement product is manufactured according to Pharmacopoeia or Formulary guidelines, then manufacture can mention on the label about it. But inclusion of these standard references does not certify about product efficacy and safety, but they only ensure that the product is manufactured according to these standards.

- Generally, herbs are not standardized for quality and quantity so the doses may vary from product to product and batch to batch. So, a label cannot ensure the accuracy of an herbal product (Coppens et al., 2006; Dwyer, Coates, & Smith, 2018).

14.2 REGULATIONS CHECK LIST FOR VARIOUS PRODUCTS

The Food and Drug Administration (FDA) is responsible for approval of all categories under food and drug products. The FDA has regulatory authority under the Federal Food, Drug, and Cosmetic Act as amended in 1994 by the Dietary Supplement Health and Education Act (DSHEA) and in 2006 by the Dietary Supplement and Non-prescription Drug Consumer Protection Act. According to DSHEA, Dietary supplements and food products are regulated by similar laws. The dietary supplement production is regulated on a federal level in the USA by Food and Drug Administration (FDA) and Federal Trade Commission (FTC) as well as by government agencies in each of the 50 states. Under FDA, both the raw material and finished product of Dietary supplements are considered. FDA has the full authority to withdraw such dietary supplement products that are adulterated or misbranded and can take legal action against these products and their manufacturers. Table 14.1 shows a checklist of various regulations under FDA & FTC for different products.

14.3 SAFETY ISSUES FOR DIETARY SUPPLEMENT

An herbal supplement is safe and can be used without medical advice, but it is not true always. There are a lot of reports available showing the ill effects of these products. So, care should be taken while consuming botanical supplement and following points to be kept in mind:

1. **Dietary Supplements are Not Claimed to Cure, Treat, Diagnose, or Lower the Symptoms of Diseases:** The supplements that are helpful in curing some diseases are generally referred to as Functional foods. Dietary supplements are not effective as vaccine to prevent any disease cause and symptoms. However, some supplements have the probability to reduce the risk of certain diseases, and it can be written on label with all indications. For example, supplement product containing Folic acid can claim to reduce the risk of brain and spinal cord birth defects.

TABLE 14.1 Regulations Check List for Various Products under FDA & FTC

FDA Regulated Products	Pre-Market Approval (FDA)	Pre-Market Notification (FDA)	Labeling (FDA)	Mandatory Adverse Event Reporting (FDA)	GMP's (FDA)	Facility Registration (FDA)	Advertising (FTC or FDA)
Foods	No	Yes	Yes	No	Yes	Yes	By FTC
Dietary supplements	No	Yes	Yes	Yes	Yes	Yes	By FTC
Drugs	Yes	No	Yes	Yes	Yes	Yes	By FDA
Biologics	Yes	No	Yes	Yes	Yes	Yes	By FDA
Medical devices	Yes	No	Yes	Yes	Yes	Yes	By FDA

2. **Improper Use of Supplements can be Risky:** It means if one is taking any previous treatment for a health problem, then he/she should not use dietary supplements before proper consultation with your doctor. Even a combination of two or more supplements may be life threatening.
3. **Unwanted Effects may be Caused by Some Dietary Supplements if Consumed Before, During, or After Surgery:** There are some side effects along with advantages of dietary supplements if used in different conditions. For example, Ginseng, Garlic, Vitamin E and *Ginkgo biloba* can cause bleeding; Kava and Valerian can cause sedation and enhance the effects of anesthetics during surgery. So, supplements should be informed to your surgeon before initiating surgery.
4. **These Are Not Recommended for All Health Problems:** As said, one cure is not for all because everybody system is different with different immunity level as well as strength. Likewise, a dietary supplement cannot be understood as safe and effective in all situations. A dietary supplement cannot be supplemented by conventional treatment for severe and chronic diseases like cancer, diabetes, depression, heart problems and hypertension. Herbs are always not prescribed for persons who may be immuno-compromised, kidney patients, with liver problems, undergone surgery or operations, pregnant or lactating women, or under age (below six years) children. So, dietary supplements should be recommended to persons according to their health situations (Mathur, 2018).

14.4 WHAT ARE THE DIFFERENT DIETARY SUPPLEMENTS?

Dietary supplements are meant to supplement our diet for various nutrients. So a dietary supplement is actually a different form of nutrition components that can strengthen our immune and body system in their own way. Here we are discussing about some dietary supplements with their role but type and dose of dietary supplement should be according to individual health condition and prescribed limit. The various dietary supplements are:

1. **Vitamins:** It is a vital nutrient required in limited quantity. These are not synthesized in sufficient amounts by the human body, so added in diet to cover the requirement. But vitamin supplements should be taken according to the body need. For example, a person who

is in direct contact with sun light for sufficient time, need not to take vitamin D supplement because his/her skin is synthesizing itself (Drouin, Godin, & Pagé, 2011). In general, a human being required 13 vitamins in their daily diet, i.e., vitamin A, B_1, B_2, B_3, B_5, B_6, B_7, B_9, B_{12}, C, D, E, and K. These all have different functions and show deficiency symptoms if not taken in adequate amount. But there are fixed dose levels for every vitamin in the form of upper intake levels (ULs) by the Institute of Medicine, USA. These ULs are the maximum tolerable amount for a vitamin (Fortmann, Burda, Senger, Lin, & Whitlock, 2013).

2. **Minerals:** These are exogenous elemental nutrients which are required in daily diet for various activities. The list of essential minerals for human include Potassium, Sodium, Phosphorus, Chlorine, Magnesium, Calcium, Manganese, Iron, Iodine, Zinc, Copper, Molybdenum, Cobalt, Chromiun, and Selenium. These are marketed as supplements, either individual or combined with vitamins. As vitamins, minerals should also be consumed according to adequate limit or recommended daily dose (Sicińska et al., 2020). They are helpful to stay healthy and reduce the risk of some diseases according to available studies, for example, calcium intake may decrease the risk of osteoporosis and Selenium intake may lower the risk of bladder cancer in females. But more studies are needed to prove these health claims (Zhang et al., 2020).
3. **Antioxidants:** An antioxidant as a dietary supplement is beneficial in lower down the unfavorable effects caused by free radicals, reactive nitrogen and reactive oxygen species on various metabolic activities in human. Dietary antioxidants are claimed to have magic power to maintain a healthy body and a long healthy life. These include Vitamin E, Flavonoid, Vitamin C, carotenoids, enzymes, and β-carotene. These all are generally obtained from vegetables and fruits. Free radicals which are produced as byproducts of the body's metabolic process can cause oxidative stress which is further responsible for many degenerative diseases related with aging. Antioxidants mainly protect our body's cells from the damage caused by free radicals (Salminen, Kauppinen, & Kaarniranta, 2014).
4. **Enzymes:** Digestive enzymes are capable of breaking larger molecules of Carbohydrates, lipids, and proteins into smaller digestible compounds. So, they are helpful to facilitate digestion of these nutrients followed by absorption. Naturally secreted digestive enzymes

include protease, lipase, and amylase for a breakdown of protein, lipid, and carbohydrate, respectively. Deficiency of these digestive enzymes may lead to digestive disorders and symptoms of stomach upset, flatulence, fullness, bloating, and belching. To prevent these problems, enzyme supplements are prescribed (Majeed et al., 2018). These exogenous enzymes are generally obtained from animals and studies are going on to obtain enzymes from micro-organisms and plants too (Ianiro, Pecere, Giorgio, Gasbarrini, & Cammarota, 2016).

5. **Amino Acids:** Essential Amino acids are also an important part of daily diet to maintain muscle strength and body immune function. These can regulate the metabolism of lipid & glucose and maintain an energy balance in the body. The essential amino acids supplements are helpful in the prevention of oxidative damage, body weight reduction, increase in synthesis of muscle protein and also promote skeletal & cardiac muscle mitochondrial biogenesis (Bifari et al., 2017). These work as building blocks for the body's proteins. The amino acids which are obtained from diet only and not synthesized in our body, are called essential amino acids, for example – leucine, isoleucine, histidine, valine, threonine, lysine, methionine, plenylalanine, and tryptophan (Dioguardi, 2011).
6. **Herbs and Extracts:** Botanicals are truly effective as dietary supplements. There is a long list available of herbs and extracts that have nutritional as well as health benefits like Spirulina, Ginseng, Green tea extract, Euphorbia extract, Fenugreek, Garlic, and many more. Use of these herbals for nutrition is popular from ancient time, and recent research have proven their health benefits too. In general, they overcome the nutrition deficiencies and help to maintain a healthy body. But care should be taken regarding quantity and combined use of these botanicals. According to traditional knowledge, herbs, and their extracts help to restore immunity, energy, spirit, and body for better health (van Breemen, 2015).
7. **Hormones:** The hormones produced by the body have an important role in growth & development. They maintain the immunity and also participate in animal reproduction. Hormones are produced endogenously from our body throughout the life. Some factors like genetics, diet, nutrition and stress level can affect hormone synthesis. Animal produces identical hormones to human; so food obtained from animal sources like meat, eggs, dairy products, and fish are good source of hormones. The naturally occurring plant hormones like phytoestrogens in food products are good for health

and comparatively safe. Phytoestrogens include lignans, isoflavones, coumestans, and phytoalexins. The main plant sources are legumes, soy products, vegetables, cereals, fruits, nuts, oilseeds, soy processed food and beverages (Palacios, Cortes, Jenks, & Maki, 2020).

8. **Homeopathic Products:** The homeopathic preparations are included in the category of "Drug" and claim to prevent or cure a disease, so these need approval from FDA before entering in market. Generally, these preparations contain small doses of natural active substances or herbs or part of herb, diluted with alcohol or water. Homeopathic medicine is based on the concept of "Like cure like" means what can cause symptoms in a healthy individual can treat the similar symptoms occurring in someone else who is unhealthy. Homeopathic preparations can heal the symptoms but not necessary that they can cure the whole disease. These preparations can cause toxic effects if taken in large amounts or not manufactured properly. As dietary supplements, these products should be used with care and thorough consultation with physician (Jonas, 2003) (Figure 14.1).

Each dietary supplement has its goods and beds. One should always discuss with your physician or any health expert before consuming them. If a person is under treatment for any complication, then it is mandatory to consult before taking a dietary supplement. These are not safe and effective for all in equal amount.

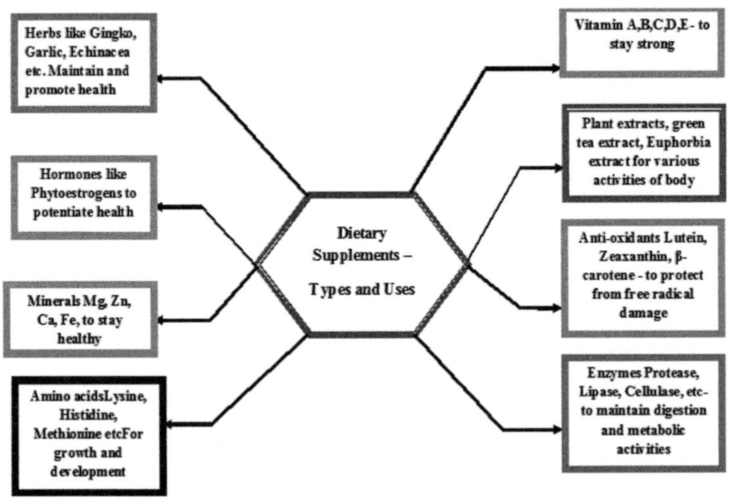

FIGURE 14.1 Different categories of dietary supplements and its health benefits.

14.5 BOTANICALS AS DIETARY SUPPLEMENTS

As we have studied earlier that dietary supplements includes a wide variety of products but still Botanicals play an important part as dietary supplement. Here we have included various studies carried out on different herbs to prove them as a dietary supplement.

14.5.1 ROLE OF SPIRULINA AS DIETARY SUPPLEMENT

Spirulina is considered as ‘Superfood’ because it provides all the nutrients including protein when consumed as a food supplement. Biologically it is a biomass of Cyanobacteria (Blue-Green algae) and can be consumed by both humans and animals. Its three species are *Arthrospira platensis*, *A. maxima,* and *A. fusiformis*. All three are used as food supplement. Spirulina can be used as a supplementary cure for malnutrition and many diseases. Its local production system works as a micronutrient complement and helps to overcome malnutrition. This gave a new rise in the development of industries for Spirulina production. According to a study carried out in Zaire from January to November 1989 on 28 children who were suffering from manifest protein-energy diseases, has shown positive effects of Spirulina on nutritional status (Mathur, 2018). The various bioactive molecules of Spirulina were studied for their beneficial effects (Table 14.2) (Bhat & Madyastha, 2000).

In one more study carried out in China, impact of Spirulina daily dose (1.5 g/day) was analyzed on health status of children and Spirulina was concluded beneficial for the same (Hassanen, Mahfouz, Farid, & Fadlullah, 2015).

TABLE 14.2 Beneficial Effects of Major Bioactive Molecules in Spirulina

Bioactive Compounds in Spirulina	Functions in Human Body
Chlorophyll, lutein	Cleansing (removal of free radicals)
β-Carotene, GLA	Protection and maintenance
Zeaxanthin	Antioxidant damage repair
C-phycocyanin (C-PC), proteins	Repair
Arginine	Hormonal balance

14.5.2 ROLE OF SOYBEAN AS DIETARY SUPPLEMENT

Soybean is an important legume of the family Leguminosae. Its scientific name is *Glycine max*. It is an important edible plant known for its seeds as a source of protein, oil, and nutraceuticals (Keservani et al., 20210a, b, 2020). Soybean contains a number of essential amino acids, carbohydrates, proteins, fats, and various secondary metabolites such as Flavones, isoflavones, phytic acids, saponins, phytosterols, peptides, and trypsin inhibitors. Soybean has been claimed for a number of health benefits, such as phytoestrogens decreases the risk of atherosclerosis by inhibiting LDL oxidation (Wiseman, 1999) and Isoflavones of Soybean are effective in diseases like cancer, bone health, menopause, obesity, cardiovascular, and diabetes (Bondesson & Gustafsson, 2010; Dixit, Antony, Sharma, & Tiwari, 2011; Kushwaha et al., 2014). Soybean is a rich source of Folic acid, which also increases its nutritional value. A number of Soy products are available for various health benefits (Shashank, Ramakrishna, Kiran, Kosturkova, & Ravishankar, 2015).

14.5.3 ROLE OF FLAX SEED AS DIETARY SUPPLEMENT

Flax is an annual herb of family Lineaceae. Scientifically it is known as *Linum usitassimum*. It is an herb with blue color flowers and golden yellow to reddish brown seeds. Its seeds are also known as Linseeds. It is cultivated for fiber as well as for medicinal and nutritional benefits (Tolkachev & Zhuchenko, 2004). It is rising as an beneficial nutritional food as it contains good amount of alpha-linolenic acid (ALA) 55%, high quality protein 28–30%, dietary fiber 35% and phytoestrogens/lignans (Carter, 1993; Rabetafika, Van Remoortel, Danthine, Paquot, & Blecker, 2011; Rubilar, Gutiérrez, Verdugo, Shene, & Sineiro, 2010). ALA is an essential polyunsaturated fatty acid and exhibits a number of activities like anti-thrombotic, anti-inflammatory, and anti-arrhythmic (Simopoulos 1999). Flaxseed is also a good source of omega-3 fatty acid, phenolic compounds and minerals. Seed and its oil can lower the growth of tumor at the later stage of cancer (Thompson, Rickard, Orcheson, & Seidl, 1996). Flaxseed is also effective as an antioxidant, hepatoprotective, and shows a significant reduction in level of LDL cholesterol and total serum cholesterol (Bhathena et al., 2003; Cunnane et al., 1993; Ridges et al., 2001). Due to presence of fibers Flaxseeds are used in the treatment of constipation, irritable bowel syndrome, lower the cholesterol level and regulate postprandial blood glucose level. Flaxseeds are available in the form of whole flaxseed, grounded, extracted oil, and mucilage. These are added as nutritional additives in a variety of dietary items and provide their health benefits (Kajla, Sharma, & Sood, 2015).

14.5.4 ROLE OF FENUGREEK AS DIETARY SUPPLEMENT

Fenugreek (Methi) is an important plant of family Leguminosae and named as *Trigonella foenum graecum*. Its leaves and seeds are famous for flavor & color in food and for a number of therapeutic properties such as antibacterial, hypocholesterolemic, gastric stimulant, lactation aid, antidiabetic, hepatoprotective, for anorexia, anticancer, and as galactagogue. Fenugreek generally contains 58% carbohydrates (of which dietary fibers are 25%), 23–26% protein, 6–7% of fat, good amount of iron & other minerals, vitamins, and phyto-constituent steroidal sapogenin. Methi is very helpful to improve digestion, and due to high fiber, gum, and protein content, it is also used as emulsifying agent, food stabilizer, and adhesive. Fenugreek seed, husk, and endosperm extract has shown 56%, 64% and 72% of antioxidant activity, respectively in free radical scavenging method (Naidu, Shyamala, Naik, Sulochanamma, & Srinivas, 2011). Fenugreek soluble dietary fiber content act as a good substrate for fermentation in the large intestine done by the microorganisms, so it acts as a probiotic in functional food products (Lee, 2009; Sowmya & Rajyalakshmi, 1999). The galactomannan composition of Fenugreek dietary fiber provides its utility in food industry as emulsifying agent and food stabilizer (Roberts, 2011; Wani & Kumar, 2016).

14.5.5 ROLE OF GINSENG AS DIETARY SUPPLEMENT

Ginseng root is commonly known for its two species *Panax ginseng* and *Panax quinquefolius*, belonging to the family Araliaceae. Ginseng contains a number of active plant constituents like ginsenosides, saponins, carbohydrates, phenolic compounds and carotenoids. These are responsible for various health benefits like antioxidant, antihyperglycemic, immunomodulator, anti-osteoporotic, anti-tumor, anti-infective, in respiratory problems and skin protecting. Ginseng has the power to alter both humoral and cellular immunity, so it is effective in the prevention of autoimmune disorders, infectious disease, cancer, allergy, in radiation protection, and as a vaccine adjuvant. According to a study, the anti-carcinogenic effect of Ginseng is due to increase in both number and action of natural killer cells (Lee, 2009). Polysaccharides found in Ginseng have been reported to improve radio sensitivity of osteo-sarcoma cells through an increase in autophagy and apoptosis (Zhang et al., 2017). Ginseng and its ginsenosides show anti-malarial effect by inhibiting the growth of *Plasmodium yoelii* in mice and boosting immunity (Han et al., 2011). So, Ginseng is having a lot of health benefits and is available in different forms for various purposes (Riaz, Rahman, Zia-Ul-Haq, Jaffar, & Manea, 2019).

14.5.6 ROLE OF GINKGO BILOBA AS DIETARY SUPPLEMENT

It is an ancient plant and also known as 'Living fossil.' It belongs to family Ginkgoaceae. Its main active constituents include terpenoids (Ginkgolides and Bilobalides), Flovonol glycosides (Quercetin and Catechin) and proanthocyanidins (Brondino et al., 2013). Its leaves are mainly used in supplements and for memory & thought problems. Ginkgo is used as a supplement for brain health and good memory. It comes in the form of extracts, tea, tablet, and capsules. Along with dementia, Ginkgo is also useful in eye problems (glaucoma), tinnitus, blood pressure problems and leg pain. Some prescribe it for benefit in depression, cancer, schizophrenia, and others, but fewer evidence is available to prove it (Kortubash et al., 2020).

14.5.7 ROLE OF GARLIC AS DIETARY SUPPLEMENT

Garlic (Lehsun) is also one of the oldest medicines of the world and has been used not only for its strong flavor but also for multiple health benefits. Scientifically it is known as *Allium sativum* and belongs to the family Liliaceae. Traditionally, garlic has been suggested for various therapeutic activities by different naturalists and researchers, such as in gastric disorders, asthma, dog & snake bites, convulsions, uterine tumors and as laxative, vermifuge & diuretic. Its activity is due to presence of organo-sulfur compounds Alliin and Allicin. Its supplements are sold in form of powder and granules. These do not contain Allicin because it is very unstable. Allicin is actually produced when garlic powder is added to water then alliin and allinase enzyme reacts. Now a number of garlic health benefits have been examined and proved such as Antiparasitic, antimicrobial, antiviral, anti-inflammatory, anticarcinogenic, cholesterol lowering, anti-thrombotic, antidiabetic, and antioxidant (Touloupakis & Ghanotakis, 2010).

14.5.8 ROLE OF ECHINACEA AS DIETARY SUPPLEMENT

Echinacea purpurea (Coneflower) is mainly known for its health benefits. It is a member of the Daisy family or Compositae or Asteraceae. It is most widely used in the treatment of the common cold due to its immune stimulatory effect. In form of supplement, it is available as Echinacea extract, dried pressed juice, freeze dried extracts, leaves, and flowers either as whole or in powder form. It is considered as an immune modulator after various searches. Other effects includes like anti-oxidant, anti-inflammatory, anti-fungal, anti-viral, anti-cancer, and anti-infective in respiratory problems (Barrett, 2003).

14.5.9 ROLE OF GREEN TEA AS DIETARY SUPPLEMENT

Green tea extract is commonly used as a dietary supplement for the purpose of weight management. It is becoming a very popular natural remedy for weight loss. It contains lesser amount of caffeine which helps the body to burn out more calories. It is also believed that green tea is effective as an antioxidant and can help to reduce the risk of cancer too. As it causes a balancing weight, so also helps in arthritis and joint pain, low the cholesterol level and improve blood circulation. But it can cause some side effects like stomach upset, vomiting, and if taken in large amounts, it can cause cardio and hepatic toxicity. So Green tea should always be used in justified amount to gain health benefit (Kortubash et al., 2020).

So, there are a lot of botanicals used as dietary supplements, but care should be taken in their use. FDA is providing data from time to time regarding any side effects or any health issues related to a dietary supplement. For example, FDA has considered some herbs as toxic such as Kava, Lobelia, Ephedra, Willow bark, Magnolia, Comfrey, and Aristolochic. FDA has reported warning signs on the use of these herbs with their possible side effects.

14.6 DIETARY FIBER

'Dietary fiber is defined as a polysaccharide containing 10 or more units of monomers which is not hydrolyzed by endogenous hormones in the small intestine.' This was defined by the World Health Organization (WHO) and Food and Agriculture Organization (FAO) along with the American Association of Cereal Chemists (AACC) (Camire & FLINT, 1991). Dietary fiber has also become an important component of our daily diet not only for its benefit in constipation problem but also due to other health benefits such as lowering the risk of heart disease, diabetes, cancer, and weight management. So, fibers are very good for health. These are found in many fruits, vegetables, legumes, and whole grains. Fibers are not digested by our food canal, but it passes as such in excreta that's why increases the bulk (Roberts, 2011). The general properties of Dietary fiber can be lined as:

- They reduce the total or LDL Cholesterol levels in blood;
- These have the capacity to be fermented by micro-flora of colon;
- They can reduce intestinal transit time and increase bulk of stool;
- They can lower the postprandial blood glucose level;
- Along with carbohydrate, they also include Lignin (A phenolic compound) if it is present naturally in plant-based food (from broccoli as fiber).

Fibers can broadly be classified on the basis of its composition of monosaccharide, attached specific sugar groups, emergence, chemical properties, solubility, gelling, and fermenting capacity. In general, fibers are broadly classified into two groups, as discussed in the following subsections.

14.6.1 SOLUBLE FIBER

These are water-soluble, well-fermented, and form a gel-like structure. These are helpful in maintaining blood sugar and cholesterol level. Various examples of soluble fibers containing items are carrots, peas, beans, citrus fruits, apples, oats, psyllium, and barley. Examples are gums, non-cellulosic polysaccharides, oligosaccharides, pectin, β-glucans, and mucilages.

14.6.2 INSOLUBLE FIBER

These are water insoluble, less fermented and generally encourage the movement of material from the digestive canal and increase the bulk of stool. So, it is helpful in prevention or relief from constipation. Examples of insoluble fiber containing food items are wheat bran, whole wheat flour, beans, nuts, green beans, cauliflower, and potatoes. Examples are lignin, cellulose, and hemicellulose (Antia, 1973; Murniece et al., 2011).

14.6.3 IMPORTANT COMPONENTS OF DIETARY FIBERS

Fibers have a wide variety of basic components. A detail about some important components of fibers is given in Table 14.3.

TABLE 14.3 Important Components of Dietary Fibers

SL. No.	Fiber Components	Type and Source	Applications	Mode of Action	References
1.	Arabinoxylan	Soluble fiber made of hemicellulose comprised of xylose backbone with side chains of arabinose, found in whole grains	Lowers blood glucose level	Slows down the rate of glucose absorption	Lu, Walker, Muir, & O'Dea (2004); Lu, Walker, Muir, Mascara, & O'Dea (2000)
2.	Inulin	Polymer of fructose monomers and is present in onions, garlic, wheat, artichokes, and bananas	Functional food ingredient	Nutritional properties	Lattimer & Haub (2010)
			Prebiotic	By restricting the growth of pathogenic bacteria	Gibson, Beatty, Wang, & Cummings (1995)
			Treat obesity	Due to short chain fatty acids and GLP-1 production	Cani, Joly, Horsmans, & Delzenne (2006)
			Increased calcium absorption	Through enhancement of vitamin D	Abrams et al. (2005); Griffin, Hicks, Heaney, & Abrams (2003)
			Decreased total serum cholesterol and LDL	Favors propionate production	Amaral, Morgan, Stephen, & Whiting (1992)
3.	β-glucan	Linear polysaccharide of glucose monomers and available in the endosperm of cereal grains, primarily barley and oats. A type of soluble fiber	Decrease in serum total and LDL cholesterol	Due to propionate production	Kim & White (2009, 2010); Naumann et al. (2006); Theuwissen & Mensink (2007)
			Lowers postprandial glucose and insulin level	Due to high viscosity and gelation property	Nazare et al. (2009)

TABLE 14.3 *(Continued)*

SL. No.	Fiber Components	Type and Source	Applications	Mode of Action	References
4.	Pectin	Linear polymer of galacturonic acid, water-soluble polysaccharide, found in citrus fruits peel	As gelling or thickening agent	–	Camire & Flint (1991)
			Cancer prevention	Due to binding of Pectin to galectin-3 and inhibiting tumor growth	Nangia-Makker et al. (2002)
			Reduction in acute intestinal infections and diarrhea	Increase growth of health friendly bacteria in large intestine	Olano-Martin, Gibson, & Rastall (2002); Rabbani et al. (2001); Triplehorn & Millard (2002)
			Improved cholesterol and lipid metabolism	Due to gelling property	Brown, Rosner, Willett, & Sacks (1999)
5.	Bran	Outermost layer of a cereal grain and consists of the nucellar epidermis, seed coat, pericarp, and aleurone	Lower serum total cholesterol level, LDL cholesterol and triglycerides.	Due to an increase in bile acid synthesis and decreased absorption of fat from the small intestine	Qureshi, Sami, & Khan (2002); Zhang et al. (1994)
			Lowers postprandial glucose level	Due to the high arabinoxylan content	Ulmius, Johansson, & Önning (2009)
6.	Cellulose	Water insoluble fiber. Linear chain of β(1→4) linked glucose monomers. It is a structural component of cell walls in green plants and vegetables	Modified cellulose shows decrease in postprandial glucose level and significant reduction in total and LDL cholesterol	Increased intestinal viscosity delays nutrient absorption and increases bile acid excretion	Maki et al. (2009); Maki et al. (2000)
7.	Resistant starch	As a starch, it is not digested in the small intestine	Shows all health benefits of dietary fiber/whole grain with the sensory feel of refined carbohydrates	–	Higgins (2004)

14.7 HEALTH BENEFITS OF FIBER DIET

A rich fiber diet is very beneficial for health, and to gain more benefit, we should eat a wide variety of foods containing fibers. Some important benefits from fibers are the following:

- Fibers help in lowering blood cholesterol level by lowering the amount of low-density lipoprotein (Brum, Ramsey, McRorie, Bauer, & Kopecky, 2018).
- Fibers are useful for smooth bowel movement. They increase the bulk of stool and make it easy to pass. If the stool is quite loose, then fiber absorbs water to solidify it and make it easy to pass (Johnson, 2004).
- Fibers help in controlling blood sugar level in diabetic patients. The soluble fibers mainly help in lowering blood sugar by decreasing its absorption and insoluble fibers may reduce the risk of type-2 diabetes (Hvidtfeldt et al., 2010).
- Fibers can be used to achieve a healthy weight because high fiber food takes more time to eat and give the feeling of a full stomach. High fiber diet gives fewer calories for the less volume of food.
- Some fibers are suggested to prevent various colon diseases like hemorrhoids and colorectal cancer (Song et al., 2018).
- Fibers play important role in maintaining an overall healthy living because of good digestion and lower risk of life-threatening diseases like heart problems and cancers.
- According to some studies, dietary fiber can interact with the phenolic compounds and help in execution of antioxidant effect jointly as antioxidant dietary fiber. Phenolic compounds bind to fiber components, which protect them from digestive enzymes and take to the microbiota in intact form, where these phenolic compounds can show antioxidant effect.

So, taking a good fiber diet is very essential but in the same way excess of fiber intake may cause problems like intestinal gas, abdominal cramps and bloating. That's why a daily dose of fiber is recommended by the Institute of Medicine as not more than 38 grams for men of the age 50 or younger and 30 grams for men of age 51 or older. For women not more than 25 grams of fiber daily up to the age 50 or younger and 21 grams daily at the age 51 or older (Lattimer & Haub, 2010).

14.8 FIBER SUPPLEMENTS

In general, fiber dose can be satisfied from daily intake of fruits, vegetables, and whole grains but some may need a fiber supplement too due to health issues and problems like improper digestion, constipation, irritable bowel syndrome, and other bowel problems. Actually, the term fiber supplement is used for the fiber products that can help in fulfillment of low dietary fiber consumption in daily diet from natural genuine sources. To cover this requirement, one should be prescribed for fiber supplements either natural or artificial. The various fiber supplements available are:

i. **From Natural Sources:** β-glucan, Psyllium, wheat bran and Inulin.
ii. **From Artificial Sources:** Methyl cellulose (obtained by wood pulp chemical treatment), Wheat dextrin (obtained from wheat starch by acid or heat treatment) and Polydextrose (obtained from polymerization of Glucose and Sorbitol).

14.9 HEALTH BENEFITS OF FIBER SUPPLEMENTS

Fiber supplements are used to satisfy the low fiber daily diet and it is assumed to have equal health benefits as dietary fiber have. But according to many clinical studies it has been proved that the fiber supplements with specific properties like solubility and viscous gel forming capacity. So, fiber supplements can be divided in four categories for clinical efficacy on the basis of the following characteristics:

- Solubility (soluble in water/about 70% solubility or not);
- Rate of fermentation (Degradation by gut bacteria and production of short chain fatty acids and gas as fermentation byproducts);
- Gelling capacity (Ability of fiber to form a cross-linked viscoelastic gel upon hydration); and
- Degree of viscosity (fibers to be viscous/thick when hydrated).

On the basis of these properties' fiber supplements are of four subtypes (Figure 14.2). According to clinical studies on fiber supplements, it was suggested that many fiber supplements are not as effective as dietary fiber; only a few, like Psyllium has shown all general benefits of fibers. So, one should take fiber supplements after consulting with a dietician or after thorough investigation for its efficacy. It is always better to consume natural fibers available in fruits, vegetables, and whole grains as such.

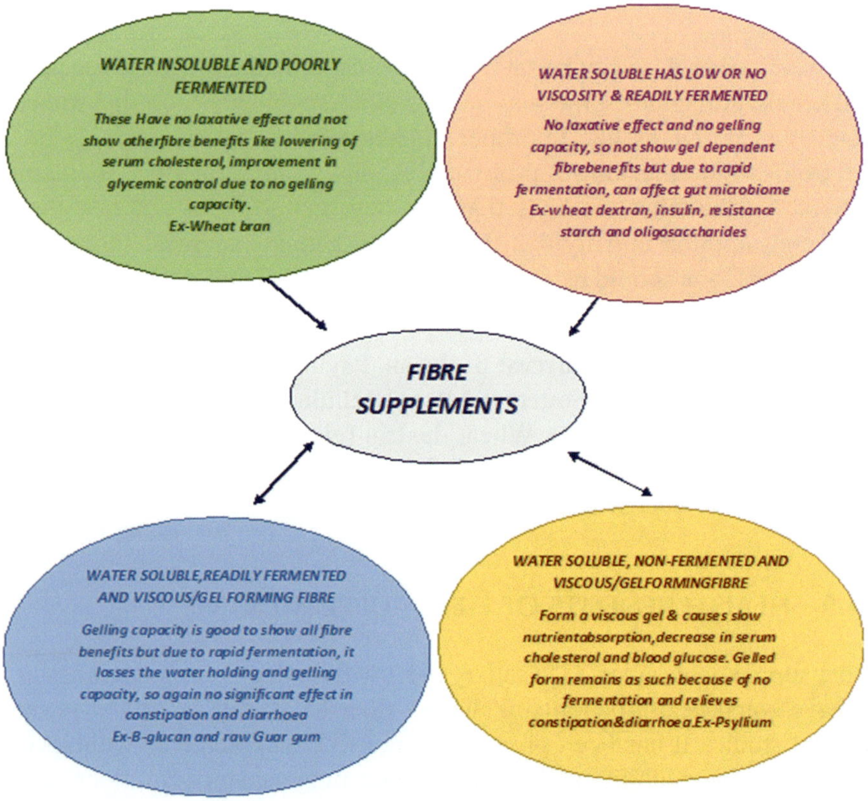

FIGURE 14.2 Various types of fiber supplements as clinical efficacy.

14.10 BOTANICALS AS DIETARY FIBERS

14.10.1 BROCCOLI

It is a member of the Cruciferae (Brassicaceae) family. Its scientific name is *Brassica oleracea*and like other vegetable of the family; it is rich in nutritional components and dietary fibers. Its bioactive components include phenolic compounds, glucosinolates, isothiocynates, vitamin C, folic acid, Vitamin K, minerals, and free sugars. The edible part of Broccoli contains about 89.3% of water, 2.82% protein, 3.29% total dietary fiber (3.00% insoluble and 0.29% soluble), 6.64% carbohydrates and 0.37% of fat. According to studies carried out, 5 g of fiber in one cup of broccoli is sufficient to support the bacteria present in the gut and makes it healthy and well balanced (Li et al., 2009; Zhang et al., 2015). Beside a dietary product, Broccoli has been found effective as antimicrobial, anti-diabetic, gastroprotective, cardioprotective, anti-inflammatory, anti-obesity, and immunomodulatory. Its glucosinolates and isothiocynates are effective as anti-cancer compound. It is recommended in the treatment of xerophthalmia, scurvy, and anemia due to its component's vitamin A, C, and folic acid, respectively (from fiber review). Not only the main broccoli flower, its leaves are highly nutritious and contain high amount of dietary fiber and phenolic compounds (Side streams of broccoli). According to a recent study, if broccoli florets are consumed with high fat diet, they it ameliorates insulin sensitivity shown by reduced serum insulin and homeostasis model assessment (HOMA)-IR index. Broccoli florets also promoted diversity of gut microbiota and low-grade strains related with inflammation.

14.10.2 BEANS

Beans are a good source of dietary fiber in the form of salad, soup, and stews. It includes many types, such as green beans, soybean, kidney beans, white beans, and lima beans. The following is approximate value of total dietary fiber (g/100 g of edible portion) present in beans like Soybean contains 15 g, Green beans 1.9 g, Kidney beans 6.3 g, White beans 17.7 g and Lima beans 4.2 g (from dietary fiber review). Along with fiber, beans have a number of nutrients like proteins, amino acid Lysine, resistant starch, polyphenols, folic acid, potassium, iron, magnesium, and zinc. A form of steamed soybean known as Edamame is a better source for fiber and protein. A half cup of Edamame provides about 9 gm of fiber. Beans are now added in bakery products due to fiber and protein content (Belghith-Fendri et al., 2016). According to a study carried out, if bean diet (Bean as fiber intake) is significantly increase by 75%, it causes an increase in satiety and also reduce feeling of hunger. The effect of bean diet was found similar to a standard diet, and it is tolerable as well as acceptable. It suggests the use of dry beans fiber in diet for weight loss (Turner et al., 2013). As per result of various clinical studies, beans are helpful in reducing blood glucose level in both normal and diabetic individuals, increasing HDL-cholesterol level, decrease energy intake, blood pressure control and low mortality risk due to its high fiber content and other active constituents (Messina, 2014).

14.10.3 AVOCADOS

Avacado (*Persea americana*) fruit contains monounsaturated fatty acids, dietary fiber, many phytochemicals and essential nutrients. As per a report, avocado contains 5.23±0.53 g soluble dietary fiber and 11.3±0.71 g of insoluble dietary fiber on a dry weight basis per 100 g of edible portion. Under insoluble fiber category, hemicellulose is found in highest amount (Hirasawa et al., 2008). The various benefits associated with avocado consumption include low body weight, waist circumference and BMI; higher HDL-cholesterol level and low risk of metabolic disorders (Sunguya et al., 2013). Avacados can be taken with toast, eggs, sauces, pizzas, and others. It can be eaten as salad and as a whole. Along with fibers, Avocados are also known for its heavy fat content. One cup of Avocado can serve 10 g of fiber. Avocados is also helpful to increase absorption of carotenoids from food, lycopene, and β-carotene from salsa, α-carotene, β-carotene, and lutein from salad, β-carotene from raw carrots and tomato sauce and also increase the bioconversion efficiency of β-carotene to vitamin A. So, it is beneficial for our eyes and brain health. This effect of avocado is due to presence of monounsaturated fatty acids (Ford & Liu, 2020).

14.10.4 BERRIES

Consumption of whole fruits is beneficial not only for nutritional purpose but also for a healthy body. The recommended daily intake of fruits is different for all age groups, such as for children of 2–8 years 1 to 1.5 cups, for adolescent boys and girls 1.5 cups, for men 2 cups and for women 1.5 to 2 cups. All of the barriers like Blueberries, raspberries, strawberries, and Blackberries are great store of fiber. The amount of fiber components is varying according to the type and quantity of berry consumed. As an estimation, one cup (144 g) of blackberries contains 5.3 g/100 g of total fiber (4.7 g insoluble and 0.6 g soluble), one cup (148 g) of blueberries contains 2.8 g/100 g of total fiber (2.4 g insoluble and 0.3 g soluble), one cup (152 g) of strawberries contains 2.0 g/100 g of total fiber (1.5 g insoluble and 0.5 g soluble), one cup (123 g) of raspberries contains 6.5 g/100 g of total fiber (5.3 g insoluble and 1.2 g soluble) and one by four cup (40 g) of cranberries contains 7.5 g/100 g of total fiber (5.0 g insoluble and 2.5 g soluble). They are also effective as antioxidant. Pectin which is a major fiber prebiotic component form approximate 35% of fruit cell wall. It is extensively studied and proved effective to promote healthy and anti-inflammatory colonic microflora ecosystem with more microbiota diversity in comparison to Inulin (Dreher, 2018). Berries contain many bioactive compounds along with fiber like polyphenols & flavonoids (Keservani & Sharma, 2014) including ellagitannins and anthocyanins. Because of good amount of soluble fiber portion, berries, and other fruits are considered superior to cereals for nutritional values (Alba, Campbell, & Kontogiorgos, 2019). These have low calories so easy to digest and good for health (Heyman et al., 2014).

14.10.5 WHOLE GRAINS

Whole grains are defined as the grains in which its anatomical components like germ, bran, and endosperm are present in the same proportions as in the intact kernel, but non-edible parts like husk and hull are removed. Wheat, rice, and oats are good source of fiber when consumed as whole grain. These are main food ingredients and are available in a number of bakery and homemade products like whole wheat bread, brown rice, whole wheat pasta and oats. According to FDA, a food product to be considered as real whole grain should be labeled whole grains as the first ingredient (Jonnalagadda et al., 2011; McKeown et al., 2010). Whole grains are more complex in comparison to refined grains and are considered as a healthier and sustainable diet because of their indigestible carbohydrates components, i.e., dietary fibers. More consumption of whole grains is recommended for everyone because they decrease the incidence and mortality risk from type-2 diabetes, cancer, and cardiovascular diseases (Keservani et al., 2016a). They can also improve the microbial flora of the digestive canal. But along with consumption of whole grain in daily diet, one should follow a healthy and physically active lifestyle to obtain more benefits (Seal, Courtin, Venema, & de Vries, 2021). Wheat contains about 9–20% of dietary fiber content on a dry weight basis; oat contains 10–37%, Barley 10–27% and Rice 3–10% of dietary fiber content. Wheat grains are rich in arabinoxylan fiber and oats & barley dietary fiber mainly contains β-glucan. Grains health benefits also depend upon their main fiber component (Joye, 2020).

14.10.6 APPLES

Apples are always said to be good for health due to its nutrition property and fiber amount. Everyone likes to eat apple any time as a healthy food. Apples contain many anti-oxidant phytochemicals like catechin, quercetin, phloridzin, and chlorogenic acid. Many epidemiological studies have shown the health benefits of apples as anticancer, anti-diabetic, anti-asthmatic, and in treatment of cardiovascular diseases. It also helps in down the cholesterol level, decrease lipid oxidation and protects our arteries (Iqbal, Khan, & Khattak, 2004). In general, an apple can provide 4 g of dietary fiber, but it depends upon apple size. The amount of dietary fiber in an apple depends upon its maturity stage too. Fiber components may vary till the ripening of fruit (Keservani et al., 2016b).

14.10.7 POPCORN

Popcorn is being liked by every age group as a tasty and light snack. Popcorn (Zea mays L.) is well known for its high fiber and phenolic content (mainly contains Ferulic acid). The popcorn pericarp is quite hard and not as porous as the other types of maize pericarps. This allows the popcorn to pop on heating because the water present inside turns to convert in steam and the hull start bursting. Popcorn has a very good antioxidant potential as compared to other grains. Due to ferulic acid content, popcorn has been found effective in reduction of the risk for heart disease, diabetes, and hypertension. Even the popped popcorn contains a similar amount of phenolic constituents, so popping does not affect its quality. According to a study, popcorn is 1.6 times more satiating as compared to potato chips which may increase oxidative stress and inflammation due to high acrylamide content (Nguyen et al., 2012). So, whole grain popcorn is an excellent choice for those who wants to reduce feeling of hunger and manage their energy intake which ultimately reduce the body weight (Coco & Vinson, 2019). Simple popcorn is better for health rather than with butter or other modifications. It is a type of whole grain with full of fiber. One cup of popcorn can provides one gram of fiber. Popcorn is also considered as the king of snack foods.

14.10.8 POTATOES

Potatoes are generally classified as 'starch containing vegetables' because their main macronutrient is Starch (A polysaccharide). Potatoes also contain a small proportion of resistant starch that does not degrade by enzymes in the small intestine. It enters in large intestine as such and is fermented by microflora to produce short chain fatty acids which are effective to lower gut pH, lower the toxic level of ammonia and promote the growth of colonic bacteria. The resistant starch may increase satiety and helps to control blood glucose and blood lipid level. With resistant starch, potatoes also contain a good amount of dietary fiber, about 2 g in 5.3 oz. Potato, found in both the skin and flesh of potato. As per a study result, more than 16% of fiber intake was associated with white potatoes for six groups of female consumers out of eight groups and similarly, more than 20% of fiber intake for six groups of male potato consumers out of 8 groups (Beals, 2019). Various types of potatoes like red potatoes, white potatoes, sweet potatoes and purple potatoes have good amount of fiber. Simple boiled or baked potatoes are better food rather than fried potatoes. About 3 g of fiber is obtained from one small potato with peel. The potatoes fiber helps to protect our food canal from harmful chemicals added during preparation of processed food (Dobrowolski et al., 2012; King & Slavin, 2013).

14.10.9 DRIED FRUITS

Dried fruits (raisins, dates, prunes, and figs) are preferred for their sweetness and long-term stability profile. Traditional dried fruits are defined as the fruits from which some extent of moisture has been removed and have no added sugar. These are rich source of fiber & potassium and also contain sugar, protein, calcium, Magnesium, carotenoids, and total phenols. For example, dates contain 6.7 g of fiber, 75 g carbohydrates, 66.5 g sugar, 1.8 g protein, 64 mg calcium, 54 mg Magnesium, 696 mg potassium, 112 mg carotenoids and 572 mg GAE total phenols per 100 g. Likewise figs contain 9.8 g fiber and raisins contain 3.7 g of fiber per 100 g of dried fruit. Raisins are highest consuming dried fruit and can be added to different food products like muffins, cookies, breads, and cereals. Daily, a balance intake of dried fruits can significantly lower the body weight, waist circumference, BMI, and sub-scapular skinfold measurements. Dried fruits also provide the nutritional benefits of fiber, minerals like calcium, iron, potassium, magnesium, zinc, copper and phosphorus and vitamins (Singh et al., 2017a) like A, C, E, riboflavin, thiamine, folate and Niacin (Carughi et al., 2015; Sadler et al., 2019). Dried fruits also help in the treatment of constipation problem because they cause easy bowel movement and give more comfort due to presence of Sorbitol sugar. But more intakes of dry fruits can cause stomach upset and diarrhea problem, so a limited amount is preferred for good digestion.

14.10.10 NUTS

Nuts are defined as dry fruits having one seed in which the ovary wall hardens on maturity. The popular edible nuts are almonds, walnuts, pistachios, hazelnuts, cashews, peanuts, and pine nuts. Nuts are often eaten as whole (fresh/roasted), as snacks, a part of meal, desserts, in spreads like peanut butter and almond paste, added in commercial food products like ice-creams, pastries, mixed dishes, bakery items and sauces; and as oils too (Kendall, Esfahani, Truan, Srichaikul, & Jenkins, 2010). Nuts are good source of dietary fiber, protein (Singh et al., 2017b), vitamins, Potassium, phytosterols, phenolic compounds, monounsaturated (oleic acid) and polyunsaturated (Linoleic and Linolenic acid) fatty acids. Consumption of nuts have proven many health benefits like low risk of cardio-vascular disease, regulation of blood glucose level, regulation of inflammation & endothelial function markers, low cancer mortality risk, and other metabolic disorders. Nuts contain dietary fiber in range from 4–11 g per 100 g. One serving of nuts is sufficient to provide 3 g of fiber. These should be eaten as raw or dry-roasted form to get high benefit (Ostadrahimi et al., 2014).

There are many other fruits and vegetables that contain a good amount of dietary fiber, only some important have been discussed here with their health benefits.

14.11 VARIOUS HEALTH CLAIMS FOR DIETARY FIBER WITH POSSIBLE MODE OF ACTION

There are a lot of health benefits from dietary fibers that have been proved by research. The dieticians and scientists working on fibers have claimed many possible activities of fibers with their mode of action. Some claims are still under investigation by approval agencies like FDA, but some are approved by FDA with their mechanism of action. Table 14.4 is a brief description of these claims and their approval status.

Both dietary supplement and dietary fiber are good for health and make us internally strong enough to fight against various diseases. These are easily available products, but precaution is mandatory as unjustified and over use can put us in great trouble.

TABLE 14.4 Various Health Claims for Dietary Fiber with Possible Mode of Action

SL. No.	Health Claims for Dietary Fiber	Approved by FDA	Possible Mode of Actions
1.	Increased consumption of dietary fiber with decreased consumption of fat (less than 30% of calories) may reduce risk of some cancers (Esposito et al., 2003).	Yes	Dietary fiber can resist fat digestion in small intestine and allowing it enter in large intestine as such, here it is fermented in short chain fatty acids which are effective against cancer (Young, Hu, Le Leu, & Nyskohus, 2005).
			Dietary fiber can increase the bulk and viscosity of feces and stop it to contact with mucosal cells (Adlercreutz et al., 1987).
			Dietary fiber can increase the binding between bile acids and carcinogens (Adlercreutz et al., 1987).
			Dietary fiber stimulates antioxidant production (Adlercreutz et al., 1987).
			Dietary fiber can enhance excretion of estrogen with feces to inhibit its absorption in the intestine (Adlercreutz et al., 1987).
2.	High fiber in diet with low saturated fat (less than 10% of calories) and cholesterol, decreases the risk of various coronary heart diseases like hypertension, hypercholesterolemia, obesity, and type-2 diabetes. Every 10 g of fiber is efficient to decrease the mortality risk of CHD by 17–35% (Hvidtfeldt et al., 2010; Streppel, Ocké, Boshuizen, Kok, & Kromhout, 2008).	Yes	Soluble dietary fiber can increase the rate of bile excretion and thus reducing serum total and LDL cholesterol (Story, Furumoto, & Buhman, 1997).
			Fiber causes the production of short chain fatty acid like propionate and it inhibits cholesterol synthesis (Amaral et al., 1992).
			Fiber reduces the risk of type-2 diabetes either through low energy intake or glycemic control (Esposito et al., 2003).

TABLE 14.4 *(Continued)*

SL. No.	Health Claims for Dietary Fiber	Approved by FDA	Possible Mode of Actions
			Dietary fiber regulates energy intake and thus encourages weight loss or maintains the optimum body weight.
			Fiber reduces pro-inflammatory cytokines such as interleukin-18 which shows plaque stability (Esposito et al., 2003).
			High fiber intake decreases the level of CRP (C-reactive protein), which act as a marker of inflammation and as a predictor for CHD (Ma et al., 2006).
3.	Increase in intake of dietary fiber causes a decrease in body weight (Tucker & Thomas, 2009).	No	Soluble fibers produce two gut hormones glucogon-like peptide (GLD-1) and peptide YY (PYY) after fermentation in the large intestine and these hormones play a role in inducing satiety (Keenan, Doria, Aiello, & King, 2006).
			Dietary fiber cause significant decrease in energy intake (Tucker & Thomas, 2009).
			Dietary fiber may reduce diet metabolizable energy which is gross energy minus the energy lost in the urine, feces, and combustible gases. It results in a decrease in fat digestibility (Baer, Rumpler, Miles, & Fahey, 1997).
4.	Dietary fiber can reduce the risk of type-2 diabetes, and this effect does not depend on other factors like family history, age, smoking, fat intake, alcohol, exercise, and others (Meyer et al., 2000; Schulze et al., 2004).	No	Insoluble dietary fiber intake can accelerate the secretion of glucose dependent insulin tropic polypeptide (GIP) and it stimulates postprandial insulin release (Weickert et al., 2005).
			Insoluble dietary fiber causes a reduction in appetite and food intake (Samra & Anderson, 2007).

TABLE 14.4 *(Continued)*

SL. No.	Health Claims for Dietary Fiber	Approved by FDA	Possible Mode of Actions
			Insoluble fiber produces short chain fatty acids which have reduced postprandial glucose response (Brighenti et al., 1995; Östman, Liljeberg Elmståhl, & Björck, 2002).
			Soluble dietary fiber causes a delay in gastric emptying and decrease absorption of macronutrients. So this results in lower postprandial blood glucose and insulin level (Jenkins et al., 1978). But according to some studies, there is no correlation between soluble fiber intake and reduced risk of type-2 diabetes (Meyer et al., 2000; Montonen, Knekt, Järvinen, Aromaa, & Reunanen, 2003; Schulze et al., 2004).

14.12 CONCLUSION

Botanicals are extensively used in the form of dietary supplements and dietary fibers throughout the world. These are available in an easily administered form for all age groups. These both come under the category of food articles, so they are free from FDA regulations before entering the market. But it is under FDA control to warn or ban any product if it causes any side effects or toxic symptoms. These are an important part of our routine food items, but it is mandatory to check for any possible side effects. One should not overuse these botanicals because quantity out of limit can be serious. So always follow the label claims and dose before taking. Meaningful use of botanicals is always good for a healthy body.

14.13 FUTURE PROSPECTIVE

- The demand for Botanicals as a dietary supplement and dietary fiber is increasing day by day. So, it emphasizes a more healthy population with a lesser risk of diseases.

- Botanicals need more standardization in terms of quality and quantity.
- One should be aware when starting any dietary supplement if he/she is under medication or has already taken any other botanical for the same purpose.
- It is the moral duty of everyone to inform the authority about any side effects or toxic symptoms caused due to the use of a dietary supplement or dietary fiber diet.

KEYWORDS

- **alpha-linolenic acid**
- **botanicals**
- **dietary fibers**
- **dietary supplements**
- **FDA regulations**
- **fiber components**

REFERENCES

Abrams, S. A., Griffin, I. J., Hawthorne, K. M., Liang, L., Gunn, S. K., Darlington, G., & Ellis, K. J., (2005). A combination of prebiotic short-and long-chain inulin-type fructans enhances calcium absorption and bone mineralization in young adolescents. *The American Journal of Clinical Nutrition, 82*(2), 471–476.

Adlercreutz, H., Hämäläinen, E., Gorbach, S., Goldin, B., Woods, M., Brunson, L. S., & Dwyer, J., (1987). Association of diet and sex hormones in relation to breast cancer. *European Journal of Cancer and Clinical Oncology, 23*(11), 1725–1726.

Alba, K., Campbell, G. M., & Kontogiorgos, V., (2019). Dietary fiber from berry-processing waste and its impact on bread structure: A review. *Journal of the Science of Food and Agriculture, 99*(9), 4189–4199.

Amaral, L., Morgan, D., Stephen, A., & Whiting, S., (1992). Effect of propionate on lipid-metabolism in healthy-human subjects. *FASEB Journal, 6*(5), A1655.

Antia, F. P., (1973). *Clinical Dietetics and Nutrition*. Oxford University Press, Ely House, 37 Dover Street, London WL.

Baer, D. J., Rumpler, W. V., Miles, C. W., & Fahey, Jr. G. C., (1997). Dietary fiber decreases the metabolizable energy content and nutrient digestibility of mixed diets fed to humans. *The Journal of Nutrition, 127*(4), 579–586.

Barrett, B., (2003). Medicinal properties of *Echinacea*: A critical review. *Phytomedicine, 10*(1), 66–86.

Beals, K. A., (2019). Potatoes, nutrition and health. *American Journal of Potato Research, 96*(2), 102–110.

Belghith-Fendri, L., Chaari, F., Kallel, F., Zouari-Ellouzi, S., Ghorbel, R., Besbes, S., & Ghribi-Aydi, D., (2016). Pea and broad bean pods as a natural source of dietary fiber: The impact on texture and sensory properties of cake. *Journal of Food Science, 81*(10), C2360–C2366.

Bhat, V. B., & Madyastha, K., (2000). C-phycocyanin: A potent peroxyl radical scavenger *in vivo* and *in vitro. Biochemical and Biophysical Research Communications, 275*(1), 20–25.

Bhathena, S. J., Ali, A. A., Haudenschild, C., Latham, P., Ranich, T., Mohamed, A. I., & Velasquez, M. T., (2003). Dietary flaxseed meal is more protective than soy protein concentrate against hypertriglyceridemia and steatosis of the liver in an animal model of obesity. *Journal of the American College of Nutrition, 22*(2), 157–164.

Bifari, F., Ruocco, C., Decimo, I., Fumagalli, G., Valerio, A., & Nisoli, E., (2017). Amino acid supplements and metabolic health: A potential interplay between intestinal microbiota and systems control. *Genes & Nutrition, 12*(1), 1–12.

Bondesson, M., & Gustafsson, J. A., (2010). Does consuming isoflavones reduce or increase breast cancer risk? *Genome Medicine, 2*(12), 1–5.

Brighenti, F., Castellani, G., Benini, L., Casiraghi, M., Leopardi, E., Crovetti, R., & Testolin, G., (1995). Effect of neutralized and native vinegar on blood glucose and acetate responses to a mixed meal in healthy subjects. *European Journal of Clinical Nutrition, 49*(4), 242–247.

Brondino, N., De Silvestri, A., Re, S., Lanati, N., Thiemann, P., Verna, A., & Politi, P., (2013). A systematic review and meta-analysis of ginkgo biloba in neuropsychiatric disorders: From ancient tradition to modern-day medicine. *Evidence-Based Complementary and Alternative Medicine, 2013*.

Brown, L., Rosner, B., Willett, W. W., & Sacks, F. M., (1999). Cholesterol-lowering effects of dietary fiber: A meta-analysis. *The American Journal of Clinical Nutrition, 69*(1), 30–42.

Brum, J., Ramsey, D., McRorie, J., Bauer, B., & Kopecky, S. L., (2018). Meta-analysis of usefulness of psyllium fiber as adjuvant anti-lipid therapy to enhance cholesterol lowering efficacy of statins. *The American Journal of Cardiology, 122*(7), 1169–1174. doi: https://doi.org/10.1016/j.amjcard.2018.06.040.

Camire, M. E., & FLINT, S. I., (1991). Thermal processing effects on dietary fiber composition and hydration capacity in corn meal, oat meal, and potato peels. *Cereal Chemistry, 68*(6), 645–647.

Cani, P., Joly, E., Horsmans, Y., & Delzenne, N. M., (2006). Oligofructose promotes satiety in healthy human: A pilot study. *European Journal of Clinical Nutrition, 60*(5), 567–572.

Carter, J., (1993). Potential of flaxseed and flaxseed oil in baked goods and other products in human nutrition. *Cereal Foods World (USA)*.

Carughi, A., Feeney, M. J., Kris-Etherton, P., Fulgoni, V., Kendall, C. W., Bulló, M., & Webb, D., (2015). Pairing nuts and dried fruit for cardiometabolic health. *Nutrition Journal, 15*(1), 1–13.

Coco, M. G., & Vinson, J. A., (2019). Analysis of popcorn (*Zea mays* L. var. everta) for antioxidant capacity and total phenolic content. *Antioxidants, 8*(1), 22.

Colombo, F., Di Lorenzo, C., Biella, S., Vecchio, S., Frigerio, G., & Restani, P., (2020). Adverse effects to food supplements containing botanical ingredients. *Journal of Functional Foods, 72*, 103990.

Coppens, P., Delmulle, L., Gulati, O., Richardson, D., Ruthsatz, M., Sievers, H., & Sidani, S., (2006). Use of botanicals in food supplements. *Annals of Nutrition and Metabolism, 50*(6), 538–554.

Cunnane, S. C., Ganguli, S., Menard, C., Liede, A. C., Hamadeh, M. J., Chen, Z. Y., & Jenkins, D. J., (1993). High α-linolenic acid flaxseed (*Linum usitatissimum*): Some nutritional properties in humans. *British Journal of Nutrition, 69*(2), 443–453.

Dioguardi, F. S., (2011). Clinical use of amino acids as dietary supplement: Pros and cons. *Journal of Cachexia, Sarcopenia and Muscle, 2*(2), 75–80.

Dixit, A. K., Antony, J., Sharma, N. K., & Tiwari, R. K., (2011). 12. Soybean constituents and their functional benefits. *Research SingPost, 37*(2), 661.

Dobrowolski, P., Huet, P., Karlsson, P., Eriksson, S., Tomaszewska, E., Gawron, A., & Pierzynowski, S. G., (2012). Potato fiber protects the small intestinal wall against the toxic influence of acrylamide. *Nutrition, 28*(4), 428–435.

Dreher, M. L., (2018). Whole fruits and fruit fiber emerging health effects. *Nutrients, 10*(12), 1833.

Drouin, G., Godin, J. R., & Pagé, B., (2011). The genetics of vitamin C loss in vertebrates. *Current Genomics, 12*(5), 371–378.

Dwyer, J., Coates, P., & Smith, M., (2018). Dietary supplements: Regulatory challenges and research resources. *Nutrients, 10*(1), 41. In: PUBMED.

Esposito, K., Nappo, F., Giugliano, F., Di Palo, C., Ciotola, M., Barbieri, M., & Giugliano, D., (2003). Meal modulation of circulating interleukin 18 and adiponectin concentrations in healthy subjects and in patients with type 2 diabetes mellitus. *The American Journal of Clinical Nutrition, 78*(6), 1135–1140.

Ford, N. A., & Liu, A. G., (2020). The forgotten fruit: A case for consuming avocado within the traditional Mediterranean diet. *Frontiers in Nutrition, 7*, 78.

Fortmann, S. P., Burda, B. U., Senger, C. A., Lin, J. S., & Whitlock, E. P., (2013). Vitamin and mineral supplements in the primary prevention of cardiovascular disease and cancer: An updated systematic evidence review for the US preventive services task force. *Annals of Internal Medicine, 159*(12), 824–834.

Gibson, G. R., Beatty, E. R., Wang, X., & Cummings, J. H., (1995). Selective stimulation of bifidobacteria in the human colon by oligofructose and inulin. *Gastroenterology, 108*(4), 975–982.

Griffin, I. J., Hicks, P. M., Heaney, R. P., & Abrams, S. A., (2003). Enriched chicory inulin increases calcium absorption mainly in girls with lower calcium absorption. *Nutrition Research, 23*(7), 901–909.

Han, H., Chen, Y., Bi, H., Yu, L., Sun, C., Li, S., & Zhou, Y., (2011). *In vivo* antimalarial activity of ginseng extracts. *Pharmaceutical Biology, 49*(3), 283–289.

Hassanen, M. R., Mahfouz, M. K., Farid, A. S., & Fadlullah, A. H., (2015). Biochemical effects of spirulina platensis against oxidative stress caused by doxorubicin. *Benha Veterinary Medical Journal, 28*(2), 147–154.

Heyman, L., Axling, U., Blanco, N., Sterner, O., Holm, C., & Berger, K., (2014). Evaluation of beneficial metabolic effects of berries in high-fat fed C57BL/6J mice. *Journal of Nutrition and Metabolism, 2014*.

Higgins, J. A., (2004). Resistant starch: Metabolic effects and potential health benefits. *Journal of AOAC International, 87*(3), 761–768.

Hirasawa, M., Shimura, K., Shimizu, A., Mura, K., Tokue, C., & Arai, S., (2008). Quantification and functional analysis of dietary fiber and polyphenols in avocado [*Persea americana*]. *Journal of the Japanese Society for Food Science and Technology (Japan)*.

Hvidtfeldt, U. A., Tolstrup, J. S., Jakobsen, M. U., Heitmann, B. L., Grønbæk, M., O'Reilly, E., & Knekt, P., (2010). Alcohol intake and risk of coronary heart disease in younger, middle-aged, and older adults. *Circulation, 121*(14), 1589–1597.

Ianiro, G., Pecere, S., Giorgio, V., Gasbarrini, A., & Cammarota, G., (2016). Digestive enzyme supplementation in gastrointestinal diseases. *Current Drug Metabolism, 17*(2), 187–193.

Iqbal, K., Khan, A., & Khattak, M., (2004). Biological significance of ascorbic acid (Vitamin C) in human health: A review. *Pakistan Journal of Nutrition, 3*(1), 5–13.

Jenkins, D., Wolever, T., Leeds, A. R., Gassull, M. A., Haisman, P., Dilawari, J., & Alberti, K., (1978). Dietary fibers, fiber analogs, and glucose tolerance: Importance of viscosity. *Br. Med. J., 1*(6124), 1392–1394.

Jiratchariyakul, W., Beerhues, L., Mahady, G. B., Kummalue, T., & Vongsakul, M., (2013). *Botanicals in Dietary Supplements*. In: Hindawi.

Johnson, L. R., (2004). *Encyclopedia of Gastroenterology* (Vol. 2). Academic Press.

Jonas, W., (2003). A critical overview of homeopathy. *Annals of Internal Medicine, 139*(8), W-76.

Jonnalagadda, S. S., Harnack, L., Hai, L. R., McKeown, N., Seal, C., Liu, S., & Fahey, G. C., (2011). Putting the whole grain puzzle together: Health benefits associated with whole grains—Summary of American society for nutrition 2010 satellite symposium. *The Journal of Nutrition, 141*(5), 1011S–1022S.

Joye, I. J., (2020). Dietary fiber from whole grains and their benefits on metabolic health. *Nutrients, 12*(10), 3045.

Kajla, P., Sharma, A., & Sood, D. R., (2015). Flaxseed—A potential functional food source. *Journal of Food Science and Technology, 52*(4), 1857–1871.

KEENAN, H., Doria, A., AIELLO, L., & KING, G., (2006). Positivity of C-peptide, GADA and IA2 antibodies in type 1 diabetic patients with extreme duration: 278-OR. *Diabetes, 55.*

Kendall, C. W., Esfahani, A., Truan, J., Srichaikul, K., & Jenkins, D. J., (2010). Health benefits of nuts in prevention and management of diabetes. *Asia Pacific Journal of Clinical Nutrition, 19*(1), 110–116.

Keservani, R. K., & Sharma, A. K., (2014). Flavonoids: Emerging trends and potential health benefits. *Journal of Chinese Pharmaceutical Sciences, 23*(12), 815.

Keservani, R. K., Kesharwani, R. K., Sharma, A. K., Vyas, N., & Chadoker, A., (2010b). Nutritional supplements: An overview. *International Journal of Current Pharmaceutical Review and Research, 1*(1), 59–75.

Keservani, R. K., Kesharwani, R. K., Vyas, N., Jain, S., Raghuvanshi, R., & Sharma, A. K., (2010a). Nutraceutical and functional food as future food: A review. *Der Pharmacia Lettre, 2*(1), 106–116.

Keservani, R. K., Sharma, A. K., & Kesharwani, R. K., (2016a). Nutraceutical and functional foods for cardiovascular health. In: *Food Process Engineering* (pp. 257–278, 291–312). Apple Academic Press, CRC Press. ISBN: 9781771884020.

Keservani, R. K., Sharma, A. K., & Kesharwani, R. K., (2020). *Nutraceuticals and Dietary Supplements: Applications in Health Improvement and Disease Management*. CRC Press. ISBN: 9781771888738.

Kim, H. J., & White, P. J., (2009). *In vitro* fermentation of oat flours from typical and high β-glucan oat lines. *Journal of Agricultural and Food Chemistry, 57*(16), 7529–7536.

Kim, H. J., & White, P. J., (2010). *In vitro* bile-acid binding and fermentation of high, medium, and low molecular weight β-glucan. *Journal of Agricultural and Food Chemistry, 58*(1), 628–634.

King, J. C., & Slavin, J. L., (2013). White potatoes, human health, and dietary guidance. *Advances in Nutrition, 4*(3), 393S–401S.

Kortubash, I., Ewing, L., Skinner, C., Nookaew, I., Avula, B., Khan, I., & Gurley, B., (2020). Green tea extract as a safe and effective dietary supplement: Lessons learned from mice. *Current Developments in Nutrition, 4*(Supplement_2), 419.

Kumadoh, D., & Ofori-Kwakye, K., (2017). Dosage forms of herbal medicinal products and their stability considerations: An overview. *J. Crit. Rev., 4*(4), 1–8.

Kushwaha, K., O'Bryan, C., Babu, D., Crandall, P., Chen, P., & Lee, S., (2014). Human health benefits of isoflavones from soybeans. *Agric. Food Anal. Bacteriol., 4*(2), 122–142.

Lattimer, J. M., & Haub, M. D., (2010). Effects of dietary fiber and its components on metabolic health. *Nutrients, 2*(12), 1266–1289.

Lee, E. L., (2009). *Genotype X Environment Impact on Selected Bioactive Compound Content of Fenugreek (Trigonella foenum-graecum L.).* Lethbridge, Alta.: University of Lethbridge, Dept. of Biological Sciences, c2009.

Li, F., Hullar, M. A., Schwarz, Y., & Lampe, J. W., (2009). Human gut bacterial communities are altered by the addition of cruciferous vegetables to a controlled fruit-and vegetable-free diet. *The Journal of Nutrition, 139*(9), 1685–1691.

Lu, Z. X., Walker, K. Z., Muir, J. G., Mascara, T., & O'Dea, K., (2000). Arabinoxylan fiber, a byproduct of wheat flour processing, reduces the postprandial glucose response in normoglycemic subjects. *The American Journal of Clinical Nutrition, 71*(5), 1123–1128.

Lu, Z., Walker, K. Z., Muir, J. G., & O'Dea, K., (2004). Arabinoxylan fiber improves metabolic control in people with type II diabetes. *European Journal of Clinical Nutrition, 58*(4), 621–628.

Ma, Y., Griffith, J. A., Chasan-Taber, L., Olendzki, B. C., Jackson, E., Stanek, III. E. J., & Ockene, I. S., (2006). Association between dietary fiber and serum C-reactive protein. *The American Journal of Clinical Nutrition, 83*(4), 760–766.

Majeed, M., Majeed, S., Nagabhushanam, K., Arumugam, S., Pande, A., Paschapur, M., & Ali, F., (2018). Evaluation of the safety and efficacy of a multienzyme complex in patients with functional dyspepsia: A randomized, double-blind, placebo-controlled study. *Journal of Medicinal Food, 21*(11), 1120–1128.

Maki, K. C., Carson, M. L., Anderson, W. K., Geohas, J., Reeves, M. S., Farmer, M. V., & Dicklin, M. R., (2009). Lipid-altering effects of different formulations of hydroxypropyl methylcellulose. *Journal of Clinical Lipidology, 3*(3), 159–166.

Maki, K. C., Davidson, M. H., Torri, S., Ingram, K. A., O'mullane, J., Daggy, B. P., & Albrecht, H. H., (2000). High-molecular-weight hydroxypropyl methylcellulose taken with or between meals is hypocholesterolemic in adult men. *The Journal of Nutrition, 130*(7), 1705–1710.

Mathur, M., (2018). Bioactive molecules of spirulina: A food supplement. *Bioactive Molecules in Food*, 1–22.

McKeown, N. M., Troy, L. M., Jacques, P. F., Hoffmann, U., O'Donnell, C. J., & Fox, C. S., (2010). Whole-and refined-grain intakes are differentially associated with abdominal visceral and subcutaneous adiposity in healthy adults: The Framingham heart Study. *The American Journal of Clinical Nutrition, 92*(5), 1165–1171.

Messina, V., (2014). Nutritional and health benefits of dried beans. *The American Journal of Clinical Nutrition, 100*(suppl_1), 437S–442S.

Meyer, K. A., Kushi, L. H., Jacobs, Jr. D. R., Slavin, J., Sellers, T. A., & Folsom, A. R., (2000). Carbohydrates, dietary fiber, and incident type 2 diabetes in older women. *The American Journal of Clinical Nutrition, 71*(4), 921–930.

Montonen, J., Knekt, P., Järvinen, R., Aromaa, A., & Reunanen, A., (2003). Whole-grain and fiber intake and the incidence of type 2 diabetes. *The American Journal of Clinical Nutrition, 77*(3), 622–629.

Murniece, I., Karklina, D., Galoburda, R., Santare, D., Skrabule, I., & Costa, H. S., (2011). Nutritional composition of freshly harvested and stored Latvian potato (*Solanum tuberosum* L.) varieties depending on traditional cooking methods. *Journal of Food Composition and Analysis, 24*(4, 5), 699–710.

Naidu, M. M., Shyamala, B., Naik, J. P., Sulochanamma, G., & Srinivas, P., (2011). Chemical composition and antioxidant activity of the husk and endosperm of fenugreek seeds. *LWT-Food SCIENCE and Technology, 44*(2), 451–456.

Nangia-Makker, P., Hogan, V., Honjo, Y., Baccarini, S., Tait, L., Bresalier, R., & Raz, A., (2002). Inhibition of human cancer cell growth and metastasis in nude mice by oral intake of modified citrus pectin. *Journal of the National Cancer Institute, 94*(24), 1854–1862.

Naumann, E., Van, R. A. B., Önning, G., Öste, R., Wydra, M., & Mensink, R. P., (2006). β-Glucan incorporated into a fruit drink effectively lowers serum LDL-cholesterol concentrations. *The American Journal of Clinical Nutrition, 83*(3), 601–605.

Nazare, J. A., Normand, S., Oste, T. A., Brac De La, P. A., Desage, M., & Laville, M., (2009). Modulation of the postprandial phase by β-glucan in overweight subjects: Effects on glucose and insulin kinetics. *Molecular Nutrition & Food Research, 53*(3), 361–369.

Nguyen, V., Cooper, L., Lowndes, J., Melanson, K., Angelopoulos, T. J., Rippe, J. M., & Reimers, K., (2012). Popcorn is more satiating than potato chips in normal-weight adults. *Nutrition Journal, 11*(1), 1–6.

Olano-Martin, E., Gibson, G. R., & Rastall, R., (2002). Comparison of the *in vitro* bifidogenic properties of pectins and pectic-oligosaccharides. *Journal of Applied Microbiology, 93*(3), 505–511.

Ostadrahimi, A., Ashrafnejad, F., Kazemi, A., Sargheini, N., Mahdavi, R., Farshchian, M., & Mahluji, S., (2014). Aflatoxin in raw and salt-roasted nuts (pistachios, peanuts and walnuts) sold in markets of Tabriz, Iran. *Jundishapur Journal of Microbiology, 7*(1).

Östman, E. M., Liljeberg, E. H. G., & Björck, I. M., (2002). Barley bread containing lactic acid improves glucose tolerance at a subsequent meal in healthy men and women. *The Journal of Nutrition, 132*(6), 1173–1175.

Palacios, O. M., Cortes, H. N., Jenks, B. H., & Maki, K. C., (2020). Naturally occurring hormones in foods and potential health effects. *Toxicology Research and Application, 4*, 2397847320936281.

Qureshi, A. A., Sami, S. A., & Khan, F. A., (2002). Effects of stabilized rice bran, its soluble and fiber fractions on blood glucose levels and serum lipid parameters in humans with diabetes mellitus types I and II. *The Journal of Nutritional Biochemistry, 13*(3), 175–187.

Rabbani, G. H., Teka, T., Zaman, B., Majid, N., Khatun, M., & Fuchs, G. J., (2001). Clinical studies in persistent diarrhea: Dietary management with green banana or pectin in Bangladeshi children. *Gastroenterology, 121*(3), 554–560.

Rabetafika, H. N., Van, R. V., Danthine, S., Paquot, M., & Blecker, C., (2011). Flaxseed proteins: Food uses and health benefits. *International Journal of Food Science & Technology, 46*(2), 221–228.

Rane, B. R., Bharath, M. S., Patil, R. R., Keservani, R. K., & Jain, A. S., (2020b). Novel approaches in nutraceuticals. In: Rajesh, K. K., Raj, K. K., & Anil, K. S., (eds.), *Enhancing the Therapeutic Efficacy of Herbal Formulations Through Novel Drug Delivery Systems* (pp. 241–266). IGI Global International Publisher, Pennsylvania, USA, Chapter 11. ISBN13: 9781799844532.

Rane, B. R., Patil, A. S., Keservani, R. K., & Jain, A. S., (2020a). Novel approaches in herbal formulation. In: Rajesh, K. K., Raj, K. K., & Anil, K. S., (eds.), *Enhancing the Therapeutic Efficacy of Herbal Formulations Through Novel Drug Delivery Systems* (pp. 43–68). IGI Global International Publisher, Pennsylvania, USA, Chapter 2. ISBN13: 9781799844532.

Rane, B. R., Tadavi, S. A., & Keservani, R. K., (2020c). Naturopathy. In: Anil, K. S., Raj, K. K., & Surya, P. G., (eds.), *Herbal Product Development* (pp. 321–347). Apple Academic Press, CRC Press, Taylor & Francis Group, Chapter 12. ISBN: 9781771888776.

Riaz, M., Rahman, N. U., Zia-Ul-Haq, M., Jaffar, H. Z. E., & Manea, R., (2019). Ginseng: A dietary supplement as an immune-modulator in various diseases. *Trends in Food Science & Technology, 83*, 12–30. doi: https://doi.org/10.1016/j.tifs.2018.11.008.

Ridges, L., Sunderland, R., Moerman, K., Meyer, B., Astheimer, L., & Howe, P., (2001). Cholesterol lowering benefits of soy and linseed enriched foods. *Asia Pacific Journal of Clinical Nutrition, 10*(3), 204–211.

Roberts, K. T., (2011). The potential of fenugreek (*Trigonella foenum-graecum*) as a functional food and nutraceutical and its effects on glycemia and lipidemia. *Journal of Medicinal Food, 14*(12), 1485–1489.

Rubilar, M., Gutiérrez, C., Verdugo, M., Shene, C., & Sineiro, J., (2010). Flaxseed as a source of functional ingredients. *Journal of Soil Science and Plant Nutrition, 10*(3), 373–377.

Sadler, M. J., Gibson, S., Whelan, K., Ha, M. A., Lovegrove, J., & Higgs, J., (2019). Dried fruit and public health–what does the evidence tell us? *International Journal of Food Sciences and Nutrition, 70*(6), 675–687.

Salminen, A., Kauppinen, A., & Kaarniranta, K., (2014). Inflammaging signaling in health span and life span regulation: Next generation targets for longevity. In: *Inflammation, Advancing Age and Nutrition* (pp. 323–332). Elsevier.

Samra, R. A., & Anderson, G. H., (2007). Insoluble cereal fiber reduces appetite and short-term food intake and glycemic response to food consumed 75 min later by healthy men. *The American Journal of Clinical Nutrition, 86*(4), 972–979.

Schulze, M. B., Liu, S., Rimm, E. B., Manson, J. E., Willett, W. C., & Hu, F. B., (2004). Glycemic index, glycemic load, and dietary fiber intake and incidence of type 2 diabetes in younger and middle-aged women. *The American Journal of Clinical Nutrition, 80*(2), 348–356.

Seal, C. J., Courtin, C. M., Venema, K., & De Vries, J., (2021). Health benefits of whole grain: Effects on dietary carbohydrate quality, the gut microbiome, and consequences of processing. *Comprehensive Reviews in Food Science and Food Safety, 20*(3), 2742–2768.

Sharma, A. K., Keservani, R. K., & Gautam, S. P., (2020). *Herbal Product Development*. Apple Academic Press, CRC Press, Taylor & Francis Group. ISBN: 9781771888776.

Shashank, A., Ramakrishna, D., Kiran, S., Kosturkova, G., & Ravishankar, G., (2015). Nutraceutical potential of soybean: Review. *Asian Journal of Clinical Nutrition, 7*(2), 22–32.

Sicińska, E., Pietruszka, B., Januszko, O., Jakubowski, S., Kielak-Biskupska, K., Rolf, K., & Kaluza, J., (2020). Intake of vitamins and minerals from voluntarily fortified foods and/or dietary supplements in school adolescents in Central-Eastern Poland. *Frontiers in Public Health, 8*, 607.

Singh, P., Kesharwani, R. K., & Keservani, R. K., (2017a). Antioxidants and vitamins: Roles in cellular function and metabolism. In: *Sustained Energy for Enhanced Human Functions and Activity* (pp. 385–407). Academic Press. ISBN:9780128054130.

Singh, P., Kesharwani, R. K., & Keservani, R. K., (2017b). Protein, carbohydrates, and fats: Energy metabolism. In: *Sustained Energy for Enhanced Human Functions and Activity* (pp. 103–115). Academic Press. ISBN:9780128054130.

Song, M., Wu, K., Meyerhardt, J. A., Ogino, S., Wang, M., Fuchs, C. S., & Chan, A. T., (2018). Fiber intake and survival after colorectal cancer diagnosis. *JAMA Oncology, 4*(1), 71–79.

Sowmya, P., & Rajyalakshmi, P., (1999). Hypocholesterolemic effect of germinated fenugreek seeds in human subjects. *Plant Foods for Human Nutrition, 53*(4), 359–365.

Story, J. A., Furumoto, E. J., & Buhman, K. K., (1997). Dietary fiber and bile acid metabolism—An update. *Dietary Fiber in Health and Disease,* 259–266.

Streppel, M. T., Ocké, M. C., Boshuizen, H. C., Kok, F. J., & Kromhout, D., (2008). Dietary fiber intake in relation to coronary heart disease and all-cause mortality over 40 y: The Zutphen study. *The American Journal of Clinical Nutrition, 88*(4), 1119–1125.

Sunguya, B. F., Poudel, K. C., Mlunde, L. B., Shakya, P., Urassa, D. P., Jimba, M., & Yasuoka, J., (2013). Effectiveness of nutrition training of health workers toward improving caregivers' feeding practices for children aged six months to two years: A systematic review. *Nutrition Journal, 12*(1), 1–14.

Theuwissen, E., & Mensink, R. P., (2007). Simultaneous intake of β-glucan and plant stanol esters affects lipid metabolism in slightly hypercholesterolemic subjects. *The Journal of Nutrition, 137*(3), 583–588.

Thompson, L. U., Rickard, S. E., Orcheson, L. J., & Seidl, M. M., (1996). Flaxseed and its Lignan and Oil Components Reduce Mammary Tumor Growth at a Late Stage of Carcinogenesis. *Carcinogenesis, 17*(6), 1373–1376.

Tolkachev, O., & Zhuchenko, A., (2004). Biologically active substances of flax: Medicinal and nutritional properties (a review). *Pharmaceutical Chemistry Journal, 34*(7), 360–367.

Touloupakis, E., & Ghanotakis, D. F., (2010). Nutraceutical use of garlic sulfur-containing compounds. In: *Bio-Farms for Nutraceuticals* (pp. 110–121). Springer.

Triplehorn, C., & Millard, P. S., (2002). A rice-based diet with green banana or pectin reduced diarrhea in infants better than a rice-alone diet. *ACP Journal Club, 136*(2), 67.

Tucker, L. A., & Thomas, K. S., (2009). Increasing total fiber intake reduces the risk of weight and fat gains in women. *The Journal of Nutrition, 139*(3), 576–581.

Turner, T. F., Nance, L. M., Strickland, W. D., Malcolm, R. J., Pechon, S., & O'Neil, P. M., (2013). Dietary adherence and satisfaction with a bean-based high-fiber weight loss diet: A pilot study. *International Scholarly Research Notices, 2013*.

Ulmius, M., Johansson, A., & Önning, G., (2009). The influence of dietary fiber source and gender on the postprandial glucose and lipid response in healthy subjects. *European Journal of Nutrition, 48*(7), 395–402.

Van, B. R. B., (2015). Development of safe and effective botanical dietary supplements: Miniperspective. *Journal of Medicinal Chemistry, 58*(21), 8360–8372.

Wani, S., & Kumar, P., (2016). Fenugreek: A review on its nutraceuticals properties and utilization in various food products. *J. Saudi Soc. Agric. Sci., 7*(2), 97–106.

Weickert, M., Mohlig, M., Koebnick, C., Holst, J., Namsolleck, P., Ristow, M., & Spranger, J., (2005). Impact of cereal fiber on glucose-regulating factors. *Diabetologia, 48*(11), 2343–2353.

Wiseman, H., (1999). The bioavailability of non-nutrient plant factors: Dietary flavonoids and phyto-oestrogens. *Proceedings of the Nutrition Society, 58*(1), 139–146.

Young, G. P., Hu, Y., Le Leu, R. K., & Nyskohus, L., (2005). Dietary fiber and colorectal cancer: A model for environment–gene interactions. *Molecular Nutrition & Food Research, 49*(6), 571–584.

Zhang, F. F., Barr, S. I., McNulty, H., Li, D., & Blumberg, J. B., (2020). Health effects of vitamin and mineral supplements. *BMJ, 369*.

Zhang, J. X., Lundin, E., Hallmans, G., Adlercreutz, H., Andersson, H., Bosaeus, I., & Dahlgren, S., (1994). Effect of rye bran on excretion of bile acids, cholesterol, nitrogen, and fat in human subjects with ileostomies. *The American Journal of Clinical Nutrition, 59*(2), 389–394.

Zhang, X. Y., Sun, K., Zhu, Q., Song, T., & Liu, Y., (2017). Ginseng polysaccharide serves as a potential radiosensitizer through inducing apoptosis and autophagy in the treatment of osteosarcoma. *The Kaohsiung Journal of Medical Sciences, 33*(11), 535–542.

Zhang, Y. J., Li, S., Gan, R. Y., Zhou, T., Xu, D. P., & Li, H. B., (2015). Impacts of gut bacteria on human health and diseases. *International Journal of Molecular Sciences, 16*(4), 7493–7519.

CHAPTER 15

REGULATORY GUIDANCE ON FOOD SUPPLEMENT AND DIETARY FIBER

ASHISH A. KARLE,[1] PRANIT S. WAGHCHAURE,[1] BHUSHAN R. RANE,[1] RAJAN V. KALAMKAR,[2] RAJ K. KESERVANI,[3] and PARIKSHIT R. SHIRODE[4]

[1]*Shri D.D. Vispute College of Pharmacy and Research Center, Devad-Vichumbe, Panvel, Navi Mumbai, Maharashtra, India*

[2]*Vivekanand Education Society's College of Pharmacy, Chembur, Mumbai, Maharashtra, India*

[3]*Faculty of B. Pharmacy, CSM Group of Institutions, Prayagraj, Uttar Pradesh, India*

[4]*Department of Shalyatantra, Parul Institute of Ayurveda, Parul University, Vadodara, Gujarat, India*

ABSTRACT

This chapter provides a short review of the main regulations concerning food supplements and dietary fibers set out by the different regulating authorities across the globe. Indian Food and Drug Administration (FDA), US FDA, European Commission, and other agencies are involved in the health and food safety authorities such as Health Canada and the US continue to develop and implement regulations aimed at ensuring consumer access to safe and effective products. A comparison between the US, EU, and other regulations, their acceptance and impact on the market is presented, together with a final suggestion to enhance the future development and distribution of functional products, which belong to an equivocal area between food and drugs. This

Food Supplements and Dietary Fiber in Health and Disease. Bhushan R. Rane, Raj K. Keservani, Durgesh Singh, Nayan A. Gujarathi, and Ashish S. Jain, (Eds.)
© 2024 Apple Academic Press, Inc. Co-published with CRC Press (Taylor & Francis)

Springer Brief aims to review and discuss the many current statutes and regulations addressing dietary ingredients, manufacturing standards, safety, labeling, and claims, all of which promote the safe use of dietary supplements and preserve continued consumer access.

15.1 INTRODUCTION

Dietary supplements are governed by different laws than conventional meals and medications by the Food and Drug Administration (FDA). Dietary supplements, on the other hand, are subject to some of the same laws that apply to ordinary meals. This chapter covers the fundamentals of dietary supplement regulation, as well as how the Dietary Supplement Health and Education Act of 1994 (DSHEA) altered the US regulatory approach, the main roles of government agencies and self-regulatory organizations involved in dietary supplement oversight, and other aspects of dietary supplement regulation. Prior to the legal classification of "dietary supplements," supplements were regulated as food products for many years. Vitamins, minerals, and meals for those on special diets were the most popular commodities.

Today, the lines aren't as clearly established. Herbs and amino acids are added to traditional cuisines. The adding of valuable additions to traditional meals can be beneficial. Herbs, extracts, and other supplements are now available in general shops, rather than just in specialty health food stores (Williams et al., 2010).

New words have been coined to go along with the new objects. Because many of these phrases in the United States lack legal definitions, their use and meaning are sometimes confusing. The phrase "nutraceutical" is a combination of the words "nutrition" and "pharmaceutical," and it refers to meals that contain a supplement or enhancement that has a specific health benefit. "Functional food" is sometimes used interchangeably with "Pharma food" and FoSHU ("Food for Specified Health Use"). The phrase "functional food," in contrast to pills, liquids, and powders, refers to traditional food products that have been changed to give particular health advantages.

Calcium-fortified orange juice and calcium-fortified yogurt are two examples of functional foods. These new terms aren't legally valid, but they do reflect the changing structure of the market. The lines between pharmaceuticals, nutritional supplements, and regular meals are becoming fragmented. To lower cholesterol, vitamin C may be added to soft drinks, plant sterols can be added to margarine and yogurt, and herbs can be added to meals (Quah et al., 2006).

Definition of a dietary supplement as per DSHEA 1994:

> "Dietary supplements are defined by the DSHEA as: a product (other than tobacco) that is intended to supplement the diet and contains one or more dietary ingredients such as vitamin, mineral, herb or other botanical, amino acid, dietary substance for use by man to supplement the diet by increasing total dietary intake, or a concentrate, metabolite, constituent, extract, or combinations of these ingredients; is intended for ingestion in pill, capsule, tablet, or powder form. When a dietary supplement is a new dietary element, supplement manufacturers are required to notify the FDA (Larissa et al., 2003)."

15.1.1 BACKGROUND OF REGULATION IN DIETARY SUPPLEMENTS

This section provides an overview of the US Food and Drug Administration's (FDA) long history of commitment to dietary supplements, as evidenced by a complex of collaborations and connections between the FDA and customers, manufacturers, trade associations, various affiliations, all levels of the government legal framework, legislators, health experts, researchers, and others (Hutt et al., 1986).

Because these commodities are utilized as food supplements as well as for other uses, they provide a more difficult regulatory task. It's critical to note that this research focuses on supplements rather than the events and guidelines for fortified food sources. Although there is indisputable overlap between the two, the main focus of the studies in this exceptional issue is on nutrients, minerals, botanicals, and amino acids created for isolated use, whether alone or in combination with other improvements.

The chapter on supplement regulation in the United States doesn't begin until the mid-20th century, partly because government regulation of consumer goods didn't appear despite long-standing endeavors until 1906, and partly because the revelations of explicit, appealing components in food responsible for wellbeing and sustenance didn't appear until the first 20 years of the 20th century (John Swann et al., 2015).

15.2 REGULATION ACT

15.2.1 REGULATION UNDER THE 1906 ACT

The distinction between food and medication was largely irrelevant under the 1906 Act. The 1906 Act was only five pages long and mostly consisted of prohibitions against debasement and misbranding. In Section 6, it differentiated between "medicine" and "food," yet the two items' guidelines were nearly indistinguishable. As a result, foods whose package had instances to qualify as a medication had lawful actions looked after under the Drug laws, unless the legitimate moves were done under the 1906 Act's food requirements. Under the 1906 Act, common instances were treated as treatment candidates for a variety of illnesses and alignments. Cases that couldn't be easily renamed and were also directed under the 1906 Act's medication arrangements were classified as misleading claims.

As the public's interest in dietary supplements grew, the need for more comprehensive guidelines arose. In 1935, the FDA launched six valid operations against vitamin claims in response to growing concerns about manufacturers profiting from the public's interest in vitamins. In the same year, it established a Vitamin Division to fight what it perceived to be vitamin market abuse. The focus was on promises, but novel ingredients or compounds with proven medicinal benefits were also highlighted. The 1906 Act, which was frequently chastised for lacking the boldness or legal authority to regulate dietary supplements, attempted to make a move (Sanchez et al., 2015).

15.2.2 REGULATION UNDER THE FEDERAL FOOD, DRUG, AND COSMETIC ACT OF 1938

During the 1930s, Congress began to adopt extended guidelines for ingested drugs, which culminated in the passage of the Federal Food, Drug, and Cosmetic Act in 1938. The FDCA replaced a 1906 statute that had become obsolete due to technical advancements in the food and drug production industries (FDA, 1981). This new display arranged a mind-boggling array of regulatory requirements for food types, drugs, cosmetics, and medical devices. The FDA was reorganized from a policing body primarily concerned with moving contaminated pharmaceuticals to an administrative office tasked with overseeing the evaluation of new medications as part of the FDCA's more substantial modifications.

The FDCA had provisions that covered foods, pharmaceuticals, and cosmetics. The applicability of these arrangements to things containing vitamins, minerals, or organic fixings (e.g., whether the item was seen as a medication or a food) was based on the item's intended use, which was not always fixed in stone by the item's labeling and marketing claims.

Except for Section 403(j), which shows that a food is misbranded if it is claimed to be "for special dietary employments" but it's label does not bear FDA-recommended proclamations about its "vitamins, mineral, and other dietary properties" adequate to advise the purchaser about its value for such uses, the first 1938 demonstration contains no specific provisions for vitamins, minerals, or botanical products (Eswaran et al., 2013).

15.2.3 VITAMIN MINERAL AMENDMENTS (1976)

Beginning in 1976, Congress began to intervene in dietary supplement guidelines. The Vitamin Mineral Amendment of 1976 was Congress's first attempt to define and govern vitamins and minerals, and it was successful. The FDA's previous attempts to set the most extreme levels of vitamins and minerals or deem vitamins or minerals medicine dependant on the edge of the extra vitamins or minerals were thwarted by the Amendment. Although the Amendment was quick to address dietary supplements, its traditionalist position limited the scope of the legislation. It was in response to the industry's mobilization against the FDA's efforts to bring an increasing number of supplements under drug restrictions (Wallace et al., 2013).

15.2.4 THE NUTRITIONAL LABELING AND EDUCATION ACT 1990

The Nutrition Labeling and Education Act of 1990 ("NLEA") was passed by Congress to bolster the FDA's legal authority to impose nutritional labeling on food. The NLEA amended Section 403 of the FDCA by adding two new subsections—(q) and (r)—creating two new food-labeling provisions. Section 403(q) establishes broad nutritional labeling requirements, but Section 403(r) prohibits food manufacturers from making unsubstantiated disease preventive or nutrient description claims. However, the NLEA required that health claims for food sources need FDA premarket approval and be based on extensive testing and logical organization. Following the passage of the NLEA in 1990, the FDA issued new food naming standards to replace the 1973 guidelines, which mandated the disclosure of any vitamin, mineral, or supplement. In most cases, the upgraded requirements necessitate a logical arrangement among trained experts regarding the health of food fixings.

15.2.5 DIETARY SUPPLEMENT HEALTH AND EDUCATION ACT OF 1994

Congress created the DSHEA in 1994 in response to "the importance of nutrients, as well as the benefits of dietary supplements to health promotion and disease prevention" and the growing reliance of customers on dietary supplements.

The Dietary Supplement Health and Education Act (DSHEA), passed in 1994, has two main goals: (a) to ensure that consumers have access to a diverse range of dietary supplements, and (b) to provide consumers with extra information regarding the intended use of dietary supplements. The long-standing order of dietary supplements as a class of food variety was not altered by DSHEA.

15.3 SAFETY STANDARDS OF STANDARDS

Dietary fibers are now used widely across the globe due to its health benefits. Its safety is important. Various regulatory provisions made for the regulation of Dietary fibers. One of the main goals of DSHEA was to create a regulatory framework for dietary supplements that would allow things that clearly had a history of safe usage to be admitted. The legislation aimed to avoid administrative roadblocks and encourage progress, while also addressing the need to ensure the safety of dietary supplement components, particularly new or innovative substances.

All dietary substances promoted in the United States before October 15, 1994, were classed as Older Dietary Ingredients by the DSHEA.

Consumers are considered safe with these "grandfathered" substances. As a result, dietary supplement products that include Older Dietary Ingredients do not need to submit additional safety data to the FDA prior to being placed on the market provided they do not cause any major harm or injury.

A dietary supplement containing an NDI is considered adulterated unless: (i) "the dietary supplement contains only nutritional ingredients that have been present in the food production as an article used for food in a form in which the NDI has been present; or (ii) the maker submits an NDI notification (NDIN) at least 75 days prior to the product's release."

The NDIN should contain information proving that the dietary component "would reasonably be anticipated to be safe" given the labeling's specified circumstances of use, a requirement that varies from that for food additives and conventional food ingredients. The NDIN approach includes gathering scientific data on the substance, such as a history of safe use of the item and substantially equivalent ingredients, as well as the NDI's dose and chemical identity, and the advised application (Menezes De et al., 2013).

15.3.1 DEVELOPMENT OF SAFETY STANDARDS

The fundamental adulteration criteria for food variety is used to determine dietary supplements. A dietary supplement is also considered adulterated if it "presents a considerable or unreasonable risk of disease or harm" whether used in the states indicated or proposed on the item label, or when used in typical states without such suggestions or ideas (Wallace et al., 2013).

15.3.2 SAFETY OF DIETARY SUPPLEMENTS

Dietary supplements, as a form of food, have security criteria that are similar to those for traditional food in a few key ways. Dietary supplement makers, in particular, are not required to register their products with the FDA or get FDA clearance prior to producing or selling them. However, before promoting a product, manufacturers should ensure that the dietary supplement and its contents are safe. Furthermore, FDA, like other FDA-directed goods, has the authority to make an authorization decision if a dietary supplement is shown to be harmful. There are also a few requirements for dietary supplements based on prior use, as well as the awareness that the security profile and intended use of dietary supplements differs from those of medicines.

Consumers are protected by these rules from potentially dangerous objects and substances. In addition to dietary supplement explicit cGMPs, FDA monitors the safety of dietary supplements by post-market monitoring of mandatory adverse event reports, which include significant injuries or illnesses that might be linked to the product. Dietary supplement labeling and claims are also scrutinized by the FDA to verify that the information is accurate and truthful. These additional security measures, in addition to the necessary legal requirements for both food and supplements, provide a balance between the FDA's need to protect the food supply and the demand for supervised consumer access to dietary supplements (Keenan et al., 2015).

The phrase "dietary supplement" had no legal definition prior to the passage of the DSHEA in 1994. Vitamins, minerals, botanicals, and other dietary supplement ingredients (and combinations of these components) were regulated by the FDA in the same way that regular food, a food added substance or GRAS fixing, or a medicine were. The DSHEA reiterated that dietary supplements should be treated as a food category and provided a specific definition for them.

This task avoided a proposal that would subject dietary supplements to a longer premarket approval process, which is reserved for things such as drugs and medical equipment. In the years leading up to DSHEA, Congress, industry, and other interested parties debated the order and the best method. In any event, it's not carved in stone that, because dietary supplements have been safely consumed by a large number of Americans for a long time, a premarket approval step akin to that of a medicine was unnecessary.

Furthermore, the added administrative requirements would effectively increase the cost of these things. Such a paradigm would not be justified for nutritional supplements, especially from an FDA assets perspective, because the health profile for these goods is anchored and immensely different from that of new, innovative medicinal components.

By specifically exempting dietary supplements from the FDCA's food additives provisions, the DSHEA indicated that constituents of dietary supplements could not be managed as food additives. Dietary supplements' role as part of a healthy lifestyle and their dedication to deterrent health goals were also recognized by Congress. Dietary supplements, when used safely and appropriately, can help to reduce the incidence of chronic infection and disease progression, reducing the need for long-term medical treatment. The present DSHEA framework places joint duty on the producers (or merchants) and the FDA for the safety of dietary supplements.

FDA has the authority to make a swift required step against a dietary supplement that has been tampered with, just as it does with any other food item (perilous). The FDCA considers an item dangerous if it "may be injurious to health," which applies to all food types and is the key viewpoint that has allowed FDA to ensure the food supply's security since 1906. However, the FDCA's additional adulteration requirements, as amended by DSHEA, provide critical security components for dietary supplement safety and the FDA's regulatory power.

Because the FDA does not regulate, require, or support dietary supplements before they are marketed, manufacturers must ensure that they do not pose a "critical or outlandish danger of illness or injury under the states of utilization suggested or proposed in the item's marking, or, on the other hand, under common states of utilization if no states of utilization are proposed or suggested in the label." This includes assurances that the components and the item meet FDA requirements for identity, purity, strength, and composition, and that the end result is safe when used together.

Furthermore, only permitted dietary components may be used in supplements, as the DSHEA mandates the FDA to issue a premarket warning for some novel dietary substances. Dietary substances that were accessible prior to the passage of the DSHEA in 1994, referred to as "old dietary ingredients," were excluded from the definition of new dietary ingredients. This premarket notification to the FDA should be sent out 75 days before the new component is advertised, and it should include evidence demonstrating that the substance "is reasonably expected to be protected."

In order for a food additive to be approved for use, a manufacturer must show that it is "not dangerous under planned usage conditions." DSHEA also provided FDA the authority to remove products from the market if the agency determines that they pose an "imminent hazard" or an "immediate security risk." Furthermore, nutritional supplements may be deemed adulterated under Section 403(g)(1) of the FDCA if they have been prepared, packed, or kept in conditions that do not satisfy cGMP criteria or, on the other hand, acceptable expiration date labeling guidelines. The resolution is clear that FDA has the weight of proof to prove that a dietary supplement is harmful, regardless of how it exercises its required power under these adulteration rules.

Finally, the FDA regulates the labeling of dietary supplements to ensure that they are accurate and not misleading, and that they follow FDA labeling requirements. This includes both the composition and the identification of dietary supplements. Products that do not fulfill these requirements are deemed misbranded and are subject to the same requirements as misbranded products (Westenbrink et al., 2013).

15.3.3 HAZARD ANALYSIS AND CRITICAL CONTROL POINT (HACCP)

The Hazard Analysis and Critical Control Point (HACCP) system has been recognized by the Codex Alimentarius Commission as a technique for assuring food safety.

Hazard Analysis Critical Control Points (HACCP) is a scientifically based approach that is directly applied to the food procurement, production, and distribution processes.

HACCP/ISO 22000 is a scientific, logical, and rigorous approach to discovering, analyzing, and managing risks in the food production, processing, manufacturing, and consumption processes.

HACCP is a food safety, pharmaceutical safety, and other preventative technique employed by the food industry that focuses on physical, chemical, and biological risks rather than completed product inspection as a means of prevention (Menezes De et al., 2013).

HACCP is a set of procedures designed to prevent issues from arising in the first place and to correct deviations in a systematic manner once they have been found.

The HACCP system regulates contaminants, pathogenic bacteria, physical items (glass, metal, and bone), chemicals (toxins, heavy metals, and pesticide residues), raw materials, processing conditions, customer usage directions, and storage conditions.

HACCP offers a great opportunity for the food industry to enhance quality while also delivering consistency and uniformity to the international market.

The Codex Alimentarius, which was issued in 1997, created a systematic HACCP process based on seven basic principles:

- Conduct a risk assessment;
- Determine the locations of the critical control points;
- Determination of critical limit values;
- Establishment of a monitoring and testing system to maintain control over a crucial point;
- When monitoring reveals that a CCP is out of control, remedial steps are taken;
- Establish measures for verifying the efficacy of the HACCP system through record-keeping; and
- Validation of the HACCP system to ensure its efficacy.

15.3.4 BENEFITS OF IMPLEMENTING HACCP/ISO 22000

- A plan to avoid foodborne illness;
- Can aid in identifying process improvements and customer complaint reductions;

- Adds value to quality management systems like ISO 9000 by lowering the need for and cost of final product testing;
- Increases client satisfaction and minimizes dissatisfaction;
- Encourages employees to be more aware of food packaging safety hazards;
- It is necessary to test data on a frequent basis;
- Helps to improve the company's image;
- Improves internal as well as external communication.

Hazard Analysis and Critical Control Points should be used in any food production process (HACCP). The whole supply chain is covered by a HACCP plan, from incoming logistics to storage, processing, sanitation, and maintenance, as well as client usage. Across all activities, protocols for internal logistics, processing needs, operating instructions, hygiene procedures, and preventative maintenance plans are required. These processes must cover all startup, shutdown, and unexpected processing halts. HACCP must be followed in order to detect the flaws in the manufacturing line and set critical limits in compliance with the legislation.

Regardless of the fact that the HACCP system was designed to generate products with zero flaws, it is impossible to produce items that are defect-free 100% of the time. However, it does establish a goal to decrease unacceptably unsafe commodities by reducing related risks throughout the manufacturing process. During HACCP implementation, it's necessary to set controls at each level of the production line where safety issues (physical, chemical, and microbiological) are likely to arise. A HACCP plan must be in place before the HACCP system can be implemented. A HACCP approach is made out of five initial phases and seven key HACCP principles.

15.4 ADVERSE EVENT REPORTING

Dietary supplement safety is also monitored by adverse reaction reporting and related record-keeping standards. Health-related events that occur after using a product, such as an allergic response, that may or may not be linked to the product are known as adverse occurrences.

Certain FDA-regulated items, such as medications, vaccines, and other biologics, medical devices, and, more recently, nutritional supplements and over-the-counter medicines, are obliged to report adverse occurrences.

There was no obligation for mandatory adverse event reporting because nutritional supplements were not before classified as a food category. The

Dietary Supplement and Non-prescription drugs Drug Consumer Protection Act was enacted by Congress on December 22, 2006, with the dietary supplement industry's backing.

Dietary supplement producers, packers, and distributors in the United States are required by law to report any significant adverse effects associated with their use to the FDA. A serious adverse event is defined as one that results in death, a life-threatening experience, inpatient hospitalization, a persistent or significant disability or incapacity; or a congenital anomaly or birth defect; or necessitates, based on reasonable medical judgment, a medical or surgical intervention to prevent an outcome described; or necessitates, based on reasonable medical judgment, a medical or surgical intervention to prevent an outcome described.

15.5 CURRENT GOOD MANUFACTURING PRACTICES

The needed methods, systems, equipment, facilities, and controls are described in cGMP standards, which apply to nutraceuticals, foodstuff, medical equipment, pharmaceutics, biologics, and veterinary goods. Dietary supplement cGMPs have been in force since June 25, 2007, when the FDA published the final regulation, Good Manufacturing Practices (gmp Practice (cGMP) in Manufacturing, Packaging, Labeling, or Holding Operations for Nutritional Supplements, in the Federal Register. The final cGMP rule establishes minimum standards for the efficacy, quality, purity, and safety of supplement products. cGMPs must be followed by anybody who imports, exports, manufactures, packages, labels, or holds a dietary supplement, and all dietary supplements sold in the United States must be made in accordance with them.

Representatives from the dietary supplement industry presented a suggested framework for the cGMP standards to FDA in November 1995, after DSHEA's authorization for FDA to develop cGMP requirements for dietary supplements. If the FDA decides to move forward with regulation to execute the rules, the plan will be a "very helpful starting point," according to the FDA. In February 1997, the agency published an ANPR asking stakeholder feedback on the industry's supplied framework, among other things. In June 2007, the FDA published the final cGMP regulation.

To guarantee that all nutritional supplements manufacturing facilities had adequate time to comply with the new rule, the cGMP requirement incorporated a staggered compliance timeline based on company size.

cGMPs are a 16-part dietary supplement that may be found in 21 CFR 111, subparts A–P, 111.1–111.610 of the Code of Federal Regulations. They encompass all standards deemed required by the FDA to assure consistent and regulated dietary supplement manufacturing, avoid adulteration or misbranding, and validate the identity, purity, quality, strength, and composition declared on the product label. It's important to note that the dietary supplement cGMPs in 21 CFR Part 111 only apply to companies who manufacture, pack, label, or store nutritional supplements for distribution in the US.

Ingredient suppliers, or those that manufacture just raw materials rather than finished items, must adhere to the food cGMPs outlined in 21 CFR Part 110; however, as a best practice, some organizations prefer to meet both cGMP standards.

Furthermore, some dietary supplement manufacturers have developed or implemented third-party systems that go beyond cGMP requirements. Because dietary supplements are governed under the "umbrella" of food, manufacturers must follow all other applicable standards. The Financial Services Modernization Act of 2010 and the Public Health Security and Bioterrorism Preparedness and Response Act of 2002 both have requirements in place.

Nutritional supplements are a one-of-a-kind mix of vitamins, minerals, and pharmaceuticals. Despite the fact that dietary supplement cGMPs are modeled after those for food, nutritional supplements and pharmaceutical cGMPs have a lot in common, such as incoming material identification checks (not required for conventional foods). Dietary supplement cGMPs include hygienic production procedures, adequate quality control activities, and adulteration prevention during manufacture, packaging, storage, and distribution, just as food cGMPs. Dietary supplement cGMPs, like drug cGMPs, include provisions for assuring the identity, purity, strength, quality, and composition of the completed product.

Unlike drug cGMPs, however, test techniques and processes do not need to be verified. Because current research only provides a limited amount of information regarding dietary supplements, only officially verified procedures are available. Producers must confirm that testing was done if they use it. The approaches adopted are scientifically sound and suitable.

The cGMPs also demand that standards be developed at any step during the manufacturing process in order to assure the quality of the dietary supplement. While cGMPs require guidelines for the materials used in dietary supplement manufacturing, labeling, and packaging, finished batches, and goods obtained from a supplier, they do not need standards for the nutritional supplement's solubility, breakdown, or bioavailability.

Product labels are also exempt from carrying an expiration or shelf date, according to the regulation. If one of the aforementioned requirements is produced, the FDA, on the other hand, requires manufacturers to have the supporting data. If a manufacturer wishes to place an expiration date on a nutritional supplement, for example, the date must first be confirmed. Additionally, each batch must contain batch production records to enable for product tracing throughout the distribution chain if necessary, such as when a product complaint has to be examined for a possible cGMP violation.

Inner standard operating procedures (SOPs) are guidelines that manufacturers must follow while carrying out a certain task or in a specific scenario. For each part of the nutritional supplement cGMP standard, SOPs must be created and followed in a consistent way. SOPs must be in writing, according to the FDA, in order to be approved. A standard SOP includes a header, purpose, scope, definitions, duties, procedure, approvals, modification history, and appendices, all of which demonstrate to the FDA that a company's system is well-controlled.

Although the dietary supplement cGMPs do not require a facility to establish and maintain documented processes for product recalls, the FDA suggests that businesses examine its Guidance for Industry: Product Recalls, Including Removal and Corrections.

It's just as important to keep track of things and have a system in place as it is to design standard SOPs. Written records must be kept for at least one year after the expiration date (if shelf-life dating is used) or two years after the last batch of nutritional supplements associated with the records was delivered. Original documents, genuine copies (e.g., microfilm or photocopies), and electronic records all need to be kept. 21 CFR Part 11 specifies the criteria under which electronic documents and electronic signatures are regarded trustworthy, reliable, and equal to paper records.

Written procedures are required for cleaning the physical plant and pest control, calibrating instruments, and monitoring and sanitizing all equipment and utensils. Quality control can include things like material assessment and quality control. Deciding on disposition; receiving components, packing, and labeling; and research lab working practices such as testing and examinations to see if specifications are met; manufacturing, packaging, and labeling processes; holding and distribution operations; and product quarantine and customer service complaints. These records contain important testing results and help the firm demonstrate to the FDA that it follows cGMPs.

Furthermore, any errors should be corrected by drawing a line across the error (where it is still readable) and adding the right individual's initials and the date (Melethil et al., 2006).

15.5.1 GMP SPECIFICATIONS FOR DIETARY SUPPLEMENTS

- A presentation has been produced for you by GMP dietary supplements specifications. The electronic manufacturing system of a small pharmaceutical company.
- Good manufacturing practices (GMP) rules now apply to all dietary supplement producers and distributors.
- The FDA had no control over it until 2007. Supplements for the diet are orally taken substances that have a dietary supplementing component.

  The FDA requires pre-market clearance for a vitamin, mineral, herb or other botanical, a concentration or extract of a plant material, and an amino acid for small pharmaceutical operations. A concentration of a vitamin, mineral, herb, or other botanical one or more of the following might be the case: a nutritional supplement ingredient in food.
- Doesn't apply to companies that just make food ingredients. The FDA's "final rule" on dietary supplements incorporates all GMP compliance requirements. Products must meet identification, purity, strength, and composition requirements, as well as contaminant limits. The master manufacturing record must be followed when it comes to packaging and labeling. The FDA requires compliance in the areas of manufacture, packaging, labeling, and storage.
- When there is a need for environmental hygiene points where cross-contamination is likely to happen to safeguard the product, certain sanitation measures must be used. Steps to cool down heating stages are necessary at every point in the manufacturing process where quality control is essential, for example: Specifications for control points.
- A small pharmaceutical company's electronic manufacturing system is a packaged and labeled product obtained from a supplier. Batch is finished, Ingredients in food (when received), in-process production, packaging components, and labels materials specifications must be developed for all materials and components used in production.

- For example, in small pharmaceutical operations, eradicating possible microbial contamination brought by a raw material. Before being tested, critical equipment must be cleaned and/or sterilized. To avoid adulteration in industrial activities, specifications must be created.
- Double-check if the products are in accordance with the purchase order. Make sure the merchandise you're getting is appropriately labeled. Labeling firms are responsible for establishing specifications. Firms that specialize in packaging and labeling are required to meet certain criteria.
- Identification, assay, appearance, odor, solubility, melting point, heavy metals, loss on drying or ignition residue are some of the characteristics of vitamins and minerals. Organic volatile impurities are organic impurities that are naturally volatile. For small pharmaceutical operations, specifications for each component utilized in manufacture are necessary.
- Botanicals may include identification (e.g., visual comparison to a standard or an image); sections of the plant (e.g., the root or leaves). Color, odor, and texture are all important factors to consider. Characteristics that distinguish the target species from its relatives.
- Research areas that are still being explored scientifically – bioavailability, dissolution, and disintegration.

  Different components that are commonly found in a natural product small pharmaceutical operations' esthetic look of dietary supplement various elements that are found naturally in a product dietary supplement's esthetic appearance.
- You explain why, in the absence of final batch testing, additional data, such as component and in-process testing, will prove that the standard is met for small pharmaceutical operations. There is no scientifically realistic means to evaluate or examine the exempted product standard at the final batch stage. The control system's ability to manufacture a nutritional supplement that fulfills the stated standard cannot be verified by the described specification.
- Sampling, safety, and handling requirements, as well as others the attribute's permissible range is defined by its limit. The approach for measuring the quality characteristic is referred to as the method. Measuring a quality feature like potency or water content with a test.

The single facility might deal with all of the aforementioned product varieties. The food supplement company may therefore employ the guideline document in accordance with the product category it works with and the procedures. (i) Health Supplements; (ii) Nutraceuticals; (iii) Food for Special Dietary Use (FSDU); (iv) Food for Special Medical Purpose (FSMP); (v) Food with Added Probiotic Ingredients; (vi) Food with Added Prebiotic Ingredients; (vii) Specialty Foods Containing Plant or Botanical Ingredients; (viii) Novel Food (Need Prior Approval as per FSS (Approval of Non-Specified Food and Food Ingredients Regulations, 2017).

The hazard analysis and HACCP plans tables, as well as the production flow diagrams, are included. It's broken down into five sections. The first section presents an overview of the Indian food supplement market, as well as the sector's expanding demand for food safety. The second section explains how to put good manufacturing and hygiene practices into practice, as outlined in Part II of Schedule 4 of the Food Safety and Standards (Licenses and Registering of Food Businesses Regulation, 2011). The chapter specifies which requirements are necessary and mandatory for food businesses, and the term "must" be used in certain instances. Furthermore, some excellent practices for food safety operations are strongly advised, and the term "should" is employed in this context.

The third section of this chapter is advisory in nature, and it gives the basic information and criteria for food businesses to use when implementing the hazard analysis and critical control point (HACCP) system alluded to in this section. Tables of Hazard Analysis are anticipated to help the industry identify the food safety hazards associated with each production phase, as well as the Critical Control Points (CCPs) and other relevant data. Sample HACCP plans were obtained from a number of well-known food supplement companies. These plans might be used as a guide by the industry, which could then change or amend them to suit its needs. An inspection checklist for food service operators to employ when auditing their facilities and operations is included in the fourth component (Phillips et al., 2011).

FBOs can evaluate themselves based on the indicated scoring. The last part offers important templates and forms for FBOs to maintain track of their data. This includes FSSAI-required documentation as well as a few layouts for tracking key food safety operations.

15.5.2 REGULATORY PROCESS FOR THE CLEARANCE

Dietary supplements are not FDA-approved as drug products; it is the manufacturer's/responsible distributor's obligation to claim the product's safety by presenting relevant documents.

The US Food and Drug Administration (USFDA) has established GMP requirements for dietary supplements that apply to both international and local enterprises. This GMP guideline outlines the requirements for dietary supplement manufacture, packaging, labeling, and storage (Cui et al., 2011).

15.6 LABELING

Dietary supplements, like traditional foods and other FDA-regulated commodities, must be appropriately labeled in order to be legally marketed in the United States. Dietary supplement labeling regulations were added to the FDCA as part of the DSHEA. Three years later, the FDA adopted laws controlling the transmission of health information. Claims for nutrient content and health in dietary supplements, including identification, nutrition labeling, component labeling, and nutrient content and health. The main distinction between dietary supplement and regular food labeling is that nutritional supplements include a Supplement Facts panel instead of the Nutrition Facts panel seen on regular foods.

The supplement facts panel (also known as the Supplement Fact box) and the Nutrition Facts panel (also known as the Nutrition Fact box) are similar in design and arrangement for consumer understanding, but the FDA has different criteria for the two types of labels. In the same way, food, and dietary supplement claims can be made. Marketers must be aware of the restrictions and limitations imposed by each of these product categories on the claims that can be made.

Dietary supplement label regulation is overseen by the FDA, which ensures that all required label components are stated accurately and that the label adequately communicates the product's ingredients. Although the FDA uses the term "labeling" to refer to any marketing materials that come with a product, the product label itself identifies it as a dietary supplement. As a result, FDA regulation of product labeling extends beyond the actual product label to include marketing, packaging, inserts, and other point-of-sale promotional materials in addition to the physical product label.

Although certain third-party information, such as articles, abstracts, or book chapters, is specifically excluded from the definition of labeling in Section 5 of the DSHEA, this information should be accurate, not misrepresenting, and published by a third-party entity other than the product's manufacturer or marketer.

The FDA and the Federal Trade Commission (FTC) share responsibility for dietary supplement advertising claims under a long-standing liaison agreement. The FDA is particularly concerned with claims made on the product label and any accompanying promotional or instructional materials, as well as the content to ensure that the claims' language meets regulatory criteria. The Federal Trade Commission focuses on advertising claims and ensures that they are accurate and not misleading. Consumers are being misled, and scientific proof to back it up is lacking. Both agencies maintain a close eye on all promises made by internet advertisements and regularly coordinate on enforcement. This is a high priority for us.

Because dietary supplements are considered foods, they must meet the same labeling requirements as food: they must be accurate, easy to understand, and unique to the product. The Dietary Supplement Health and Education Act (DSHEA), as amended by the FDCA Section 403(s) 60, specifies the basic labeling standards for dietary supplements. The FDA rules that implement this statute provide additional particular criteria, such as typeface, print size, and label positioning. All dietary supplement labels must have a statement of identity, the net amount of contents, nutrition information, including the Supplement Facts panel, a comprehensive list of product components, and the name and location of the producer, packer, or distributor.

If a dietary supplement label fails to provide the required information in the proper manner, the FDA can consider the product misbranded. The FDA may also require additional label information and/or disclaimer statements for nutritional supplements that meet certain conditions.

15.6.1 US NUTRACEUTICAL MARKET

In the United States, dietary supplements constitute a $32 billion business. All of these goods are referred to as "dietary supplements" in the United States, including vitamins, minerals, botanicals, sports nutrition supplements, weight management supplements, and specialized supplements. Nearly 150 million Americans consume dietary supplements each year. Sales of nutritional products reached $11.5 billion in 2012 and are predicted to hit $15.5 billion in 2017.

There are two types of nutraceuticals in the Indian market: functional foods and beverages and dietary supplements:

1. **Foods and Drinks with a Purpose:** This category makes up more than 60% of the entire market. According to the World Health

Organization, fortified food is defined as processed foods that have been supplemented with micronutrients. This includes all sports drinks, fortified drinks, fortified juices, fortified meals, and energy drinks.

2. **Nutritional Supplements:** In India, this category accounts for the remaining 40% of the Nutraceutical market. This category includes vitamin and mineral supplements, herbal supplements, protein supplements, and Chyawanprash.

15.7 REGULATORY STATUS OF NUTRACEUTICALS

A variety of organizations, including government agencies, have promoted nutraceuticals and functional foods, and public awareness of their use has expanded. In many countries, there are no specific standards for the manufacture and use of nutraceuticals. The Dietary Supplement Health and Education Act (DSHEA), approved by Congress in 1994 and implemented in 1995 in the United States, has several requirements. Similarly, Poland's Food and Nutrition Safety Act was approved in 2006, and the Food and Drugs Act of Canada has precise requirements. Proper regulatory recognition of these things will result in a slew of new products for the pharmaceutical industry, as well as a market growth.

The majority of nations have yet to adopt nutraceutical regulatory requirements, which might result in a flood of low-quality items flooding the healthcare industry, especially in developing countries. As a result, the global health community must create nutraceutical regulatory regulations as soon as possible in order to protect the market from counterfeit and low-quality drugs. Furthermore, intensive scientific study is necessary in both the fields of functional foods and nutraceuticals to uncover their specific mechanisms of action and negative effects.

15.8 NUTRACEUTICAL REGULATIONS

The laws governing nutraceuticals differ widely from nation to country. Regardless of jurisdiction, industry standards regularly stray into a gray region where data and obligations can be ambiguous, misleading, and, in some cases, lethal. Both makers and buyers should be aware of their country's nutraceutical regulations in order to make safe and informed selections and decisions.

15.8.1 EUROPEAN REGULATIONS (EFSA)

Nutraceuticals are food supplements that include a concentrated quantity of nutrients to complement regular dietary consumption and provide nutritional and/or physiological advantages, as defined and regulated by the European Food Safety Authority (EFSA). The major focus is on the supplement's contents, such as vitamins, minerals, and amino acids, as well as the amounts at which they are present. Under Directive 2002/46/EC, nutraceuticals created in the EU must only include substances that have been authorized and published by the European Commission. Any firm that wishes to incorporate a vitamin, mineral, or other ingredient that isn't on this list can apply for authorization from the European Commission.

Regulation (EC) No 1924/2006, issued by the European Commission, established Union norms on nutrition and health claims. On July 1, 2007, the regulation entered into force.

This regulation outlines the legal framework that food manufacturers must adhere to when highlighting the unique health and nutritional advantages of their products on product labels or in advertising. The rules of the Regulation apply to both nutrition and health claims (for example, "low fat" and "high fiber") (such as "Vitamin D is needed for the normal growth and development of bone in children").

The purpose of these laws is to guarantee that just about every claim made on a food is generally labeling, presentation or advertising in the European Union is true, clear, and scientifically supported. Food with claims that might mislead buyers is forbidden on the EU market.

This protects consumers while also stimulating innovation and guaranteeing a level playing field. The standards ensure that commodities bearing claims can freely circulate within the European Union, as any food company can make the same claims on its products wherever it is located (Keenan et al., 2015).

15.8.2 USA REGULATIONS (DSHEA AND FDA)

Nutraceuticals are classified as dietary supplements by the US Food and Medication Administration (FDA), which imposes regulations on both finished supplements and dietary components that differ from those that apply to conventional food and drug products. The Nutritional Supplement Health and Education Act (DSHEA) was enacted in 1994 with widespread public support and debate. The DSHEA effectively defined and regulated dietary supplements in the United States for the first time, prohibiting nutraceutical manufacturers from making certain claims without proof and requiring them to fulfill specific FDA requirements.

According to the DSHEA, a "product (other than tobacco) designed to supplement the diet that carries or includes one or more of the essential nutritional elements." A food product for use by man to supplement the diet by significantly increasing dietary intake; or a concentration, metabolite, component, extract, or combination of any of the aforementioned elements.

15.8.3 REGISTRATION OF DIETARY SUPPLEMENTS IN US

Dietary supplements are governed by 21 CFR 190, which divides their contents under two categories for registration in the United States: active and inactive substances. The product's active ingredient must fulfill the DSHEA's 1994 definition. If it meets the criterion, it can be registered as a dietary ingredient.

The nutritional ingredient is divided into two sorts for legal registration reasons. A product that was on the market on or before October 15, 1994, is referred to as "grandfathered" or "old dietary ingredient" (ODI). These items are permitted to stay on the market since its safety signal has been validated.

Products released on the market after October 15, 1994, or changes to the ODI, are considered new dietary ingredients (NDI). The manufacturer must first get FDA premarket clearance before selling the products in the United States. The Center for Food Safety and Applied Nutrition is the NDI's competent entity (CFSAN).

For premarket authorization for the NDI, send the paperwork to the Office of Nutrition Products, Labeling, and Dietary Supplements (HFS-820), Center for Food Safety and Applied Nutrition, Food, and Drug, 5100 Paint Branch Pkwy, College Park, MD 20740.

- The product's name (including any binomial names if it's an herb/ botanical).
- The following is the product description:
  - o The NDI level of the product;
  - o The labeling statement/conditions for permitted usage.
- Proof of Safety (may include history of use, in case of changed ODI; published articles for NDI).
- The Dietary Supplement's maker or distributor's signature of concerned authorities.

15.8.4 REGISTRATION OF DIETARY SUPPLEMENTS IN INDIA

A product should first be licensed as a nutraceutical before it can be sold in India. The FSS Act outlines the procedures for registering a business (2006).

Nutraceutical products are available, but there is no standard format for them. Due to a lack of a defined pathway for product registration, nutraceutical companies in India struggle to have their products licensed. In May of 2011, the Food Safety and Standard Authority of India (FSSAI) released the Food Safety and Standard Rules, 2011. Food goods, food enterprises, packaging, and labeling systems, food standards, and food additives are all covered by this law. The FSS guidelines have been in effect across the country since August 5, 2011. This establishes a single legal framework within which competent authorities can regulate the sale, manufacture, and distribution of commodities across the country (Phillips et al., 20111).

15.9 SPECIFICATIONS FOR DIETARY SUPPLEMENTS AND NUTRACEUTICALS

15.9.1 PHARMACOPEIAL SPECIFICATIONS

Nutraceuticals are regulated by a multitude of regulations, each with its own terminology that differs from country to country. Different countries classify nutraceuticals and dietary supplements differently, and some governments classify nutraceuticals as food. In general, a dietary supplement is a substance that is used orally and contains a nutritious element to complement one's diet. Nutraceuticals are known by many different names and classifications all over the world. In the United States, it's called a dietary supplement; in Canada, it's called a Natural Health Product; in Australia, it's called complementary medicine; and in the European Union, it's called food.

15.9.2 DIETARY SUPPLEMENT HEALTH EDUCATION ACT (DSHEA) 1994

Senator Orrin G. Hatch presented a bill in the Senate that defines a dietary supplement and establishes legal standards for the marketing of food supplements in the US. A dietary supplement, according to the law, is a product that contains one or more of the following necessary elements:

- Vitamin;
- Mineral;
- Herb or other botanical;
- Amino acid;
- Food substance for use by humans to supplement the diet by increasing the total daily intake of that ingredient;
- Concentration, metabolite, constituent, extract, or combination of any of the above;
- Dietary supplements must also be commodities designed for oral administration, according to the DSHEA.

The Dietary Supplement Health and Education Act (DSHEA) creates a regulatory framework for the production and marketing of dietary supplements that contain dietary components in the United States (Public Law 103,417, October 25, 1994). (Vitamin, mineral, herb or other botanical, amino acid, or a concentrate, metabolite, constituent, or extract, or combination of any of these ingredients).

DSHEA not only made supplementation available to consumers with the objective of improving and maintaining health, but it also allowed the supplement industry in the United States to grow from a low point of around $4 billion in 1994 to an estimated $35 billion in 2015. DS producers are responsible for evaluating a product's safety and quality under the DSHEA, but they are not obligated to communicate that information with the FDA prior to its distribution unless the product contains a new dietary ingredient (NDI) that was issued after October 15, 1994.

For all NDIs, manufacturers must file a 75-day premarket notice to the FDA, outlining the information that led to a reasonable expectation of safety being determined. The FDA has the authority to remove a product from the market if it creates a "significant or unreasonable risk of disease or injury." The FDA, on the other hand, is responsible for demonstrating that the product poses a significant risk to public health, which is a lengthy process. Taking legal action necessitates a concerted effort involving personnel from many agencies, with the Department of Justice leading the charge. It's unclear whether similar procedures to monitor compliance will be conducted on a regular basis. Due to the FDA's lack of resources for detecting hazard, products of dubious quality are allowed to remain on the market without penalties. Furthermore, prescription drugs and analogs posing as DS have been improperly introduced utilizing the DSHEA's premarketing monitoring requirements. There have also been claims that the present surveillance system has faults.

The FDA was given permission by the DSHEA to prescribe and apply existing GMPs for DS in order to solve quality difficulties. Around 13 years after DSHEA was established, 21 CFR Part 111 (Current Good Manufacturing Practice in Manufacturing, Packaging, Labeling, or Holding Operations for Dietary Supplements) became a requirement in the Code of Federal Regulations (CFR). When it comes to DS quality, GMPs demand manufacturers to develop their own criteria for dietary ingredients, other components, in-process materials, and finished dietary supplements. The application of GMP requirements through the manufacturer's own specifications has resulted in a lack of uniformity in the industry. Even though two items from different manufacturers have the same label, they may be made to quite different quality standards. According to GMP rules, endproduct testing utilizing just one of the established requirements might also serve as a proxy for all quality aspects of the final DS (21 CFR 111.75). As a result, manufacturers may employ multiple methods to assess the quality of DS, even if they contain the same component or are labeled with the same generic name.

Manufacturers must ensure that laboratory examination and testing methodologies are appropriate for their intended use, as well as recognize and then use appropriate empirically rational method(s) for each established configuration for which checking or examination is required (21 CFR 111.320), but this rule does not apply to analytical methods used as part of these specifications.

Adulteration of completed DS items in the following categories was cited as a major problem in Dr. Hamburg's letter:

- Enhancement of sexual performance;
- Weight reduction;
- Boosting athletic performance.

15.9.3 FOOD SAFETY STANDARD AND STANDARDS ACT (FSSA): 2006

This law was passed in 2006 to create the Financial Services and Markets Authority (FSSA), a government organization that regulates the financial industry, manufacture, storage, distribution, sale, and import to ensure food supply and safety. Nutraceutical goods are included in the category of foods under the FSS Act 2006, Rules and Regulations 2011. Foods for particular dietary objectives, functional foods, nutraceutical or health supplements are defined in Section 22(1) of the FSSA as:

(1) "Foods for special dietary uses" means: (a) foods that are specially processed or formulated to satisfy specific dietary requirements that exist due to a particular physical or physiological condition or specific diseases and disorders and that are presented as such, wherein the composition of these foodstuffs must differ significantly from that of ordinary foods of comparable nature, if applicable. (i) botanicals or plants in the form of powder, concentrate, or extract in ethyl alcohol, water, or hydro alcoholic extract, alone or in combination; (ii) minerals, vitamins, proteins, metals, or their compounds, or amino acids (in amounts not exceeding the Recommended Daily Allowance for Indians) or enzymes (within permissible limits); (iii) substances with animal origins; (iv) does not include a narcotic drug or a psychotropic substance.
(2) "Genetically engineered or modified food" refers to food and food ingredients created from but not incorporating genetically modified or engineered organisms obtained through modern biotechnology.
(3) "Organic food" refers to foodstuffs produced in compliance with predetermined organic production criteria;
(4) "Proprietary and Novel Food" refers to a food product for which no standards have been established but which is safe.

KEYWORDS

- **dietary supplements**
- **Food and Drug Administration**
- **food supplements**
- **hazard analysis and critical control point**
- **psychotropic substance**
- **standard operating procedures**

REFERENCES

Anderson, J. W., Baird, P., Davis, R. H., Ferreri, S., Knudtson, M., Koraym, A., Waters, V., & Williams, C. L., (2009). Health benefits of dietary fiber. *Nutr. Rev., 67*, 188e205.

Asp, N. G., Furda, I., Schweizer, T. F., & Prosky, L., (1988). Dietary fiber definition and analysis. *Am. J. Clin. Nutr., 48*, 688e190.

Asp, N. G., Johansson, C. G., Hallmer, H., & Siljestrom, M., (1983). Rapid enzymatic assay of insoluble, and soluble dietary fiber. *J. Agric Food Chem., 31*, 476e482.

Baker, D., (1981). Notes on the neutral detergent fiber method. In: James, W. P. T., & Theander, O., (eds.), *The Analysis of Dietary Fiber in Food* (pp. 159e162). New York: Marcel Dekker.

Bird, A. R., Conlon, M. A., Christophersen, C. T., & Topping, D. L., (2010). Resistant starch, large bowel fermentation and a broader perspective of prebiotics and probiotics. *Benef. Mirbobes., 1*, 423e431.

Bonnema, A. L., Kohlberg, L. W., Thomas, W., & Slavin, J. L., (2010). Gastrointestinal tolerance to chicory inulin products. *J. Am. Diet. Assoc., 110*, 865e868.

Chawla, R., & Patil, G. R., (2010). Soluble dietary fiber. *Compr. Rev. Food Sci. Food Saf., 9*, 178e196.

Codex Alimentarius., (2008). *Report of the 30th Session of the Codex Committee on Nutrition and Foods for Special Dietary Uses*. Cape Town, South Africa.

Cui, S. W., (2011). An introduction: Evolution and finalization of the regulatory definition of dietary fiber. *Food Hydrocoll., 25*, 139e143.

De Menezes, E. W., Giuntini, E. B., Dan, M. C., Sarda, F. A., Lajolo, F. M., Lanza, E., & Jones, D. Y., (2013). Codex dietary fiber definition justification for inclusion of carbohydrates from 3 to 9 degrees of polymerization. *Food Chem., 140*, 581e585.

De Vries, J. W., (2004). Dietary fiber: The influence of definition on analysis and regulation. *J. AOAC Int., 87*, 682e706.

DeVries, J. W., (2010). Validation official methodology commensurate with dietary fiber research and definitions. In: van der Kamp, J. W., Jones, J., McCleary, B., & Topping, D. (Eds.), *Dietary Fiber: New Frontiers for Food and Health* (pp. 29–48). Wageningen. The Netherlands: Wageningen Academic Publishers.

Elleuch, M., Bedigian, D., Roiseux, O., Besbes, S., Blecker, C., & Attia, H., (2011). Dietary fiber and fiber-rich by-products of food processing: Characterization, technological functionality and commercial applications: A review. *Food Chem., 124*, 411e421.

Elmstahl, H. L., (2002). Resistant starch content in a selection of starchy foods on the Swedish market. *Eur. J. Clin. Nutr., 56*, 500e505.

Englyst, H. N., Kingman, S. M., & Cummings, J. H., (1992). Classification and measurement of nutritionally starch fractions. *Eur. J. Clin. Nutr., 46*, 33e50.

Englyst, K., Liu, S., & Englyst, H., (2007). Nutritional characterization and measurement of dietary carbohydrates. *Eur. J. Clin. Nutr., 61*(1), 19e39.

Eswaran, S., Muir, J., & Chey, W. D., (2013). Fiber and functional gastrointestinal disorders. *Am. J. Gastroenterol., 108*(5), 718e727.

Food and Drug Administration, Ministry of Health, and Welfare. Regulations on nutrition labeling for prepackaged food products. Available at: https://drive.google.com/file/d/0B0ncnWxYYhkgOWdnOEZFNC1zQ2M/view (accessed on 28 January 2023).

Fuentes-Zaragoza, E., Riquelme-Navarrete, M. J., Sanchez-Zapata, E., & Alvarez, J. A., (2010). Resistant starch as functional ingredient: A review. *Food Res Int., 43*, 931e942.

Furda, I., (1981). Simultaneous analysis of soluble and insoluble dietary fiber. In: James, W. P. T., & Theander, O., (eds.), *The Analysis of Fiber in Foods* (pp. 163e172). New York: Marcel Dekker.

Gallagher, P., & O'Mahony, D., (2009). Constipation in old age. *Best Pract. Res. Clin. Gastroenterol., 23*, 875e887.

Grabitske, H. A., & Slavin, J. L., (2008). Low-digestible carbohydrates in practice. *J. Am. Diet. Assoc., 108*, 1677e1681.

Gralak, M. A., Leontowicz, M., Morawiec, M., Bartinkowska, E., & Kulasek, G. W., (1996). Comparison of the influence of dietary fiber sources with different proportions of soluble and insoluble fiber on Ca, Mg, Fe, Zn, Mn and Cu apparent absorption in rats. *Arch Anim. Nutr., 49*, 293e299.

Guillon, F., & Champ, M., (2000). Structural and physical properties of dietary fiber, and consequence of processing on human physiology. *Food Res. Int., 33*, 233e245.

Gunness, P., & Gidley, M. J., (2010). Mechanisms underlying the cholesterol-lowering properties of soluble dietary fiber polysaccharides. *Food Funct., 1*, 149e155.

Heckman, M. M., & Lane, S. A., (1981). Comparison of dietary fiber methods for food. *J. AOAC Int., 64*, 1339e1343.

Ho, K. S., Tan, C. Y., MohdDaud, M. A., & Seow-Choen, F., (2012). Stopping or reducing dietary fiber intake reduces constipation and its associated symptoms. *World J. Gastroenterol., 18*, 4593e4596.

Keenan, M. J., Zhou, J., Hegsted, M., Pelkman, C., Durham, H. A., Coulon, D. B., & Martin, R. J., (2015). Role of resistant starch in improving gut health, adiposity, and insulin resistance. *Adv. Nutr. Int. Rev. J., 6*, 198e205.

Marlett, J. A., McBurney, M. I., & Slavin, J. L., (2002). Position of the American dietetic Association: Health implications of dietary fiber. *J. Am. Diet. Assoc., 102*, 993e1000.

McCance, R. A., & Lawrence, R. D., (1929). *The Carbohydrate Content of Foods*. London: Medical Research Council Special Report Series 135 Her Majesty's Stationery Office.

McCleary, B. V., (2014). Modification to AOAC official methods 2009.01 and 2011.25 to allow for minor over estimation of low molecular weight soluble dietary fiber in samples containing starch. *J. AOAC Int., 97*, 896e901.

Mudgil, D., & Barak, S., (2013). Composition, properties and health benefits of indigestible carbohydrate polymers as dietary fiber: A review. *Int. J. Biol. Macromol., 61*, 1e6.

Muller-Lissner, S. A., Kamm, M. A., Scarpignato, C., & Wald, A., (2005). Myths and misconceptions about chronic constipation. *Am. J. Gastroenterol., 100*, 232e242.

Mussamatto, S. I., & Mancilha, I. M., (2007). Nondigestible oligosaccharides: A review. *Carbohydr. Polym., 68*, 587e597.

Nair, K. K., Kharb, S., & Thompkinson, D. K., (2010). Inulin dietary fiber with functional and health attributes: A review. *Food Rev. Int., 26*, 189e203.

Nugent, A. P., (2005). Health properties of resistant starch. *Br. Nutr. Foundation Nutr. Bull., 30*, 27e54.

Quah, H. M., Ooi, B. S., Seow-Choen, F., Sng, K. K., & Ho, K. S., (2006). Prospective randomized crossover trial comparing fiber with lactulose in the treatment of idiopathic chronic constipation. *Tech Coloproctol., 10*, 111e114.

Roberfroid, M. B., (2007). Inulin-type fructans: Functional food ingredients. *J. Nutr., 137*, 2493e2502.

Schweizer, T. F., & Wursch, P., (1979). Analysis of dietary fiber. *J. Sci. Food Agric., 30*, 613e619.

Slavin, J., (2013). Fiber and prebiotics: Mechanisms and health benefits. *Nutrients, 5*, 1417e1435.

Southgate, D. A. T., (1977). The definition and analysis of dietary fiber. *Nutr. Rev., 35*, 31e7.

Theander, O., & Aman, P., (1979). Studies on dietary fibers. I. Analysis and chemical characterization of water-soluble and water-insoluble dietary fibers. *Swedish J. Agric. Research, 9*, 97.

Trowell, H. C., (1972). Crude fiber, dietary fiber, and atherosclerosis. *Atherosclerosis, 16*, 138e148.

Westenbrink, S., Brunt, K., & Van, D. K. J. W., (2013). Dietary fiber: Challenges in production and use of food composition data. *Food Chem., 140*, 562e567.

Williams, R. D., & Olmstead, W. D., (1996). A biochemical method for determining indigestible residue (crude fiber) in feces: Lignin, cellulose, and non-water soluble hemicellulose. *J. Biol. Chem., 108*, 653e666.

INDEX

D

F

H

J

K

L

X

Y

For Product Safety Concerns and Information please contact our
EU representative GPSR@taylorandfrancis.com Taylor & Francis
Verlag GmbH, Kaufingerstraße 24, 80331 München, Germany